ENDOCRINE ONCOLOGY

CONTEMPORARY ENDOCRINOLOGY

P. Michael Conn, SERIES EDITOR

ENDOCRINE ONCOLOGY

Edited by

STEPHEN P. ETHIER, PhD

Department of Radiation Oncology,
University of Michigan Cancer Center,
Ann Arbor, MI

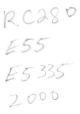

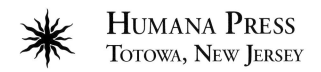

HUMANA PRESS
TOTOWA, NEW JERSEY

PREFACE

Endocrine oncology is a broad subject that would be difficult, if not impossible, to cover adequately in a single book. Cancers of endocrine tissues, such as breast and prostate, are very important from a public health point of view because of their increasing prevalence; they have also been the focus of intensive research, which has expanded dramatically in recent years. In order to keep this book to a manageable size and still have it be useful to the reader with an interest in this subject, I decided to focus primarily on the endocrinology of cancers of the breast, prostate, endometrium, and ovary. As a result, there is very little information in this book on the molecular genetics of endocrine cancers, and such information is available in other excellent books.

Despite the great advances in our understanding of the genetics of endocrine cancers, important and controversial issues relating to the endocrinology and cell biology of malignancies of endocrine tissues remain to be resolved, and I have tried to cover these issues in detail in *Endocrine Oncology*. For example, while it has been known for many years that steroid hormones, particularly estradiol, influence breast cancer development and progression, many issues remain to be resolved regarding the true role of estradiol in breast cancer progression. Indeed, it is still not clear how to predict response of breast cancer patients with estrogen receptor-positive disease to antiestrogen therapy. Of further importance to the field is the relatively limited understanding, still, of how steroid hormones function to regulate normal mammary gland homeostasis in humans. For that reason, the first six chapters of this book focus on that specific area of research, and the first three chapters focus primarily on the role of estrogen and progesterone receptors in normal mammary gland function. The recent observations that estrogens and progestins signal normal mammary epithelial cell proliferation via paracrine mechanisms to neighboring cells, which are steroid hormone receptor-negative, are exciting and may help to shed light on many aspects of human breast carcinogenesis. These findings are relevant to the question of how many pathways or precursor cells are able to give rise to human breast cancers that either express or do not express steroid hormone receptors, and this important topic is the subject of Chapter 4. As is discussed in Chapter 5, expression of certain growth factor receptors can modify the expression of steroid hormone receptors, which in turn can influence breast cancer progression. These receptors may also influence the response of steroid hormone receptor-positive breast cancer cells to antiestrogens. A detailed discussion of factors that influence response to antiestrogens is presented in Chapter 6. Thus, the first part of this book attempts to cover several important and intertwined issues in ways that may help to clarify the important issues that remain to be resolved in the field.

As is evident from Chapters 7 and 8, steroids are not the only hormones important in breast cancer development. Prolactin, which is clearly important in rodent models of breast carcinogenesis, may play a similar role in human breast cancer development. In addition, peptide hormones such as chorionic gonadotropin may play important roles in modifying breast cancer progression.

With a similar approach, the second part of the book examines the role of steroid hormones in prostate cancer development and treatment. In many ways, breast and pros-

tate cancers are parallel diseases in that they are both influenced by steroid hormones, both give rise to what is initially hormone receptor-positive disease that responds to endocrine therapy, and both eventually progresses to a hormone-independent state. These issues are discussed in Chapters 13 through 15, which also demonstrates that, while there are many parallels between breast and prostate cancers, there are many distinguishing features as well.

The next two chapters focus on epithelial ovarian cancer and endometrial cancer. Once again, the emphasis of these chapters is on the endocrinology of these diseases. Since the pathogenesis of endometrial cancer appears to be influenced by certain antiestrogens that are used in breast cancer therapy, the issue of how estrogens affect different target tissues is critically important to our understanding of disease progression and the use of antiestrogen therapy.

Having focused on the role of hormones in the development of breast, prostate, ovarian, and endometrial cancer in the first 13 chapters of the book, the next four chapters present an in-depth discussion of the role of growth factors in endocrine neoplasia. A wealth of data in the literature points to an intimate interaction between hormones and growth factors in mediating normal tissue homeostasis and in pathological processes involving endocrine tissues. In particular, members of the epidermal growth factor family, the insulin-like growth factors and their binding proteins, and the fibroblast growth factors have all been implicated in the progression of endocrine neoplasia. Clearly, a book that focuses on endocrine aspects of cancers of endocrine tissues would be incomplete without a detailed discussion of the role of growth factors in the progression of these diseases.

It has recently become clear that the ability of steroid hormone receptors to influence gene expression is modified by the repertoire of transcriptional co-activators and co-repressors present in target cells. Furthermore, some of the genes that code for these proteins may function as oncogenes in breast and other cancers. It is also now known that hormones can directly affect the expression of proteins that modify the cell death response of epithelial cells under both physiologic and pathologic conditions. Finally, while it is well known that inactivation of tumor suppressor genes is important in cancer progression, endocrine tissues such as breast and ovary seem to have their own special suppressor genes, *BRCA1* and *BRCA2*. Thus, these three subjects, which are of particular importance to the development of endocrine malignancies, are covered in the final three chapters of this book.

As I mentioned at the outset, no book on endocrine oncology can be complete, since this subject encompasses a vast area of clinical medicine and cancer biology research. It was my intention, and it is my hope, that in developing this book, some of the most important issues relating to the endocrinology and cell biology of endocrine neoplasia have been appropriately identified and thoroughly discussed. It is also my hope that the readers of this book learn as much as I did from the outstanding contributions made by the authors, to whom I am greatly indebted for their hard work and dedication.

Stephen P. Ethier, PhD

CONTENTS

CONTRIBUTORS

CRAIG ALLRED, MD, *Division of Medical Oncology, Department of Pathology, University of Texas Health Science Center, San Antonio, TX*

ELIZABETH ANDERSON, PhD, *Clinical Research Department, Christie Hospital NHS Trust Manchester, UK*

VICKI V. BAKER, MD, *Department of Obstetrics and Gynecology, University of Michigan Medical Center, Ann Arbor, MI*

ROSEMARY L. BALLEINE, PhD, FRCPA, *Westmead Institute for Cancer Research, University of Sydney at Westmead Hospital, Westmead, Australia*

RICHARD R. BARAKAT, MD, *Gynecology Service Academic Office, Memorial Sloan-Kettering Cancer Center, New York, NY*

DAVID R. BEIDLER, PhD, *Department of Medicine, University of Adelaide, Adelaide, South Australia*

CATERINA BIANCO, MD, PhD, *Tumor Growth Factor Section, Laboratory of Tumor Immunology and Biology, National Cancer Institute, National Institutes of Health, Bethesda, MD*

POWEL BROWN, MD, PhD, *Division of Medical Oncology, Department of Medicine, University of Texas Health Science Center, San Antonio, TX*

CHRISTINE L. CLARKE, PhD, *Westmead Institute for Cancer Research, University of Sydney at Westmead Hospital, Westmead, Australia*

ROBERT B. CLARKE, MD, PhD, *Departments of Clinical Research and Medical Oncology, Christie Hospital NHS Trust, Manchester, UK*

R. C. COOMBES, MD, PhD, *Department of Cancer Medicine, Imperial College School of Medicine, Charing Cross Hospital, London, UK*

AMANDA COUTTS, PhD, *Department of Biochemistry and Molecular Biology, University of Manitoba, Winnipeg, Manitoba, Canada*

MARTA DE SANTIS, PhD, *Tumor Growth Factor Section, Laboratory of Tumor Immunology and Biology, National Cancer Institute, National Institutes of Health, Bethesda, MD*

HELMUT DOTZLAW, PhD, *Department of Biochemistry and Molecular Biology, University of Manitoba, Winnipeg, Manitoba, Canada*

ANDREAS D. EBERT, MD, PhD, *Department of Obstetrics and Gynecology, Laboratory of Tumor Biology and Microcirculation, Medical Center Benjamin Franklin, Fee University Berlin, Berlin, Germany*

SUZANNE FUQUA, PhD, *Division of Medical Oncology, Department of Medicine, University of Texas Health Science Center, San Antonio, TX*

J. GOMM, PhD, *Department of Cancer Medicine, Imperial College School of Medicine, Charing Cross Hospital, London, UK*

W. J. GULLICK, PhD, *ICRF Molecular Oncology Unit, Imperial College School of Medicine, Hammersmith Hospital, London, UK*

ANTHONY HOWELL, MD, *Departments of Clinical Research and Medical Oncology, Christie Hospital NHS Trust, Manchester, UK*

AIHUA HUANG, MSc, *Department of Pathology, University of Manitoba, Winnipeg, Manitoba, Canada*

SYBILLE M. N. HUNT, PhD, *Westmead Institute for Cancer Research, University of Sydney at Westmead Hospital, Westmead, Australia*

HELEN C. HURST, PhD, *ICRF Molecular Oncology Unit, Imperial College School of Medicine, Hammersmith Hospital, London, UK*

C. JOHNSTON, PhD, *Department of Cancer Medicine, imperial College School of Medicine, Charing Cross Hospital, London, UK*

V. CRAIG JORDAN, PhD, DSC, *Lynn Sage Breast Cancer Research Program, Robert H. Lurie Comprehensive Cancer Center, Chicago, IL*

JEFFREY M. KAMRADT, MD, *Division of Endocrinology, Metabolism, and Hypertension, Wayne State University School of Medicine, Detroit, MI*

DOLORES J. LAMB, PhD, *Division of Reproductive Medicine and Surgery, Scott Department of Urology and Department of Cell Biology, Baylor College of Medicine, Houston, TX*

ADRIAN V. LEE, PhD, *Division of Medical Oncology, Department of Medicine, University of Texas Health Science Center, San Antonio, TX*

K. E. LEVERTON, PhD, *ICRF Molecular Oncology Unit, Imperial College School of Medicine, Hammersmith Hospital, London, UK*

ETIENNE LEYGUE, PhD, *Department of Biochemistry and Molecular Biology, University of Manitoba, Winipeg, Manitoba, Canada*

BIAO LU, MSc, *Department of Biochemistry and Molecular Biology, University of Manitoba, Winnipeg, Manitoba, Canada*

MARCO MARCELLI, PhD, *Department of Psychiatry and Behavioral Sciences, Emory University School of Medicine, Atlanta, GA*

S. MARSH, FRCS, MD, *Department of Cancer Medicine, Imperial College School of Medicine, Charing Cross Hospital, London, UK*

ISABEL MARTINEZ-LACACI, PhD, *Tumor Growth Factor Section, Laboratory of Tumor Immunology and Biology, National Cancer Institute, National Institutes of Health, Bethesda, MD*

EILEEN M. MCGOWAN, MSc, *Westmead Institute for Cancer Research, University of Sydney at Westmead Hospital, Westmead, Australia*

PAUL S. MELTZER, MD, PhD, *Cancer Genetics Branch, National Human Genome Research Institute, National Institutes of Health, Bethesda, MD*

SOFIA D. MERAJVER, MD, *Division of Hematology and Oncology, Department of Internal Medicine, University of Michigan Health Systems, University of Michigan Comprehensive Cancer Center, Ann Arbor, MI*

GIUSEPPE MINNITI, MD, *Department of Pediatrics, Oregon Health Sciences University, Portland, OR*

PATRICIA A. MOTE, BSc, *Westmead Institute for Cancer Research, University of Sydney at Westmead Hospital, Westmead, Australia*

LEIGH C. MURPHY, PhD, *Department of Biochemistry and Molecular Biology, University of Manitoba, Winnipeg, Manitoba, Canada*

YOUNGMAN OH, PhD, *Department of Pediatrics, Oregon Health Sciences University, Portland, OR*

KENNETH J. PIENTA, MD, *University of Michigan Medical Center, Ann Arbor, MI*

I. H. RUSSO, MD, *Breast Cancer Research Laboratory, Fox Chase Cancer Center, Philadelphia, PA*

JOSE RUSSO, MD, *Breast Cancer Research Laboratory, Fox Chase Cancer Center, Philadelphia, PA*

DAVID S. SALOMON, PhD, *Tumor Growth Factor Section, Laboratory of Tumor Immunology and Biology, National Cancer Institute, National Institutes of Health, Bethesda, MD*

MARA DE SANTIS, MD, *Department of Psychiatry and Behavioral Sciences, Emory University School of Medicine, Atlanta, GA*

YUKIO SONODA, MD, *Gynecology Service, Department of Surgery, Memorial Sloan-Kettering Cancer Center, New York, NY*

VENIL N. SUMANTRAN, PhD, *Division of Endocrinology, Metabolism, and Hypertension, Wayne State University School of Medicine, Detroit, MI*

KENNETH L. VAN GOLEN, MD, *Division of Hematology and Oncology, Department of Internal Medicine, University of Michigan Health System, University of Michigan Comprehensive Cancer Center, Ann Arbor, MI*

BARBARA K. VONDERHAAR, PhD, *Molecular and Cellular Endocrinology Section, Laboratory of Tumor Immunology and Biology, National Cancer Institute, Bethesda, MD*

PETER H. WATSON, MD, *Department of Pathology, University of Manitoba, Winnipeg, Manitoba, Canada*

CHRISTIAN WECHSELBERGER, PhD, *Tumor Growth Factor Section, Laboratory of Tumor Immunology and Biology, National Cancer Institute, National Institutes of Health, Bethesda, MD*

NANCY L. WEIGEL, PhD, *Department of Cell Biology, Baylor College of Medicine, Houston, TX*

MAX S. WICHA, MD, *Department of Internal Medicine and University of Michigan Comprehensive Cancer Center, University of Michigan, Ann Arbor, MI*

KATHY YAO, MD, *Department of Surgery and the Robert H. Lurie Comprehensive Cancer Center, Northwestern University Medical School, Chicago, IL*

DOUGLAS YEE, PhD, *Division of Medical Oncology, Department of Medicine, University of Texas Health Science Center, San Antonio, TX*

1

Estrogen Receptor in Mammary Gland Physiology

Elizabeth Anderson, PHD,
Robert B. Clarke, PHD, and Anthony Howell, MD

CONTENTS

INTRODUCTION

It is taken for granted that the ovarian steroid, estrogen, is required for normal human breast development and tumorigenesis, but we still do not know exactly how this steroid exerts its effects, or even exactly what these effects are. These questions are not just academic: The mammary epithelium is the tissue from which most breast tumors arise, and understanding how processes such as its proliferation and differentiation are controlled may lead to an increased understanding of how cancers arise. Elucidation of normal breast function and physiology may also identify new targets and/or strategies for

From: *Contemporary Endocrinology: Endocrine Oncology*
Edited by: S. P. Ethier © Humana Press Inc., Totowa, NJ

preventing breast cancer (BC), a disease that affects more than 1/12 women in the Western world. This chapter reviews what is known about the role of the estrogen receptor (ER) in controling mammary gland physiology in human female breast tissue, although animal models will be referred to when appropriate.

STRUCTURE OF THE HUMAN MAMMARY GLAND

The mammary gland is an unusual organ in that is not fully developed at birth. There is further development at puberty, and the gland becomes fully differentiated and functional only at the time of pregnancy and subsequent lactation. The various stages of human mammary gland development have been elegantly and comprehensively described by Russo and Russo (1). Briefly, the major histological unit of the human breast is the lobular structure arising from a terminal duct. These ductal and lobular structures are lined by a continuous layer of luminal epithelial cells (ECs), which are, in turn, surrounded by a second layer of myo-ECs. In the adult nonpregnant, nonlactating breast, these myo-ECs are in direct contact with the basement membrane, and the whole structure is then surrounded by delimiting fibroblasts and a specialized intralobular stroma. Most human breast tumors are not only morphologically similar to the luminal EC population, but they also retain many of their biochemical characteristics (2). For example, most tumors express the same cytokeratin profile as luminal ECs, they contain steroid receptors, and they express polymorphic epithelial mucin (3,4). This leads to the conclusion that it is the luminal ECs in the mammary gland that are the major targets for malignant transformation and subsequent tumor formation. Consequently, an increased understanding of the mechanisms controling growth and differentiation of this population may identify new targets and strategies for early detection and prevention of BC in women.

ESTROGEN IS REQUIRED
FOR BREAST DEVELOPMENT AND TUMORIGENESIS

In terms of biological activity, the most important circulating estrogen in women is estradiol (E_2). From the advent of menarche until the menopause, E_2 is synthesized and secreted in a cyclical manner by the ovaries under the control of the pituitary gonadotrophins. The clinical and epidemiological evidence for an obligate role of estrogen in human mammary gland development and tumor formation is considerable. Observation of girls with estrogen deficiency through, e.g., gonadal dysgenesis or gonadotrophin deficiency, demonstrates that the steroid is strictly necessary (although probably not sufficient) for pubertal breast development (5). The incidence of BC in men is 1% of the incidence in women. Reducing exposure of the mammary gland to the fluctuating E_2 levels of the menstrual cycle, through an early natural or artificially induced menopause, substantially lowers the risk of developing BC. Conversely, increasing exposure through early menarche, late menopause, or late age at first full-term pregnancy raises the risk of cancer (6). The paramount role of E_2 in mammary gland development and tumorigenesis has been confirmed in several rat and mouse models, and perhaps the most compelling evidence comes from studies on mice in which the gene for the ER, the mediator of E_2 action, has been disrupted or knocked out. The mammary glands in these ER knockout (ERKO) mice comprise rudimentary ducts without terminal end buds or alveolar buds. These structures are confined to the nipple area, and cannot be induced to develop further (7). The rudimentary mammary glands of these ERKO mice are resistant to malignant tumor formation caused by introduction of the *wnt*-1 oncogene through transgenic manipulation, which provides very strong evidence for the role of estrogen and its cognate receptor in tumor promotion *(7)*. Finally, a large number of studies on rat models of mammary carcinogenesis show that administration of exogenous estrogens greatly enhances tumor formation; reduction of endogenous estrogen levels through, for example, ovariectomy or administration of inhibitors of E_2 synthesis, reduces or even eliminates tumor incidence *(8,9)*.

EFFECTS OF E_2 ARE MEDIATED BY ER

Like the other steroids, E_2 is lipophilic and enters cells and their nuclei primarily by diffusing through plasma and nuclear membranes. Once in the nucleus, E_2 encounters proteins known as ERs, because they bind E_2 with high affinity and specificity. Until relatively recently, only one ER gene (now called the ERα) was thought to be present in either humans or rodents. However, in 1996, a second species, or ERβ, was isolated and cloned from rat prostate and ovary, closely followed by the human homolog in the same year *(10,11)*. Both ERα and ERβ are members of the steroid/thyroid hormone nuclear receptor superfamily, and may be described as ligand-dependent nuclear transcription factors. Both proteins have the modular structure that typifies the nuclear receptor superfamily comprising six functional domains designated A–F, which include regions involved in steroid binding and interaction with DNA. The ERβ gene shows a high degree of sequence homology with the ERα in its hormone-binding (96%) and DNA-binding (58%) domains *(11)*. However, the ERβ gene is smaller than the ERα gene, has a different chromosomal location, and encodes a shorter protein (477 vs 595 amino acids for the ERβ and ERα, respectively) *(12)*. These features, together with the overlapping but distinctly different tissue distribution of ERβ, compared to ERα mRNA, have led many workers to suggest that the ERβ mediates some of the nonclassical effects of the estrogens and antiestrogens *(13)*. Alternatively, the fact that the ERβ is expressed in some of the same tissues as ERα has led to speculation that ERβ might interact with and modulate the actions of the ERα *(14)*. Much progress has been made recently toward understanding how binding of E_2 to either ERα or ERβ enhances specific gene transcription: This is described later in this volume.

As far as the human mammary gland is concerned, ERβ mRNA can be detected, but ERα mRNA appears to be present in greater amounts *(12)*. Furthermore, mice in which the ERβ gene has been knocked out have fully developed and functional mammary glands, but ERα knockout mice, as mentioned above, have only vestigial ductal structures *(15)*. Taken together, these data imply that the ERβ might not play a major role in the physiology of either the human or the mouse mammary gland, and the remainder of this chapter presents findings related only to the ERα.

ESTROGEN STIMULATES PROLIFERATION OF NORMAL HUMAN NONPREGNANT, NONLACTATING BREAST EPITHELIUM

The first studies on the effects of estrogen on the adult human mammary epithelium examined proliferative activity and other parameters throughout the menstrual cycle. It is difficult to obtain truly normal breast tissue for investigations of this type. To study normal physiology and function, it is highly desirable to use breast tissue from women who are not at increased risk of cancer, or who do not have a pre-existing malignant lesion. This means that most groups, including the authors, have used tissue from reduction mammoplasties or tissue adjacent to fibroadenomas, because these lesions were thought not to be associated with an increased risk of cancer. More recently, the relationship between the presence of a fibroadenoma and subsequent risk of BC has become less certain *(16)*, but material from women with these lesions still represents the most normal tissue that can be obtained, and it continues to be used in the authors' and other studies.

The proliferative activity of normal breast tissue taken at different times of the menstrual cycle was first assessed by labeling with tritiated thymidine ($[^3H]$-dT). The tissue, once removed from the patient, is incubated with the $[^3H]$-dT, then fixed and sectioned. Autoradiography reveals the cells that have incorporated $[^3H]$-dT and a thymidine-labeling index (TLI) can then be calculated as the percentage of ECs labeled with the radioactive nucleotide. One very striking finding is the variation in the TLI measurements between individual patients, which cannot be attributed to experimental variability. Whether this has any biological significance in terms of breast tissue estrogen sensitivity and risk of BC remains to be seen. Despite the high level of interindividual variation, the consensus is that the proliferative activity of human breast ECs is elevated in the luteal phase of the menstrual cycle *(17–23)*. Detailed analysis of other kinetic parameters, such as the mitotic and apoptotic indices, shows a similar pattern of change, because they also are higher in the second half of the cycle, compared to the first, although the apoptotic index reaches a peak around 3 d after the peak of proliferative activity *(19)*. Cyclical variation in epithelial expression of other proteins related to the proliferative and apoptotic processes has also been shown. For example, the antiapoptotic protein, Bcl-2, reaches peak levels in the middle of the menstrual cycle, and falls to a nadir at the time when apoptosis is greatest *(24)*.

Cyclical variation in mammary gland activity is not restricted to humans: The mouse mammary gland also undergoes cycles of proliferation and quiescence within the 5 d of the estrous cycle, so that the epithelial TLI is 3–4× higher during estrous, compared to proestrous *(25)*.

The obvious candidates for the control of these changes in the human and mouse mammary epithelia are E_2 and progesterone (P), because they are produced cyclically by the ovaries, and maximal breast proliferative activity in humans coincides with the mid-luteal phase peaks of E_2 and P secretion. In contrast, proliferation of the human endometrium, regarded as the classical estrogen target tissue, is highest in the follicular phase, and declines when P levels rise in the second half of the menstrual cycle. These observations have led several groups to suggest that, for the human breast epithelium, P is the major stimulatory steroid, either alone or after estrogen priming *(21)*. This suggestion has been investigated further, using a variety of different experimental approaches and models.

The simplest approach is the establishment of breast EC cultures in which the effects of E_2 and P can be determined under strictly defined conditions. However, it has proved difficult to establish luminal ECs in culture without them losing their original characteristics and steroid responsiveness. There is only one study *(26)* in which reasonably normal ECs have been cultured, but this does show that E_2 and not P enhances proliferative activity.

Because cultures of human breast ECs appear to be poor models for the study of steroid responsiveness, the other approach adopted by many workers is an in vivo system in which human breast tissue is implanted into athymic nude mice. This approach was first devised in the 1980s, and involved implanting several small pieces of normal human breast tissue subcutaneously into female athymic nude mice *(27)*. The mice were then treated with E_2, P, thyroxine, or human placental lactogen, either singly or in combination, and breast tissue pieces were removed at various time points thereafter for measure-

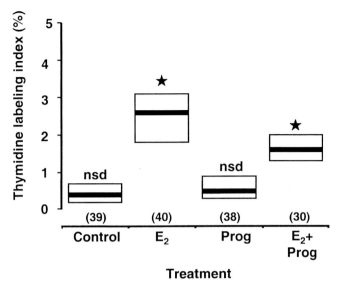

Fig. 1. Estradiol, but not P, stimulates the proliferative activity of normal human breast tissue implanted into athymic nude mice. This figure summarizes the results of measuring the proliferative activity of tissue implanted into athymic mice 14 d after the insertion of pellets containing either no steroid (Control), 2 mg estradiol (E_2), 4 mg P (Prog), or 4 mg P inserted after priming for 7 d with a 2-mg E_2 pellet (E_2 + Prog). Proliferative activity was assessed by determining the uptake of [^{3}H]-dT, and the data are the thymidine labeling indices (TLIs) calculated as the percentage of luminal ECs containing radiolabel. The open columns indicate the interquartile ranges; the horizontal bars indicate the median values; the numbers in parentheses along the abscissa indicate the number of observations in each group. *, significantly different ($P < 0.05$) from the pretreatment value by the Mann-Whitney U test.

ment of proliferative activity by [^{3}H]-dT labeling. This first study showed that human breast EC proliferation was stimulated by E_2. Thyroxine also stimulated proliferation, but human placental lactogen alone was without effect, although it did enhance the effects of E_2 when given in combination. In contrast, P did not alter the proliferative activity of the implanted tissue either alone or in combination with the other agents. Other investigators *(28–30)* used variations of this model in which, e.g., the human breast tissue was partially enzymatically digested before being implanted into either intact mammary fat pads of the athymic mice or into pads that had been cleared of their parenchyma. Yet another variation involved embedding human mammary ECs into extracellular matrices (type I collagen or reconstituted basement membrane) before subcutaneous implantation into the athymic mice *(31)*. Few of these studies addressed the effects of the ovarian steroids, but, when these were investigated, E_2 was shown to stimulate proliferation *(29)*.

Although informative, some of the early in vivo experiments used tissue taken from the periphery of diffuse benign breast lesions, and most of the studies used treatment schedules that resulted in the delivery of uncertain amounts of E_2, P, and other hormones. The authors' studies, using the in vivo model as originally conceived, tried to address these problems by ensuring that the tissue to be implanted was confirmed as histologically normal by a pathologist. The authors also calibrated the slow-release steroid-silastic pellets used, so that they delivered serum levels of E_2 and P similar to those seen in women during the menstrual cycle *(32)*. The results of these experiments are summarized in Fig. 1, and the most important take-home points are that E_2 stimulates the proliferative activity of normal human breast ECs, as measured by [^{3}H]-dT uptake, and that P, either alone or after E_2 priming, has no effect on EC proliferation. Further experiments have shown that the response to E_2 is dose-dependent between median E_2 serum concentrations of 400–1300 pmol/L, which are representative of those seen in the menstrual cycle. However, raising E_2 levels to those of early pregnancy (a median of 4400 pmol/L) does not further increase the levels of proliferative activity. The conclusion of these studies is that E_2 is the major steroid mitogen for the nonpregnant, nonlactating human breast, but other factors, in addition to E_2, must be required to enhance breast EC proliferation to the early pregnancy levels reported by other groups.

ESTROGEN INDUCES PROGESTERONE RECEPTOR EXPRESSION IN HUMAN BREAST EPITHELIUM

Because it seemed clear that human breast epithelium was an estrogen target tissue in terms of the control of proliferation, interest developed in other potential effects of estrogen on this tissue. Again, the first studies examined the expression of the ER and products of ER action, such as the progesterone receptor (PR) in breast tissue obtained at different times through the menstrual cycle. Using immunohistochemistry (IHC) on frozen sections of breast tissue, the authors, and others, demonstrated that approx 5% of luminal ECs contained ER (33–36). Moreover, the number of cells expressing ER was highest in the follicular phase of the cycle, lowest in the luteal phase, and, consequently, was inversely related to proliferative activity. In contrast, IHC detection of PR expression on adjacent frozen sections revealed that 15–20% of ECs contained PRs, and that this proportion did not vary appreciably during the cycle. Comparison with the endometrium, where PR is an estrogen-inducible protein, led to the suggestion that the PR may be constitutively expressed in the human breast. Again, the cell culture models proved disappointing, although, in the single report (26) of estrogen-responsive normal ECs in culture, E_2 treatment was shown to increase expression of both ER and PR. The in vivo model of human breast tissue implanted into athymic mice has provided more information on the control of steroid receptor content. First, it was found that the percentage of normal ECs expressing the ER fell from ~5%, at removal from the patients, to <1% 2 wk after being implanted into untreated mice (32). Administration of E_2 or P, either singly or in combination, had no effect on ER expression, but it is now known that these rather low levels of ER expression resulted from the insensitivity of the IHC technique for ER detection in frozen sections, especially after it had been adapted for use in the xenograft experiments. Second, the proportion of ECs expressing PR was also <1% 2 wk after being implanted into untreated mice, but the percentage of cells expressing PR was increased 15–20-fold by E_2 treatment at luteal-phase concentrations. This provided firm evidence that PR expression in human breast epithelium was controlled by estrogen, at least when the tissue is implanted into athymic mice.

The early studies on human breast EC proliferation and steroid receptor expression suggested that, although these processes may be controlled by ovarian steroids, the mechanisms involved could be appreciably different from those in the endometrium. However, later studies, using experimental models such as the implantation of human tissue into athymic mice, demonstrated that both mammary EC proliferation and PR expression are under estrogenic control. One explanation for the differences between the early and late studies may lie in the differential sensitivity of proliferation and PR expression to estrogen stimulation.

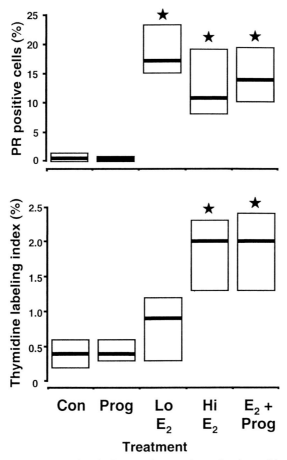

Fig. 2. Proliferation and PR expression in human breast tissue implanted into athymic mice are differentially sensitive to the effects of E_2. This figure summarizes the results of experiments in which PR expression (upper panel) and proliferation (lower panel) were determined 7 d after the insertion of pellets containing either no steroid (Con), 4 mg P (Prog); 0.5 mg E_2 (Lo E_2), which increased serum E_2 concentrations to the equivalent of those in the human follicular phase, 2 mg E_2 (Hi E_2), which gave the equivalent of human luteal-phase levels, and 2 mg E_2 combined with a 4-mg P pellet (E_2 + Prog) as in Fig. 1. The open columns represent the interquartile ranges of the data; the horizontal bars indicate the medians. *, significantly different from the control by Mann-Whitney U test.

PROLIFERATION AND PR EXPRESSION
ARE DIFFERENTIALLY SENSITIVE TO ESTROGEN STIMULATION

The suggestion that maximal induction of proliferation and PR expression may require exposure to differing concentrations of estrogen came from studies using human tissue implanted into athymic mice *(37)*. The upper panel of Fig. 2 shows the results of IHC detection of PR in sections cut from fixed and paraffin-embedded specimens of breast tissue xenografts removed from mice treated with follicular- or luteal-phase levels of E_2. These measurements show that the low E_2 levels of the follicular phase are sufficient to maximally induce PR expression, because the higher luteal-phase concentrations do not further enhance PR expression. However, follicular-phase E_2 levels are not sufficient to stimulate proliferative activity above that of the untreated breast tissue, and it is only when luteal-phase E_2 concentrations are reached that the TLI is significantly increased (lower panel, Fig. 2). These findings indicate that PR expression is far more sensitive to estrogen than proliferation, and explain the discrepancy between the data on PR expression during the cycle and those obtained from the model of normal human breast tissue implanted into athymic mice: Even the lowest levels of E_2 seen in serum or in breast tissue itself during the menstrual cycle are sufficient to completely induce PR expression, but proliferation is only enhanced when luteal-phase levels are reached.

STEROID RECEPTOR EXPRESSION
AND PROLIFERATION ARE DISSOCIATED IN LUMINAL ECs

The above findings lead to the question of whether PR expression and proliferation occur in the same cell that is differentially sensitive to two concentrations of E_2, or whether the two processes take place in separate populations of ECs. Dual labeling techniques, in which steroid receptor expression and proliferation were detected simultaneously in sections of human breast tissue, provided the answer to this question (38). In the first experiments, sections of [³H]-dT-labeled breast tissue, taken at different times of the menstrual cycle, were stained by IHC, to reveal the PR-expressing cells, then autoradiographed to determine which cells had taken up [³H]-dT. Figure 3A shows an example of this labeling, and indicates separation of the PR-expressing and -proliferating cells. Quantitation of the number of PR-positive cells, those that were [³H]-dT-labeled, and those in which labeling was coincident (see Table 1), confirmed the existence of two separate populations of estrogen-responsive luminal ECs. However, an alternative explanation suggested by studies on cultured human BC cells is that PR synthesis was downregulated during the S-phase of the cell cycle detected by [³H]-dT labeling. In order to confirm the existence of the two separate populations of luminal ECs, dual fluorescent-label IHC was used to simultaneously detect the Ki-67 proliferation-associated antigen (Ag) and steroid receptor expression. The Ki-67 antigen has been reported as being present in cell nuclei at all stages of the cell cycle, except G0, and should be co-localized with the PR, if, as suggested above, the receptor is downregulated during S-phase (39). Dual immunofluorescent labeling of normal tissue showed that very few cells contained both the PR and the Ki-67 Ag, and this was confirmed by counting the numbers of cells expressing these two Ags in many representative samples of normal human breast tissue (Table 1).

Since both the PR-expressing and proliferative cells are responsive to estrogen, it seems reasonable to assume that both populations would contain the ER. Accordingly, analysis of the coincidence of ER and PR expression and of ER and Ki-67 expression, was carried out using the same methods and samples as above. The results from these experiments show, first, that the proportion of luminal cells containing the ER is higher than would be predicted from the previous studies on ER expression in the normal breast, because of the greater sensitivity of the IHC method for detecting ER and Ki-67 expression in fixed paraffin-embedded tissue, which involves a microwave Ag retrieval step. Second, and as expected, there is almost complete coincidence of labeling for the ER and PR, in that 96% of cells labeled with the anti-PR antibody also contain ER (Fig. 3B and Table 1). However, the third and most surprising finding was the almost complete dissociation between ER expression and proliferation within the luminal epithelium. A representative photomicrograph is shown in Fig. 3C, and quantitation of the proportion of

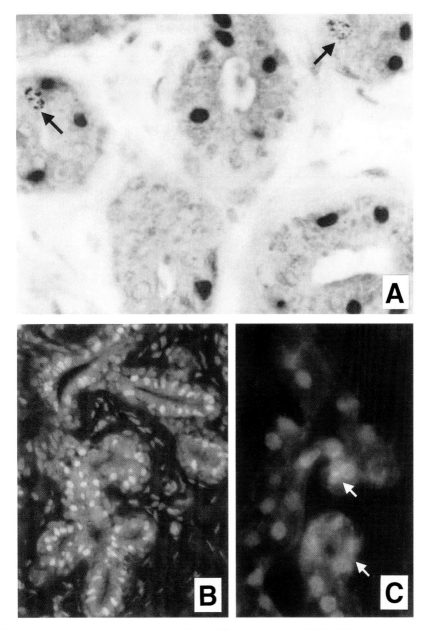

Fig. 3. Steroid receptors are not expressed in proliferating luminal ECs. These are representative photomicrographs obtained from dual-label IHC and autoradiography. (**A**) Section of [^{3}H]-dT-labeled normal human breast tissue, in which PR-expressing cells have been revealed by IHC (brown nuclei), followed by autoradiography, to show the proliferating cells (black grains overlying cell nuclei, as indicated by the arrows). (**B**) Section of normal human breast tissue in which ER and PR expression have been determined using a dual-label immunofluorescent technique. In this particular case, all the ER-expressing cells (which would fluoresce green) also express the PR (which would fluoresce red), to give a yellow color. The section has also been counterstained with the blue fluorochrome, DAPI. (**C**) section of normal human breast tissue in which ER and Ki-67 expression has been determined using a dual-label immunofluorescent technique. In this case, ER expressing cells are labeled with the red fluorochrome, and those cells expressing the Ki-67 Ag are labeled green. The arrows indicate areas in which proliferating cells are adjacent to those expressing the ER.

Table 1
Data from the Simultaneous Estimation of Proliferation
and Steroid Receptor Expression in Samples of Normal Human Breast Tissue

No. samples	Cells counted	ER+ve	PR+ve	[^{3}H]-dT+ve	Ki-67+ve	No. cells dual-labeled	% dual labeled[a]
10	10,026	1735		46		1	2
25	25,302		3232	382		17	4.5
25	28,395	2107			639	9	1.4
25	28,018		3231		391		1.8
13	13,895	1792	1765				96

[a] Percentage of proliferating cells (as indicated by the cells labeled with [^{3}H]-dT or the Ki-67 antibody), also containing steroid receptors.

doubly and singly labeled cells (Table 1) shows that far fewer cells than would be expected contain both ER and the Ki-67 Ag. Also, as demonstrated in Fig. 3C, many of the proliferating cells are adjacent to cells expressing steroid receptors, which appear to be evenly distributed throughout the luminal epithelium. This dissociation between luminal cell steroid receptor expression and proliferation in the human breast has been confirmed by at least one other group (40). It also appears that a similar situation may occur in rodents, because these authors have observed separate populations of PR expressing and [^{3}H]-dT-labeled cells in the rat mammary gland (40). In the mouse mammary gland, there is dissociation between ER expression and [^{3}H]-dT uptake in the terminal end buds during both pubertal growth and estrous-cycle-associated proliferation (25).

It appears that the processes of PR expression and proliferation in human luminal ECs are differentially sensitive to the effects of E_2. Expression of the PR is exquisitely sensitive, which means that, in vivo, there is always sufficient E_2, either in the circulation or in the breast tissue itself, to ensure that the receptor is maximally expressed. It is also clear that steroid receptor expression and proliferation occur in separate populations of luminal ECs, although proliferating cells are usually adjacent to those containing steroid receptors. The implication of these findings is that proliferation is not controlled directly by E_2, although other processes, such as PR expression, are. These findings raise many questions about the hormonal control of normal breast physiology and function.

ARE EFFECTS OF ESTROGEN MEDIATED BY PARACRINE GROWTH FACTORS?

The studies described above provide some clues about how E_2 may control EC proliferation indirectly, and these have been incorporated into the model illustrated in Fig. 4. The fact that ER-negative but proliferative cells are often adjacent to those that are ER-positive suggests that the ER-positive cells act as E_2 sensors, which secrete juxtacrine and/or paracrine factors that trigger proliferation of the ER-negative cells, once a threshold E_2 concentration is reached. Studies on cultured BC cell lines provide indirect support for this model. These show that medium conditioned by E_2-treated ER-positive BC cells stimulates proliferation of ER-negative cell lines growing in culture or as xenografts in athymic mice (41). Conversely, conditioned medium from ER-positive BC cells treated with antiestrogens inhibits proliferation when applied to ER-negative BC cells (42). Further analysis of the conditioned medium suggests that peptide growth factors, such as

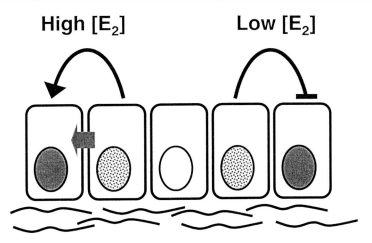

Fig. 4. Model for the indirect estrogenic control of normal human breast EC proliferation. In this model, the cells capable of proliferation are ER-negative (as indicated by the dark nuclei), but are situated very close or adjacent to those containing the receptor (represented by the speckled nuclei). The ER-containing cells act as estrogen sensors and secrete paracrine or juxtacrine growth factors, which influence the activity of the ER-negative proliferative cells. In this model, the ER-containing cells secrete growth stimulatory factors when E_2 levels are high, as shown in the lefthand part of this scheme, and growth inhibitory peptides when E_2 levels are low, as on the righthand side of the diagram.

insulin-like growth factor-I, and transforming growth factors-α and -β, are involved in mediating these paracrine effects. A final piece of evidence for a paracrine mechanism of controling proliferation in the mammary gland comes from tissue recombination studies *(43)*, in which epithelium isolated from ERKO mice is combined with stroma (in this case, the fat pads) from wild-type mice, and cultured in the subrenal capsules of E_2-treated athymic mice. The results of this experiment and its reverse, in which wild-type epithelium is combined with ERKO fat pads, demonstrate that, in the mouse, E_2 stimulates epithelial proliferation indirectly via a paracrine mechanism. However, the estrogen-sensing cells appear to be in the stromal compartment, because wild-type epithelium does not respond to E_2 treatment when combined with ERKO stroma (or fat pads). In humans, the ER has never been detected in the stroma surrounding the mammary epithelium, leading to the conclusion that the estrogen-sensing cells are in the epithelial compartment. It is not as yet clear how separate populations of ER-expressing and -proliferating mammary ECs might arise. The authors' working hypothesis is that the ER-negative proliferating cells represent precursor or stem cells, which eventually differentiate to become nonproliferative, ER-positive cells.

BIOLOGICAL CONSEQUENCES OF INDIRECT MECHANISM OF E_2 ACTION

This chapter reviews the role of the ER in controling proliferation and other processes in the normal human nonpregnant, nonlactating breast. Both ER and its ligand, E_2, are necessary for the development of mammary epithelial structures. However, it is becoming clear that the ER is not expressed in the proliferating population of cells, which suggests that the effects of E_2 are mediated by paracrine and/or juxtacrine factors. Why does

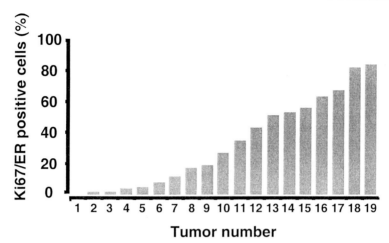

Fig. 5. The dissociation between steroid receptor expression and proliferation is maintained in some human breast tumors, but lost in others. This figure indicates the proportion of ER-containing cells that are also labeled with an antibody against the Ki-67-proliferation-associated Ag in 19 human breast tumors.

E_2 exert its effects on the mammary epithelium by this indirect mechanism? The authors have established that the human breast is an estrogen target tissue, as is the endometrium, but, unlike the epithelial elements of the endometrium, the proliferative activity of the breast epithelium is not highly sensitive to estrogen. This makes biological sense, because it would be undesirable for the breast to undergo changes in proliferation of the magnitude and speed as those seen in the endometrium during each menstrual cycle. Therefore an indirect or paracrine method of controlling breast EC proliferation may have evolved to attenuate sensitivity to E_2. During pregnancy, when more extensive proliferative activity is required, circulating levels of E_2 are much higher, and there are large numbers of other factors that could enhance estrogen sensitivity.

If breast EC proliferative activity is so insensitive to E_2, why is PR expression so exquisitely sensitive to the hormone? The authors' hypothesis is that the ER- and PR-expressing cells are a differentiated population, and, if this is correct, it is possible that P has a role in maintaining or even inducing this differentiation. In biological terms, induction of differentiation would be an additional means of preventing undesirable proliferative activity in the luminal population of breast ECs.

Breast tumor formation also requires E_2, and a large proportion of cancers (~70%) express the ER, often at high levels. Examination of ER and Ki-67 expression in human breast tumors, using the techniques described above, reveals that some tumors maintain complete dissociation between receptor expression and proliferation, but others contain large populations of proliferating cells that also express the ER (Fig. 5; *38*). The implications of this finding are not yet clear, but the authors' favored explanation is that these dual-labeled tumor cells have partially differentiated, so that they express the ER, retain the capacity to divide, and are still being controled by paracrine mechanisms. The alternative explanation is that the ER in the dual-labeled cells is driving proliferation via a more direct mechanism. Whichever explanation is correct, it seems likely that increasing ER content would be one way in which tumors enhance their sensitivity to E_2 stimulation, which may, in turn, accelerate their progression.

CLINICAL CONSEQUENCES
OF INDIRECT MECHANISM OF E_2 ACTION

An increased understanding of the role of the ER in mammary gland physiology has important clinical implications. First, there is considerable interindividual variation in breast EC proliferative activity, but it is not yet known whether women with high rates of proliferation are at increased risk of BC. Current interpretation of the mechanisms of carcinogenesis suggests that this may be the case, and it should be remembered that most of the endocrinological BC risk factors increase the number of times that the breast epithelium undergoes a cyclical increase in proliferation. If it could be shown that estrogen sensitivity of the luminal ECs does correlate with BC risk, individual risk prediction might be envisaged, based on measuring products of E_2 action in samples obtained by relatively noninvasive techniques, such as nipple or fine-needle aspiration.

In the future, noninvasive functional scanning techniques, such as positron emission tomography, based on the use of E_2 or thymidine isotopes, may be used to detect breast epithelial activity. In terms of BC prevention, strategies that reduce or prevent the cyclical variation in EC proliferation should be effective. This could be achieved by administering antiestrogens, such as tamoxifen or raloxifene, both of which have been shown to reduce BC incidence in clinical trials *(44,45)*. An alternative approach that is also being tested is the use of gonadotrophin-releasing hormone agonists to inhibit ovarian steroid secretion, combined with very small replacement doses of estrogen and androgen to protect the cardiovascular and skeletal systems *(46)*. A final approach, which may be more specific with fewer associated side effects, could be the induction of differentiation within the luminal epithelium. Early first full-term pregnancy protects against BC, presumably because a large number of ECs undergo terminal differentiation and become, therefore, resistant to malignant transformation *(6)*. Furthermore, pregnancy-associated hormones, such as human chorionic gonadotrophin, protect against induction of mammary tumors in rodents, but only if they are administered in early reproductive life, when the gland is most susceptible to carcinogenic agents *(4,7)*. Unfortunately, the age at which first full-term pregnancy occurs in women is increasing rapidly, which means that encouraging early pregnancy is unlikely to succeed as a BC prevention strategy. However, short-term administration of a differentiating agent early in reproductive life could be an effective and acceptable means of achieving the same aim.

SUMMARY

It is now clear that the ER and its ligand, E_2 are obligatory for the growth and development of the mammary gland in both humans and rodents. E_2 is also the stimulus for the cyclical increases in mammary EC proliferation during the menstrual cycle in women and during the estrous cycle in mice. However, the ER probably does not interact directly with the intracellular mechanisms controlling proliferation, instead, ER containing cells appear to alter the activity of adjacent proliferative ER-negative cells via the secretion of paracrine or juxtacrine growth factors. The authors postulate that this indirect effect on proliferation combined with the exquisite sensitivity of processes thought to be associated with differentiation (e.g., PR expression) is one way of preventing unwanted proliferation in the mammary gland in the absence of pregnancy. In some human breast tumors, the dissociation between steroid receptor expression and proliferation is lost. In these cases, it is not clear whether E_2 continues to drive proliferation by the indirect mechanisms that occur in the normal breast, or whether an alternative, more direct, effect of the ER has arisen during the process of malignant transformation. Thus, detailed characterization of EC ER expression in relation to proliferation, and other processes at various stages during development, has enhanced understanding of the role of the receptor in mammary gland physiology. Future studies of this type should lead to the identification of new targets, which, in turn, could form the basis of novel strategies for prevention and early detection of human BC.

REFERENCES

1. Russo J, Russo IH. Development of the human mammary gland. In: Neville MC, Daniel CW, eds. The Mammary Gland. Development, Regulation and Function. Plenum, New York, 1987, pp. 67–93.
2. Wellings SR, Jensen HM, Marcum RG. An atlas of subgross pathology of the human breast with special reference to possible precancerous lesions. J Natl Cancer Inst 1975;55:231–273.
3. Taylor-Papadimitriou J, Millis R, Burchell J, Nash R, Pang L, Gilbert J. Patterns of reaction of monoclonal antibodies HMFG-1 and 2 with benign breast tissues and breast carcinomas. J Exp Pathol 1986;2:247–260.
4. Taylor-Papadimitriou J, Stampfer M, Bartek J, Lewis A, Boshell M, Lane EB, Leigh IM. Keratin expression in human mammary epithelial cells cultured from normal and malignant tissue: relation to in vivo phenotypes and influence of medium. J Cell Sci 1987;94:403–413.
5. Laron Z, Pauli R, Pertzelan A. Clinical evidence on the role of oestrogens in the development of the breasts. Proc Roy Soc Edin B 1989;95:13–22.
6. Key TJA, Pike MC. The role of oestrogens and progestagens in the epidemiology and prevention of breast cancer. Eur J Cancer Clin Oncol 1988;24:29–43.
7. Bocchinfuso WP, Korach KS. Mammary gland development and tumorigenesis in estrogen receptor knockout mice. J Mammary Gland Biol Neoplasia 1997;2:323–334.
8. Nandi S, Guzman RC, Yang J. Hormones and mammary carcinogenesis in mice, rats and humans: a unifying hypothesis. Proc Natl Acad Sci USA 1995;92:3650–3657.
9. Lubet RA, Steele VE, DeCoster R, Bowden C, You M, Juliana MM, Eto I, Kelloff GJ, Grubbs CJ. Chemopreventive effects of the aromatase inhibitor vorozole (R 83842) in the methylnitrosourea-induced mammary cancer model. Carcinogenesis 1998;19:1345–1351.
10. Kuiper GGJM, Enmark E, Pelto-Huikko M, Nilsson S, Gustafsson J-A. Cloning of a novel estrogen receptor expressed in rat prostate and ovary. Proc Natl Acad Sci USA 1996;93:5925–5930.
11. Mosselman S, Polman J, Dijkema R. ERβ: identification and characterization of a novel human estrogen receptor. FEBS Lett 1996;392:49–53.
12. Enmark E, Pelto-Huikko M, Grandien K, Lagercrantz S, Lagercrantz J, Fried G, Nordenskjold M, Gustafsson J-A. Human estrogen receptor β-gene structure, chromosomal location and expression pattern. J Clin Endocrinol Metab 1997;82:4258–4265.
13. Kuiper GGJM, Carlsson B, Grandien K, Enmark E, Haggblad J, Nilsson S, Gustafsson J-A. Comparison of the ligand binding specificity and transcript tissue distribution of estrogen receptors α and β. Endocrinology 1997;138:863–870.
14. Katzenellenbogen BS, Korach KS. Editorial: A new actor in the estrogen receptor drama—enter ERβ. Endocrinology 1997;138:861,862.
15. Krege JH, Hodgin JB, Couse JF, Enmark E, Warner M, Mahler JF, et al. Generation and reproductive phenotypes of mice lacking oestrogen receptor β. Proc Natl Acad Sci USA 1998;95:15,677–15,682.
16. Dupont WD, Page DL, Parl FF, Vnencak-Jones CL, Plummer WD Jr, Rados MS, Schuyler PA. Long term risk of breast cancer in women with fibroadenoma. N Engl J Med 1994;331:10–15.
17. Masters JRW, Drife JO, Scarisbrook JJ. Cyclic variation of DNA synthesis in human breast epithelium. J Natl Cancer Inst 1977;58:1263–1265.
18. Meyer JS. Cell proliferation in normal human breast ducts, fibroadenomas and other ductal hyperplasias measured by nuclear labeling with tritiated thymidine. Effects of menstrual phase, age and oral contraceptive hormones. Hum Pathol 1977;8:67–81.
19. Anderson TJ, Ferguson DJP, Raab GM. Cell turnover in the "resting" human breast: influence of parity, oral contraceptive pill, age and laterality. Br J Cancer 1982;46:376–382.
20. Going JJ, Anderson TJ, Battersby S, MacIntyre CCA. Proliferative and secretory activity in human breast tissue during natural and artificial menstrual cycles. Am J Pathol 1988;130:193–204.

21. Potten CS, Watson RJ, Williams GT, Tickle S, Roberts SA, Harris M, Howell A. The effect of age and menstrual cycle upon proliferative activity of the normal human breast. Br J Cancer 1988;58:163–170.
22. Olssen H, Jernstrom H, Alm P, Kreipe H, Ingvar P, Jonssen E, Ryden S. Proliferation of the breast epithelium in relation to menstrual cycle phase, hormonal use and reproductive factors. Breast Cancer Res Treat 1996;40:187–196.
23. Soderqvist G, Isaksson E, von Schoultz B, Carlstrom K, Tani E, Skoog L. Proliferation of breast epithelial cells in healthy women during the menstrual cycle. Am J Obstet Gynecol 1997;176:123–128.
24. Sabourin JC, Martin A, Baruch J, Truc JB, Gompel A, Poitout P. *bcl*-2 expression in normal human breast tissue during the menstrual cycle. Int J Cancer 1994;59:1–6.
25. Zeps N, Bentel JM, Papadimitriou JM, D'Antuono MF, Dawkins HS. Estrogen receptor-negative epithelial cells in mouse mammary gland development and growth. Differentiation 1998;62:221-226.
26. Malet C, Gompel A, Yaneva H, Cren H, Fidji N, Mowszowicz I, Kutenn F, Mauvai-Jarvis P. Estradiol and progesterone receptors in cultured normal human breast epithelial cells and fibroblasts: immunocyto-chemical studies. J Clin Endocrinol Metab 1991;73:8–17.
27. McManus MJ, Welsch CW. The effect of estrogen, progesterone, thyroxine and human placental lacto-gen on DNA synthesis of human breast ductal epithelium maintained in athymic nude mice. Cancer 1984;54:1920–1927.
28. Gusterson BA, Williams J, Bunnage H, O'Hare MJ, Dubois JD. Human breast epithelium transplanted into nude mice. Proliferation and milk protein production in response to pregnancy. Virchows Arch A Pathol Anat Histopathol 1984;404:325–333.
29. Sheffield LG, Welsch CW. Transplantation of human breast epithelia to mammary-gland free fat pads of athymic nude mice: influence of mammotrophic hormones on growth of breast epithelia. Int J Cancer 1988;41:713–719.
30. Dubois JD, O'Hare MJ, Monaghan P, Bartek J, Norris R, Gusterson BA. Human breast epithelial xeno-grafts: an immunocytochemical and ultrastructural study of differentiation and lactation. Differentiation 1987;35:72–82.
31. Popnikolov NK, Yang J, Guzman RC, Nandi S. Reconstituted human normal breast in nude mice using collagen gel or Matrigel. Cell Biol Int 1995;19:539–546.
32. Laidlaw IJ, Clarke RB, Howell A, Owen AWMC, Potten CS, Anderson E. Proliferation of normal human breast tissue implanted into athymic nude mice is stimulated by estrogen and progesterone. Endocrinology 1995;136:164–171.
33. Williams G, Anderson E, Howell A, Watson R, Coyne J, Roberts SA, Potten CS. Oral contraceptive use increases proliferation and decreases oestrogen receptor content of epithelial cells in the normal human breast. Int J Cancer 1991;48:206–210.
34. Ricketts D, Turnbull L, Ryall R, Bakhshi R, Rawson NS, Gazet JC, Nolan C, Coombes RC. Estrogen and progesterone receptors in the normal female breast. Cancer Res 1991;51:1817–1822.
35. Soderqvist G, von Schoultz B, Tani E, Skoog L. Estrogen and progesterone receptor content in breast epithelial cells from healthy women during the menstrual cycle. Am J Obstet Gynecol 1993;168:874–879.
36. Boyd M, Hildebrandt RH, Bartow SA. Expression of the estrogen receptor gene in developing and adult human breast. Breast Cancer Res Treat 1996;37:243–251.
37. Clarke RB, Howell A, Anderson E. Estrogen sensitivity of normal human breast *in vivo* and implanted into athymic nude mice: analysis of the relationship between estrogen-induced proliferation and proges-terone receptor expression. Breast Cancer Res Treat 1997;45:121–133.
38. Clarke RB, Howell A, Potten CS, Anderson E. Dissociation between steroid receptor expression and cell proliferation in the human breast. Cancer Res 1997;57:4987–4991.
39. Gerdes J, Lemke H, Baisch H, Wacker HH, Schwab U, Stein H. Cell cycle analysis of a cell proliferation associated human nuclear antigen defined by the monoclonal antibody Ki-67. J Immunol 1984;133:1710–1715.
40. Russo IH, Russo J. Role of hormones in mammary cancer initiation and progression. J Mammary Gland Biol Neoplasia 1998;3:49–61.
41. Clarke R, Dickson RB, Lippman ME. Hormonal aspects of breast cancer. Growth factors, drugs and stromal interactions. Crit Rev Oncol Hematol 1992;12:1–23.
42. Knabbe C, Lippman ME, Wakefield LM, Flanders KC, Kasid A, Derynck R, Dickson RB. Evidence that transforming growth factor β is a hormonally regulated negative growth factor in human breast cancer cells. Cell 1987;48:417–428.
43. Cunha GR, Young P, Hom YK, Cooke PS, Taylor JA, Lubahn DB. Elucidation of a role for stromal steroid hormone receptors in mammary gland growth and development using tissue recombination experiments. J Mammary Gland Biol Neoplasia 1997;2:393–402.

44. Fisher B, Costantino JP, Wickerham DL, Redmond CK, Kavanah M, Cronin WM, et al. Tamoxifen for prevention of breast cancer: report of the National Surgical Adjuvant Breast and Bowel Project P-1 study. J Natl Cancer Inst 1998;90:1371–1388.
45. Husten L. Raloxifene reduces breast cancer risk. Lancet 1999;353:44.
46. Pike MC, Daniels JR, Spicer DV. A hormonal contraceptive approach to reducing breast and ovarian cancer risk: an update. Endocr-Related Cancer 1997;4:125–133.
47. Russo J, Russo IH. Role of differentiation in the pathogenesis and prevention of breast cancer. Endocr-Related Cancer 1997;4:7–21.

2

Multiple Facets of Estrogen Receptor in Human Breast Cancer

Leigh C. Murphy, PHD, Etienne Leygue, PHD, Helmut Dotzlaw, PHD, Amanda Coutts, PHD, Biao Lu, MSC, Aihua Huang, MSC, and Peter H. Watson, MB

CONTENTS

INTRODUCTION

Estrogen is a major regulator of mammary gland development and function, and affects the growth and progression of mammary cancers *(1,2)*. In particular, the growth responsiveness of breast cancer (BC) cells to estrogen is the basic rationale for the efficacy of the so-called endocrine therapies, such as antiestrogens. Estrogens mediate their action via the estrogen receptor (ER), which belongs to the steroid/thyroid/retinoid receptor gene superfamily *(3)*. The protein products of this family are intracellular, ligand-activated transcription factors regulating the expression of several gene products, which ultimately elicit a target tissue-specific response *(4)*. Indeed, ER, together with progesterone receptor (PR), expression in human breast tumors, are important prognostic indicators, as well as markers of responsiveness to endocrine therapies *(5,6)*. However, although the majority of human BCs are thought to be initially hormone-responsive, it is well appreciated that alterations in responsiveness to estrogen occurs during breast tumorigenesis. During BC progression, some ER-positive BCs are *de novo* resistant to endocrine therapies, and of those that originally respond to antiestrogens, many develop resistance. This progression from hormonal dependence to independence is a significant clinical problem,

From: *Contemporary Endocrinology: Endocrine Oncology*
Edited by: S. P. Ethier © Humana Press Inc., Totowa, NJ

because it limits the useful of the relatively nontoxic endocrine therapies, and is associated with a more aggressive disease phenotype *(7)*. This occurs despite the continued expression of ER, and often PR *(8,9)*. The ER is pivotal in estrogen and antiestrogen action in any target cell, but the nature of the ER is clearly multifaceted.

Until recently, it was thought that only one ER gene existed. However, a novel ER, now referred to as ERβ, has recently been cloned and characterized *(10,11)*. Moreover, it has recently been shown that ERβ mRNA is expressed in both normal and neoplastic human breast tissue *(12–14)*. This suggests that ERβ may have a role in estrogen action in both normal and neoplastic human breast tissue. Furthermore, it has now become apparent that several variant mRNA species of both the classical ERα and ERβ can be expressed in human breast tissues, and may therefore have roles in estrogen and antiestrogen signal transduction *(13,15–18)*. The current data suggest that an evaluation of estrogen interaction with human breast tissue needs to include ERα, ERβ, and any variant forms of these receptors that may be expressed. The following chapter focuses on the multifaceted nature of the ER in human breast tissues.

ERα AND ITS VARIANTS

Identification of ERα Variant mRNAs in Human Breast Tissues

A large body of data has accumulated supporting the existence of ERα variants *(19,20)*. The majority of the data supporting the expression of ERα variants has been at the mRNA level. Two main structural patterns of ERα variant mRNAs have been consistently identified: the truncated ERα mRNAs *(21)* and the exon-deleted ERα mRNAs *(22)*. The truncated ERα mRNAs were originally identified, by Northern blot analysis, as fairly abundant smaller-sized mRNA species in some human BC biopsy samples *(23)*. The cDNAs of several truncated ERα mRNAs have been cloned and found to contain authentic polyadenylation signals followed by poly(A) tails. The exon-deleted ERα mRNAs have been identified mostly from reverse transcription polymerase chain reaction (RT-PCR) products, using targeted primers.

Multiple ERα variant mRNAs are often detected in individual tumor specimens. In order to determine the relative frequency and pattern of variant expression in a particular sample, an RT-PCR approach was developed that allowed the simultaneous detection of all deleted ERα variant mRNAs containing the primer annealing sites in exons 1 and 8, at levels that represent their initial relative representation in the RNA extract. Since truncated transcripts do not have exon 8 sequences, they will not be measured by this technique. Examples of the results obtained are shown (Fig. 1), and serve to illustrate that

Fig. 1. Top panel. Schematic representation of WT ERα (WT-ER) cDNA and primers allowing co-amplification of most of the described exon-deleted ERα variants. ERα cDNA contains eight different exons coding for a protein divided into structural and functional domains (A–F). Region A/B of the receptor is implicated in transactivating function (AF-1). The DNA-binding domain is located in the C region. Region E is implicated in hormone binding and another transactivating function (AF-2). 1/8U and 1/8L primers allow amplification of 1381-bp fragment corresponding to WT ERα mRNA. Co-amplification of all possible exon-deleted or -inserted variants, which contain exon 1 and 8 sequences, can occur. Amplification of the previously described ERα variant mRNAs deleted in exon 3 (D3-ER), exon 4 (D4-ER), exon 7 (D7-ER), both exons 3 and 4 (D3–4-ER), exons 2 and 3 (D2–3-ER), exons 4 and exon 7 (D4/7-ER), would generate 1264-, 1045-, 1197-, 928-, 1073-, and 861-bp fragments, respectively. **Bottom panel.** Co-amplification of WT ERα and deleted variant mRNAs in breast tumor samples. Total RNA extracted from ER-positive (+) and ER-negative (−) breast tumors was reverse-transcribed and PCR-amplified, as described *(24)*, using 1/8U

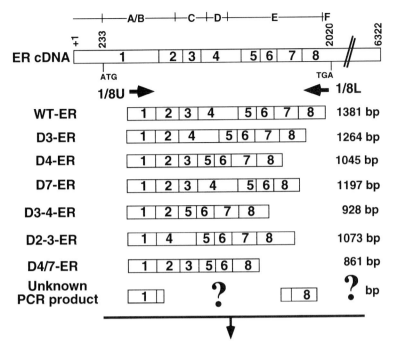

PCR Co-amplification of WT-ER
and all known and unknown
deleted-ER variant mRNAs

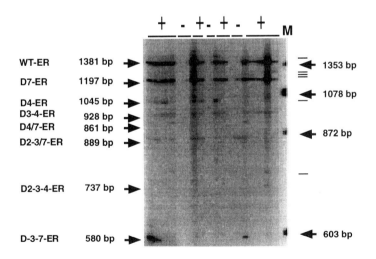

and 1/8L primers. Radioactive PCR products were separated on a 3.5% acrylamide gel, and visualized by autoradiography. Bands reproducibly obtained within the set of tumors studied, and which migrated at 1381, 1197, 1045, 928, 889, 861, 737, and 580 bp, were identified as corresponding to WT-ER mRNA and variant mRNAs deleted in exon 7 (D7-ER), exon 4 (D4-ER), both exons 3 and 4 (D3–4-ER), exons 2, 3, and 7 (D2–3/7-ER), both exons 4 and 7 (D4/7-ER), exons 2, 3, and 4 (D2–3–4-ER), and within exon 3 to within exon 7 (D-3–7-ER), respectively. PCR products indicated by dashes (-), barely detectable within the tumor population, i.e., present in less than or equal to three particular tumors, have not yet been identified. M, Molecular weight marker (phi174, Gibco-BRL, Grand Island, NY). Adapted with permission from ref. *24*.

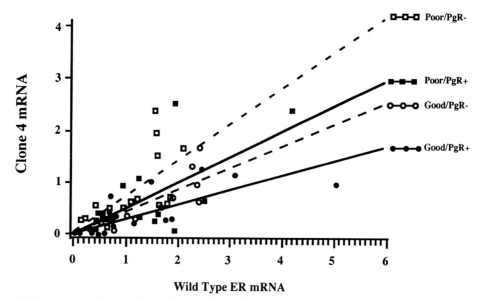

Fig. 2. Linear regression analysis of the relationship between the clone-4-truncated ERα mRNA and the WT ERα mRNA in the various groups. Closed circles represent the good prognosis/ER-positive–PR-positive group; open circles represent the good prognosis/ER-positive–PR-negative group; closed squares represent the poor prognosis/ER-positive–PR-negative group; open squares represent the poor prognosis/ER-positive–PR-negative group. Good vs Poor, $P = 0.0004$; PR-negative vs PR-positive. $P = 0.011$. Reproduced with permission from ref. *25*.

a complex pattern of exon-deleted variant ERα transcripts are expressed in any one tumor, that the pattern and relative frequency of detection of ERα variant mRNAs may vary between tumors, and that, in some cases, the relative frequency of detection of individual ERα variant mRNAs may be correlated with known prognostic markers *(24)*.

An example of such a correlation is shown in Fig. 2 *(25)*. The expression of the truncated clone-4 ERα variant mRNA was measured relative to the wild-type (WT) ERα mRNA in a group of breast tumors. The relative expression of the clone-4 variant was significantly increased in those tumors with characteristics of poor prognosis, compared to those tumors with good prognostic characteristics, i.e., clone-4 expression was higher in large tumors with high S-phase fraction, and from patients with nodal involvement, compared to small tumors with low S-phase fraction from patients without nodal involvement. Also, in this group, the relative expression of clone-4 was significantly higher in PR-negative tumors vs PR-positive tumors, suggesting a correlation of increased truncated variant expression and markers of endocrine resistance.

Data support the possibility that ERα variant proteins exist, and that their pattern and frequency are different from different individuals. In some cases, the expression of single ERα variant mRNA species was correlated with known markers of prognosis and endocrine sensitivity. This, in turn, suggested the hypothesis that altered expression of ERα variants may be a mechanism associated with progression to hormone independence.

Putative Biological Significance of ERα Variant mRNAs

Expression of ERα Variant mRNAs in Normal and Neoplastic Human Breast Tissue

Most studies investigating ERα variant mRNAs have used human BC tissues or cell lines *(19)*. However, it is now known that both truncated and exon-deleted ERα variant mRNAs can be detected in other tissues, including normal tissues *(19)*. In particular, ERα variant mRNAs have been identified in normal human breast tissue and cells *(26–29)*. Therefore, ERα variant mRNAs are not tumor-specific, are not found in the complete absence of the WT ERα mRNA, and are probably generated by alternative splicing mechanisms.

These observations raised the question of whether the expression of ERα variant mRNAs is altered during breast tumorigenesis and/or progression. When the level of expression of individual variant ERα mRNAs was measured relative to the level of the WT ER transcript, differences between normal and breast tumor tissues were found. The relative expression of clone-4-truncated ERα variant mRNA and the exon-5-deleted ERα variant mRNA, but not the exon-7-deleted ERα variant mRNA, was significantly increased in breast tumors, compared to normal breast tissues obtained from both reduction mammoplasties and normal tissues adjacent to breast tumors *(26,27)*. Preliminary data suggests that this is also true for samples of ER-positive breast tumors and their matched, adjacent normal tissues *(29a)*; there is also evidence suggesting that an exon-3-deleted ERα variant mRNA is decreased in BCs, compared to normal human breast epithelium *(29)*. Because this ERα variant mRNA encodes a protein that can inhibit WT ERα transcriptional activity *(30)* and causes growth suppression when stably overexpressed in ER-positive MCF-7 human BC cells *(29)*, it was concluded that the exon-3-deleted ERα variant may function to attenuate estrogenic effects in normal mammary epithelium. This function is markedly reduced via decreased exon-3-deleted ERα expression during breast tumorigenesis. In preliminary studies of ER-positive human breast tumor samples and their matched adjacent normal tissues, a statistically significant decreased relative expression of the exon-3-deleted ERα mRNA in the tumor, compared to the normal breast tissues, was noted *(29a)*.

The available data provide evidence for an extensive and complex pattern of alternative splicing associated with the ERα gene, which may be altered during breast tumorigenesis.

SPECIFICITY OF ERα SPLICE VARIANTS IN HUMAN BREAST TUMORS

It is unlikely that the mechanisms generating alternatively spliced forms of ERα result from a generalized deregulation of splicing processes within breast tumors, since similar variants for the glucocorticoid receptor *(16,28)*, the retinoic acid receptors-α and -γ *(28)*, and vitamin D_3 receptor *(16)* have not been found in breast tumor tissues. However, similar splice variants of PR (*see* subheading Expression of Other Steroid Hormone Receptors, below) were found in both normal and neoplastic breast tissues *(31,32)*.

EXPRESSION OF ERα VARIANT mRNAS DURING BC PROGRESSION

As described above, the relative expression of at least one ERα variant mRNA, i.e., clone-4-truncated ERα mRNA, is significantly higher in primary breast tumors with characteristics of poor prognosis (including the presence of concurrent lymph node metastases), compared to primary tumors with good prognostic markers (including lack of concurrent lymph node metastases) *(25)*. An increased relative expression of exon-5-deleted ERα mRNA has been found in locoregional BC relapse tissue (in the same breast as the original primary tumor, but no lymph node metastases) obtained from patients following a median disease-free interval of 15 mo, compared to both the corresponding primary breast tumor *(33)* and the primary breast tumor tissue of patients who did not relapse during this period. Although the difference did not reach statistical significance, these same authors reported a trend toward higher relative expression of exon-5-deleted ERα mRNA in primary tumors of women who relapsed, compared to primary tumors of those that did not relapse. Together, these data suggest that, in addition to altered expression of ERα variant mRNA, which occurs during breast tumorigenesis, further changes in ERα variant expression may occur during BC progression. However, another study *(34)* has recently found no significant differences in the relative expression of clone-4-truncated, exon-5-deleted, and exon-7-deleted ERα mRNAs, between a series of primary breast tumors and their matched concurrent lymph node metastasis, suggesting that altered expression of ERα variant mRNAs probably occurs prior to the acquisition of the ability to metastasize, and therefore may be a marker of future metastatic potential. This hypothesis remains to be tested.

EXPRESSION OF ERα VARIANT mRNAS AND ENDOCRINE RESISTANCE

The hypothesis that altered forms of ERα may be a mechanism associated with endocrine resistance has been suggested for some time. Moreover, the identification of ERα variant mRNAs in human breast biopsy samples *(23,35,36)* provided good preliminary data for the hypothesis. In addition, preliminary functional data of the recombinant exon-5-deleted ERα protein suggested that it possessed constitutive, hormone-independent transcriptional activity that was about 15% that of the WT ER *(36)*. The data using a yeast expression system were also consistent with the correlation of relatively high levels of exon-5-deleted ERα mRNA in several human BC biopsy samples classified as ER-negative and PR-positive and/or pS2-positive *(36–38)*. It was also found that the exon-5-deleted ERα mRNA was often co-expressed at relatively high levels with the WT ERα in many human BC that were ER-positive *(38)*. It has been observed that transiently expressed exon-5-deleted ERα has an inhibitory effect on endogenously expressed WT ERα in MCF-7 human BC cells *(39)*, although it does not decrease the WT activity to the same extent as hydroxytamoxifen. In contrast, in human osteosarcoma cells, exon-5-deleted ERα was shown to have little effect alone, but significantly enhanced estrogen-stimulated gene expression by transiently co-expressed WT ERα *(40)*. The limitations of transient expression analysis were addressed by two groups who stably overexpressed the exon-5-deleted ERα in MCF-7 human BC cells *(41,42)*. However, different phenotypes were obtained by the two groups. No effect of the recombinant exon-5-deleted ERα on growth or estrogen/antiestrogen activity in MCF-7 cells was found in one study *(41)*; in the other study *(42)*, the overexpression of recombinant exon-5-deleted ERα in MCF-7 cells was associated with estrogen-independent and antiestrogen-resistant growth. The reasons for the differences between the two studies are unclear, but may be the result of different MCF-7 variants, or changes that could have occurred in the transfectants in addition to transgene expression. The transgene in the Rea and Parker study *(41)* was episomally maintained; in the study by Fuqua et al. *(42)*, the transgene was presumably integrated into the host chromosomes in a random fashion.

Several laboratories have developed cell culture models of estrogen independence and antiestrogen resistance. Variable results have been obtained when the association of altered ERα variant mRNA expression with estrogen/antiestrogen responsiveness was investigated. An increased relative expression of an exon-3 + 4-deleted ERα variant mRNA was found in an estrogen-independent MCF-7 cell line (T5-PRF) derived by long-term growth in estrogen-depleted medium *(43,44)*. However, this cell line was still sensitive to antiestrogens *(43)*. Although one cell line that was tamoxifen (TAM)-resistant had differential expression of an exon-2-deleted ERα and an exon-5-deleted ERα mRNA, compared to the parental cell line *(45)*, other independently derived antiestrogen-resistant clones showed no major differences in the expression of ERα variant mRNAs *(46,47)*.

Investigation of ERα splice variants, using clinical tissue samples, has also led to variable conclusions. The relative expression of the clone-4-truncated ERα variant mRNA was significantly increased in primary breast tumors with characteristics of poor prognosis, compared to tumors with good prognostic characteristics *(25)*. Similarly, the relative expression of clone 4 was significantly higher in PR-negative vs PR-positive tumors, suggesting a correlation of increased truncated variant expression and markers of endocrine resistance *(25)*. Furthermore, an increased frequency of detection of ERα variant mRNAs deleted in exons 2–4 and 3–7 was associated with high tumor grade, but an increased detection of an exon-4-deleted ERα variant mRNA was associated with low tumor grade *(24)*. The presence of exon-5-deleted ERα mRNA was found in one study *(39)* to be associated with increased disease-free survival. However, no difference in the relative expression of an exon-5-deleted ERα variant mRNA was found between all TAM-resistant tumors and primary control breast tumors *(37)*, although, in the subgroup of TAM-resistant tumors that were ER-positive/pS2-positive, the relative expression of the exon-5-deleted ERα was significantly greater than the control TAM-sensitive group.

Although increased expression of any one ERα variant does not correlate with TAM resistance of BCs overall, its association with, and therefore possible involvement in, endocrine resistance in some tumors cannot be excluded. Moreover, the presence of multiple types of ERα variant mRNAs in any one tumor or normal tissue sample has been well documented *(24,28)*, but no data have been published in which total ERα splice variant expression has been analyzed in relationship to endocrine resistance and prognosis. Although mutations have been found in the ERα gene in human breast tumors, they are rare and are not more frequent in TAM-resistant tumors *(48)*.

IDENTIFICATION OF ERα VARIANT PROTEINS

The detection of proteins that correspond to ERα variant mRNAs remains an important issue. It is relevant, therefore, to understand the structure of these proteins. The predicted proteins of some of the most frequently detected ERα variant transcripts are shown schematically in Fig. 3. All of the variant transcripts would encode ERα proteins missing some structural/functional domains of the WT ERα. Although the ERα variant transcripts encode several different types of protein, there are some common themes that emerge. A common feature of these putative proteins is the universal presence of the A/B region, which is known to contain the cell and promoter specific AF-1 function. Exon-4-deleted and exon-3 + 4-deleted ERα mRNAs are in frame and encode proteins that do not bind ligand. However, the majority of the most abundantly expressed variant transcripts, i.e, exon-7-deleted, an exon-4 + 7-deleted, and the clone-4-truncated ERα mRNAs, encode proteins that are C-terminally truncated, and cannot bind ligand. Thus, a common feature of these variants is the inability to bind ligand. The results obtained, in which recombinant techniques were used to measure the function of individual ERα variants in vitro, are variable, and often depend on co-expression of the WT receptor. It is difficult to make general conclusions, but many recombinant ERα variant proteins have been observed to modulate the activity of the WT receptor. However, the relevance of the relative levels of expression of WT and variant ERα proteins that are achieved under the experimental conditions used is unclear, because limited data have been published on the

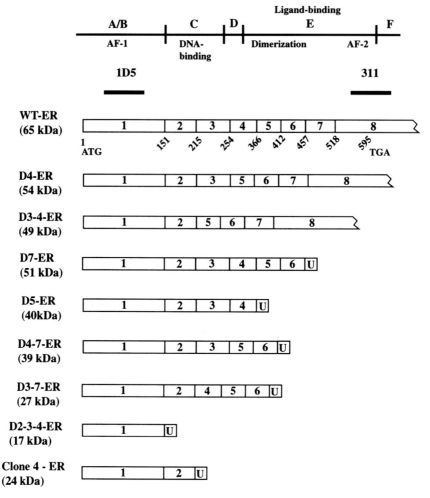

Fig. 3. Schematic representation of the ERα variant proteins predicted to be encoded by ERα variant mRNAs. Identical sequence is depicted by numbered exons. U, amino acid sequence unrelated to WT human ERα amino acid sequence. U sequences are unique to any particular variant. The position of N- and C-terminal epitopes, recognized by 1D5 and AER311 Abs, respectively, are indicated.

detection of ERα variant proteins encoded by known ERα variant mRNAs in tissues or cells in vivo.

From a different perspective, the prediction that the majority of ERα variant proteins are C-terminally truncated has implications for the determination of clinical ER status. Early detection, and changes in clinical practice, have resulted in smaller amounts of breast tumor tissue being available for assay. For this and other reasons, the use of immunohistochemistry (IHC) methods to assess ER status is becoming more common. Therefore, depending on the antibodies (Abs) used, the presence of C-terminally truncated ERα variant proteins could theoretically influence determination of ER status of the tumor sample. The authors have tested this experimentally, by transiently transfecting WT ERα and clone-4-truncated ERα expression vectors into Cos-1 cells, and determining ER status of the cells, using Abs either to the N-terminus of the ERα (Fig. 3, 1D5, Dako) or Abs to the C-terminus (Fig. 3, AER311, Neomarkers). Preliminary data, using different combinations of WT ERα and variant ERα expression vectors transfected into Cos-1 cells, indicate that the signals (expressed as H-scores, which take into account the intensity of staining and the number of positively staining cells) obtained with the N-terminal and C-terminal Abs, become increasing discrepant (N-terminal > C-terminal signal) with increasing variant expression, presumably because of increased ERα-like proteins containing the N-terminal region, but not the C-terminal region. These preliminary data suggest that increased expression of C-terminally truncated ERα variant proteins could interfere with the IHC determination of ER status.

This possibility was investigated in human breast tumor tissues *(49)*. A series of breast tumors was assayed for ERα, using the set of Abs described above, and the H-scores from each Ab were compared for each tumor. The tumors fell into two distinct groups: one in which the H-scores obtained with each Ab were consistent and not significantly different from each other; and another group, in which the H-scores obtained with each Ab were inconsistent and significantly different from each other. Further, in all but one case, the H-score was higher for the N-terminal Ab, compared to the C-terminal Ab *(50)*. In preliminary experiments using a subset of the original tumor set, the authors found similar results, using another set of N-terminal and C-terminal ERα Abs. Together with the previous experimental data, one interpretation of the tumor data would be that the discrepant tumors had higher levels of C-terminally truncated ERα-like proteins.

To address the hypothesis that the C-terminally truncated ERα-like proteins could correspond to proteins encoded by ERα variant transcripts, the authors compared expression of ERα variant mRNAs in the consistent and inconsistent tumors. The results show a significantly higher relative expression and detection of ERα variant mRNAs that would encode C-terminally truncated proteins in the inconsistent vs the consistent tumors *(50)*. These results suggest that, irrespective of function, the expression of significant amounts of C-terminally truncated ERα variant proteins could interfere with the IHC determination of ER status, which, in turn, might underlie some of the inconsistencies between ER status and clinical response to endocrine therapy. These data are consistent with the hypothesis that ERα variant mRNAs may be stably translated in vivo. However, such data are indirect, and other mechanisms, e.g., altered epitope detection, increased proteolytic activity, and so on, may underlie the discrepant ERα H-scores found in some human breast tumors.

More recently, data published from several independent groups support the detection of ERα-like proteins in cell lines and tissues in vivo, which could correspond to those predicted to be encoded by previously identified ERα variant mRNAs. The presence of an exon-5-deleted ERα protein was demonstrated immunohistochemically in some human breast tumors, using a monoclonal Ab specific to the predicted unique C-terminal amino acids of the exon-5-deleted ERα protein *(39)*. However, although there was a correlation between IHC detection and presence or absence of exon-5-deleted ERα mRNA determined by RT-PCR, the group was unable to detect any similar protein by Western blotting, suggesting either very low levels, compared to WT ERα, or differential stability of the variant protein relative to the WT ERα during the extraction procedure. In addition, an ERα-like protein, consistent with that predicted to be encoded by the exon-5-deleted ER mRNA, is expressed in some BT 20 human BC cell lines, as determined by Western blot analysis *(51)*. Western blotting of ovarian tissue has identified both a 65-kDa WT ERα protein and a 53-kDa protein recognized by ERα Abs to epitopes in the N-terminus and C-terminus of the WT protein, but not with an Ab recognizing an epitope encoded

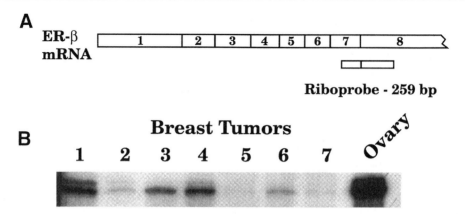

Fig. 4. Detection of ERβ mRNA in human breast tumors by RNase protection assay. (**A**) Schematic representation of hERβ mRNA showing various exon sequences, and identifying the riboprobe position and size of the expected protected fragment (259 bp). (**B**) Total RNA was isolated from seven breast tumor samples, and 25 μg was used in an RNase protection assay, as previously described *(21)*. Ovarian RNA was used as a positive control.

by exon 4 *(52)*. These results correlated with the presence of both WT and exon-4-deleted ERα mRNAs in these tissues, and suggested that the 53-kDa protein was derived from the exon-4-deleted ERα mRNA.

More recently, a 61-kDa ERα-like protein and a more abundant 65-kDa WT ERα protein were identified in MCF-7 cells *(29)*. The 61-kDa protein is thought to be encoded by an exon-3-deleted ERα mRNA expressed at low levels in these cells, and its co-migration, both before and after dephosphorylation with the recombinant exon-3-deleted ERα protein, when expressed at higher levels after stable transgene expression in another MCF-7 clone, was thought to strongly suggest its identity with the recombinant exon-3-deleted ERα protein.

There is accumulating evidence suggesting that variant ERα proteins, which correspond to those predicted to be encoded by some of the ERα variant mRNAs, can be detected by conventional technologies in clinical specimens.

ERβ AND ITS VARIANTS

Identification of ERβ mRNA in Human Breast Tissues

With the discovery of ERβ, which had properties similar to, yet distinct from, ERα *(10, 11,53,54)*, and can interact with the ERα *(55,56)*, it became important to know whether ERβ was expressed in human breast tumors, and, if so, what role it plays in estrogen/ antiestrogen action.

The authors have detected the presence of ERβ mRNA, both by RT-PCR *(12,14)* and by RNase protection assay (Fig. 4; *14*), in some human BC biopsy samples and some human BC cell lines. *In situ* hybridization analysis suggested that expression of ERβ mRNA could be detected in the BC cells of a human BC biopsy sample *(14)*. Using an RT-PCR approach to analyze both ERβ and ERα mRNA expression in a range of breast tumors *(12)*, the following was observed: There was no correlation between ERβ expression and ERα expression in breast tumors; in some cases, both ERβ and ERα mRNA were expressed in the same tumor; in those tumors in which both ER mRNAs were expressed, the relative expression appeared to vary widely among tumors. Furthermore, ERβ mRNA can be detected in normal human breast tissues by RT-PCR *(13)* and RNase protection assay *(14)*. Although there are no data reporting the expression of ERβ protein(s) in human breast tissues as yet, the available information suggest that ERβ may be expressed in both normal and neoplastic human breast tissues, and may have a role in these tissues.

Expression of ERβ mRNA During Breast Tumorigenesis

The demonstration of ERβ mRNA expression in both human breast tumors and normal human breast tissue suggests that the well-documented role of estrogen in breast tumorigenesis *(1,57)* may involve both receptors. Using a multiplex RT-PCR approach, it has been shown that the ERα:ERβ ratio in a small group of ER-positive human breast tumors was significantly higher than the ratio in their adjacent normal breast tissues *(58)*. The increase in ERα:ERβ ratio in breast tumors was primarily the result of a significant upregulation of ERα mRNA in all ER-positive tumors, in conjunction with a lower ERβ mRNA expression in the tumor, compared to the normal compartment in some, but not all, ER-positive cases. Preliminary data suggest that the level of ERβ mRNA in breast tumors may be correlated with the degree of inflammation (unpublished data). Because *in situ* hybridization data suggest that expression of ERβ mRNA could be detected in the cancer cells of a human BC biopsy sample *(14)*, and that human lymphocytes in lymph nodes can also express ERβ mRNA *(14)*, it is possible that the cell type contributing to the expression of ERβ mRNA may be heterogeneous, depending on the tumor characteristics. If the RNA studies reflect the protein levels of the two ERs, results to date provide evidence to suggest that the role of ERα- and ERβ-driven pathways, and/or their interaction, probably changes during breast tumorigenesis.

Identification of ERβ Variant mRNAs in Human Breast Tissues

The presence of multiple ERα variant mRNAs in both normal and neoplastic human breast tissues has led to the question of the expression of ERβ variant mRNAs. Several ERβ variant mRNAs have been detected. The authors have identified an exon-5 + 6-deleted ERβ mRNA in human breast tumors *(59)*. This transcript is in-frame, and would be expected to encode an ERβ-like protein deleted of 91 amino acids within the hormone binding domain. A human ERβ variant mRNA, deleted in exon 5, was identified in MDA-MB231 human BC cells and in some human breast tumor specimens *(18)*. Although that group was unable to detect an exon-5-deleted ERβ mRNA in normal human breast tissue, the authors have detected both exon-5-deleted ERβ mRNA and an exon-6-deleted ERβ mRNA, as well as an an exon-5 + 6-deleted ERβ mRNA, in normal human breast tissue samples *(13)*, and in some human breast tumors. The exon-5-deleted ERβ mRNA and the exon-6-deleted ERβ mRNA are out-of-frame and predicted to encode C-terminally truncated ERβ-like proteins, which would not bind ligand.

More recently, several exon-8-deleted human ERβ mRNAs have been identified *(17)* from a human testis cDNA library, and by RT-PCR from the human BC cell line MDA-MB435. These variants have been named human ERβ2–5. It should be noted that human ERβ2 is not the equivalent of the ERβ variant mRNA with an in-frame insertion of 54 nucleotides between exons 5 and 6 identified in rodent tissues *(13,60,61)*, and also named ERβ2. The authors have been unable to detect an equivalent of the rodent ERβ2 mRNA in any normal or neoplastic human tissue so far studied *(13)*.

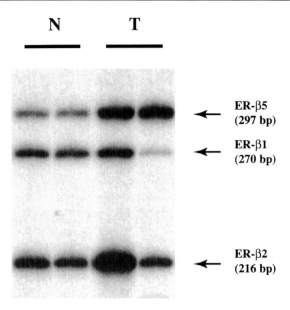

Fig. 5. RT-triple primer PCR analysis *(26)* of the relative expression of human ERβ1, human ERβ5, and human ERβ2 mRNAs in normal (N) and breast tumor (T) tissue samples.

Several of the human ERβ variants deleted in exon 8, specifically hERβ2 and hERβ5, can be detected in normal human mammary gland and in several human BC cell lines *(17)*. The predominant type of hERβ exon-8-deleted mRNA present varies among the different cell lines. The authors have confirmed the presence of the hERβ2 and the hERβ5 variant mRNAs in several normal human breast tissue samples from both reduction mammoplasties and normal tissue adjacent to breast tumors (Fig. 5; unpublished data). Moreover, the authors have identified both hERβ2 and the hERβ5 variant mRNAs in several human breast tumor samples (Fig. 5; unpublished data). Using a semiquantitative RT-triple primer PCR approach *(26)*, which simultaneously measures the relative expression of the WT hERβ1 and the two variant hERβ2 and hERβ5 mRNAs, it appears that, in most, but not all, cases, the level of the variant mRNA species exceeds that of the WT hERβ1 (Fig. 5; unpublished data) in both normal and neoplastic human breast tissues. The known sequence of all human ERβ-like transcripts is shown schematically in Fig. 6; also shown in this figure are the proteins predicted to be encoded by these variant hERβ mRNAs. All the hERβ variant mRNAs identified to date are predicted to encode proteins that are altered in the C-terminus in some fashion, and are unlikely to bind ligand *(62)*. However, published data *(17)* suggest that some of these variant receptors can form homo- or heterodimers among themselves and with WT hERβ and hERα, and may preferentially inhibit hERα DNA-binding transcriptional activity *(62)*.

Putative Role of ERβ and Its Variants in Breast Cancer

Transient transfection studies have provided data which suggest that ERβ1, i.e., the WT ERβ, can only mediate an antagonist response when bound to TAM-like agents, in contrast to the TAM-bound WT ERα, which can mediate either an antagonist or agonist activity on a basal promoter linked to a classical estrogen response element *(53,63)*. This suggests the possibility that altered relative expression of the two ERs may underlie

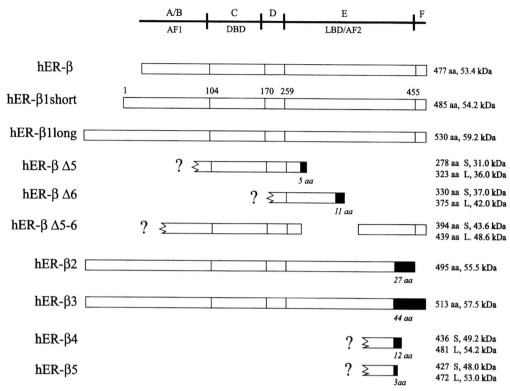

Fig. 6. Human ERβ isoforms. All hERβ isoforms are aligned. White boxes indicate identity of amino acid between sequences. Amino acid positions of the different structural domains are indicated for the hERβ1 short *(14)*, which contains eight extra N-terminal amino acids, compared to the first hERβ described *(10)*. hERβ1 long (Genbank AF051427) contains 45 additional N-terminal amino acids. hERβ1Δ5 *(13,18)*, hERβ1Δ6 *(13)*, hERβ2 (Genbank AF051428, AB006589cx), hERβ3 (Genbank AF060555), hERβ4 (Genbank AF061054), and hERβ5 (Genbank AF061055) are truncated, and contain different C-terminal amino acids (black boxes). hERβΔ5–6 *(13)* (Genbank AF074599) is missing 91 amino acids within the LBD/AF-2 domain. For each receptor, the length (aa) and the calculated molecular mass (kDa), when known or corresponding to the short (S) or the long (L) forms of the putative proteins, are given. Broken boxes and question marks indicate that flanking amino acid sequences are unknown.

altered responses to antiestrogens, and could be a mechanism of altered responsiveness to antiestrogens in human BC. The activity of the estrogen-bound ERβ1 on activating protein 1 (AP-1)-containing promoters is inhibitory, in contrast to that of estrogen-bound ERα, which stimulates transcription *(54)*. Furthermore, antiestrogens of all types demonstrated marked transcriptional activity through ERβ1 on promoters that contained AP-1 sites *(54)*. A nonligand-binding hERβ variant protein, encoded by the variant hERβ2 (also named hERβcx), can heterodimerize with ERβ1, but preferentially heterodimerizes with ERα, and shows a dominant-negative activity only against ERα-mediated transactivation *(17,62)*. It is possible, therefore, that ERβ1 and its variants could have a direct regulatory role on ERα activity. Since the authors have observed an increased ratio of ERα:ERβ mRNA in human breast tumors, compared to their adjacent matched normal tissues, which primarily results from increased expression of ERα mRNA in the breast tumor component *(58)*, it is possible that this may translate into unregulated ERα activity and unregulated growth responses mediated through ERα.

However, there are several issues that must be addressed before anyone can begin to develop rational pathophysiologically relevant hypotheses regarding the role of ERβ and/or its variants in human breast tissues. First, it is not yet known whether ERβ and ERα are expressed together in the same breast cells, or separately in different normal or neoplastic cell populations. Second, studies so far have only measured mRNA levels. No studies of ERβ protein expression in human breast have been published to date. Therefore, the pathophysiological relevance of the relative levels of ERβ and ERα expression achieved in transient expression studies, and the resulting functional outcome, are unknown. Third, some in vitro studies have been done using an N-terminally truncated ERβ1 *(64)*, and the functional impact of this is also unknown.

EXPRESSION OF OTHER STEROID HORMONE RECEPTORS AND THEIR VARIANTS IN HUMAN BC

The observation that the PR gene showed a complex pattern of alternative splicing similar to, although not as extensive as, that of ERα, led to the further characterization of PR variants *(16,31,32)*. Two commonly expressed variant transcripts identified in human breast tumors and normal human breast tissue were cloned and sequenced. Variant PR mRNAs with either a precise deletion of exon 6 or exon 4 were identified in most breast tumors examined. PR transcripts deleted in exon 2, exons 3 + 6, or exons 5 + 6, were also found in a few breast tumors *(31,32)*. The exon-6-deleted transcript was the most abundant and frequently expressed PR variant mRNA in the human breast tumors examined, and specific PCR primers were designed to determine the expression of this transcript, relative to the WT PR, using RT-PCR analysis *(27)*. Altered expression of ERα variant mRNAs was observed previously between normal and neoplastic breast tissue; therefore, it was of interest to determine if exon-6-deleted PR mRNA expression was altered during breast tumorigenesis. Using an approach similar to that described previously *(27)*, the relative expression of the exon-6-deleted variant PR mRNA to the WT PR mRNA was examined in 10 normal reduction mammoplasty samples and 17 breast tumors. The relative expression of the exon-6-deleted PR variant to the WT PR mRNA was found to be significantly lower ($P < 0.01$) in normal breast tissues (median = 4.8%) than in breast tumors (median = 13.9%) (unpublished data).

The exon-2-deleted PR mRNA encodes a C-terminally truncated PR-like protein without a DNA or a ligand-binding domain *(32)*. The exon-4-deleted PR mRNA is in-frame, but encodes a protein deleted in exon 4 sequences, missing a nuclear localization signal, and the recombinant protein representing exon-4-deleted PR-A did not bind DNA and had little effect on WT PR-A function *(32)*. Exon-6-deleted PR variant mRNA is out-of-frame and encodes a C-terminally truncated PR-like protein lacking the hormone-binding domain, and the exon-5 + 6-deleted PR variant mRNA is in-frame, but encodes a protein deleted in exon 5 + 6 sequences of the hormone-binding domain *(32)*. Richter et al. *(32)* have demonstrated that recombinant proteins, representing the exon-6-deleted PR-A and the exon-5 + 6-deleted PR-A are dominant-negative transcriptional inhibitors of both the WT PR-A and PR-B *(32)*. It is possible, therefore, that the presence of PR variant proteins encoded by the identified PR variant mRNAs could modify WT PR activity and influence responses to endocrine therapies. Small, variant PR-like proteins have been identified by Western blotting in some breast tumors *(32,65,66)*, which correspond in size to some of the proteins predicted to be encoded by some of the exon-deleted PR mRNAs. However,

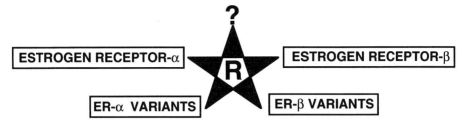

Fig. 7. Schematic representation of the known and unknown (?) multiple facets of the estrogen receptor (R).

some data *(66)* suggest that the presence and abundance of PR variant mRNAs may not correlate with the detection of these smaller-sized PR immunoreactive species in human breast tumors.

The measurement of PR is an important tool in clinical decision-making with respect to prognosis and treatment of human BC. Furthermore, the level of PR expression provides important clinical information *(67)*. As the use of enzyme-linked immunosorbent assays and IHC assays for PR detection increases, it is likely that variant PR expression will interfere with these assays, whatever their function. PR Ab (AB-52 Ab) used in such assays detect epitopes in the N-terminal region of the WT molecule, which is shared by truncated PR-like molecules. If any or all of the deleted PR variant mRNAs so far identified are translated into stable proteins, they will be co-detected with the WT PR in such assays. Presence of PR variants may also be a factor contributing to discrepancies between biochemical measurement and immunological detection of PR. Indeed, the potential for ERα variant expression to interfere with the IHC assessment of ER status has been documented *(49,50,68)*.

CONCLUSIONS AND CONTROVERSIES

The multifaceted nature of the ER is suggested by the expression of ERα mRNA, ERβ mRNA, and their variant mRNAs in both normal and neoplastic human breast tissues (Fig. 7). There is a large body of molecular data that support at least the potential for the multifaceted nature of the ER, and therefore estrogen/antiestrogen signaling in both normal and neoplastic human breast tissues. Alterations in the relative expression of several ER-like mRNAs have been shown to occur during breast tumorigenesis, and the relative frequency of detection and expression of individual ER-like mRNAs can be correlated with different prognostic characteristics in BC. This, in turn, suggests a possible role in breast tumorigenesis and possibly hormonal progression in BC. However, there are still major gaps that need to be filled before there can be a clear idea of the pathophysiological and functional relevance of the experimental results so far in hand. Unequivocal data are required to support the in vivo detection of variant ERα, variant ERβ, and WT ERβ proteins, which correspond to the variant ERα, variant ERβ, and WT ERβ mRNA species, respectively. There is a need to experimentally determine putative function, using expression levels that reflect pathophysiological levels of expression. There is a need to know if the two WT ERs and/or their variants are co-expressed in the same cells within heterogeneous normal and neoplastic breast tissues. Further, given the detection of multiple forms of variant ER-like species in any one breast tissue sample, the limitations in interpreting data from experimental systems, in which only one variant species is considered in the presence or absence of WT protein, needs to be understood.

ACKNOWLEDGMENTS

This work was supported by grants from the Canadian BC Research Initiative (CBCRI) and the U.S. Army Medical Research and Materiel Command (USAMRMC). The Manitoba Breast Tumor Bank is supported by funding from the National Cancer Institute of Canada (NCIC). LCM is a Medical Research Council of Canada (MRC) Scientist, PHW is a MRC Clinician-Scientist, EL is a recipient of a USAMRMC Postdoctoral Fellowship, AC is a recipient of a Manitoba Health Research Council (MHRC) Studentship.

REFERENCES

1. Vorherr H. Breast Cancer. Urban & Schwarzenberg, Baltimore, 1980.
2. Clarke R, Skaar T, Baumann K, Leonessa F, James M, Lippman M, et al. Hormonal carcinogenesis in breast cancer: cellular and molecular studies of malignant progression. Breast Cancer Res Treat 1994;31: 237–248.
3. Green S, Kumar V, Krust A, Walter P, Chambon P. Structural and functional domains of the estrogen receptor. Cold Spring Harbor Symp Quant Biol 1986;51:751–758.
4. Tsai MJ, O'Malley BW. Molecular mechanisms of action of steroid/thyroid receptor superfamily. Annu Rev Biochem 1994;63:451–486.
5. Horwitz KB, McGuire WL, Pearson OH, Segaloff A. Predicting response to endocrine therapy in human breast cancer: a hypothesis. Science 1975;189:726,727.
6. Horwitz K, Koseki Y, McGuire W. Estrogen control of progesterone receptor in human breast cancer: role of estradiol and antiestrogen. Endocrinology 1978;103:1742–1751.
7. Murphy L. Mechanisms associated with the progression of breast cancer from hormone dependence to independence. Pezcoller Foundation J 1995;2:6–16.
8. Taylor R, Powles T, Humphreys J, Bettelheim R, Dowsett M, Casey A, Neville A, Coombes R. Effects of endocrine therapy on steroid-receptor content of breast cancer. Br J Cancer 1982;45:80–84.
9. Katzenellenbogen B. Antiestrogen resistance: mechanisms by which breast cancer cells undermine the effectiveness of endocrine therapy. J Natl Cancer Inst 1991;83:1434,1435.
10. Mosselman S, Polman J, Dijkema R. ER-beta: identification and characterization of a novel human estrogen receptor. FEBS Lett 1996;392:49–53.
11. Kuiper G, Enmark E, Pelto-Huikko M, Nilsson S, Gustafsson J-A. Cloning of a novel estrogen receptor expressed in rat prostate and ovary. Proc Natl Acad Sci USA 1996;93:5925–5930.
12. Dotzlaw H, Leygue E, Watson P, Murphy L. Expression of estrogen receptor-beta in human breast tumors. J Clin Endocrinol Metab 1997;82:2371–2374.
13. Lu B, Leygue E, Dotzlaw H, Murphy LJ, Murphy LC, Watson PH. Estrogen receptor-beta mRNA variants in human and murine tissues. Mol Cell Endocrinol 1998;138:199–203.
14. Enmark E, Pelto-Huikko M, Grandien K, Lagercrantz S, Lagercrantz J, Fried G, Nordenskjold M, Gustafsson J-A. Human estrogen receptor β gene structure, chromosomal localization and expression pattern. J Clin Endocrinol Metab 1997;82:4258–4265.
15. Murphy L, Leygue E, Dotzlaw H, Douglas D, Coutts A, Watson P. Oestrogen receptor variants and mutations in human breast cancer. Ann Med 1997;29:221–234.
16. Murphy L, Dotzlaw H, Leygue E, Coutts A, Watson P. The Pathophysiological role of estrogen receptor variants in human breast cancer. J Steroid Biochem Mol Biol 1998;65:175–180.
17. Moore J, McKee D, Slentz-Kesler K, Moore L, Jones S, Horne E, et al. Cloning and characterization of human estrogen receptor β isoforms. Biochem Biophys Res Commun 1998;247:75–78.
18. Vladusic E, Hornby A, Guerra-Vladusic F, Lupu R. Expression of estrogen receptor β messenger RNA variant in breast cancer. Cancer Res 1998;58:210–214.
19. Murphy L, Dotzlaw H, Leygue E, Douglas D, Coutts A, Watson P. Estrogen receptor variants and mutations: a review. J Steroid Biochem Mol Biol 1997;62:363–372.
20. McGuire WL, Chamness GC, Fuqua SA. Estrogen receptor variants in clinical breast cancer. Mol Endocrinol 1991;5:1571–1577.
21. Dotzlaw H, Alkhalaf M, Murphy LC. Characterization of estrogen receptor variant mRNAs from human breast cancers. Mol Endocrinol 1992;6:773–785.
22. Fuqua SA, Allred DC, Auchus RJ. Expression of estrogen receptor variants. J Cell Biochem 1993; 17G(Suppl):194–197.

23. Murphy LC, Dotzlaw H. Variant estrogen receptor mRNA species detected in human breast cancer biopsy samples. Mol Endocrinol 1989;3:687–693.
24. Leygue E, Huang A, Murphy L, Watson P. Prevalence of estrogen receptor variant messenger RNAs in human breast cancer. Cancer Res 1996;56:4324–4327.
25. Murphy LC, Hilsenbeck SG, Dotzlaw H, Fuqua SAW. Relationship of clone 4 estrogen receptor variant messenger RNA expression to some known prognostic variables in human breast cancer. Clin Cancer Res 1995;1:155–159.
26. Leygue E, Murphy L, Kuttenn F, Watson P. Triple primer polymerase chain reaction. A new way to quantify truncated mRNA expression. Am J Pathol 1996;148:1097–1103.
27. Leygue ER, Watson PH, Murphy LC. Estrogen receptor variants in normal human mammary tissue. J Natl Cancer Inst 1996;88:284–290.
28. Pfeffer U, Fecarotta E, Vidali G. Coexpression of multiple estrogen receptor variant messenger RNAs in normal and neoplastic breast tissues and in MCF-7 cells. Cancer Res 1995;55:2158–2165.
29. Erenburg I, Schachter B, Lopez RM, Ossowski L. Loss of an estrogen receptor isoform (ER-alpha deleted 3) in breast cancer and the consequences of its reexpression: interference with estrogen-stimulated properties of malignant transformation. Mol Endocrinol 1997;11:2004–2015.
29a. Leygue E, Dotzlaw H, Watson PH, Murphy LC. Altered expression of estrogen receptor-α variant messenger RNAs between adjacent normal breast and breast tumor tissues. Breast Cancer Res 1999;51:2–10.
30. Wang Y, Miksicek RJ. Identification of a dominant negative form of the human estrogen receptor. Mol Endocrinol 1991;5:1707–1715.
31. Leygue E, Dotzlaw H, Watson PH, Murphy LC. Identification of novel exon-deleted progesterone receptor variant mRNAs in human breast tissue. Biochem Biophys Res Commun 1996;228:63–68.
32. Richter J, Lange C, Wierman A, Brooks K, Tung L, Takimoto G, Horwitz KB. Progesterone receptor variants found in breast cells repress transcription by wild type receptors. Breast Cancer Res Treat 1998; 48:231–241.
33. Gallacchi P, Schoumacher F, Eppenberger-Castori S, Landenberg EV, Kueng W, Eppenberger U, Mueller H. Increased expression of estrogen receptor exon 5 deletion variant in relapse tissues of human breast cancer. Int J Cancer 1998;79:44–48.
34. Leygue E, Hall R, Dotzlaw H, Watson P, Murphy L. Estrogen receptor-alpha variant mRNA expression in primary human breast tumors and matched lymph node metastases. Br J Cancer 1999;79:978–983.
35. Garcia T, Lehrer S, Bloomer WD, Schachter B. A variant estrogen receptor messenger ribonucleic acid is associated with reduced levels of estrogen binding in human mammary tumors. Mol Endocrinol 1988; 2:785–791.
36. Fuqua SA, Fitzgerald SD, Chamness GC, Tandon AK, McDonnell DP, Nawaz Z, O'Malley BW, McGuire WL. Variant human breast tumor estrogen receptor with constitutive transcriptional activity. Cancer Res 1991;51:105–109.
37. Daffada AA, Johnston SR, Smith IE, Detre S, King N, Dowsett M. Exon 5 deletion variant estrogen receptor messenger RNA expression in relation to tamoxifen resistance and progesterone receptor/pS2 status in human breast cancer. Cancer Res 1995;55:288–293.
38. Zhang QX, Borg A, Fuqua SA. An exon 5 deletion variant of the estrogen receptor frequently coexpressed with wild type estrogen receptor in human breast cancer. Cancer Res 1993;53:5882–5884.
39. Desai A, Luqmani Y, Coope R, Dagg B, Gomm J, Pace P, et al. Presence of exon 5 deleted oestrogen receptor in human breast cancer: functional analysis and clinical significance. Br J Cancer 1997;75: 1173–1184.
40. Chaidarun S, Alexander J. A tumor specific truncated estrogen receptor splice variant enhances estrogen stimulated gene expression. Mol Endocrinol 1998;12:1355–1366.
41. Rea D, Parker MG. Effects of an exon 5 variant of the estrogen receptor in MCF-7 breast cancer cells. Cancer Res 1996;56:1556–1563.
42. Fuqua SA, Wolf DM. Molecular aspects of estrogen receptor variants in breast cancer. Breast Cancer Res Treat 1995;35:233–241.
43. Coutts A, Davie J, Dotzlaw H, Murphy L. Estrogen regulation of nuclear matrix-intermediate filament proteins in human breast cancer cells. J Cell Biochem 1996;63:174–184.
44. Coutts A, Leygue E, Murphy L. Mechanisms of hormone independence in human breast cancer cells. Abstract. 1998. In: 88th Annual Meeting of the American Association for Cancer Research pp. 296, San Diego, CA, 1997.
45. Madsen MW, Reiter BE Lykkesfeldt AE. Differential expression of estrogen receptor mRNA splice variants in the tamoxifen resistant human breast cancer cell line, MCF-7/TAMR-1 compared to the parental MCF-7 cell line. Mol Cell Endocrinol 1995;109:197–207.

46. Madsen MW, Reiter BE, Larsen SS, Briand P, Lykkesfeldt AE. Estrogen receptor messenger RNA splice variants are not involved in antiestrogen resistance in sublines of MCF-7 human breast cancer cells. Cancer Res 1997;57:585–589.

47. Brunner N, Boysen B, Jirus S, Skaar T, Holst-Hanson C, Lippman J, et al. MCF7/LCC9: an antiestrogen resistant MCF 7 variant in which acquired resistance to the steroidal antiestrogen ICI 182780 confers an early cross resistance to the nonsteroidal antiestrogen tamoxifen. Cancer Res 1997;57:3486–3493.

48. Karnik PS, Kulkarni S, Liu XP, Budd GT, Bukowski RM. Estrogen receptor mutations in tamoxifen-resistant breast cancer. Cancer Res 1994;54:349–353.

49. Huang A, Pettigrew N, Watson P. Immunohistochemical assay for oestrogen receptors in paraffin wax sections of breast carcinoma using a new monoclonal antibody. J Pathol 1996;180:223–227.

50. Huang A, Leygue E, Snell L, Murphy L, Watson P. Expression of estrogen receptor variants mRNAs and determination of estrogen status in human breast cancer. Am J Pathol 1997;150:1827–1833.

51. Castles CG, Fuqua SA, Klotz DM, Hill SM. Expression of a constitutively active estrogen receptor variant in the estrogen receptor-negative BT-20 human breast cancer cell line. Cancer Res 1993;53:5934–5939.

52. Park W, Choi J, Hwang E, Lee J. Identification of a variant estrogen receptor lacking exon 4 and its coexpression with wild type estrogen receptor in ovarian carcinomas. Clin Cancer Res 1996;2:2029–2035.

53. Tremblay G, Tremblay A, Copeland N, Gilbert D, Jenkins N, Labrie F, Giguere V. Cloning, chromosomal localization, and functional analysis of the murine estrogen receptor β. Mol Endocrinol 1997;11: 353–365.

54. Paech K, Webb P, Kuiper G, Nilsson S, Gustafsson JA, Kushner PJ, Scanlan TS. Differential ligand activation of estrogen receptors ER alpha and ER beta at AP1 sites. Science 1997;277:1508–1510.

55. Cowley S, Hoare S, Mosselman S, Parker M. Estrogen receptors alpha and beta form heterodimers on DNA. J Biol Chem 1997;272:19,858–19,862.

56. Pettersson K, Grandien K, Kuiper GG, Gustafsson JA. Mouse estrogen receptor beta forms estrogen response element-binding heterodimers with estrogen receptor alpha. Mol Endocrinol 1997;11:1486–1496.

57. Colditz G. Relationship between estrogen levels, use of hormone replacement therapy, and breast cancer. J Natl Cancer Inst 1998;90:814–823.

58. Leygue E, Dotzlaw H, Watson P, Murphy L. Altered estrogen receptor alpha and beta mRNA expression during human breast tumorigenesis. Cancer Res 1998;58:3197–3201.

59. Leygue E, Dotzlaw H, Hare H, Watson P, Murphy L. Expression of estrogen receptor beta variant mRNAs in human breast tumors. Breast Cancer Res Treat 1997;46,48(Abstract).

60. Chu S, Fuller P. Identification of a splice variant of the rat estrogen receptor β gene. Mol Cell Endocrinol 1997;132:195–199.

61. Petersen D, Tkalcevic G, Koza-Taylor P, Turi T Brown T. Identification of estrogen receptor β2, a functional variant of estrogen receptor β expressed in normal rat tissues. Endocrinology 1998;139:1082–1092.

62. Ogawa S, Inoue S, Watanabe T, Orimo A, Hosoi T, Ouchi Y, Muramatsu M. Molecular cloning and characterization of human estrogen receptor βcx: potential inhibitor of estrogen action in human. Nucleic Acids Res 1998;26:3505–3512.

63. Watanabe T, Inoue S, Ogawa S, Ishii Y, Hiroi H, Ikeda K, Orimo A, Muramatsu M. Agonistic effect of tamoxifen is dependent on cell type, ERE-promoter context and estrogen receptor subtype: functional differences between estrogen receptors α and β. Biochem Biophys Res Commun 1997;236:140–145.

64. Leygue E, Dotzlaw H, Lu B, Glor C, Watson P, Murphy L. Estrogen receptor-beta: mine is longer than yours? J Clin Endocrinol Metab 1998;83:3754–3755.

65. Graham J, Yeates C, Balleine R, Harvey S, Milliken J, Bilou M, Clarke C. Characterization of progesterone A and B expression in human breast cancer. Cancer Res 1995;55:5063–5068.

66. Yeates C, Hunt S, Balleine R, Clarke C. Characterization of a truncated progesterone receptor protein in breast tumors. J Clin Endocrinol Metab 1998;83:460–467.

67. Clark GM, McGuire WL, Hubay CA, Pearson OH, Marshall JS. Progesterone receptors as a prognostic factor in stage II breast cancer. N Engl J Med 1983;309:1343–1347.

68. Huang A, Leygue E, Dotzlaw H, Murphy L, Watson P. Estrogen receptor-α mRNA variants influence the determination of estrogen receptor status in human breast cancer. Breast Cancer Res Treat 1999; 58:219–225.

3

Progesterone Receptors in Normal and Neoplastic Breast

Rosemary L. Balleine, PHD, FRCPA,
Patricia A. Mote, BSC,
Sybille M. N. Hunt, PHD,
Eileen M. McGowan, MSC,
and Christine L. Clarke, PHD

INTRODUCTION

The ovarian steroid hormone, progesterone (P), being fat-soluble, gains access to the intracellular compartment by diffusion through the lipid bilayer cell membrane. In target tissues such as the breast, it interacts with a specific receptor protein, progesterone receptor (PR), and induces formation of receptor dimers, which bind to palindromic hormone response elements in DNA and affect gene transcription *(1,2)*. By these means, P plays a fundamental role in the development and function of the normal breast, and, in this process, PR is a critical intermediate.

In normal mouse mammary gland development, and also in pregnancy, P is required for the development of the lobuloalveolar structures involved in lactation *(3–5)*. P also affects the nonlactating mature breast, as evidenced by increase in breast lobule size, epithelial mitoses, secretory activity, and stromal edema, seen in the P-rich luteal phase of the menstrual cycle *(6)*. The role of P in development and/or progression in breast cancer (BC) is less clear, but PR is expressed in a significant proportion of breast tumors, and its presence is associated with a higher likelihood of response to endocrine agents *(7)*. Breast tumors that contain PR are also likely to display features of good prognosis *(8–10)*.

This chapter reviews current knowledge on the expression, regulation, and function of PR in the normal breast and in BC, with particular emphasis on evidence that the two PR isoforms, PR-A and PR-B, may be expressed and regulated differently in breast tumors.

From: *Contemporary Endocrinology: Endocrine Oncology*
Edited by: S. P. Ethier © Humana Press Inc., Totowa, NJ

PROGESTERONE RECEPTOR

PR-A and PR-B

The PR protein exists as two isoforms, designated PR-A and PR-B, which are identical, except that the smaller PR-A protein has a 164-amino acid truncation at the N-terminus, compared to the larger protein PR-B *(14)*. The two proteins are products of a single gene that spans over 90 kb on chromosome 11q22-q23, and is divided into eight exons *(12,13)*. PR-A and PR-B are translated from separate transcripts formed under the control of distinct promoters in the 5' flanking region *(14)*, which allows expression of the two isoforms to be independently regulated *(15)*.

Other PR Proteins

In addition to PR-A and PR-B, there is suggestive evidence for the existence of other smaller PR isoforms, although the significance of these in vivo remains to be determined. Wei and Miner *(16)* and Wei et al. *(17)* have identified a 60-kDa PR protein in the T47D BC cell line, which may be an N-terminally truncated isoform that arises from a translation start site at methionine 595, compared with the full-length PR. Constructed in vitro, this protein, designated PR-C, was able to form heterodimers with PR-B, and apparently enhanced the transcriptional activity of the other PR isoforms in transfection studies *(17,18)*. Studies from this laboratory, examining the expression of PR-A and PR-B in breast tumor extracts by Western blot analysis, have revealed a third immunoreactive protein with a mol wt of approx 78 kDa. This protein, designated PR78kDa, was seen only in a proportion of cases, and, in 26% of all tumors, was present at levels greater than 20% of total PR concentration *(19)*. Examination of PR at the mRNA level has also suggested the possibility that additional truncated forms of the receptor may exist. In studies analogous to those performed on the estrogen receptor (ER), the existence of PR transcripts, from which exon sequences have been specifically deleted by alternative splicing, has recently been described *(20)*, and in vitro functional studies have provided evidence that PR variants, lacking exon 6 and exons 5 + 6 of the PR sequence, may have dominant-negative activity relative to the wild-type receptor *(21)*. It is unlikely that the PR78kDa corresponds to one of these truncated transcripts *(22)*, and the extent to which they are translated in vivo is uncertain.

Function of PR-A and PR-B

Both PR-A and PR-B function as ligand-activated transcription factors, but it has been suggested, on the basis of in vitro studies, that the two proteins are not functionally equivalent. Transient co-expression of PR-B or PR-A and progestin-sensitive reporter genes has shown that, in general, PR-B is transcriptionally the more active of the two isoforms *(23,24)*. Furthermore, PR-A can act as a dominant repressor of PR-B activation *(24–26)*, and similarly inhibits the transcriptional activity of receptors for androgens, glucocorticoids and mineralocorticoids *(26,27)*. PR-A has also been implicated in inhibition of ER activity: co-expression of PR-A, ER, and transfection of estrogen-sensitive reporters has shown a striking diminution of ER transactivation *(23,27,28)*.

Insight into the basis of the different functions of PR-A and PR-B has come from studies that have examined the specific functions of previously uncharacterized domains of the receptor protein. Consistent with the observation that PR-B is the principal effector isoform, a third transactivation function region, TAF 3, has been identified in the N-terminal region of the receptor unique to PR-B *(29)*, and the repressor activity of PR-A has been attributed to a region in the common amino terminus, which has inhibitory function operative only in the context of the PR-A *(24,30)*. Differences in phosphorylation of PR-A and PR-B may also play a role in distinguishing the function of the two receptors *(31–33)*.

Co-regulators of PR Action

In recent years, it has become clear that there are numerous accessory molecules involved in the control of steroid hormone receptor action. In the case of PR, co-repressors, such as nuclear receptor co-repressor and silencing mediator for retinoid and thyroid human receptor, are associated with the inactive receptor complex, and function to limit access of the receptor to DNA by a process of hypoacetylation of histone proteins *(34,35)*. On binding of P, multiple co-activator proteins with acetyltransferase activity, such as SRC-1 and CBP/p300, are recruited and facilitate PR activity *(36–39)*. It is likely, therefore, that the presence and levels of various co-regulatory molecules are important determinants of the nature of P responses.

PR AND THE NORMAL MAMMARY GLAND

PR Expression in the Normal Breast

Given the hormone-responsive character of the normal breast, it is remarkable that ER and PR are detectable in only a small proportion of epithelial cells (ECs). In studies that have reported immunohistochemical staining of tissue sections, it is consistently observed that a minority of cells express receptors, and that there is considerable variability in the number of positively stained cells in different lobules of the same breast *(40)*.

Battersby et al. *(40)* described two patterns of PR staining in terminal duct lobular units: sporadic, in which 5–30% of cells were positive; and ring-like, in which PR expression was detected in more than 30% of nuclei. The co-existence of receptor-positive and -negative cells in the normal mammary gland epithelium is intriguing, and there is recent evidence to suggest that these may represent distinct cell subpopulations. In mice, a morphological distinction between receptor-positive and -negative cells has been observed as luminal ECs, which are sometimes PR-positive; are large, with round nuclei; and have been compared with undifferentiated mammary epithelial progenitor cells *(41,42)*. In contrast, cells with small, irregular nuclei and compact chromatin, resembling differentiated ductal cells, are always PR-negative *(42)*.

Regulation of PR Expression

PR can be detected in ECs of the breast at all stages of the menstrual cycle *(40,43–45)*, and there is no evidence in the human that its levels change in the fluctuating hormonal environment of the cycle, despite the unequivocal evidence, derived from other target tissues, that PR expression is under hormonal control *(11)*. The number of PR-positive cells in the breast must be subject to some degree of hormonal regulation, however: In premenopausal women, PR is the predominant receptor, found in 12–29% of ECs, compared with ER, which is found in 4–10% of cells *(45–47)*. Yet, in the relatively hormone-impoverished circumstance of postmenopause, ER expression is increased in the normal breast, and few cells are PR-positive *(46)*.

In addition to the regulation of PR levels by ovarian hormones in some circumstances, there is evidence of a reduction in PR expression coincident with functional differentiation, because PR, present in the mammary gland of nonpregnant female mice, is reduced during pregnancy, and is virtually undetectable during established lactation *(42)*. Furthermore, in humans, there is a relative reduction in PR expression in the more complex lobules of the breast, compared with simple, less well differentiated structures *(48)*.

Paracrine Action of PR

The relative paucity of receptor-positive cells in the breast, despite its hormone-respon-sive nature has focused attention on whether ovarian hormones act only in cells that express ER and/or PR. Recent data have shown that, in the human breast, ECs that expressed ER and PR did not proliferate, but were in close proximity to receptor-negative cells that proliferated *(49)*, and it has been postulated that receptor-positive cells may influence neighboring PR-negative cells by a paracrine mechanism *(50)*. In support of this hypothesis is the demonstration that chimeric mammary epithelium, comprised of epithelium derived from PR-null mice in close proximity to cells containing wild-type PR, underwent complete alveolar development *(5)*.

Mechanisms of PR Action in the Mammary Gland

The effects of P in the mammary gland have been described as both proliferative and differentiating, and, in support of this, a number of genes involved in cell cycle control, steroid and growth factor action, and differentiation have been shown to be directly or indirectly responsive to progestins in in vitro studies *(51*; Table 1). For example, using a differential display technique in the T47D BC cell line, Kester et al. *(52)* identified the progestin-sensitive nature of a number of genes involved in differentiation, and found also that estrogen treatment could repress expression of some of these. Consistent with this, treatment of T47D cells in culture with estradiol was associated with morphological dedifferentiation, an effect that could be abrogated by simultaneous treatment with progestin *(52)*.

P has been implicated in cell proliferation in the mammary gland, as peak mitotic activity of breast epithelium is seen during the luteal phase of the menstrual cycle, when serum P levels are high *(6,53,54)*. In addition, high proliferation rates in the breast were seen in women taking progestin-only oral contraceptive preparations *(55)*, and animal studies have demonstrated DNA synthesis in response to P in the mammary gland *(56)*. Despite this, in vivo studies have, in the main, supported the view that the principal mitogenic stimulus in the breast is estrogen *(55,57–62)*. At a molecular level, P can both stimulate and inhibit cell cycle progression. Studies of the effects of progestins on the growth of BC cell lines have shown that the response is bi-phasic, with a transient acceleration of cells through the G1-phase, and consequent increase in the S-phase fraction, followed by cell cycle arrest and growth inhibition *(63)*. These effects are accompanied by alteration in the expression and activity of cell cycle regulatory proteins *(64)*. A recent study by Groshong et al. *(65)*, using BC cell lines, suggests that P is neither inherently inhibitory or proliferative, but that its effects are dependent on length of treatment, when sustained exposure to P inhibits, and transient exposure stimulates, cell growth *(65)*.

PR Expression in the Normal Mammary Gland: Summary

PR is expressed in the ECs of the normal mammary gland, and PR-positive cells may represent distinct cell populations. The number of cells expressing PR is relatively low,

Table 1
Recently Described Progestin Regulated Genes

Regulation of cell cycle:	
Cyclin D1 and cyclin-dependent kinase 4	*(65,94,95)*
Cyclin-dependent kinase inhibitors p21 and p27[Kip1]	*(65)*
Leukemia inhibitory factor: a pleiotropic inflammatory cytokine	*(96)*
Type 1 insulin-like growth factor receptor	*(97)*
PRG1: gene with strong homology to 6-phosphofructo-2-kinase/fructose-2,6-biphosphatase	*(98)*
Regulation of differentiation:	
CD-9, CD-59, and Desmoplakin	*(52)*
Regulation of gene expression:	
TSC-22: a putative transcriptional regulator	
Ptg-12: a putative zinc finger protein	
Ptg-11: a gene with homology with members of the SR protein family of spicing factors	
FKBP51: an immunophilin	*(52)*
Oncogenes and tumor suppressors:	
p53	*(99)*
BRCA1	*(100)*
Genes involved in tumor invasion:	
Tumor inhibitor of metalloproteinase-2	*(101)*
Vascular endothelial growth factor	*(102)*
Genes with other functions:	
Na^+/K^+-ATPase a1 subunit	*(52)*
Annexin-VI	*(52)*
Pepsinogen C	*(103)*
Flavin-containing mono-oxygenase 5	*(104)*
Prostate specific antigen	*(105)*

Other progestin regulated genes are described in *(51)*.

and is unchanged during the hormonal fluctuations in the ovarian cycle, but PR levels in the gland decrease upon functional differentiation of the mammary gland, during pregnancy, lactation, and after the menopause. P plays a role in mammary gland function and lobuloalveolar development, and the underlying mechanisms mediating these effects are likely to include a number of molecular pathways, including those involved in cell cycle progression, growth factor activity, and differentiation. A proportion of the effects of P may be mediated by paracrine mechanisms, because there are emerging suggestions that ovarian hormones influence mammary gland biology by influencing the behavior of receptor-negative cells in the vicinity of cells that express receptors.

PR IN BC

PR Expression and Regulation in Premalignant and Invasive BC

Evidence from studies *(66)* of breast histopathology and epidemiology shows that cancer of the breast may evolve through a series of hyperplastic, then dysplastic, changes in the epithelium. Further support for this model has come from loss of heterozygosity studies reported by O'Connell et al. *(67)*, which showed that premalignant disease commonly

Table 2
Relative Expression of PR-A and PR-B
in Primary BC Specimens Determined
by Western Blot Analysis of Tumor Cytosol Extracts

PR-A:B Ratio	No. of tumors	Total (%)
0–1	88	43.6
1–2	36	17.8
2–3	16	7.9
3–4	12	5.9
4–5	14	6.9
>5	36	17.9

Adapted with permission from ref. *19* and *73*.

shared the same genetic lesions as concurrent invasive cancer. There is little published information about the expression of PR in the process of malignant transformation, and inconsistencies in histopathological classification make the few available studies difficult to compare. The available evidence suggests that PR expression may be increased in premalignant lesions, compared with the normal breast, and, similarly, expression of ER and the estrogen-responsive protein, pS2, may also be higher *(46,66,68,69)*. There is, however, clearly a need for more detailed studies in this area.

The rate of PR positivity in invasive BC ranges from 54 to 70%, compared with 69–81% for ER *(9,10,70)*. A relationship between receptor expression and the hormonal environment of a tumor indicates that a degree of hormonal regulation of receptor expression is retained in some breast tumors. It is further noted that alterations in tumor receptor profiles under this influence are similar to those described in normal breast epithelium. In premenopausal women, rates of ER positivity in breast tumors were highest in the follicular phase of the menstrual cycle. Although there was no significant difference in PR positivity between different phases, a tendency for higher PR expression at about the time of ovulation was found *(71)*. It also has been consistently reported that tumors of younger or premenopausal women are more likely to be PR-positive, and to contain higher levels of PR, than those of older women; conversely, tumors of older or postmenopausal patients are more likely to be ER-positive and to contain higher levels of ER *(8,9,71,72)*.

Expression of PR-A and PR-B in BC

In tumors that do express PR, the relative expression of the two PR isoforms, A and B, is variable, and may influence the degree and nature of P responsiveness. In a series of 202 primary BC specimens, the ratio of PR-A to PR-B was measured on Western blots of tumor cytosol extracts. In the majority of cases, the two proteins were present in similar quantities, with the median ratio of PR-A:B being 1.26, and 61% of cases having a ratio of PR-A:B between 0 and 2 (Table 2). In 25% of the cohort, however, the ratio of PR-A:B was greater than 4, indicating a particular excess of PR-A *(19,73)*. Because the relative expression of the two PR isoforms in the normal breast is not currently known, the extent to which this variability in the levels of PR-A and PR-B reflects a pathological dysregulation of receptor expression is uncertain. In vitro evidence, discussed earlier, which indicates that the functions of the two PR isoforms are disparate, and that PR-A may repress the function of PR-B and other hormone receptors, including ER, suggests that a relative overexpression of PR-A may influence hormone responsiveness in BC. These issues form the basis of on-going studies at this laboratory.

Clinical Correlates of PR Expression in BC

The biological significance of receptor expression in breast tumors is reflected by the fact that primary BCs that are receptor positive are likely to be smaller, less highly prolif- erative, and more highly differentiated than those that fail to express receptors (8–10). Receptor expression may also influence the pattern of metastatic spread, because it has been reported that ER/PR-positive tumors have a propensity to recur in bone (74).

In ductal carcinoma *in situ* of the breast, there is an inverse relationship between expression of ER and PR, and grade (75). In a recent report by Querzoli et al. (76) 92–100% of cribriform carcinoma *in situ* cases were PR-positive and 71–79% of other noncomedo ductal carcinoma *in situ* variants were PR-positive. In contrast, only 26–27% of comedo carcinoma *in situ* cases expressed PR. The pattern of ER expression in these lesions was similar, but it was notable that, although all of the cases of lobular carcinoma *in situ* were ER-positive, only 47–50% of these expressed PR (76).

PR as a Clinical Marker in BC

In BC, PR is used clinically as a marker of hormone responsiveness and the likely success of endocrine manipulation as a form of treatment. Because the most commonly used therapeutic endocrine agent in BC, Tamoxifen, acts by binding to ER, the signifi- cance of PR derives principally from the fact that PR is synthesized in response to estro- gen activation of its cognate receptor, and the presence of PR in ER-positive breast tumors is therefore evidence of an intact estrogen-response pathway (77). Consistent with this, rates of response to endocrine therapy in BC are higher for patients whose tumors express both ER and PR, compared with those that express ER alone (7,78) and, in patients whose tumor PR levels have been monitored during tamoxifen therapy, fluctuations in PR levels in response to this treatment have been associated with favorable treatment outcome (79,80). The synthetic P analog, medroxyprogesterone acetate, is also used as a therapeu- tic agent in BC, and PR is likely to play a more direct role in mediating response to this form of treatment (81).

Association of PR Expression with Progression in BC

Although malignant tumors represent a monoclonal proliferation of cells, when sec- tions of receptor-positive BC are stained for ER or PR by immunohistochemistry, con- siderable variation in receptor expression within a tumor mass is seen. This heterogeneity is of two types: variation in the signal from different cells within a tumor cell clump; and regional differences across the section, with tumor cells in one area staining strongly, but in another, little or no staining is seen (47,82). The clinical significance of this intrigu- ing observation is uncertain. It suggests the possibility that disease progression may be accompanied by loss of receptor expression in BC, which, in turn, may be a potential mechanism for the acquisition of resistance to hormonal therapy in this disease. Studies that have compared ER and PR in primary tumors with simultaneously or subsequently sampled secondary tumor deposits have reported, however, that, in the majority of cases, the receptor phenotype of a tumor is not altered with disease progression (83–92).

Moreover, recent studies from this group have shown that secondary tumor deposits from postmenopausal women specifically lack PR. Because the ER and PR status of the primary tumor is largely maintained in secondary deposits, this suggests that primary tumors lacking PR are more likely to progress to a secondary site than tumors that contain PR *(83)*, and implicates absence of PR with disease progression.

Function of PR in BC

The observation that primary tumors lacking PR are more likely to progress to a secondary site than tumors that contain PR suggests that PR may play a role in BC other than as a marker of likely response to endocrine agents. P plays a role in inhibition of estrogen action in the normal uterus, through downregulation of ER and induction of estrogen metabolism *(93)*, and also has these effects in BC cells in culture *(93)*. Based on in vitro studies, PRA may inhibit ER function *(23,27,28)*, and a proportion of BCs contain very high relative levels of this protein *(19)*. By these means, P may limit or inhibit estrogen action in breast tumors, and therefore serve a direct beneficial function on progression of the disease. However, whether PR mediates any antiestrogenic effects in BC in vivo is not known, and further studies in this area are urgently needed.

PR in BC: Summary

PR is expressed in primary invasive BCs, and approx 50–70% of cases are positive. Primary and *in situ* BCs containing PR express markers of good prognosis, including small size and low grade. There is little information on expression of PR in premalignant breast lesions, but there is a suggestion that receptor levels are increased, compared with the normal breast. Within PR-positive cases, the relative expression of PR-A and PR-B is not normally distributed, with a significant proportion of cases expressing one predominant isoform. Notably, 25% of cases have a fourfold excess of PR-A, which may be associated with altered hormone responsiveness in a proportion of tumors.

Tumors containing PR are more likely to respond to endocrine agents, reflecting in part the estrogen-responsive nature of PR, and the fact that presence of PR is taken as a marker of an intact estrogen-response pathway. In postmenopausal women, primary tumors that lack PR, however, are more likely to progress to secondary sites, suggesting that PR expression may be implicated with disease progression in BC.

CONCLUSION AND FUTURE PERSPECTIVES

P plays a major role in the growth and differentiation of the normal mammary gland, and PR expression in this tissue is indicative of this. However, there is still a great deal to be learned about P action in the normal breast. Notably, the relative levels of the two PR isoforms, PR-A and PR-B, in the normal breast are not known, and elucidation of this feature is essential to understanding the physiological significance of the postulated differences in the activities of these proteins in vitro. Furthermore, many of the molecular targets on which PR acts in the normal breast, in order to mediate its effects, remain to be defined. There is a suggestion that P may act by paracrine mechanisms in the normal breast, and future studies, aimed at examining the mechanisms through which such paracrine effects could be mediated, are needed.

The role of P and the presence of PR in premalignant lesions of the breast are poorly defined and the role played by P in breast carcinogenesis unknown. The presence of PR in breast tumors is held to be a marker of a functional ER, but there is evidence that presence of PR in breast tumors may have a role outside of its utility as a marker. There is an association between expression of PR and biological features associated with favorable clinical outcome in BC, and also an apparent relationship between failure of PR expression and disease progression. Given the differentiating and estrogen inhibitory effects of P in physiological circumstances, it is possible that these associations are a consequence of a facility to control cellular processes in PR-positive breast tumors, which is lost when PR is not expressed. Future studies aimed at further elucidating the molecular mechanisms that determine the regulation and nature of P responses will allow the relationship between PR expression and BC biology to be more fully understood.

REFERENCES

1. Evans RM. The steroid and thyroid hormone receptor superfamily. Science 1988;240:889–895.
2. Mangelsdorf DJ, Thummel C, Beato M, Herrlich P, Schutz G, Umesono K, et al. The nuclear receptor superfamily: the second decade. Cell 1995;83:835–839.
3. Lydon JP, DeMayo FJ, Funk CR, Mani SK, Hughes AR, Montgomery CA Jr, et al. Mice lacking progesterone receptor exhibit pleiotropic reproductive abnormalities. Genes Dev 1995;9:2266–2278.
4. Humphreys RC, Lydon J, O'Malley BW, Rosen JM. Mammary gland development is mediated by both stromal and epithelial progesterone receptors. Mol Endocrinol 1997;11:801–810.
5. Brisken C, Park S, Vass T, Lydon JP, O'Malley BW, Weinberg RA. Paracrine role for the epithelial progesterone receptor in mammary gland development. Proc Natl Acad Sci USA 1998;95:5076–5081.
6. Longacre TA, Bartow SA. A correlative morphologic study of human breast and endometrium in the menstrual cycle. Am J Surg Pathol 1986;10:382–393.
7. McGuire WL, Chamness GC, Fuqua SAW. Estrogen receptor variants in clinical breast cancer. Mol Endocrinol 1991;5:1571–1577.
8. Clark GM, Osborne CK, McGuire WL. Correlations between estrogen receptor, progesterone receptor, and patient characteristics in human breast cancer. J Clin Oncol 1984;2:1102–1109.
9. Thorpe SM, Rose C. Oestrogen and progesterone receptor determinations in breast cancer: technology and biology. Cancer Surv 1986;5:505–525.
10. Wenger CR, Beardslee S, Owens MA, Pounds G, Oldaker T, Vendely P, et al. DNA ploidy, S-phase, and steroid receptors in more than 127,000 breast cancer patients. Breast Cancer Res Treat 1993;28:9–26.
11. Clarke CL. Ovarian steroid hormone receptors and their mechanisms of action. In: Rice GE, Brennecke SP, eds. Molecular Aspects of Placental and Fetal Membrane Autocoids, CRC, Boca Raton, 1993, pp. 27–54.
12. Mattei M-G, Krust A, Stropp U, Mattei J-F, Chambon P. Assignment of the human progesterone receptor to the q22 band of chromosome 11. Hum Genet 1988;78:96,97.
13. Misrahi M, Venencie P-Y, Saugier-Veber P, Sar S, Dessen P, Milgrom E. Structure of the human progesterone receptor gene. Biochem Biophys Acta 1993;1216:289–292.
14. Kastner P, Krust A, Turcotte B, Stropp U, Tora L, Gronemeyer H, Chambon P. Two distinct estrogen-regulated promoters generate transcripts encoding the two functionally different human progesterone receptor isoforms. EMBO J 1990;9:1603–1614.
15. Graham JD, Roman SD, McGowan E, Sutherland RL, Clarke CL. Preferential stimulation of human progesterone receptor B expression by estrogen in T-47D human breast cancer cells. J Biol Chem 1995; 270:30,693–30,700.
16. Wei LL, Miner R. Evidence for the existence of a third progesterone receptor protein in human breast cancer cell line T47D. Cancer Res 1994;54:340–343.
17. Wei LL, Hawkins P, Baker C, Norris B, Sheridan PL, Quinn PG. An amino-terminal truncated progesterone receptor isoform, PR_c, enhances progestin-induced transcriptional activity. Mol Endocr 1996; 10:1379–1387.
18. Wei LL, Norris BM, Baker CJ. An N-terminal truncated third progesterone receptor forms heterodimers with PR B but interferes in PR B-DNA binding. J Steroid Biochem Mol Biol 1997;62:287–297.
19. Graham JD, Yeates C, Balleine RL, Harvey SS, Milliken JS, Bilous AM, Clarke CL. Characterization of progesterone receptor A and B expression in human breast cancer. Cancer Res 1995;55:5063–5068.

20. Leygue E, Dotzlaw H, Watson PH, Murphy LC. Identification of novel exon-deleted progesterone receptor variant mRNAs in human breast cancer. Biochem Biophys Res Commun 1996;228:63–68.
21. Richer JK, Lange CA, Wierman AM, Brooks KM, Tung L, Takimoto GS, Horwitz KB. Progesterone receptor variants found in breast cells repress transcription by wild-type receptors. Breast Cancer Res Treat 1998;48:231–241.
22. Yeates C, Hunt SMN, Balleine RL, Clarke CL. Characterization of a truncated progesterone receptor protein in breast tumours. J Clin Endocrinol Metab 1998;83:460–467.
23. Wen DX, Xu YF, Mais DE, Goldman ME, McDonnell DP. The A and B forms of the human progesterone receptor operate through distinct signalling pathways within target cells. Mol Cell Biol 1994; 14:8356–8364.
24. Giangrande PH, Pollio G, McDonnell DP. Mapping and characterization of the functional domains responsible for the differential activity of the A and B isoforms of the human progesterone receptor. J Biol Chem 1997;272:32,889–32,900.
25. Tung L, Mohamed MK, Hoeffler JP, Takimoto GS, Horwitz KB. Antagonist-occupied human progesterone receptor B-receptors activate transcription without binding to progesterone response elements and are dominantly inhibited by A receptors. Mol Endocrinol 1993;7:1256–1265.
26. Vegeto E, Shahbaz MM, Wen DX, Goldman ME, O'Malley BW, McDonnell DP. Human progesterone receptor A form is a cell- and promotor-specific repressor of human progesterone receptor B function. Mol Endocrinol 1993;7:1244–1255.
27. McDonnell DP, Shahbaz MM, Vegeto E, Goldman ME. The human progesterone receptor A-form functions as a transcriptional modulator of mineralocorticoid receptor transcriptional activity. J Steroid Biochem Mol Biol 1994;48:425–432.
28. Kraus WL, Weis KE, Katzenellenbogen BS. Inhibitory cross-talk between steroid hormone receptors: differential targeting of estrogen receptor in the repression of its transcriptional activity by agonist- and antagonist-occupied progestin receptors. Mol Cell Biol 1995;15:1847–1857.
29. Sartorius CA, Melville MY, Hovland AR, Tung L, Takimoto GS, Horwitz KB. A third transactivation function (AF3) of human progesterone receptors located in the unique N-terminal segment of the B-isoform. Mol Endocrinol 1994;8:1347–1360.
30. Rudie Hovland A, Powell RL, Takimoto GS, Tung L, Horwitz KB. N-terminal inhibitory function, IF, suppresses transcription by the A-isoform but not the B-isoform of human progesterone receptors. J Biol Chem 1998;273:5545–5560.
31. Kazmi SMI, Visconti V, Plante RK, Ishaque A, Lau C. Differential regulation of human progesterone receptor A and B form-mediated transactivation by phosphorylation. Endocrinology 1993;133: 1230–1238.
32. Zhang Y, Beck CA, Poletti A, Edwards DP, Weigel NL. Identification of phosphorylation sites unique to the B form of human progesterone receptor. J Biol Chem 1994;49:31,034–31,040.
33. Zhang Y, Beck CA, Poletti A, Clement JP IV, Prendergast P, Yip T-T, et al. Phosphorylation of human progesterone receptor by cyclin-dependent kinase 2 on three sites that are authentic basal phosphorylation sites in vivo. Mol Endocrinol 1997;11:823–832.
34. Wagner BL, Norris JD, Knotts TA, Weigel NL, McDonnell DP. The nuclear corepressors NCor and SMRT are key regulators of both ligand- and 8-bromo-cyclic AMP-dependent transcriptional activity of the human progesterone receptor. Mol Cell Biol 1998;18:1369–1378.
35. Wong C-W, Privalsky ML. Transcriptional repression by the SMRT-mSin3 corepressor: multiple interactions, multiple mechanisms, and a potential role for TFIIB. Mol Cell Biol 1998;18:5500–5510.
36. Onate SA, Tsai SY, Tsai M-J, O'Malley BW. Sequence and characterization of a coactivator for the steroid hormone receptor superfamily. Science 1995;270:1354–1357.
37. Onate SA, Boonyaratanakornkit V, Spencer TE, Tsai SY, Tsai M-J, Edwards DP, O'Malley BW. The steroid receptor coactivator-1 contains multiple receptor interacting and activation domains that cooperatively enhance the activation function 1 (AF1) and AF2 domains of stroid receptors. J Biol Chem 1998;273:12,101–12,108.
38. Yao T-P, Ku G, Zhou N, Scully R, Livingston DM. The nuclear hormone receptor coactivator SRC-1 is a specific target of p300. Proc Natl Acad Sci USA 1996;93:10,626–10,631.
39. Migliaccio A, Piccolo D, Castoria G, Di Domenico M, Bilancio A, Lombardi M, et al. Activation of the Src/p21^{ras}/ERK pathway by progesterone receptor via cross-talk with estrogen receptor. EMBO J 1998;17:2008–2018.
40. Battersby S, Robertson BJ, Anderson TJ, King RJB, McPherson K. Influence of menstrual cycle, parity and oral contraceptive use on steroid hormone receptors in normal breast. Br J Cancer 1992;65:601–607.

41. Smith GH. A morphologically distinct candidate for an epithelial stem cell in mouse mammary gland. J Cell Science 1988;89:173–183.
42. Shyamala G. Roles of estrogen and progesterone in normal mammary gland development. Trends Endocrinol Metab 1997;8:34–39.
43. Joyeux C, Chalbos D, Rochefort H. Effects of progestins and menstrual cycle on fatty acid synthetase and progesterone receptor in human mammary glands. J Clin Endocrinol Metab 1990;70:1438–1444.
44. Soderqvist G, Von Schoultz B, Tani E, Skoog L. Estrogen and progesterone receptor content in breast epithelial cells from healthy women during the menstrual cycle. Am J Obstet Gynecol 1993;168:874–879.
45. Williams G, Anderson E, Howell A, Watson R, Coyne J, Roberts SA, Potten CS. Oral contraceptive (OCP) use increases proliferation and decreases oestrogen receptor content of epithelial cells in the normal human breast. Int J Cancer 1991;48:206–210.
46. Jacquemier JD, Hassoun J, Torrente M, Martin P-M. Distribution of estrogen and progesterone receptors in healthy tissue adjacent to breast lesions at various stages: immunohistochemical study of 107 cases. Breast Cancer Res Treat 1990;15:109–117.
47. Zeimet AG, Muller-Holzner E, Marth C, Daxenbichler G. Immunocytochemical versus biochemical receptor determination in normal and tumorous tissues of the female reproductive tract and the breast. J Steroid Biochem Mol Biol 1994;49:365–372.
48. Calef G, Alvarado MV, Bonney GE, Amfoh KK, Russo J. Influence of lobular development on breast epithelial cell proliferation and steroid hormone receptor content. Int J Oncol 1995;7:1285–1288.
49. Clarke RB, Howell A, Potten CS, Anderson E. Dissociation between steroid receptor expression and cell proliferation in the human breast. Cancer Res 1997;57:4987–4991.
50. Silberstein GB, Van Horn K, Shyamala G, Daniel CW. Progesterone receptors in the mouse mammary duct: distribution and developmental regulation. Cell Growth Differ 1996;7:945–952.
51. Graham JD, Clarke CL. Physiological action of progesterone in target tissues. Endocr Rev 1997;18:502–519.
52. Kester HA, van der Leede BM, van der Saag PT, van der Burg B. Novel progesterone target genes identified by an improved differential display technique suggest that progestin-induced growth inhibition of breast cancer cells coincides with enhanced differentiation. J Biol Chem 1997;272:16,637–16,643.
53. Going JJ, Anderseon TJ, Battersby S, MacIntyre CCA. Proliferative and secretory activity in human breast during natural and artificial menstrual cycles. Am J Pathol 1988;130:193–204.
54. Ferguson DJP, Anderson TJ. Morphological evaluation of cell turnover in relation to the menstrual cycle in the "resting" human breast. Br J Cancer 1981;44:177–181.
55. Anderson TJ, Battersby S, King RJB, McPherson K, Going J. Oral contraceptive use influences resting breast proliferation. Hum Pathol 1989;20:1139–1144.
56. Haslam SZ. Progesterone effects on deoxyribonucleic acid synthesis in normal mouse mammary glands. Endocrinology 1988;122:464–470.
57. Laidlaw IJ, Clarke RB, Howell A, Owen AW, Potten CS, Anderson E. The proliferation of normal human breast tissue implanted into athymic nude mice is stimulated by estrogen but not progesterone. Endocrinology 1995;136:164–171.
58. Anderson E, Clarke RB, Howell A. Changes in the normal breast throughout the menstrual cycle: relevance to breast carcinogenesis. Endocrine-Related Cancer 1997;4:23–33.
59. Clarke RB, Howell A, Anderson E. Estrogen sensitivity of normal human breast tissue in vivo and implanted into athymic nude mice: Analysis of the relationship between estrogen-induced proliferation and progesterone receptor expression. Breast Cancer Res Treat 1997;45:121–133.
60. McManus MJ, Welsch CW. Hormone-induced ductal DNA synthesis of human breast tissues maintained in the athymic nude mouse. Cancer Res 1981;41:3300–3305.
61. McManus MJ, Welsch CW. The effect of estrogen, progesterone, thyroxine, and human placental lactogen on DNA synthesis of human breast ductal epithelium maintained in athymic nude mice. Cancer 1984;54:1920–1927.
62. Silberstein GB, Van Horn K, Shyamala G, Daniel CW. Essential role of endogenous estrogen in directly stimulating mammary growth demonstrated by implants containing pure antiestrogens. Endocrinology 1994;134:84–90.
63. Musgrove EA, Lee CSL, Sutherland RL. Progestins both stimulate and inhibit breast cancer cell cycle progression while increasing expression of transforming growth factor a, epidermal growth factor receptor, c-fos and c-myc genes. Mol Cell Biol 1991;11:5032–5043.
64. Musgrove EA, Swarbrick A, Lee CSL, Cornish AL, Sutherland RL. Mechanisms of cyclin-dependent kinase inactivation by progestins. Mol Cell Biol 1998;18:1812–1825.

65. Groshong SD, Owen GI, Grimison B, Schauer IE, Todd MC, Langan TA, et al. Biphasic regulation of breast cancer cell growth by progesterone: role of the cyclin-dependent kinase inhibitors, p21 and p27Kip1. Mol Endocrinol 1997;11:1593–1607.

66. Allred DC, O'Connell P, Fuqua SAW, Osborne CK. Immunohistochemical studies of early breast cancer. Breast Cancer Res Treat 1994;32:13–18.

67. O'Connell P, Pekkel V, Fuqua SAW, Osborne CK, Clark GM, Allred DC. Analysis of loss of heterozygosity in 399 premalignant breast lesions at 15 genetic loci. J Natl Cancer Inst 1998;90:697–703.

68. Jacquemier JD, Rolland PH, Vague D, Lieutaud R, Spitalier JM, Martin PM. Relationships between steroid receptor and epithelial cell proliferation in benign fibrocystic disease of the breast. Cancer 1982;49:2534–2536.

69. Luqmani YA, Campbell T, Soomro S, Shousha S, Rio MC, Coombes RC. Immunohistochemical localisation of pS2 protein in ductal carcinoma *in situ* and benign lesions of the breast. Br J Cancer 1993;67: 749–753.

70. Pichon MF, Broet P, Magdelenat H, Delarue JC, Spyratos F, Basuyan JP, et al. Prognostic value of steroid receptors after long term follow-up of 2257 operable breast cancers. Br J Cancer 1996;73:1545–1551.

71. Pujol P, Daures J-P, Thezenas S, Guilleux F, Rouanet P, Grenier J. Changing estrogen and progesterone receptor patterns in breast carcinoma during the menstrual cycle and menopause. Cancer 1998;83: 698–705.

72. Romain S, Laine Bidron C, Martin PM, Magdelenat H. EORTC Receptor Study Group Report: steroid receptor distribution in 47 892 breast cancers. A collaborative study of 7 European laboratories. Eur J Cancer 1995;31A:411–417.

73. Graham JD, Yeates C, Balleine RL, Harvey SS, Milliken JS, Bilous AM, Clarke CL. Progesterone receptor A and B protein expression in human breast cancer. J Steroid Biochem Mol Biol 1996;56:93–98.

74. Kamby C, Andersen J, Ejlertsen B, Birkler NE, Rytter L, Zedeler K, et al. Histological grade and steroid receptor content of primary breast cancer: impact on prognosis and possible modes of action. Br J Cancer 1988;58:480–486.

75. Millis RR, Bobrow LG, Barnes DM. Immunohistochemical evaluation of biological markers in mammary carcinoma in situ: correlation with morphological features and recently proposed schemes for histological classification. Breast 1996;5:113–122.

76. Querzoli P, Albonico G, Ferretti S, Rinaldi R, Beccati D, Corcione S, Indelli M, Nenci I. Modulation of biomarkers in minimal breast carcinoma. A model for human breast carcinoma progression. Cancer 1998;83:89–97.

77. Horwitz KB, McGuire WL, Pearson OH, Segaloff A. Predicting response to endocrine therapy in human breast cancer: a hypothesis. Science 1975;189:726,727.

78. Ravdin PM, Green S, Dorr TM, McGuire WL, Fabian C, Pugh RP, et al. Prognostic significance of progesterone receptor levels in estrogen receptor-positive patients with metastatic breast cancer treated with tamoxifen: results of a prospective Southwest Oncology Group study. J Clin Oncol 1992; 10:1284–1291.

79. Howell A, Harland RNL, Barnes DM, Baildam DM, Wilkinson MJS, Hayward E, Swindell R, Sellwood RA. Endocrine therapy for advanced carcinoma of the breast: relationship between the effect of tamoxifen upon concentrations of progesterone receptor and subsequent response to treatment. Cancer Res 1987;47:300–304.

80. Murray PA, Gomm J, Ricketts D, Powels T, Coombes RC. The effect of endocrine therapy on the levels of oestrogen and progesterone receptor and transforming growth factor-b1 in metastatic human breast cancer: an immunocytochemical study. Eur J Cancer 1994;30A:1218–1222.

81. Horwitz KB. The molecular biology of RU486. Is there a role for antiprogestins in the treatment of breast cancer? Endocr Rev 1992;13:146–163.

82. Kommoss F, Pfisterer J, Idris T, Giese E, Sauerbrei W, Schafer W, Thome M, Pfleiderer A. Steroid receptors in carcinoma of the breast. Results of immunocytochemical and biochemical determination and their effects on short-term prognosis. Anal Quant Cytol Histol 1994;16:203–210.

83. Balleine RL, Earl MJ, Greenberg ML, Clarke CL. Absence of progesterone receptor associated with secondary breast cancer in postmenopausal women. Br J Cancer, 1998; in press.

84. Jakesz R, Dittrich CH, Hanusch J, Kolb R, Lenzhofer R, Moser K, et al. Simultaneous and sequential determinations of steroid hormone receptors in human breast cancer. Ann Surg 1984;201:305–310.

85. Gross GE, Clark GM, Chamness GC, McGuire WL. Multiple progesterone receptor assays in human breast cancer. Cancer Res 1984;44:836–840.

86. Allegra JC, Barlock A, Huff K, Lippman ME. Changes in multiple or sequential estrogen receptor determinations in breast cancer. Cancer 1980;45:792–794.

87. Paridaens R, Sylvester RJ, Ferrazzi E, Legros N, Leclercq G, Heuson JC. Clinical significance of the quantitative assessment of estrogen receptors in advanced breast cancer. Cancer 1980;46:2889–2895.

88. Peetz ME, Nunley DL, Moseley HS, Keenan EJ, Davenport CE, Fletcher WS. Multiple simultaneous and sequential estrogen receptor values in patients with breast cancer. Am J Surg 1982;143:591–594.

89. Hull DF III, Clark GM, Osborne CK, Chamness GC, Knight WA III, McGuire WL. Multiple estrogen receptor assays in human breast cancer. Cancer Res 1983;43:413–416.

90. Crawford DJ, Cowan S, Fitch R, Smith DC, Leake RE. Stability of oestrogen receptor status in sequential biopsies from patients with breast cancer. Br J Cancer 1987;56:137–140.

91. Spataro V, Price K, Goldhirsch A, Cavalli F, Simoncini E, Castiglione M, et al. Sequential estrogen receptor determinations from primary breast cancer and at relapse: prognostic and therapeutic relevance. Ann Oncol 1992;3:733–740.

92. Kuukasjarvi T, Kononen J, Helin H, Holli K, Isola J. Loss of estrogen receptor in recurrent breast cancer is associated with poor response to endocrine therapy. J Clin Oncol 1996;14:2584–2589.

93. Clarke CL, Sutherland RL. Progestin regulation of cellular proliferation. Endocr Rev 1990;11:266–301.

94. Said TK, Conneely OM, Medina D, O'Malley BW, Lydon JP. Progesterone, in addition to estrogen, induces cyclin D1 expression in the murine mammary epithelial cell in vivo. Endocrinology 1997;138: 3933–3939.

95. Musgrove EA, Lee CSL, Cornish AL, Swarbrick A, Sutherland RL. Antiprogestin inhibition of cell cycle progression in T47D breast cancer cells is accompanied by induction of the CDK inhibitor p21. Mol Endocrinol 1997;11:54–66.

96. Bamberger AM, Thuneke I, Schulte HM. Differential regulation of the human 'leukemia inhibitory factor' (LIF) promoter in the T47D and MDA-MB 231 breast cancer cells. Breast Cancer Res Treat 1998;47:153–161.

97. Clarke RB, Howell A, Anderson E. Type I insulin-like growth factor receptor gene expression in normal human breast tissue treated with oestrogen and progesterone. Br J Cancer 1997;75:251–257.

98. Hamilton JA, Callaghan MJ, Sutherland RL, Watts CKW. Identification of PRG1, a novel progestin-responsive gene with sequence homology to 6-phosphofructo-2-kinase/fructose-2,6-bisphosphatase. Mol Endocr 1997;11:490–502.

99. Hurd C, Khattree N, Alban P, Nag K, Jhanwar SC, Dinda S, Moudgil VK. Hormonal regulation of the p53 tumor suppressor protein in T47D human breast carcinoma cell line. J Biol Chem 1995;270: 28,507–28,510.

100. Rajan JV, Marquis ST, Perry Gardner H, Chodosh LA. Developmental expression of Brca2 colocalizes with Brca1 and is associated with proliferation and differentiation in multiple tissues. Dev Biol 1997; 184:385–401.

101. van den Brule F, Engel J, Stetler-Stevenson WG, Liu F-T, Sobel ME, Castronovo V. Genes involved in tumor invasion and metastasis are differentially modulated by estradiol and progestin in human breast-cancer cells. Int J Cancer 1992;52:653–657.

102. Hyder SM, Murthy L, Stancel GM. Progestin regulation of vascular endothelial growth factor in human breast cancer cells. Cancer Res 1998;58:392–395.

103. Balbin M, Lopez-Otin C. Hormonal regulation of the human pepsinogen C gene in breast cancer cells. J Biol Chem 1996;271:15,175–15,181.

104. Miller MM, James RA, Richer JK, Gordon DF, Wood WM, Horwitz KB. Progesterone regulated expression of flavin-containing monooxygenase 5 by the B-isoform of progesterone receptors: implications for tamoxifen carcinogenicity. J Clin Endocrinol Metab 1997;82:2956–2961.

105. Zarghami N, Grass L, Diamandis EP. Steroid hormone regulation of prostate-specific antigen gene expression in breast cancer. Br J Cancer 1997;75:579–588.

4

Pathogenesis of Estrogen-Receptor-Positive and -Negative Breast Cancer

Powel Brown, MD, PHD,
Suzanne Fuqua, PHD, and Craig Allred, MD

CONTENTS

INTRODUCTION

Over the last 20 years, there have been major advances in the treatment and prevention of breast cancer (BC), including the development and widespread use of mammography to detect cancer at an early stage, and the use of adjuvant chemotherapy or hormonal therapy to treat these early cancers to improve survival. Most recently, it has been shown that intervening at an even earlier stage is possible. Thus, clinical trials have demonstrated that it is possible to reduce BC incidence by treating women at high risk of developing BC with antiestrogens. Although all of these advances have improved the outcome for women with BC or women at high risk, cancer remains the leading cause of death in women aged 40–79 yr, with BC being the most common cause of cancer-related death in this age group, and the second most common cause of cancer-related death in women overall *(1)*. In addition, hormonal therapies using antiestrogens may be ineffective in

From: *Contemporary Endocrinology: Endocrine Oncology*
Edited by: S. P. Ethier © Humana Press Inc., Totowa, NJ

women who develop estrogen-receptor (ER)-negative BC. To continue to make progress in the treatment and prevention of this disease, it will be important to elucidate the steps in the genesis of BC. Detailed knowledge of the molecular events that occur to transform normal human mammary epithelial cells into invasive cancer will provide the clues for future efforts to irradicate this disease.

IMPORTANCE OF ESTROGEN AND ER IN GENESIS OF BREAST CANCER

One of the most important features of breast cells is their sensitivity and response to the hormone, estrogen. Epidemiologic studies have demonstrated that increased exposure to estrogen is associated with a high risk of developing BC (2). In addition, the ER is an important target for the treatment and prevention of BC, and the antiestrogen, tamoxifen (TAM), is the most commonly used drug for the treatment of BC. While TAM effectively inhibits the growth of BCs expressing the ER, many BCs do not express the receptor, and thus are resistant to antiestrogen therapy. Furthermore, although ER-positive cancers initially respond to antiestrogens, they invariably develop resistance to antiestrogen therapy. Thus, a better understanding of the processes responsible for the development of ER-positive and -negative BCs will facilitate the development of effective ways to treat this disease.

EFFECT OF ESTROGEN ON NORMAL GLAND DEVELOPMENT

Estrogens are critical regulators of normal development of the breast and genital organs (reviewed in ref. 3). The physiologic role of these hormones in the breast is to stimulate the growth of the ductal epithelium, and to induce the formation of lobules and ultimately terminal duct-lobular units. As described below, breast epithelial cells at these different stages of differentiation express ERs and respond to estrogen.

ESTROGEN RECEPTORS

ERs are proteins of the nuclear steroid hormone receptor family, which bind estrogens, translocate to the nucleus, and bind DNA. These DNA-binding proteins then regulate transcription and activate the expression of genes that have estrogen-responsive elements (ERE) within their promoters. Two ERs are now known to exist; ERα and ERβ.

ERα was initially cloned in 1985 by Walter et al. (4) and, in 1986, by Greene et al. (5). This gene was found to have several domains now typical of proteins of the steroid hormone receptor family. It contains two transactivation domains: a DNA-binding domain, and a hormone-binding domain (structural features shown in Fig. 1; reviewed in ref. 6). This protein is expressed in normal breast epithelium, as well as in other estrogen-responsive tissues, such as the ovaries, uterus, liver, and brain. It is also expressed in malignant tumors of the breast, ovary, and uterus. In the case of BC, approx 50–70% of all BC expresses ERα. Many studies (7–11) have demonstrated that the expression of this protein is an important prognostic marker, and most of these studies found that patients whose tumors express ERα have an improved disease-free survival; many also show improved overall survival as well. Results from studies from San Antonio and National Surgical and Adjuvant Breast and Bowel Project (NSABP) suggest that this disease-free survival advantage is approx 10% at 5 yr (12). ERα is also an important predictive marker, predicting a response to antiestrogen therapy such as TAM (11).

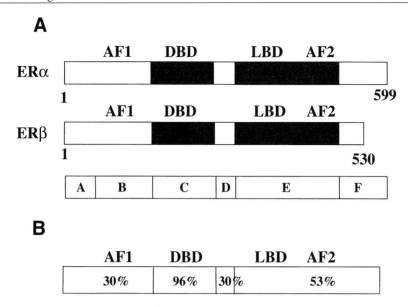

Fig. 1. Schematic map of ERα and ERβ: (**A**) The two transactivation domains (AF-1 and AF-2), the DNA-binding domain (DBD), and the ligand-binding domain (LBD) are shown. Also shown are the homology regions of ER (A, B, C, D, E, and F regions). (**B**) The percent homology between human ERα and ERβ. Note the similarity in the DBD and LBD domains.

The existence of ERα has been known for many years, but the existence of a second ER, ERβ has been appreciated only for the last 3 yr *(13–15)*. ERβ is very similar to ERα: The ERβ protein has the same overall structure, with two transactivation domains (AF-1 and AF-2), DNA-binding domain, and a hormone-binding domain (Fig. 1). In the human, ERβ and ERα share 30% homology at the amino acid level in the A/B domains, which contain AF-1, 96% homology in the DNA-binding domain, and 53% homology in the E and F domains, which contain the ligand-binding and AF-2 domains *(16)*. Like ERα, the ERβ protein is expressed in estrogen-responsive tissues. However, these two genes show differential expression in estrogen-responsive tissues in mice, with ERα being highly expressed in mammary, uterus, testis, pituitary, ovary, kidney, epididymis, and adrenal tissues; ERβ is highly expressed in prostate, ovary, lung, bladder, brain, and testis tissues *(17)*. Other investigators have shown expression of ERβ in normal and malignant breast and ovary cells *(13,18–22)*. However, many BCs and ovarian cancers do not express ERβ *(18,21,22)*. Other studies have suggested that these two proteins may have different functions: They both respond to estrogen by inducing gene expression, buy they appear to activate a different set of genes. In breast cells, estrogen binds to either ERα or ERβ, and activates the expression of genes with classical EREs within their promoters *(6)*. When bound to ERα, but not to ERβ, estrogen can also activate the expression of genes with nonclassical response elements, such as genes with activating protein 1 (AP-1) responsive elements *(23,24)*. Thus, the expression of these estrogen-responsive genes can be modulated by the relative amounts of ERα and ERβ. ERα and ERβ also can bind the antiestrogen, TAM, which can antagonize the effect of estrogen and inhibit the expression of genes with classical EREs within their promoters. However, TAM can also function as an agonist in some cells, when bound to either ERα or ERβ, and induce the expression of genes with AP-1 sites within their promoters *(23,24)*. In addition to the different forms of ERs, the expression of estrogen-responsive genes is regulated by

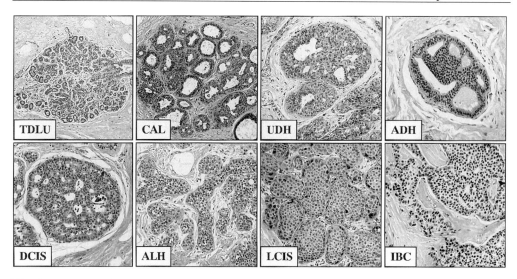

Fig. 2. Representative examples of premalignant breast lesions. All proliferative breast disease, benign or malignant, is thought to arise from stem cells in normal terminal duct lobular units (TDLU). Commonly, through proliferation of their lining epithelium, TDLUs unfold and enlarge, a process referred to a columnar alteration of lobules (CAL), because of the tall columnar appearance of the activated epithelium. Through continued proliferation, CAL often gives rise to more cellular, but still benign, lesions, referred to as usual ductal hyperpasias (UDH), and the more clonal-appearing atypical ductal hyperplasias (ADH). Ductal carcinoma *in situ* (DCIS) is a malignant but noninvasive precursor that may arise from ADH. Atypical lobular hyperplasia (ALH) and lobular carcinoma *in situ* (LCIS) are clinically somewhat analagous to ADH and DCIS, but have distinct histological appearances. All these lesions are epidemilogic risk factors, and also probably precursors of invasive BCs (IBC), which are histologically very diverse.

several different co-factors, termed co-activators or co-repressors *(25)*. These proteins bind the ERs and modulate the expression of estrogen-responsive genes. Thus, the specific response to estrogen and TAM depends on the specific cell type, the levels of ERα and ERβ, and the levels of co-activator and co-repressor proteins within a cell.

ER EXPRESSION DURING BREAST CANCER EVOLUTION

Invasive BC is thought to arise from benign premalignant lesions. A model of BC evolution has been proposed, based primarily on epidemiologic data *(26,27)*. In this model, stem cells within normal terminal ductal lobular units (TDLUs) are hypothesized to evolve through a series of increasingly abnormal proliferative breast lesions, from usual hyperplasia (UH), to atypical hyperplasia (AH), to carcinoma *in situ* (CIS), and finally to invasive carcinoma. Examples of these lesions are shown in Fig. 2. TDLUs contain benign ECs that line the terminal ducts and lobules. These cells show generally low levels of proliferation and ER expression. Columnar alteration of lobules (CAL lesions also known as unfolded lobules) contain benign ECs that have begun to proliferate and are strongly ER-positive. Benign-appearing lesions showing more proliferation are termed UH. More atypical proliferative lesions are termed atypical ductal or atypical lobular hyperplasias (ADH or ALH). These lesions are associated with an increased risk of invasive BC (an approximate fivefold increase risk of a normal women) *(28)*. Unequivocal premalignant lesions include ductal carcinoma *in situ* (DCIS) and lobular carcinoma *in situ* (LCIS). These lesions are more highly associated with risk of invasive BC (an approximate 10-fold increase) *(28)*. Although most investigators recognize this theory of BC evolution as imperfect and oversimplified, particularly for early stages of tumor progression, some elements of the model are almost certainly relevant, and it has been very useful in designing experimental studies into the biological mechanisms of BC evolution, which still are in their infancy.

Recent molecular data support this model by demonstrating that synchronous UH, AH *(29)*, and CIS share identical genetic abnormalities *(30–32)*. It is also known that women with these premalignant lesions carry an increased risk of eventually developing invasive BC. Several investigators have examined ER expression in these lesions. ER is expressed in most normal TDLUs, but its expression is usually very low, with no more than 10% of cells expressing at any one time *(33–35)*. This may be in part, because ER levels fluctuate during the menstrual cycle, with highest levels seen during the follicular phase of the cycle *(36,37)*. In contrast to that seen in normal cells, about 60% of UH and 80% of AH express ER, usually in a large proportion of cells *(38–40)*. Similarly, low grade/noncomedo DCIS cells express generally high levels of ER *(41)*. In contrast, in high grade/comedo DCIS, only about 30% of the lesions express ER *(41)*. Finally, between 50 and 70% of invasive BCs express ER, similar to that reported for UH, AH, and low- grade DCIS premalignant lesions.

An elegant case-control study *(42,43)* has examined ER and progesterone receptor (PR) expression in patients with invasive BC, compared to benign breast disease controls. Those authors found that elevated ER expression in benign epithelium was a significant risk factor for BC development, and also suggest that overexpression of ER in TDLUs augments normal estrogen sensitivity. Since prolonged estrogen exposure is an important risk factor for BC, abnormal ER expression in the benign epithelium may contribute to and increase the risk of progression to cancer.

GENESIS OF BREAST CANCER

Estrogen and progesterone and their receptors, ER and PR, are clearly important in the genesis of BC. These hormones control the proliferation and differentiation of normal mammary ECs, and also are critical regulators of the growth of ER-positive BC cells. However, peptide growth factors (GF), receptors, and tumor suppressor genes are also important for the genesis of BC. These include GFs, such as epidermal growth factor (EGF), transforming growth factor α, heregulins, and insulin-like growth factors (IGFs), and their receptors, such as EGFR, erb-2, -3, and -4, and IGFR; and the tumor suppressor genes, *p53*, *Rb*, *BRCA1*, and *BRCA2*. These proteins and their role in breast carcinogenesis are discussed later in Chapter 5, and in recent reviews *(44)*. However, it should be noted that many of these GFs and GFRs are altered in more undifferentiated cells, which typically do not express ER. For example, breast cells that express high levels of erbB-2 typically are ER-negative *(45)*. A similar inverse relationship exists for EGFR *(46)*. In addition, recent studies have suggested that tumors arising in individuals with *BRCA1* or -2 mutations more commonly are high-grade *(47–49)*, lack ER *(47,50)*, and contain *p53* mutations *(51)*, than do sporadic BCs. In general, well-differentiated breast tumors express the ER, and are stimulated to grow by estrogen; poorly differentiated breast tumors often do not express ER, and instead may have high expression of EGFR or erbB-2, and have tumor-suppressor gene mutations.

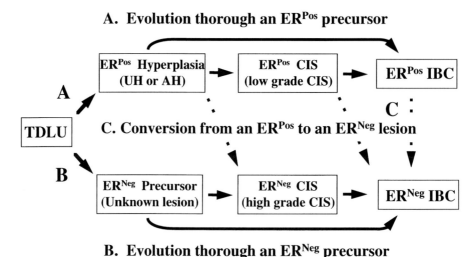

A. Evolution thorough an ER^Pos precursor

C. Conversion from an ER^Pos to an ER^Neg lesion

B. Evolution thorough an ER^Neg precursor

Fig. 3. Proposed models of evolution of ER-positive and -negative invasive BC. The normal precursor to BC is presumed to be the ER-heterogeneous TDLU. ER-positive BCs may evolve through the pathway marked "A": through ER-positive hyperplasias, ER-positive CIS lesions to invasive ER-positive BC (it is possible that some BCs do not evolve through CIS lesions, as marked by the curved arrow). ER-negative BCs may evolve through the pathway marked "B": through an ER-negative precursor lesion, to ER-negative CIS lesions, typically seen with high-grade CIS, to invasive ER-negative BC. Alternatively, ER-negative BCs can evolve from ER-positive precursor lesions (conversion from ER-positive to -negative lesions), as marked by the dotted arrows and by "C".

EVOLUTION OF ER-NEGATIVE BREAST CANCERS

To fully understand the genesis of BC, it will be important to understand how both ER-positive and -negative BCs arise. One critical question that remains unanswered is whether ER-negative BCs arise from ER-positive or -negative stem cells. The answer to this question is of paramount importance, because it will affect understanding of breast oncogenesis as well as drive future drug development for the prevention and treatment of BC. If ER-negative cancers arise independently of ER-positive cells, than it would be predicted that antiestrogen therapies would be ineffective at preventing the development of ER-negative BCs. In that case, antiestrogen drugs may actually select for the development of ER-negative tumors. On the other hand, if ER-negative BCs arise from ER-positive precursors, then antiestrogen drugs would be expected to suppress the development of both ER-positive and -negative BCs.

Figure 3 shows proposed pathways for the genesis of ER-positive and -negative invasive BCs. As shown in the top portion of the model, ER-positive BCs may arise from the ER-heterogenous TDLU through an ER-positive precursor (ER-positive hyperplasias, such as UH and AH, and/or through ER-positive CIS lesions; marked A in Fig. 3). As shown in the lower portion of the model, ER-negative invasive BCs may evolve from TDLUs through precursors that are ER-negative (marked B in Fig. 3). In this case, ER-negative tumors would evolve independently of ER-positive cells. Shown in the middle of Fig. 3 is the conversion from ER-positive precursors to ER-negative lesions (marked C in Fig. 3). In this case, ER-negative cancers would arise from ER-positive precursors. As discussed below, data exist to support both models of ER-negative BC evolution.

Thus, it is possible that ER-negative BCs can evolve either independently of ER-positive cells, or through a pathway involving an ER-positive precursor.

STUDIES SUPPORTING THE HYPOTHESIS THAT ER-NEGATIVE CANCERS ARISE FROM ER-POSITIVE PRECURSOR

Epidemiologic Studies

Data from epidemiologic studies, clinical trials, and in vitro studies of BC cell lines all provide support of the hypothesis that ER-negative cancers can arise from ER-positive cells. A vast amount of data from these epidemiologic studies suggest that the most important risk factor for BC development is the cumulative exposure to estrogen and possibly also P hormones *(52)*. Such studies demonstrate that BC risk is increased with early menarche *(53–56)*, late menopause *(57,58)*, obesity in postmenopausal women *(59, 60)*, hormone replacement therapy (meta-analysis performed in refs. *61–63*), all of which lead to increased exposure to estrogen or progesterone. In addition, studies have shown that factors that decrease exposure to estrogen or progesterone reduce BC risk. Well-established factors associated with reduced incidence of BC include early first-term pregnancy *(64)*, lactation *(65,66)*, and increased physical activity *(67,68)*. In addition, premenopausal women who have had bilateral oophorectomy or pelvic radiation have markedly reduced risk of BC, up to a 50% reduction in risk, compared to the general population *(69,70)*.

These epidemiologic data have led researchers to suggest that the driving force behind these associations is the proliferative effect of estrogens on breast epithelial cells (presumably ER-positive breast cells). These proliferating cells then acquire genetic damage, resulting in mutation and amplification of oncogenes, mutation and loss of tumor-suppressor genes, and ultimately causing transformation of these cells into a fully malignant phenotype. If all BC evolve through this oncogenic pathway dependent on the tumor-promoting properties of estrogen, then it is likely that these cancers will arise from an ER-positive precursor. Since few, if any, of the epidemiologic studies distinguish between the risk of developing ER-positive or -negative BC, it is not possible to definitely conclude from the epidemiologic data that all BCs evolve from an ER-positive precursor. However, the strong association of overall BC risk with cumulative exposure to estrogen is supportive of the hypothesis that most BCs evolve from an ER-positive precursor.

Studies of Primary vs Metastatic Tumors

Results of studies of metastatic BC also suggest that ER-negative BC cells can evolve from ER-positive breast cells. It is possible that evolution of ER-negative cells can occur either spontaneously or through selection after treatment with antiestrogens. Although apparently an infrequent event, spontaneous evolution of ER-negative cancer cells has been observed when the level of ER was measured in BC metastases arising in patients with known ER-positive primary tumors. Thus, several studies *(71–73)* have noted that the ER status of recurrent or metastatic lesions can be discordant with the ER status of the primary tumor. In another study*(74)*, sequential biopsies of primary tumors revealed conversion of ER-positive tumors into ER-negative tumors in 19% of the cases. The most compelling data was presented in a recent study reported by Kuukasjarvi et al. *(71)*, who reported the ER status of primary and matched asynchronous metastatic lesions from patients who had not received any adjuvant therapy. In this study, 70% of the primary

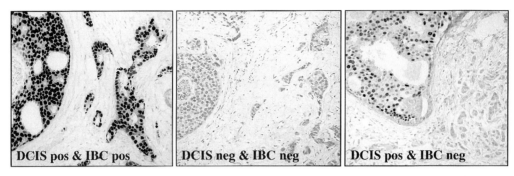

Fig. 4. Representative examples of tumors composed of both ductal carcinoma in situ (DCIS) and invasive BC (IBC) immunostained for estrogen receptor (ER) (DCIS is on the left and IBC on the right in each panel). The most common (60–70%) phenotype consists of ER-positive DCIS associated with ER-positive IBC. In the next most common (30–40%) phenotype, the DCIS and IBC components are both ER-negative. Rarely (<5%), cases are observed in which ER is positive in the DCIS, but negative in the IBC. The opposite phenotype is almost never observed.

tumors were positive for ER; only 54% of the metastatic tumors were positive for ER. In the matched tumors, 46% of the tumors were ER-positive at both the primary site and the metastatic site; 24% of the tumors showed discordance, with the primary site tumors being ER-positive and the metastatic sites being ER-negative.

This evolution from an ER-positive phenotype to an ER-negative phenotype can also occur at the preinvasive stage, e.g., ER-positive DCIS can evolve to ER-negative invasive BC, but this occurs rarely. An example of this conversion during evolution is shown in Fig. 4. Shown are three examples of DCIS and closely associated invasive BC. In the first example, both lesions express ER; in the second example, neither the DCIS nor the invasive BC express ER. The third example shows a ER-positive DCIS lesion with a closely approximated ER-negative invasive BC. The frequency of ER-positive DCIS lesions with ER-negative invasive cancer is low, but this example demonstrates that this discordance can occur at the level of preinvasive disease. These data are consistent with the hypothesis that ER-positive primary tumors can evolve into ER-negative tumors when they become metastatic.

In patients who have been treated with antiestrogens such as TAM, it is possible that the therapy selects for evolution of ER-negative cells. However, the majority of BCs retain ER when they acquire resistance to TAM: Only approx 10–20% of resistant tumors lose either ER or PR *(75)*. It is thought that TAM resistance is probably multifactorial, with mutation of ER *(76)*, alternative splicing to form truncated isoforms of ER *(77–79)*, and other signaling pathway alterations all contributing to the resistant phenotype. Recently, truncated ERβ isoforms have been detected in a number of ER-negative breast tumors and cell lines *(80–83)*. The existence of ERβ isoforms in ER-negative BC, which are incapable of binding hormone, but nonetheless have potential modulatory effects on ER activity, could prove to have important clinical implications for BC progression. Their role in TAM resistance is currently not known.

These clinical data support the hypothesis that ER-negative tumors can evolve from ER-positive primary tumors. However, it should be noted that these data are also consistent with an alternate possibility that the primary tumors contain a heterogeneous mixture of ER-positive and -negative tumor cells, and that the ER-negative tumor cells have a growth advantage that allows them to metastasize and recur. Indeed, most ER-positive invasive BCs typically show a heterogeneous staining pattern for ER, with both ER-positive and -negative cells being present. Thus, the available data do not provide definitive proof that ER-negative cells necessarily evolve from the ER-positive cells, but only that both can occur in the same patient.

In Vitro Conversion
of ER-Positive Breast Cancer to ER-Negative Breast Cancer

Studies of BC cell lines also provide data to suggest that ER-negative BCs can arise from ER-positive cells. Previous studies *(84–89)* have demonstrated that overexpression of peptide GFs and their receptors is associated with the ER-negative phenotype. Several investigators *(87,90)* have demonstrated that breast tumors that have high expression of EGFR are more commonly ER-negative, but many other studies have shown that high expression of erbB-2 or HER2/neu is associated with ER negativity *(84,85,88,89)*. Overexpression of the fibroblast growth factors (FGF) peptide GFs is also associated with the ER-negative phenotype *(91,92)*. These clinical observations led researchers to investigate the effect of over-expression of these peptide GFs, their receptors, or molecules, which transduce mitogenic signals in ER-positive cells. Thus, gene encoding EGFR, erbB-2, and FGF have all been transfected into ER-positive MCF-7 BC cells. In each of these cases, over-expression of these peptide GFs or their receptors interferes with estrogen signaling. In the case of EGFR, Miller et al. *(93)* demonstrated that overexpression of EGFR in MCF-7 cells resulted in enhanced growth in vitro, without loss of the ER. Overexpression of erbB-2 also induced loss of responsiveness to estrogen and resistance to antiestrogens, without loss of the ER *(94,95)*.

Data to support the hypothesis that ER-negative cells can arise from ER-positive cells also comes from studies overexpressing the molecules that transduce peptide mitogenic signals. Such mitogenic transducers include the *raf* proto-oncogene, which is an important transducer of signals that activate the Ras/Raf/MAP kinase cascade, and the c-Jun protein, which is a component of the AP-1 transcription factor, a transcription factor activated by the stress activated kinases, SAP kinase and p38, as well as by protein kinase C-dependent signals. In studies of MCF-7 cells transfected with the *raf* proto-oncogene, El-Ashry et al. *(96)* have shown that overexpression of an activated Raf protein causes ER-positive MCF-7 cells to downregulate ER, and become ER-negative. Concomitantly, these cells no longer respond to estrogen, and fail to be inhibited by antiestrogens. Those investigators then demonstrated that overexpression of an activated *raf* gene in these cells causes transcriptional downregulation of ER, effectively transforming these cells into ER-negative BC cells. Similar results were observed by Wise et al. *(97)*, when the c-Jun protein was overexpressed in MCF-7 cells. ER-positive MCF-7 cells were stably transfected with the c-*jun* gene, and their response to estrogen and TAM was investigated. These studies showed that the c-Jun-overexpressing cells no longer expressed ER protein, and that they failed to respond to estrogen, as assessed by estrogen-dependent reporter assays or by estrogen-induced mitogenic assays. As with the Raf-overexpressing cells, these c-Jun overexpressing MCF-7 cells grew in the absence of estrogen, were not growth-stimulated by estrogen, and were insensitive to antiestrogens. Those investigators also demonstrated that the c-Jun-overexpressing ER-negative MCF-7 cells grew in nude mice, as xenografts in an estrogen-independent manner *(97)*. Thus, in at least some cases, overexpression of molecules that transduce peptide GF signals can cause ER-positive BC cells to lose expression of the ER and become estrogen-independent.

Another example of ER-positive MCF-7 cells becoming ER-negative is the selection of clones of MCF-7 cells that lack ER. One such subclone is the Adriamycin-resistant MCF-7 cell line, MCF-7 ADR, isolated by Fairchild et al. *(98)*. This subclone was isolated by growing MCF-7 cells in the presence of the chemotherapeutic agent, Adriamycin (doxyrubicin). A subclone of the parental MCF-7 cells grew in the presence of Adriamycin, which was found to overexpress the multidrug resistance gene, *mdr*-1. In addition, these cells were noted to have lost ER expression. In subsequent studies, Vickers et al. *(99)* showed that these cells no longer responded to estrogen, and that they were unaffected by antiestrogens.

In all of the above examples of ER-positive BC cells becoming ER-negative, the cells have been transfected with GFs, receptors, or transcription factors, or have had a strong selection pressure to select for drug resistance. There have been no examples of spontaneous loss of ER in any commonly used BC cell lines, with the exception of T47-D, which was originally shown to express both ER and PR *(100)*. This cell line is well known for exhibiting a high degree of genetic instability, and loss of ER has been shown to occur with simple dilution cloning without further selection *(100–103)*. More recent data show that T47-D cells can also be induced to lose their expression of ER by selection in estrogen-deficient media *(104,105)*. Murphy et al. *(105)* isolated subclones of T47-D cells that do not express ER or PR, by culturing the cells for extended times in media lacking estrogen. After more than 1 yr, an ER-negative/PR-negative clone grew, which, when subcloned, stably retained an ER-negative phenotype. These ER-negative T47-D cells no longer respond to estrogen, and are unaffected by antiestrogens.

These in vitro studies demonstrate that it is possible for ER-negative cells to arise from ER-positive BC cell lines. Although these in vitro experiments do not demonstrate that the ER-negative cells necessarily evolve from ER-positive cells, the data do demonstrate that, under certain conditions, it is possible for ER-positive cells to lose expression of ER, and thus become ER-negative.

STUDIES SUPPORTING THE HYPOTHESIS THAT ER-NEGATIVE CANCERS ARISE INDEPENDENT OF ER-POSITIVE CELLS

The data discussed above support the hypothesis that ER-negative breast tumors can evolve from ER-positive tumors, but other data support the alternate hypothesis, that ER-positive and ER-negative tumors evolve independently. Data suggesting that these two forms of BC arise independently include epidemiologic data, studies of primary breast tumors compared with paired metastases, and in vivo and in vitro studies of BC cells.

Epidemiologic Studies

Most studies of the epidemiology of BC have found associations between exposure to estrogen or progesterone and risk of BC. However, these studies typically report an association with overall BC, and do not investigate whether there exists similar associations between estrogen exposure and risk of ER-positive or ER-negative BC. ER-positive BCs make up 50–70% of all BCs, depending on the assay used to measure ER. Therefore, if a positive association exists between estrogen exposure and risk of ER-positive BC only (i.e., no association with ER-negative BC), there still may be an observable association between estrogen exposure and risk of overall BC. Thus, the available epidemiologic data does not specifically address whether the risk of ER-negative BCs is associated with chronic estrogen or P exposure.

One recent report of alcohol consumption and risk of BC investigated the relationship between the amount of alcohol consumed and the risk of ER-positive and -negative BC *(106)*. The results demonstrated that the risk of ER-positive BC was increased with increasing consumption of alcohol; the risk of ER-negative BC was not related to consumption of alcohol. This effect of alcohol has been proposed to result from an increase in plasma estrogen levels in women consuming alcohol *(107)*. Those studies suggest that ER-positive and -negative BCs may have different risk factors, and that ER-negative BCs may be less dependent on exposure to estrogen than ER-positive BCs. It will be important to analyze the risk of both ER-positive and -negative BCs in future epidemiologic studies, to clarify whether estrogen exposure influences the risk of ER-negative BC.

In Vivo Stability of ER Expression in BCs

As discussed above, there exist reports that ER-positive primary BCs can be associated with ER-negative primary or metastatic lesions, either sponateously or after antiestrogen treatment *(71–73,108,109)*. However, although such discordant cases are seen, the frequency of discordant ER expression in the breast carcinomas is less than 40%. Discordance in the expression of ER between multiple intratumoral assays are performed range from 12 to 32% *(73,110,111)*; discordance between primary and metastatic lesions range from 15 to 36% *(71,73,74,112)*. True discordance is likely to be much less than 30%, since many of these studies were conducted using ligand-binding assays to measure ER expression *(73,110,111)*. The discordance seen in these older studies probably results from the high false-negative rate of ligand-binding assay, and not from true discordance of ER expression. Thus, concordance in the expression of ER in multiple intratumoral biopsies and between primary and metastatic lesions is much more common. This is true even in cases in which the metastatic lesions have arisen after antiestrogen treatment. The concordance between ER-negative primary and recurrent tumors is also common, particularly in studies using immunohistochemistry to measure ER expression. Thus, in their study, Kuukasjarvi et al. *(71)* observed that ER-negative primary tumors all developed ER-negative recurrences; Johnston et al. *(108)* found only 1/37 ER-negative primary tumors was ER-positive on recurrence. All of these data demonstrate that, although discordance in ER expression can occur between primary and recurrent tumors, concordance between primary and recurrent tumors is more common.

The data from these studies of paired primary and metastatic tumor samples can also be interpreted to support the concept of tumor heterogeneity at the primary tumor, as discussed above and by Osborne *(73)*. It is possible, in women whose primary tumor is ER-positive and whose metastatic tumor is ER-negative, that the original primary tumor contained both ER-positive and -negative malignant cells. Thus, the results from studies of ER expression in primary and recurrent tumors do not prove that ER-negative tumors arose from an ER-positive precursor. The results are equally consistent with the hypothesis that ER-positive and -negative tumors arise independently, and that, rarely, some individuals have primary tumors which are heterogeneous for the expression of ER.

In Vitro Stability of ER-Positive BC Phenotype

Examples of ER-positive BC cell lines converting to an ER-negative phenotype, either spontaneously or through selection, have been described above. However, this conversion is a rare event. With the exception of the T47-D BC cell line, no other BC cell line has been reported to have spontaneously converted to an ER-negative phenotype. Given the fact that many of the current widely studied BC cell lines have been in culture for more than 20 yr, it is remarkable that almost all of the originally ER-positive cell lines have retained the expression of the ER over this time. This observation suggests that, although loss of ER expression in previously ER-positive BC cells can occur, it is a rare event (at least in cells grown in culture). This stability of the ER-positive phenotype provides support to the hypothesis that BC cells do not commonly spontaneously convert to an ER-negative phenotype.

Extensive effort has also been made to select ER-negative MCF-7 clones that have been grown in the absence of estrogen, or in the presence of antiestrogens. In many of these studies, estrogen-independent and/or antiestrogen resistant cells have been isolated *(113–115)*. However, in each case, expression of the ER is retained. Other events have taken place in these cells that result in estrogen-independent growth, but in all cases, the ER is still expressed. Thus, in MCF-7 cells, it is difficult to select for the loss of ER. As mentioned above, ER-negative MCF-7 BC cells have been isolated only when the cells were forced to overexpress signal transduction molecules (such as Raf or c-Jun), or when they were selected for resistance to chemotherapeutic agents.

Data from Chemoprevention Trials Using Antiestrogens

As discussed above, data from epidemiologic studies, clinical studies of metastases, and in vitro studies of cell lines can be used to support either hypothesis for the genesis of ER-negative BC. However, results from recent clinical chemoprevention trials may be able to provide the most conclusive evidence to support either one or the other of these proposed mechanisms of carcinogenesis. These chemoprevention trials tested the ability of antiestrogens to prevent BC. Results from three trials in which the antiestrogen, TAM, was used, were published last year *(116–118)*. In addition, other clinical trials using the second-generation selective ER modulator (SERM), raloxifene, to prevent bone fractures in women with osteoporosis, were also published recently *(119)*. This same cohort of women is being studied for the incidence of BC to determine whether this other antiestrogen also reduces the incidence of BC.

The results from the three TAM chemoprevention trials were reported at interim analysis, and are shown in Table 1. The largest of the three trials, the NSABP P-1 Breast Cancer Prevention Trial, was stopped early, because results of an interim analysis showed a significant reduction in the incidence of BC in women taking TAM, compared to those who took placebo *(116)*. In this trial, over 13,000 women at high risk of developing BC (e.g., women who had greater or equal to the risk of a 60-yr-old women as determined by the Gail model *[120]*), were treated with either TAM or placebo for a planned period of 5 yr. At interim analysis, the women had received an average of 4 yr of study drug. The analysis at time of publication demonstrated a 49% reduction in the incidence of BC in the women who took TAM (*see* Table 1). These results were highly significant, and represent the most convincing evidence that antiestrogens suppress the development or clinical appearance of BC in women without a previous history of BC.

The results of the two other TAM chemoprevention trials, which were reported to be negative, are also shown in Table 1. These studies include the trial conducted at the Royal Marsden Hospital in the UK, in which 2471 women were randomized to receive either TAM or placebo *(117)*, and the trial done in Italy, in which 5408 women who had a hysterectomy were treated with TAM or placebo *(118)*. Both of these trials showed no significant difference in the incidence of BC in women taking TAM, compared to placebo.

Table 1
TAM BC Chemoprevention Trials

Trial	Sample size	Woman-yr follow-up	Median follow-up (mo)	Results					
				No. Breast cancer		Breast cancer/1000 woman yr		% Reduction	Ref.
				Placebo	TAM	Placebo	TAM		
NSABP P-1	13,388	52,401	55 mo	175	89	6.76	3.43	49%	(116)
England	2471	12,355	70 mo	36	34	5.0	4.7	No significant reduction	(117)
Italian	5408	20,731	46 mo	22	19	2.3	2.1	No significant reduction	(118)

Table 2
Incidence of ER-Positive and -Negative BCs in NSABP P-1

Trial	Cancer	No. of BCs		% Reduction	Ref.
		Placebo	TAM		
NSABP P-1	All BC	175	89	49	*(116)*
(*N* = 13,388)	ER-positive	130	41	69	
	ER-negative	31	38	No reduction	
	ER unknown	14	10	29	

These two negative trials had different eligibility criteria, compared to the NSABP P-1 trial, and also had other features that may account for the difference in the results. Among these differences, allowing the use of hormone replacement, and the difference in patient population (e.g., the Royal Marsden trial recruited women who were more likely to have familial BC than those enrolled in the NSABP P-1 trial), may contribute to the different results, compared to that reported in the NSABP P-1 trial.

The results of a clinical trial using the second-generation antiestrogen SERM, raloxifene, in women with osteoporosis, were also reported recently *(119)*. In this clinical trial, the efficacy of raloxifene was studied to determine whether this antiestrogen would reduce bone fractures in women with osteoporosis. A secondary end point in this trial was the incidence of BC. It was hypothesized that, in addition to preventing bone fractures and slowing the progression of bone loss in these women, raloxifene would reduce BC incidence. The results from this trial demonstrated that raloxifene slowed the progression of bone loss *(119)*, and also reduced the incidence of bone fractures and BC *(121)*. Thus, this trial supports the finding of the NSABP P-1 trial that antiestrogens can reduce the incidence of BC in women who have not previously been diagnosed with BC.

The data from these clinical trials, suggesting that antiestrogens reduce BC incidence, support the proposal that BCs evolve from a precursor that is sensitive to antiestrogens (and thus are likely to be ER-positive). However, it is important to consider two additional important features of these data. First, it must be noted that the follow-up of patients on these trials is short (average and median time of follow-up on the P-1 trial is 48 and 55 mo, respectively *[116]*). Thus, the BCs that did arise probabaly arose from small BCs that were present, but clinically undetectable. Some of the BCs that were prevented were likely to also be clinically cryptic BCs whose growth was suppressed by the antiestrogen treatment. Thus, the data do not yet conclusively demonstrate that the reduction in incidence in BC in the antiestrogen-treated groups is the result of blocking the transformation of normal ER-positive precursor breast ECs into malignant BC cells. However, additional analysis of the NSABP P-1 data demonstrates that antiestrogens significantly reduced the incidence of preinvasive BC. Thus, these investigators also found a 50% reduction in the incidence of DCIS and LCIS lesions in the cohort of women taking TAM. These data suggest that antiestrogens also suppress the development of preinvasive BC.

A second important feature of the data from both the NSABP P-1 and the raloxifene trials is the effect that antiestrogen treatment had on the incidence of ER-positive and -negative BCs in women taking these antiestrogens. Antiestrogen-treatment caused an approx 50% reduction in the incidence of overall BC, but this suppression of BC resulted totally from a reduction in ER-positive BCs (*see* Table 2). Thus, in the NSABP P-1 trial, 175 vs 89 cases of invasive BC were seen in the placebo vs TAM-treated groups. There was a 69% reduction in ER-positive BCs (there were 130 ER-positive BCs in the placebo group and 41 ER-positive cancers in the TAM group). However, as shown in Table 2, there was no reduction in the incidence of ER-negative BCs (there were 31 ER-negative BCs in the placebo group and 38 ER-negative cancers in the TAM group) *(116)*. Similar results were seen in trials using raloxifene *(121)*. These data suggest that antiestrogens do not affect the development of ER-negative BC. Alternatively, this lack of effect on ER-negative BC could be the result of lack of effect on established, but clinically undetectable ER-negative BCs. If ER-negative BCs evolve from ER-positive precursors, then longer follow-up should eventually show a reduction in both ER-positive and -negative BCs. However, at this time, the above data are consistent with the hypothesis that ER-negative BCs evolve through an estrogen-independent process.

CONCLUSIONS

The above discussion points out that the mechanisms by which ER-negative BCs arise are still mostly unknown. As presented, there exist data to suggest that ER-negative BCs can arise either independently from ER-positive breast cells or through a pathway involving an ER-positive precursor cell. These two apparently opposing oncogenic pathways are not necessarily mutually exclusive. Thus, it is possible that some ER-negative BCs evolve from ER-positive cells; others evolve independently. Further study of premalignant human breast cells, and the mechanisms by which they become transformed into both ER-positive and -negative BCs, will be needed before these questions can be resolved. However, with recent exciting clinical trial data demonstrating the effectiveness of antiestrogens in suppressing the development of BC (especially ER-positive BC), there has been a renewed interest in developing effective chemopreventive strategies for the prevention of ER-negative BC. Future laboratory and clinical studies will probably focus on the question of how best to prevent the development of ER-negative BC. Through such studies, major reductions in the incidence and mortality of BC are likely.

REFERENCES

1. Landis S, Murray T, Bolden S, Wingo P. Cancer Statistics 1999. CA J 1999;49:8–31.
2. Henderson BE, Ross R, Bernstein L. Estrogens as a cause of human cancer: the Richard and Hindau Rosenthal Foundation Award Lecture. Cancer Res 1988;48:246–253.
3. Osborne M. Breast anatomy and development. In: Harris J, Lippman M, Morrow M, Hellman S, eds. Diseases of the Breast. Lippincott-Raven, Philadelphia, 1996, pp. 1–14.
4. Walter P, Green S, Greene G, Krust A, Bornert J, Jeltsch J, et al. Cloning of the human estrogen receptor cDNA. Proc Natl Acad Sci USA 1985;82:7889–7893.
5. Greene G, Gilna P, Waterfield M, Baker A, Hort Y, Shine J. Sequence and expression of human estrogen receptor complementary DNA. Science 1986;231:1150–1154.
6. Fuqua S. Chapter title. In: Harris J, Lippman M, Morrow M, Hellman S, eds. Diseases of the Breast. Lippincott-Raven, Philadelphia, 1996, pp. 261–271.
7. Knight W, Livingston R, Gregory E, McGuire W. Estrogen receptor as an independent prognostic factor for early recurrence in breast cancer. Cancer Res 1977;37:4669–4671.
8. Adami H, Graffman S, Lindgren A, Sallstrom J. Prognostic implication of estrogen receptor content in breast cancer. Breast Cancer Res Treat 1985;5:293–300.
9. Clark G, Osborne C, McGuire W. Correlations between estrogen receptor, progesterone receptor, and patient characteristics in human breast cancer. J Clin Oncol 1984;2:1102–1109.
10. Foekens J, Portengen H, Putten WV Peters H, Krijnen H, Alexieva-Figusch J, Klijn J. Prognostic value of estrogen and progesterone receptors measured by enzyme immunoassays in human breast tumor cytosols. Cancer Res 1989;49:5823–5828.

11. Clark G. Prognostic and predictive factors. In: Harris J, Lippman M, Morrow M, Hellman S, eds. Diseases of the Breast. Lippincott-Raven, Philadelphia, 1996, pp. 461–485.
12. Clark G, McGuire W. Steroid receptors and other prognostic factors in primary breast cancer. Semin Oncol 1988;15:20–25.
13. Kuiper G, Enmark E, Pelto-Huikko M, Nilsson S, Gustafsson J-A. Cloning of a novel estrogen receptor expressed in rat prostate and ovary. Proc Natl Acad Sci USA 1996;93:5925–5930.
14. Mosselman S, Polman J, Dijkema R. ERβ: identification and characterization of a novel human estrogen receptor. FEBS 1996;392:49–53.
15. Tremblay G, Tremblay A, Copeland N, Gilbert D, Jenkins N, Labrie F, Giguere V. Cloning, chromosomal localization, and functional analysis of the murine estrogen receptor beta. Mol Endocrinol 1997; 11:353–365.
16. Ogawa S, Inoue S, Watanabe T, Hiroi H, Orimo A, Hosoi T, Ouchi Y, Muramatsu M. The complete primary structure of human estrogen receptor β (hERβ) and its heterodimerization with ER α in vivo and in vitro. Biochem Biophys Res Commun 1998;243:122–126.
17. Kuiper G, Gustafsson J-A. The novel estrogen receptor-β subtype: potential role in the cell- and promoter-specific actions of estrogens and anti-estrogens. FEBS Lett 1997;410:87–90.
18. Dotzlaw H, Leygue E, Watson P, Murphy L. Expression of estrogen receptor-beta in human breast tumors. J Clin Endocrinol Metab 1996;82:2371–2374.
19. Enmark E, Pelto-Huikko M, Grandien K, Lagercrantz S, Lagercrantz J, Fried G, Nordenskjold M, Gustafsson J. Human estrogen receptor beta-gene structure, chromosomal localization, and expression pattern. J Clin Endorcrinol Metab 1997;82:4258–4265.
20. Lu B, Leygue E, Dotzlaw H, Murphy L, Murphy L, Watson P. Estrogen receptor-β mRna variants in human and murine tissues. Mol Cell Endocrinol 1998;138:199–203.
21. Leygue E, Dotzlaw H, Watson P, Murphy L. Altered estrogen receptor α and β messenger RNA expression during human breast tumorigenesis. Cancer Res 1998;58:3197–3201.
22. Brandenberger A, Tee M, Jaffe R. Estrogen receptor alpha (ER-alpha) and beta (ER-beta) mRNAs in normal ovary, ovarian serous cystadenocarcinoma and ovarian cancer cell lines: down-regulation of ER-beta in neoplastic tissues. J Clin Endocrinol Metab 1998;83:1025–1028.
23. Watanabe T, Inoue S, Ogawa S, Ishii Y, Hiroi H, Ikeda K, Orimo A, Muramatsu M. Agnostic effect of tamoxifen is dependent on cell type, ERE-promoter context, and estrogen receptor subtype: functional difference between estrogen receptors alpha and beta. Biochem Biophys Res Commun 1997; 236:140–145.
24. Paech K, Webb P, Kuiper G, Nilsson S, Gustafsson J-A, Kushner P, Scanlan T. Differential ligand activation of estrogen receptors ERα and ERβ at AP1 sites. Science 1997;277:1508–1510.
25. Shibata H, Spencer T, Onate S, Jenster G, Tsai S, Tsai M, O'Malley B. Role of co-activators and co-repressors in the mechanism of steroid/thyroid receptor action. Recent Prog Horm Res 1997;52: 141–164.
26. Dupont WD, Page DL. Risk factors for breast cancer in women with proliferative breast disease. N Engl J Med 1985;312:146–151.
27. Dupont WD, Parl FF, Hartmann WH, Brinton LA, Winfield AC, Worrel JA, Schuyler AP, Plummer WD. Breast cancer risk associated with proliferative breast disease and atypical hyperplasia. Cancer 1993;71:1258–1265.
28. Morrow M, Schnitt S, Harris F. In situ carcinomas. In: Harris J, Lippman M, Morrow M, Hellman S, eds. Diseases of the Breast. Lippincott-Raven, Philadelphia, 1996, pp. 355–376.
29. Rosenberg CL, Larson PS, Romo JD, De Las Morenas A, Faller DV. Microsatellite alterations indicating monoclonality in atypical hyperplasias associated with breast cancer. Human Pathol 1997;28: 214–219.
30. O'Connell P, Pekkel V, Fuqua S, Osborne CK, Allred DC. Molecular genetic studies of early breast cancer evolution. Breast Cancer Res Treat 1994;32:5–12.
31. O'Connell P, Pekkel V, Fuqua SAW, Osborne CK, Allred DC. Analysis of loss of heterozygosity in 399 premalignant breast lesions at 15 genetic loci. J Natl Cancer Inst 1998;90:697–703.
32. Lakhani SR, Slack DN, Hamoudi RA, Collins N, Stratton MR, Sloane JP. Detection of allelic imbalance indicates that a proportion of mammary hyperplasia of usual type are clonal neoplastic proliferations. Lab Invest 1996;74:129–135.
33. Ricketts D, Turnbull L, Tyall G, Bakhshi R, Rawson NSB, Gazet JC, Nolan C, Coombes RC. Estrogen and progesterone receptors in the normal female breast. Cancer Res 1991;51:1817–1822.

34. Peterson OW, Hoyer PE, van Deurs B. Frequency and distribution of estrogen receptor-positive cells in normal, nonlactating human breast tissue. J Natl Cancer Inst 1986;77:343–349.
35. Allegra JC, Lippman ME, Green L, Barlock A, Simon R, Thompson EB, Hugg KK, Griffin W. Estrogen receptor values in patients with benign breast disease. Cancer 1979;44:228–231.
36. Battersby S, Robertson BJ, Anderson TJ, King RJB, McPherson K. Influence of menstrual cycle, parity, and oral contraceptive use on steroid hormone receptors in normal breast. Br J Cancer 1992;65: 601–607.
37. Markopoulos C, Berder U, Wilson P, Gazet JC, Coombes RC. Oestrogen receptor content of normal breast cells and breast carcinoma throughout the menstrual cycle. Br Med J 1988;296:1149–1351.
38. Giri DD, Dundas AC, Nottingham JF, Underwood JCE. Oestrogen receptors in benign epithelial lesions and intraduct carcinomas of the breast: an immunohistological study. Histopathology 1989;15: 575–584.
39. Karayiannakis AJ, Bastounis EA, Chatzigianni EB, Makri GG, Alexiou D, Karamanakos P. Immuno-histochemical detection of oestrogen receptors in ductal carcinoma in situ of the breast. Eur J Surg Oncol 1996;22:578–582.
40. Zafrani B, Leroyer A, Fourquet A, Laurent M, Torphilme D, Validire P, Sastre-Garau A. Mammo-graphically detected ductal in situ carcinoma of the breast analyzed with a new classification. A study of 127 cases: correlation with estrogen and progesterone receptors, p53, and c-erbB-2 proteins, and proliferative activity. Semin Diagn Pathol 1994;11:208–214.
41. Burr M, Zimarowski M, Schnitt S, Baker S, Lew R. Estrogen receptor immunohistochemistry in carcinoma in situ of the breast. Cancer 1992;69:1174–1181.
42. Khan S, Rogers M, Khurana K, Meguid M, Numann P. Estrogen receptor expression in benign breast epithelium and breast cancer risk. J Natl Cancer Inst 1998;90:37–42.
43. Khan S, Rogers M, Obando J, Tamsen A. Estrogen receptor expression of benign breast epithelium and its association with breast cancer. Cancer Res 1994;54:993–997.
44. Dickson R, Lippman M. Oncogenes and suppressor genes. In: Harris J, Lippman M, Morrow M, Hellman S, eds. Diseases of the Breast. Lippincott-Raven, Philadelphia, 1996, pp. 221–234.
45. Allred D, Harvey J, Berardo M, Clark G. Prognostic and predictive factors in breast cancer by immuno-histochemical analysis. Mod Pathol 1998;11:155–168.
46. Mansour O, Zekri A, Harvey J, Teramoto Y, el-Ahmady O. Tissue and serum c-erbB-2 and tissue EGFR in breast carcinoma: three years follow-up. Anticancer Res 1997;17:3101–3106.
47. Johannsson O, Idvall I, Anderson C, Borg A, Barkardottir R, Egilsson V, Olsson H. Tumour biological features of BRCA1-induced breast and ovarian cancer. Eur J Cancer 1997;33:362–371.
48. Consortium BCL. Pathology of familial breast cancer: differences between breast cancers in carriers of BRCA1 or BRCA2 mutations and sporadic cases. Breast Cancer Linkage Consortium. Lancet 1997; 349:1505–1510.
49. Eiseinger F, Jacquemier J, Charpin C, Stoppa-Lyonnet D, Paillerets BB.-d, Peyrat J, et al. Mutations at BRCA1: the medullary breast carcinoma revisited. Cancer Res 1998;58:1588–92.
50. Sourvinos G, Spandidos D. Decreased BRCA1 expression levels may arrest the cell cycle through activation of p53 checkpoint in human sporadic breast tumors. Biochem Biophys Res Commun 1998; 245:75–80.
51. Rhei E, Bogomolniy F, Federici M, Maresco D, Offit K, Robson M, Saigo P, Boyd J. Molecular gene-tic characterization of BRCA1- and BRCA2-linked hereditary ovarian cancers. Cancer Res 1998;58: 3193–3196.
52. Henderson B, Bernstein L. Endogenous and exogenous hormonal factrors. In: Harris J, Lippman M, Morrow M, Hellman S, eds. Diseases of the Breast. Lippincott-Raven, Philadelphia, 1996, pp. 185–200.
53. Henderson B, Ross R, Judd H, Krailo M, Pike M. Do regular ovulatory cycles increase breast cancer risk? Cancer 1985;56:1206–1208.
54. Henderson B, Gerkins V, Rosario I, Casagrande J, Pike M. Elevated serum levels of estrogen and prolactin in daughters of patients with breast cancer. N Engl J Med 1975;293:790–795.
55. Trichopoulus D, Brown J, Garas J, Papaioannou A, MacMahon B. Elevated urine estrogen and preg-nanediol levels in daughters of breast cancer patients. J Natl Cancer Inst 1981;67:603–606.
56. MacMahon B, Trichopoulos D, Brown J, Andersen A, Aoki K, Cole P, et al. Age at menarche, prob-ability of ovulation and breast cancer risk. Int J Cancer 1982;29:13–16.
57. Trichopoulos D, MacMahon B, Cole P. Menopause and breast cancer risk. J Natl Cancer Inst 1972;48: 605–613.

58. Henderson B, Ross R, Pike M, Casagrande J. Endogenous hormones as a major factor in human cancer. Cancer Res 1982;42:3232–3239.
59. DeWaard F, Cornelis J, Aoki K, Yoshida M. Breast cancer incidence according to weight and height in two cities of the Netherlands and in Aichi prefecture, Japan. Cancer 1977;40:1269–1275.
60. Hunter D, Willet W. Nutrition and breast cancer. Cancer Causes Control 1996;7:56–68.
61. Steinberg K, Thacker S, Smith S, Stroup D, Zack M, Flanders W, Berkelman R. A meta-analysis of the effect of estrogen replacement therapy on the risk of breast cancer. JAMA 1991;265:1985–1990.
62. Sillero-Arenas M, Delgado-Rodriguez M, Rodigues-Canteras R, Bueno-Cavanillas A, Galvez-Vargas R. Menopausal hormone replacement therapy and breast cancer: a meta-analysis. Obstet Gynecol 1992;79:286–294.
63. Collaborative Group on Hormonal Factors in Breast Cancer, I.C.E.U., Radcliffe Infirmary, Oxford, UK. Breast cancer and hormonal contraceptives: collaborative reanalysis of individual data on 53 297 women with breast cancer and 100 239 women without breast cancer from 54 epidemiological studies. Lancet 1996;347:1713–1727.
64. Yuan J, Yu M, Ross R, Gao Y, Henderson B. Risk factors for breast cancer in Chinese women in Shanghai. Cancer Res 1988;48:1949–1953.
65. Enger S, Ross R, Henderson B, Bernstein L. Breastfeeding history, pregnancy experience and risk of breast cancer. Br J Cancer 1997;76:118–123.
66. Newcomb P, Storer B, Longnecker M, Mittendorf R, Greenberg E, Clapp R, et al. Lactation and a reduced risk of premenopausal breast cancer. N Engl J Med 1994;330:81–87.
67. Bernstein L, Ross R, Lobo R, Hanisch R, Krailo M, Henderson B. The effects of moderate physical activity on mentrual cycle patterns in adolescence: implications for breast cancer prevention. Br J Cancer 1987;55:681–685.
68. Bernstein L, Henderson B, Hanisch R, Sullivan-Halley J, Ross R. Physical exercise and reduced risk of breast cancer in young women. J Natl Cancer Inst 1994;86:1403–1408.
69. Parazzini F, Braga C, Vecchia CL, Negri E, Acerboni S, Franceschi S. Hysterectomy, oophorectomy in premenopause, and risk of breast cancer. Obstet Gynecol 1997;90:453–456.
70. Schairer C, Persson I, Falkeborn M, Naessen T, Troisi R, Brinton L. Breast cancer risk associated with gynecologic surgery and indications for such surgery. Int J Cancer 1997;70:150–154.
71. Kuukasjarvi T, Kononen J, Helin H, Holli IG, Isola J. Loss of estrogen receptor in recurrent breast cancer is associated with poor response to endocrine therapy. J Clin Oncol 1996;14:2584–2589.
72. Holdaway I, Bowditch F, Bowditch J. Variation in receptor status between primary and metastatic breast cancer. Cancer 1983;52:479–485.
73. Osborne C. Heterogeneity in hormone receptor status in primary and metastatic breast cancer. Semin Oncol 1985;12:317–326.
74. Hull D, Clark G, Osborne C, Chamness G, Knight W, McGuire W. Multiple estrogen receptor assays in human breast cancer. Cancer Res 1983;43:413–416.
75. Encarnacion C, Ciocca D, McGuire W, Clark G, Fuqua S, Osborne C. Measurement of steroid hormone receptors in breast cancer patients on tamoxifen. Breast Cancer Res Treat 1993;26:237–246.
76. Zhang Q, Borg A, Wolf D, Oesterreich S, Fuqua S. Estrogen receptor mutant with strong hormone-independent activity from a metastatic breast cancer. Cancer Res 1997;57:1244–1249.
77. Zhang Q, Hilsenbeck S, Fuqua S, Borg A. Multiple splicing variants of the estrogen receptor are present in individual human breast tumors. J Steroid Biochem Mol Biol 1996;59:251–260.
78. Murphy L, Leygue E, Dotzlaw H, Douglas D, Coutts A, Watson P. Oestrogen receptor variants and mutations in human breast cancer. Ann Med 1997;29:221–234.
79. McGuire W, Chamness G, Fuqua S. Estrogen receptor variants in clinical breast cancer. Mol Endocrinol 1991;5:1571–1577.
80. Moore J, McKee D, Slentz-Kesler K, Moore L, Jones S, Horne E, et al. Cloning and characterization of human estrogen receptor beta isoforms. Biochem Biophys Res Commun 1998;247:75–78.
81. Ogawa S, Inoue S, Watanabe T, Orimo A, Hosoi T, Ouchi Y, Muramatsu M. Molecular cloning and characterization of human estrogen receptor bcx: a potential inhibitor of estrogen action in humans. Nucleic Acids Res 1998;26:3505–3512.
82. Vladusic E, Hornby A, Guerra-Vladusic F, Lupu R. Expression of estrogen receptor beta messenger RNA variant in breast cancer. Cancer Res 1998;58:210–214.
83. Lu B, Leygue E, Dotzlaw H, Murphy L, Murphy L, Watson P. Estrogen receptor-beta mRNA variants in human and murine tissues. Mol Cell Endocrinol 1998;138:199–203.

84. Elledge R, Green S, Ciocca D, Pugh R, Allred D, Clark G, et al. HER-2 expression and response to tamoxifen in estrogen receptor-positive breast cancer: a Southwest Oncology Group Study. Clin Cancer Res 1998;4:7–12.

85. Allred D, Clark G, Molina R, Tandon A, Schnitt S, Gilchrist K, et al. Overexpression of HER-2/neu and its relationship with other prognostic factors change during the progression of in situ to invasive breast cancer. Hum Pathol 1992;23:974–979.

86. Carlomagno C, Perrone F, Gallo C, Laurentiis MD, Lauria R, Morabito A, et al. c-erb B2 over-expression decreases the benefit of adjuvant tamoxifen in early-stage breast cancer without axillary lymph node metastases. J Clin Oncol 1996;14:2702–2708.

87. Schroeder W, Biesterfeld S, Zillessen S, Rath W. Epidermal growth factor receptor-immunohistochemical detection and clinical significance for treatment of primary breast cancer. Anticancer Res 1997;17:2799–2802.

88. Zeillinger R, Kury F, Czerwenka K, Kubista E, Sliutz G, Knogler W, et al. HER-2 amplification, steroid receptors and epidermal growth factor receptor in primary breast cancer. Oncogene 1989;4:109–114.

89. Adnane J, Gaudray P, Simon M, Simony-Lafontaine J, Jeanteur P, Theillet C. Proto-oncogene amplification and human breast tumor phenotype. Oncogene 1989;4:1389–1395.

90. Harris A, Nicholson S, Sainsbury R, Wright C, Farndon J. Epidermal growth factor receptor and other oncogenes as prognostic markers. J Natl Cancer Inst Monogr 1992;11:181–187.

91. Eppenberger U, Kueng W, Schlaeppi J, Roesel J, Benz C, Mueller H, et al. Markers of tumor angiogenesis and proteolysis independently define high- low-risk subsets of node-negative breast cancer patients. J Clin Oncol 1998;16:3129–3136.

92. Yiangou C, Gomm J, Coope R, Law M, Luqmani Y, Shousha S, Coombes R, Johnston C. Fibroblast growth factor 2 in breast cancer: occurrence and prognostic significance. Br J Cancer 1997;75:28–33.

93. Miller D, El-Ashry D, Cheville A, Liu Y, McLeskey S, Kern F. Emergence of MCF7 cells overexpressing a transfected epidermal growth factor receptor (EGFR) under estrogen-depleted conditions: evidence for a role of EGFR in breast cancer growth and progression. Cell Growth Differ 1994;5:1263–1274.

94. Liu Y, El-Ashry D, Chen D, Ding I, Kern F. MCF7 breast cancer cells overexpressing transfected c-erbB2 have an in vitro growth advantage in estrogen-depleted conditions and reduced estrogen-dependence and tamoxifen-sensitivity in vivo. Breast Cancer Res Treat 1995;34:97–117.

95. Benz C, Scott G, Sarup J, Johnson R, Tripathy D, Coronado E, Shepard H, Osborne C. Estrogen-dependent, tamoxifen-resistant tumorigenic growth of MCF-7 cells transfected with HER2/neu. Breast Cancer Res Treat 1993;24:85–95.

96. El-Ashry D, Miller D, Kharbanda S, Lippman M, Kern F. Constitutive Raf-1 kinase activity in breast cancer cells induces both estrogen-independent growth and apoptosis. Oncogene 1997;15:423–435.

97. Wise S, Smith L, Hendricks D, Sabichi A, Bober M, Brown P, Birrer M. Over-expression of the cJun oncoprotein in the human breast cancer cell line MCF-7 results in tamoxifen resistance and increased invasiveness. Proc Am Assoc Cancer Res 1997;38:173.

98. Fairchild C, Ivy S, Kao-Shan C, Whang-Peng J, Rosen N, Israel M, et al. Isolation of amplified and overexpressed DNA sequences from adriamycin-resistant human breast cancer cells. Cancer Res 1987;47:5141–5148.

99. Vickers P, Dickson R, Shoemaker R, Cowan K. A multidrug-resistant MCF-7 human breast cancer cell line which exhibits cross-resistance to antiestrogens and hormone-independent tumor growth in vivo. Mol Endocrinol 1988;2:886–892.

100. Reddel R, Alexander I, Koga M, Shine J, Sutherland R. Genetic instability and the development of steroid hormone insensitivity in cultured T 47D human breast cancer cells. Cancer Res 1988;48:4340–4347.

101. Graham M, Smith J, Jewett P, Horwitz K. Heterogeneity of progesterone receptor content and remodeling by tamoxifen characterize subpopulations of cultured human breast cancer cells: analysis by quantitative dual parameter flow cytometry. Cancer Res 1992;52:593–602.

102. Sartorius C, Groshong S, Miller L, Powell R, Tung L, Takimoto G, Horwitz K. New T47D breast cancer cell lines for the independent study of progesterone B- and A-receptors: only antiprogestin-occupied B-receptors are switched to transcriptional agonists by cAMP[1]. Cancer Res 1994;54:3868–3877.

103. Graham M, Dalquist K, Horwitz K. Simultaneous measurement of progesterone receptors and DNA indices by flow cytometry: analysis of breast cancer cell mixtures and genetic instability of the T47D line. Cancer Res 1989;49:3943–3949.

104. Horwitz K, Mockus M, Lessey B. Variant T47D human breast cancer cells with high progesterone-receptor levels despite estrogen and antiestrogen resistance. Cell 1982;28:633–642.

105. Murphy C, Pink J, Jordan V. Characterization of a receptor-negative hormone-nonresponsive clone derived from a T47D human breast cancer cell line kept under estrogen-free conditions. Cancer Res 1990;50:7285–7292.

106. Nasca P, Liu S, Baptiste M, Kwon C, Jacobson H, Metzger B. Alcohol consumption and breast cancer: estrogen receptor status and histology. Am J Epidemiol 1994;140:980–988.

107. Reichman M, Judd J, Longcope C, Schatzkin A, Clevidence B, Nair P, Campbell W, Taylor P. Effects of alcohol consumption on plasma and urinary hormone concentrations in premenopausal women. J Natl Cancer Inst 1993;85:722–727.

108. Johnston SR, Saccani-Jotti G, Smith I, Salter J, Newby J, Coppen M, Ebbs S, Dowsett M. Changes in estrogen receptor, progesterone receptor, and pS2 expression in tamoxifen-resistant human breast cancer. Cancer Res 1995;55:3331–3338.

109. Raemaekers J, Beex L, Koenders A, Pieters G, Smals A, Benraad T, Kloppenborg P. Concordance and discordance of estrogen and progesterone receptor content in sequential biopsies of patients with advanced breast cancer: relation to survival. Eur J Cancer Clin Oncol 1984;20:1011–1018.

110. Tilley W, Keightley D, Cant E. Inter-site variation of oestrogen receptors in human breast cancers. Br J Cancer 1978;38:544–546.

111. Davis B, Zava D, Locher G, Goldhirsch A, Hartmann W. Receptor heterogeneity of human breast cancer as measured by multiple intratumoral assays of estrogen and progesterone receptor. Eur J Cancer Clin Oncol 1984;20:375–382.

112. Allegra J, Barlock A, Huff K, Lippman M. Changes in multiple or sequential estrogen receptor determinations in breast cancer. Cancer 1980;45:792–794.

113. Welshons W, Jordan V. Adaptation of estrogen-dependent MCF-7 cells to low estrogen (phenol red-free) culture. Eur J Cancer Clin Oncol 1987;23:1935–1939.

114. Herman M, Katzenellenbogen B. Response-specific antiestrogen resistance in a newly characterized MCF-7 human breast cancer cell line resulting from long-term exposure to transhydroxytamoxifen. J Steroid Biochem Mol Biol 1996;59:121–134.

115. Katzenellenbogen B, Kendra K, Norman M, Berthois Y. Proliferation hormonal responsiveness and estrogen receptor content of MCF-7 human breast cancer cells grown in the short-term and long-term absence of estrogens. Cancer Res 1987;47:4355–4360.

116. Fisher B, Costantino JP, Wickerham DL, Redmond CK, Kavanah M, Cronin WM, et al. Tamoxifen for prevention of breast cancer: report of the National Surgical Adjuvant Breast and Bowel Project P-1 study. J Natl Cancer Inst 1998;90:1371–1388.

117. Powles T, Eeles R, Ashley S, Easton D, Chang J, Dowsett M, et al. Interim analysis of the incidence of breast cancer in the Royal Marsden Hospital tamoxifen randomised chemoprevention trial. Lancet 1998;352:98–101.

118. Veronesi U, Maisonneuve P, Costa A, Sacchini V, Maltoni C, Roberson C, Rotmensz N, Boyle P. Prevention of breast cancer with tamoxifen: preliminary findings from the Italian randomised trial among hysterectomised women. Lancet 1998;352:93–97.

119. Delmas P, Bjarnason H, Mitlak B, Ravoux A, Shah A, Huster W, Draper M, Christiansen C. Effects of raloxifene on bone mineral density, serum cholesterol concentrations, and uterine endometrium in postmenopausal women. N Engl J Med 1997;337:1641–1647.

120. Gail M, Benichou J. Validation studies on a model for breast cancer risk. J Natl Cancer Inst 1994; 86:573–575.

121. Cummings S, Norton L, Eckert S, Grady D, Cauley J, Knickerbocker R, et al. Raloxifene reduces the risk of breast cancer and may decrease the risk of endometrial cancer in postmenopausal women. Two-year findings from the Multiple Outcomes of Raloxifene Evaluation trial. Proc Am Soc Clin Oncol 1998;17:2a.

5

Regulation of EGFR and *ERBB2* Expression by Estrogen Receptor in Breast Cancer

Helen C. Hurst, PHD

CONTENTS

INTRODUCTION

The epidermal growth factor receptor (EGFR/*ERBB1*) and the *ERBB2* (*HER2/neu*) genes are both members of the type I family of growth factor receptors, and encode transmembrane receptor tyrosine kinase proteins expressed on the epithelia of a number of tissues during mammalian embryogenesis. Thus, these proteins play key roles during development as demonstrated by the lack of viability of mice homologously deleted for either gene *(1,2)*. However, expression of these genes in most adult tissues is much less marked, with the significant exception of certain solid tumors. The potential import of these findings lies in the fact that both genes can act as oncogenes in a variety of in vitro and in vivo assays *(3,4)*. There is therefore a large literature documenting the incidence of overexpression of these proteins in a range of human carcinomas, including those from endocrine and nonendocrine tissues. For completeness, summarized below are the key features of expression of these genes in the normal breast and during tumorigenesis which are relevant to this chapter.

EXPRESSION IN NORMAL AND BREAST TUMOR TISSUE

Epidermal Growth Factor Receptor

Studies in mice have shown that, in adult mammals, marked expression of EGFR is confined to the mammary gland of pregnant animals. Expression peaks during the

From: *Contemporary Endocrinology: Endocrine Oncology*
Edited by: S. P. Ethier © Humana Press Inc., Totowa, NJ

Table 1
Relative Levels of ER, EGFR,
and *ERBB2* in Breast Tumor-Derived Cell Lines

Cell Line	ER	EGFR	ERBB2
MCF7	+++	+/−	−
T47D	++	+/−	+/−
ZR 75-1	+	+/−	+
BT474	+/−	+	+++[a]
SKBR3	−	+	+++[a]
BT-20	−	++	−
MDA-MB231	−	++	−
MDA-MB468	−	+++[a]	−
MDA-MB453	−	-	++

[a]Overexpression associated with gene amplification.
Data compiled from references *12*, *13*, and *15*.

proliferative phase and declines later in pregnancy and during lactation *(5)*. In humans, EGFR is expressed at variable levels in lobular, ductal, stromal, and myoepithelial cells of the normal breast, and is infrequently overexpressed in mammary carcinoma, in which it is associated with a poor clinical response *(3)*. Tumor expression of EGFR is also generally associated with a loss of the estrogen receptor (ER) *(6)*. However, co-expression of these two receptors can be observed both in tumor samples and derived cell lines, although a clear inverse linear relationship between levels of expression clearly exists (Table 1). Amplification of the EGFR gene is only observed sporadically in about 2% of breast carcinomas *(7)*, and, consequently, most deregulation of expression levels is thought to occur at the level of transcription.

ERBB2

Studies on the rodent homolog, *neu*, indicate that this gene is expressed in complex patterns at all stages of mammary differentiation *(8)*. Overexpression of *ERBB2* is found in 20–30% of human carcinomas, and this is frequently accompanied by a moderate (up to 8–10 copies) amplification of the gene *(4)*. Because this is easily sampled in clinical tissue, this feature of *ERBB2* overexpression is the most frequently documented. However, overexpression can also occur from a single copy gene, and, whether or not the gene is amplified, the transcriptional activity of *ERBB2* is increased about fivefold in cells with the overexpressing phenotype. This applies both to clinical specimens *(9–11)* and tumor-derived cell lines *(12–14)*. Tumor expression of this gene is again associated with a poor clinical outcome and resistance to chemo- and endocrine therapy *(4)*. The latter observation has also been associated with a loss of ER expression in *ERBB2*-positive tumors and cell lines (Table 1).

Expression studies have therefore shown that there is often an inverse relationship between ER status and tumor expression of either EGFR or *ERBB2*, suggesting that estrogens act to repress transcription of these two genes. Because their expression is also associated with poor prognosis, the interest in taking these studies further lies in whether understanding the mechanistic details can lead to improved patient care. Experimentally, the majority of hard data about how estrogens may regulate the expression of these two genes has come from studies in breast-tumor-derived cell lines, but clearly the biological relevance of these observations can only come from clinical data. The in vitro and in vivo information currently available is reviewed below, and these observations are brought together in a final discussion.

REGULATION OF EGFR AND *ERBB2* BY ER IN CELL LINES

EGFR

It has proven difficult to establish that the estrogen-bound ER can directly repress expression from the EGFR gene. Indeed, the majority of studies have shown the opposite effect. Thus, in three ER-positive cell lines, addition of estradiol (E$_2$) following several days of estrogen withdrawal, led to a transient 2–3-fold induction of EGFR mRNA and protein levels *(16)*. This effect was abolished in the presence of antiestrogens. The rapid downregulation of EGFR mRNA levels following stimulation indicated that the ER may induce factor(s) to limit EGFR expression in these cells. Although the authors noted imperfect ER DNA-binding sites within the 5' flanking regions of the EGFR gene, these are highly speculative. Indeed, other data from the same group provide stronger evidence that the real determinants of estrogen regulation of EGFR may lie elsewhere. By examining the chromatin structure around the EGFR gene in a number of breast tumor lines, using the DNase I hypersensitive site assay, Chrysogelos *(15)* made a number of interesting findings. First, ER-positive lines with low levels of EGFR exhibited a strong hypersensitive site at the exon 1–intron 1 boundary, which may indicate the binding of an ER-inducible repressor that blocks EGFR transcription. In other lines with the reverse phenotype (high EGFR, low ER), additional hypersensitive sites were mapped within the first intron, which may indicate the presence of positively acting enhancers that are not active in ER positive lines. Unfortunately, none of these potentially interesting observations has so far been investigated further. Parallel studies, in which ER has been transfected into EGFR-positive lines, have also failed to demonstrate conclusively that the ER alone can act to repress EGFR expression with the overexpressing phenotype in cell lines *(17)*.

ERBB2

In contrast to the cell line studies on EGFR, it has been relatively straightforward to demonstrate estrogen repression of *ERBB2* expression. Two groups first showed that culturing ER-positive breast tumor lines with 1–10 nM E$_2$ led to progressive loss of *ERBB2* mRNA and protein (about fourfold over 48 h), and this was reversed on withdrawal of estrogen or addition of antiestrogens *(18,19)*. Furthermore, similar results could also be replicated in mouse xenografts *(20)* and lines with amplified copies of the *ERBB2* gene *(21,22)*. Because ER-positive cells tend to arrest their growth and differentiate in the absence of estrogen, it was also shown, using other growth modulalory molecules, that the effect of E$_2$ on *ERBB2* levels was specific and not directly related to the growth status of the cells *(23)*.

These cell line studies have now been extended to examine if the effect of estrogen is at the level of gene transcription, and what the mechanism may be. Nuclear run experiments have shown that ER-positive cell lines exhibit a 3–4-fold reduced level of *ERBB2* transcription when grown in E$_2$, compared to when steroid is withdrawn or antiestrogens are added to the culture medium *(24,25)*. This level of effect closely mirrors the change in expression monitored by Northern blots, and indicates that the majority of the effect of estrogens is indeed at the level of transcription. However, it is more difficult to

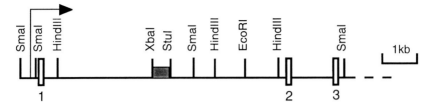

Fig. 1. The diagram shows the 5' end (first 3 exons, numbered) of the *ERBB2* gene, with an arrow marking the major transcriptional start site. The position of the 400 bp XbaI/StuI restriction fragment within the first intron, which acts as an estrogen-repressible enhancer *(25)*, is indicated with a grey box.

establish whether this is a direct transcriptional response or one requiring the synthesis of an intermediate factor, i.e., perhaps a labile repressor encoded by a gene stimulated by the estrogen-bound ER. Cycloheximide blockade of protein synthesis certainly prevented estrogen repression of *ERBB2* expression *(24)*, but this could also be explained by loss of the ER protein itself, which has a half-life of 6 h.

Transcriptional regulation of genes is most commonly found to be at the level of initiation, and further work has therefore used reporter assays and transient transfection experiments to search for elements within the *ERBB2* gene capable of mediating the response to estrogen. The author's studies have led to the conclusion that estrogen repression of *ERBB2* transcription is mediated primarily by an enhancer that maps within the first intron of the gene (Fig. 1) and overlaps a DNase I hypersensitive site found prominently only in *ERBB2*-expressing breast lines *(25)*. This enhancer was able to repress expression from a minimal (to −86) *ERBB2* proximal promoter in estrogenic conditions in ER-positive breast cells and in ER-negative cells, when co-transfected with an ER expression plasmid. Furthermore, the enhancer was also able to repress the activity of a heterologous promoter in estrogenic conditions. Consequently, three different types of transfection experiment demonstrated the importance of this intronic element for estrogen repression. In contrast, reporter constructs carrying just 5' flanking sequences (from −86 bp to −6 kbp) failed to reveal an estrogen-related element 5' of the *ERBB2* transcription start site.

These findings disagree with two other reports *(21,24)*, in which *ERBB2* promoter activity did appear to be suppressed by estrogens. It is likely, however, that this reflects differences in the experimental systems used. One study examined the rodent *neu* promoter activity in NIH-3T3 mouse fibroblasts and CV-1 monkey fibroblasts co-transfected with an ER expression plasmid *(21)*. Because the *neu* promoter is not well conserved with its human counterpart, e.g., it lacks a TATA box, this may account for the discrepancy. The use of fibroblasts, rather than breast epithelial cells, is probably also significant. The second experimental system also employed the *ERBB2* promoter and an ER-positive breast cancer cell line, but transcriptional repression by estrogens could only be shown when ER levels were raised further by co-transfection of an ER expression construct *(24)*. Those authors have more recently *(26)* localized the estrogen-responsive sequence in their experiments to the binding site for the transcription factor AP-2, which maps at −213 in the promoter, relative to the transcriptional start site *(27)*. Because estrogen repression from promoters lacking AP-2 sites can be seen providing that the intron 1 enhancer is also present, this observation is again at variance with the author's work (*see* below). In the final analysis, it is possible that both the promoter and the intronic enhancer may be required for full estrogen repression of *ERBB2* expression.

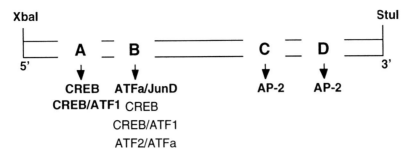

Fig. 2. Diagram of the 400 bp *Xba*I/Stu I restriction fragment from the *ERBB2* first intron, which acts as an estrogen-suppressible enhancer. The four footprinting sites, A–D, are indicated with the names of transcription factors that bind at the various sites, listed below each one in bold. Factors that bind weakly to FPB are also listed *(40)*.

The author's recent studies have involved in vitro and in vivo footprinting of the smallest DNA (400 bp) that retains full enhancer activity. This has allowed mapping of four (termed FPA–D) transcription factor binding sites within this region (Fig. 2), consistent with a role as a transcriptional enhancer. Mutagenesis of the individual factor binding sites has shown that three of the four sites are required for estrogen-regulated enhancer activity: two sites (FPC and D) play a minor role, and FPB appears to be the major site. FPC and D bind AP-2 proteins; FPB is related to a cAMP response element sequence and binds CREB and activating transcription factor (ATF)-1 weakly, but shows a strong interaction with a complex that is a heterodimer between ATFa and JunD. Examination of the DNA-binding activity and phosphorylation status of these factors, in extracts from cells grown in estrogenic or antiestrogenic conditions, has failed to reveal any changes that might account for the conditional activity of this enhancer. Therefore, the author has turned attention to the ER itself, and the current hypothesis is that there is competition between the ER and factors bound at the intronic enhancer for the recruitment of limiting, shared co-factors. A number of co-activators have been found to interact with the ER in a ligand-dependent manner. In estrogenic conditions, the ER might preferentially bind these co-factors, thus depleting the *ERBB2* enhancer and reducing its activity. However, addition of antiestrogen releases co-activators from the ER, and these may then be available for recruitment by the enhancer-bound proteins, thereby increasing *ERBB2* transcription levels *(40)*.

A number of cell-based studies have also addressed the wider question of whether expression of *ERBB2* in ER-positive cells alters their growth properties. Stable introduction of an *ERBB2* expression plasmid into ER-positive cells seems to result in cells that may continue to respond to E_2 *(28)*, but now fail to arrest their growth in the presence of tamoxifen (TAM) *(28,29)*. These cells therefore apparently mimic the clinical phenomenon of acquired TAM resistance, but this needs to be examined more closely using clinical material.

DOES ER REGULATE EGFR AND *ERBB2* EXPRESSION IN BREAST TUMORS?

There have been relatively few detailed clinical analyses into how ER may directly regulate either EGFR or *ERBB2* in breast cancers, and the studies that have been carried out yielded contradictory results. Thus, although highly significant ($P = 0.0032$) inverse relationships between ER and EGFR status can be documented in a series of tumor specimens *(6),* this is not corroborated in other studies. For example, when paired samples were taken from a series of patients before and after short-term (7 d) treatment with the antiestrogen ICI 182780 (100 nM), ER protein levels were found to fall ($P = 0.009$), but levels of EGFR were unaltered *(30),* when they might have been expected to rise.

There have been several clinical correlations between *ERBB2* expression and a poor response to endocrine therapy in both node-positive *(31,32)* and node-negative *(33)* disease. This has led to the idea that *ERBB2* may contribute to the phenomenon of TAM resistance. However, this is a highly controversial area, and one recent study *(34)* examining ER-positive patients only (i.e., ones more likely to respond to TAM therapy) found that, although *ERBB2* positivity was again associated with lower ER values, there was no link with a poorer response to TAM or a more aggressive clinical course. Consequently, it would be an advantage to more directly examine the effect of antiestrogen treatment on the *ERBB2* status in clinical samples. This has been attempted in two studies in which *ERBB2* levels in tumor samples from small patient groups were examined pre- and post-short-term (2–3 wk), preoperative TAM treatment. In the first of these, *ERBB2* levels were not significantly altered in the ER-positive cases, but they were unexpectedly reduced in the ER-negative tumors *(35).* The second study did find significant upregulation of *ERBB2* expression in TAM-treated, ER-positive samples, and the pattern of *ERBB2* immunoreactivity observed was consistent with the activation of a single copy gene *(36).* Obviously, the second study more closely reflects the findings in cultured cells and the conclusions from the majority of the clinical studies, but both of these reports suffer from low patient numbers and limited treatment times.

Also at issue is the nature of the phenomenon being studied. TAM resistance has two manifestations: *de novo* resistance, in which patients never respond, and acquired resistance, in which an initial response is followed by a relapse while on therapy. There is also a third scenario, in which adjuvant TAM, given postoperatively, is followed by relapse, usually at a distant site, which may reflect either *de novo* or acquired resistance. A recent study *(37)* has examined EGFR and *ERBB2* expression in patients separated into groups based on the nature of their response to TAM. Interestingly, there was a correlation between the expression of either receptor with *de novo* resistance, with the patients expressing either *ERBB2* and/or EGFR having a much poorer chance of response than double negatives ($P = 0.0039$). However, the data argued against the expression of either receptor playing a role in acquired resistance *(37).*

DISCUSSION

Many of the studies examining the relationship between the expression of these receptor kinases and the ER in breast tumors and derived cell lines have been done in an attempt to find a molecular basis for the apparent progression of breast disease. The acquired expression of growth hormone receptors could thus provide an attractive explanation for how the cells become hormone-independent for growth. However, the concept of tumor progression itself is controversial, with several observers providing persuasive arguments that ER status does not actually alter at all and tumors are either positive or negative from the outset, arising by completely separate mechanisms *(38;* Chapter 4). Given this background, it is thus not surprising that the question of whether ER can modulate EGFR and *ERBB2* expression is still unresolved.

Overall, there is perhaps more evidence, both from clinical material and cell lines, that expression of *ERBB2* is more likely than EGFR to be genuinely downregulated by the estrogen-bound ER. However, in both cases, the models being examined may be too simplistic, and thus the final interpretation of the data could be confounded. Certainly, there is evidence that EGFR may be regulated differently in ER-positive vs –negative cells *(26)*. Moreover, the expression in the same cells of potential ligands and/or dimerization partners for both receptors must also be considered. Thus, it has been shown that transcription of the *ERBB3* family member can also be downregulated by estrogens, and apparently upregulated by antiestrogen *(25)*. *ERBB3* and *ERBB2* are thought to form preferential dimerization partners in breast epithelia for the binding of their ligands, the neuregulins, and they are also known to cooperate in in vitro transformation assays *(39)*. Given their similar response to antiestrogens, it is therefore possible that tumors with dual expression of these two proteins may have a completely different prognosis and response to therapy from ones that express just one of them. However, this aspect, particularly with reference to ER status, has not been examined in clinical material, to date.

Consequently, more detailed analyses of clinical specimens, particularly of samples from patients before and after antiestrogen treatment, need to be performed. to determine if estrogens can really regulate EGFR and *ERBB2* expression. This has become a pressing issue, given the publicity that has surrounded the administration of TAM prophylatically to women with a genetic predisposition to breast cancer. If these women are to be properly counseled about the relative risks of their genetic inheritance vs the possible side effects of the long-term use of this drug, then it is vital to determine the true in vivo effect of estrogens on the expression levels of these proto-oncogenes.

REFERENCES

1. Sibilia M, Wagner EF. Strain-dependent epithelial defects in mice lacking the EGF receptor. Science 1995;269:234–238.
2. Lee KF, Simon H, Chen H, Bates B, Hung MC, Hauser C. Requirement for neuregulin receptor *ERBB2* in neural and cardiac development. Nature 1995;378:394–398.
3. Chrysogelos SA, Dickson RB. EGF receptor expression, regulation, and function in breast cancer. Breast Cancer Res Treat 1994;29:29–40.
4. Hynes NE, Stern DF. The biology of erbB2/neu/Her-2 and its role in cancer. Biochim Biophys Acta 1994;1198:165–184.
5. Edery M, Pang K, Tarson L, Colosi T, Nandi S. Epidermal growth factor receptor levels in mouse mammary glands in various physiological states. Endocrinology 1985;117:405–411.
6. Fox SB, Smith K, Hollyer J, Greenall M, Hastrich D, Harris AL. The epidermal growth factor receptor as a prognostic marker: results of 370 patients and review of 3009 patients. Breast Cancer Res Treat 1994;29:41–49.
7. Klijn JGM, Look MP, Portengen H, Alexieva-Figusch J, Vanputten WLJ, Foekens JA. The prognostic value of epidermal growth factor receptor (EGFR) in primary breasts cancer: results of a 10-year follow-up study. Breast Cancer Res Treat 1994;29:73–83.
8. Dati C, Maggiora P, Puech C, De Bortoli M, Escot C. (1996) Expression of the *ERBB2* protooncogene during differentiation of the mammary gland in the rat. Cell Tissue Res 1996;285:403–410.
9. King CR, Swain SM, Porter L, Steinberg SM, Lippman ME, Gelmann EP. Heterogeneous expression of erbB-2 messenger RNA in human-breast cancer. Cancer Res 1989;49:4185–4191.
10. Kury FD, Schneeberger C, Sliutz G, Kubista E, Salzer H, Medl M. Determination of Her-2/*neu* amplification and expression in tumor tissue and cultured cells using a simple, phenol free method for nucleic acid isolation. Oncogene 1990;5:1403–1408.
11. Parkes HC, Lillicrop K, Howell A, Craig RK. c-*erb*B-2 mRNA expression in human breast tumors: comparison with c-*erb*B-2 DNA amplification and correlation with prognosis. Br J Cancer 1990;61:39–45.

12. Kraus MH, Popescu NC, Amsbaugh C, King CR. Overexpression of the EGF receptor-related proto-oncogene *erb*B-2 in human mammary tumor lines by different molecular mechanisms. EMBO J 1987; 6:605–610.

13. Hollywood DP, Hurst HC. Novel transcription factor, OB2-1, is required for overexpression of the protooncogene c-erbB-2 in mammary tumor lines. EMBO J 1993;12:2369–2375.

14. Pasleau F, Grooteclaes M, Golwinkler R. Expression of the c-erbB2 gene in the BT474 human mammary tumor cell line: measurement of c-erbB2 messenger RNA half-life. Oncogene 1993;8:849–854.

15. Chrysogelos SA. Chromatin structure of the EGFR gene suggests a role for intron-1 sequences in its regulation in breast-cancer cells. Nucleic Acids Res 1993;21:5736–5741.

16. Yarden RI, Lauber AH, Elashry D, Chrysogelos SA. Bimodal regulation of epidermal growth factor receptor by estrogen in breast-cancer cells. Endocrinology 1996;137:2739–2747.

17. Miller DL, Elashry D, Cheville AL, Liu YL, McLeskey SW, Kern FG. Emergence of MCF7 cells overexpressing a transfected epidermal growth factor receptor (EGFR) under estrogen-depleted conditions: evidence for a role of EGFR in breast-cancer growth and progression. Cell Growth Differ 1994;5: 1263–1274.

18. Dati C, Antoniotti S, Taverna D, Perroteau I, De Bortoli, M. Inhibition of c-erbB-2 oncogene expression by estrogens in human breast-cancer cells. Oncogene 1990;5:1001–1006.

19. Read LD, Keith D, Slamon DJ, Katzenellenbogen BS. Hormonal modulation of Her-2/*neu* protoonco-gene messenger-ribonucleioc acid and p185 protein expression in human breast cancer cell lines. Cancer Res 1990;50:3947–3951.

20. Warri AM, Laine AM, Majasuo KE, Alitalo KK, Harkonen PL. Estrogen suppression of erbB2 expression is associated with increased growth rate of ZR-75-1 human breast cancer cells *in vitro* and in nude mice. Int J Cancer 1991;49:616–623.

21. Russell KS, Hung MC. Transcriptional repression of the *neu* protooncogene by estrogen stimulated estrogen-receptor. Cancer Res 1992;52:6624–6629.

22. Grunt TW, Saceda M, Martin MB, Lupu R, Dittrich E, Krupitza G, et al. Bidirectional interactions between the estrogen-receptor and the c-erbs-2 signaling pathways: heregulin inhibits estrogenic effects in breast cancer cells. Int J Cancer 1995;63:560–567.

23. Taverna D, Antoniotti S, Maggiora P, Dati C, De Bortoli M, Hynes NE. ErbB2 expression in estrogen-receptor-positive breast tumor cells is regulated by growth-modulatory reagents. Int J Cancer 1994;56: 522–528.

24. Antoniotti S, Taverna D, Maggiora P, Sapei ML, Hynes NE, De Bortoli M. Estrogen and epidermal growth factor down-regulate erbb-2 oncogene protein expression in breast cancer cells by different mechanisms. Br J Cancer 1994;70:1095–1101.

25. Bates NP, Hurst HC. An intron 1 enhancer element mediates oestrogen-induced suppression of ERBB2 expression. Oncogene 1997;15:473–481.

26. De Bortoli M, Dati C. Hormonal regulation of Type I receptor tyrosine kinase expression in the mammary gland. J Mammary Gland Biol Neoplasia 1997;2:175–185.

27. Bosher JM, Williams T, Hurst HC. (1995) The developmentally regulated transcription factor AP-2 is involved in c-erbb-2 overexpression in human mammary-carcinoma. Proc Natl Acad Sci USA 1995;92: 744–747.

28. Benz CC, Scott GK, Sarup JC, Johnson RM, Tripathy D, Coronado E, Shepard HM, Osborne CK. Estrogen-dependent, tamoxifen-resistant tumorigenic growth of MCF-7 cells transfected with Her2/*neu*. Breast Cancer Res Treat 1992;24:85–95.

29. Pietras RJ, Arboleda J, Reese DM, Wongvipat N, Pegram MD, Ramos L, et al. Her-2 tyrosine kinase pathway targets estrogen-receptor and promotes hormone-independent growth in human breast-cancer cells. Oncogene 1995;10:2435–2446.

30. McClelland RA, Gee JMW, Francis AB, Robertson JFR, Blamey RW, Wakelilng AE, Nicholson RI. Short-term effects of pure antiestrogen IC1182780 treatment on estrogen-receptor, epidermal growth-factor receptor and transforming growth-factor-alpha protein expression in human breast cancer. Eur J Cancer 1996;32A:413–416.

31. Sjogren S, Inganas M, Lindgren A, Holmberg L, Bergh J. Prognostic and predictive value of c-erbB-2 overexpression in primary breast cancer, alone and in combination with other prognostic markers. J Clin Oncol 1998;16:462–469.

32. Borg A, Baldetorp B, Ferno M, Killander D, Olsson H, Ryden S, Sigurdsson H. Erbb2 amplification is associated with tamoxifen resistance in steroid-receptor positive breast cancer. Cancer Lett 1994;81:137–144.

33. Carlomagno C, Perrone F, Gallo C, Delaurentiis M, Lauria R, Morabito A, et al. c-erbB2 overexpression decreases the benefit of adjuvant tamoxifen in early-stage breast cancer without axillary lymph-node metastases. 1996.
34. Elledge RM, Green S, Ciocca D, Pugh R, Allred DC, Clark GM, et al. Her-2 expression and response to tamoxifen in estrogen receptor-positive breast cancer: a Southwest Oncology Group study. Clin Can Res 1998;4:7–12.
35. Le Poy X, Escot C, Brouillet JP, Theillet C, Maudelonde T, Simony-Lafontaine J, Pujol H, Rochefort H. Decrease of c-erbb-2 and c-myc RNA levels in tamoxifen-treated breast-cancer. Oncogene 1991;6: 431–437.
36. Johnston SRD, MvLennan KA, Salter J, Sacks NM, McKinna JA, Baum M, Smith IE, Dowsett M. Tamoxifen induces the expression of cytoplasmic c-erbB2 immunoreaticivity in oestrogen-receptor-positive breast carcinomas in vivo. Breast 1993;2:93–99.
37. Newby JC, Johnston SRD, Smith IE, Dowsett M. Expression of epidermal growth-factor receptor and c-erbb2 during the development of tamoxifen resistance in human breast-cancer. Clin Cancer Res 1997; 3:1643–1651.
38. Robertson JFR. Oestrogen-receptor: a stable phenotype in breast cancer. Br J Cancer 1996;73:5–12.
39. Alimandi M, Romano A, Curia MC, Muraro R, Fedi P, Aaronson SA, Difiore PP, Kraus MH. Cooperative signaling of Erbb3 and Erbb2 in neoplastic transformation and human mammary carcinomas. Oncogene 1995;10:1813–1821.
40. Newman SP, Bates NP, Vernimmen D, Parker MG, Hurst HC. Cofactor competition between the ligand-bound oestrogen receptor and an intron 1 enhancer leads to oestrogen repression of ERBB2 expression in breast cancer. Oncogene 2000;19:490–497.

6

Tamoxifen and Other Antiestrogens in Prevention and Therapy of Breast Cancer

Kathy Yao, MD, and V. Craig Jordan, PHD, DSC

INTRODUCTION

In 1936, Lacassagne *(1)* suggested that, if breast cancer (BC) was caused by a special hereditary sensitivity to estrogen, then an antagonist to estrogen action could be used to prevent the disease. However, at the time, there was no antagonist to estrogen action, other than oophorectomy.

In 1962, Jensen and Jacobson *(2)* described the selective binding and retention of radiolabeled estradiol in the estrogen target tissues of the immature rat. Jensen reasoned that estrogen action required an estrogen receptor (ER) in its target tissue. The ER was subsequently isolated as a soluble protein by Gorski's group *(3,4)*, and both Jensen *(5)* and Gorski *(6)* developed subcellular models to describe how estrogen could initiate estrogen action in the nucleus of target cells. However, Jensen took the concept one step further by suggesting that the measurement of the ER in breast tumors could be used to identify hormone-responsive BCs for endocrine therapy *(7)*. This work, in the 1960s and 1970s, can now be viewed as an example of successful translational research in endocrinology *(8)*.

From: *Contemporary Endocrinology: Endocrine Oncology*
Edited by: S. P. Ethier © Humana Press Inc., Totowa, NJ

The discovery of the ER as the mechanism of estrogen action in target tissues by Jensen, and the use of ER assays to predict the hormone sensitivity of breast tumors (7), also opened the door to therapeutic opportunities. Nonsteroidal antiestrogens block estrogen action, but were initially evaluated for a variety of clinical applications. One compound, ICI 46,474, the trans isomer of a substituted triphenylethylene, was discovered during research on infertility (9,10), and was initially marketed as a profertility drug (11). ICI 46,474 blocked estrogen action in the rat uterus and vagina, and produced an effective contraceptive effect in rodents. One of the discoverers of ICI 46,474, the late Dr. Arthur Walpole at ICI Pharmaceuticals division (now Zeneca), was the head of the fertility control program, but promoted the testing of ICI 46,474 as a treatment for advanced BC (12). However, the development of the drug over the next 20 yr led to the selection of tamoxifen (TAM) (ICI 46,474) as the endocrine agent of choice for the treatment of all stages of BC.

TAM is a triumph of rational clinical testing based on successful translational research. Principles, established in the laboratory over the past 30 yr, can now be evaluated for their benefit in lives saved. Through this process, progress can be measured and new agents can be evaluated, through the same method of translational research, to predict whether an advantage can be anticipated over and above the gold standard, TAM.

TAM AS AN ANTITUMOR AGENT

TAM is the endocrine agent of choice for the treatment of all stages of BC. However, two features of the drug have set it apart from other anticancer agents. First, adjuvant TAM is the only single agent that confers a survival advantage with a minimum of side effects. Second, women who have had one BC are at increased risk for a second BC in the opposite breast, but TAM is the only agent that has been shown to decrease the incidence of contralateral BC. The process of proving the efficacy of TAM has involved numerous randomized clinical trials, with different designs (plus/minus chemotherapy) in different countries over the past twenty 20 yr. Fortunately, it is now easy to evaluate the impact of TAM as a BC therapy. All of the world's randomized clinical trials are periodically reviewed at Oxford, and the resulting reports provide clinicians with an overview analysis as a guide for the standards of patient care.

The 1998 Oxford Overview Analysis (13) involved any randomized trial that was started before 1990. The analysis included 55 trials of adjuvant TAM vs no TAM before recurrence. The study population was 37,000 women, thus comprising 87% of world evidence. Of these women, fewer than 8000 had a very low or zero level of ER, and 18,000 were classified as ER-positive. The remaining nearly 12,000 women were unknown for ER, but it is estimated that two-thirds would be ER-positive. The 10-yr analysis was therefore able to establish response rates based on receptor status, the effect of age on response, the impact of the duration of therapy on decreases in death rate, and the impact on contralateral BC. Contralateral BC incidence is a surrogate end point for the prevention of BC.

The overview shows that the proportional mortality reductions were similar for women with node-positive or -negative disease. However, the absolute reductions in mortality were much greater in node-positive than -negative disease. Additionally, patients with ER-positive disease have an increased reduction in death rate with longer duration of TAM treatment; patients who are ER-negative do not benefit from TAM, regardless of the duration of therapy.

Table 1
Comparison of Proportional Risk Reduction
of Adjuvant TAM Therapy Based on ER Status

Estrogen receptor poor	Percent reduction in recurrence rates (±SD)	Percent reduction in death rates (±SD)
Duration of TAM (yr)		
1	6 ± 8	6 ± 8
2	13 ± 5	7 ± 5
5	6 ± 11	−3 ± 11
Estrogen receptor positive		
1	21 ± 5	14 ± 5
2	28 ± 3	18 ± 4
5	50 ± 4	28 ± 5

Nearly 8000 patients are ER poor and 18,000 patients ER-positive. Adapted with permission from ref. *13*.

This clinical trial database *(13)* was also used to answer the questions raised over the past two decades by laboratory results and hypotheses. In the 1970s, three laboratory observations *(14,15)* emerged that merited evaluation in clinical trial: TAM blocks estrogen binding to the ER, so that patients with ER-positive disease would be more likely to respond than those with ER-negative disease. TAM prevents mammary cancer in rats *(13,14)*, so that the drug could reduce the incidence of primary BC; and long-term treatment was better than short-term treatment to prevent rat mammary carcinogenesis, so longer adjuvant therapy with TAM should be superior to short-term adjuvant therapy *(15–17)*, i.e., 5 yr of TAM should be superior to 1 yr of TAM. In summary, the Overview Analysis provides compelling clinical evidence for the value of TAM as a therapeutic agent.

ER STATUS AND DURATION OF TAM

The ER status of a patient is highly predictive of a treatment response to long-term TAM therapy. The treatment effect, based on receptor status, is is summarized in Table 1. The recurrence reductions produced by TAM in ER-positive patients are all highly significant ($2 P < 0.00001$), and the trend between them is also highly significant ($\chi^2 = 45.5$, $2 P < 0.00001$). By contrast, the therapeutic effect of TAM on ER-negative patients is minimal. Additionally, the question could be asked, does more ER give a better response to TAM? In the trials of about 5 yr of TAM, the proportional reductions of recurrence were $43 \pm 5\%$ and $60 \pm 6\%$ for patients with below or above 100 fmol/mg cystol protein. This translated to a reduction in mortality of $23 \pm 6\%$ and $36 \pm 7\%$, respectively. Clearly, one can conclude that ER is a powerful predictor of TAM response, a conclusion consistent with TAM's proven mechanism of action as an estrogen antagonist in BC *(18)*.

The Overview Analysis also provides unequivocal proof of the laboratory principle *(15–17)* that longer adjuvant TAM therapy was predicted to provide more benefit. Five yr of TAM was superior to 2 yr or 1 yr in the population of pre- and postmenopausal women, which excluded known ER-poor patients. TAM was virtually without benefit in ER poor patients (Fig. 1). The duration of TAM was critical for ER-positive women who were premenopausal. One yr of TAM was without benefit, but 5 yr of adjuvant TAM

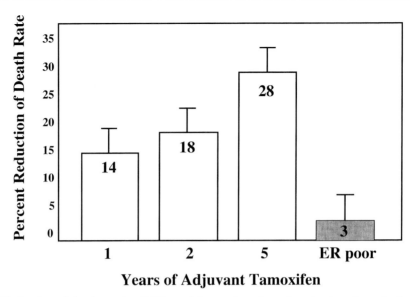

Fig. 1. Reduction of death rate in all ER-positive patients based on the duration of adjuvant TAM therapy (solid black histograms). By contrast, ER-poor patients (grey histogram) have little benefit from TAM. Adapted with permission from ref. *13*.

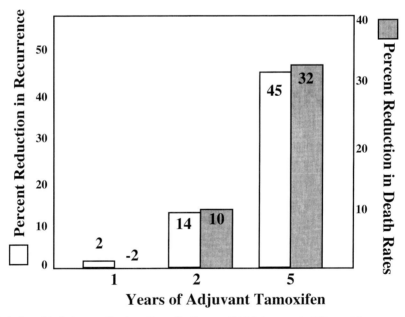

Fig. 2. Relationship between the duration of adjuvant TAM therapy in ER-positive premenopausal patients and reduction in recurrence and death rate. Longer duration has a dramatic effect on patient survival. Adapted with permission from ref. *13*.

produced the same proportional benefits in pre- and postmenopausal women. The powerful benefit of increasing the duration of TAM in premenopausal patients is illustrated in Fig. 2. It is also important to point out that the reduction of death rates in women under 50 yr of age and over 60 yr of age, treated with 5 yr of TAM, is identical, at around 33% (Table 2). By contrast, the effect of TAM duration on women over the age of 60 yr is less

Table 2
Proportional Risk Reductions
in 60–69-yr-old Women When the Known ER Poor Patients are Excluded

Duration of TAM (yr)	Percent reduction in recurrence rates (±SD)	Percent reduction in death rates (±SD)
1	26 ± 6	12 ± 6
2	33 ± 3	12 ± 6
5	54 ± 5	33 ± 6

The duration of TAM is 1, 2, or 5 yr. Adapted with permission from ref. *13*.

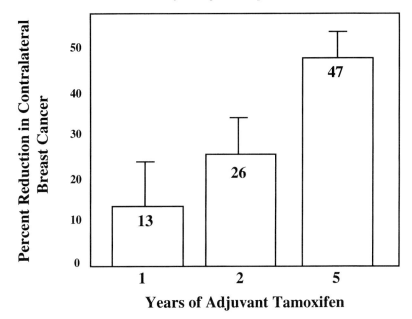

Years of Adjuvant Tamoxifen

Fig. 3. Relationship between the duration of adjuvant TAM and the reduction in contralateral BC (white histogram). Longer duration is clearly superior and 5 yr of TAM produces a 47% reduction in contralateral BC. Adapted with permission from ref. *13*.

dramatic, because 1 yr of TAM is much more effective in postmenopausal women. These data are illustrated in Table 2, which shows a 2–3-fold increase in the effectiveness of TAM by increasing the duration from 1 to 5 yr; there is a 20-fold increase in TAM's effectiveness for premenopausal women with an increased duration of 1–5 yr (Fig. 2).

CONTRALATERAL BC

TAM consistently reduced the risk of contralateral BC, independent of age, in the Overview Analysis. Moreover, extending the duration of TAM has an increasing benefit on the decreasing incidence of contralateral (new) BC. These data are illustrated in Fig. 3, and show that 1 yr of TAM produces only a 13% (SD 13) in the proportional reduction in contralateral BC, but 5 yr of TAM produces a 47% (SD 9) reduction However, the benefit of TAM is maintained until 10 yr after the diagnosis of the first BC, i.e., TAM administered as a five-yr pulse, confers long-term breast protection for the 5 yr after treatment stops. These data have important implications for the prevention BC in well women, because long-term benefit must accrue from the random application of preventive application.

Table 3
Results of the 1998 Overview Analysis

Decreased mortality in node-negative and -positive patients	Decreased contralateral BC in pre- and post-menopausal women
Decreased recurrence and mortality in ER-positive patients	• Longer TAM therapy has increasing benefit on decreasing contralateral
• No significant effect in ER-negative patients 5 yr of TAM superior to 1 or 2 yr	cancers
• Greater effect seen for premenopausal women Benefit of TAM is maintained out to 10 yr	Increased incidence of endometrial cancer

The analysis includes 55 trials of adjuvant TAM vs no TAM before recurrence. The study population was 37,000 women. Adapted with permission from ref. *13*.

Finally, the proportional reduction in contralateral BC appears to be similar in women with ER-poor tumors (29 ± 15%), compared with the rest of the study population (30 ± 6%). This is an important result for the potential application of TAM for the reduction of contralateral BC in the woman with a primary BC that is unequivocally ER-negative.

ENDOMETRIAL CANCER

The overall increase in the incidence of endometrial cancer was 2–3-fold in the Overview Analysis. There was no association with dose; however, there was a suggestion that 1 and 2 yr of TAM doubled the incidence of endometrial cancer, and 5 yr quadrupled incidence. However, the side effect is so rare (i.e., the numbers are very small) that the ratios are not significantly different from one another for each duration of TAM. It is, however, important to state that the absolute increase in endometrial cancer was only half as big as the absolute decrease in contralateral BC.

The Overview Analysis was able to identify 3673 women who took 5 yr of adjuvant TAM. With 26,400 woman-years of follow-up before BC recurrence in this group, there were seven endometrial cancer deaths. It is estimated that, during the whole first decade, the cumulative risk was 2 deaths per 1000 women. It is important to state that the current knowledge about the association of TAM with endometrial cancer will improve these statistics. In general, the reported trials were conducted without awareness of the endometrial side effects of TAM. This is no longer the situation, and early detection will improve mortality figures associated with TAM.

CONCLUSIONS

TAM has been extensively tested in clinical trials of adjuvant therapy for 20 yr. It is clear that TAM benefits the treatment of BC unlike anly other breast cancer agent, as demonstrated in the recent Overview Analysis (Table 3). The value of a long duration of treatment is most important for the premenopausal patient (Fig. 2). This latter finding is new, because the results for premenopausal women could not be ascertained with certainty in earlier overviews. The Oxford Overview Analysis has established the veracity of the laboratory concepts that TAM would be most effective in ER-positive disease, longer duration would be more beneficial, and TAM would prevent primary BC, in this case contralateral disease.

Overall, the absolute improvement in recurrence was greater during the first 5 yr following surgery, but improvement in survival increased steadily throughout the first

10 yr. There is an accumulation of the tumoristatic/tumoricidal actions of TAM for at least the first 5 yr of treatment, but the benefit continues after therapy stops. This is also true for the reduction in contralateral BC; the breast seems to be protected, so that the value remains after therapy stops. This observation is important for the application of TAM as a preventive, because a 5-yr pulse of TAM would be expected to protect a woman from BC for many years afterwards.

Finally, the risk:benefit ratio of TAM therapy can be stated to be strongly in the benefit category. The risk of endometrial cancer, a concept derived from laboratory studies *(19)*, is of concern, but the benefits clearly outweigh the risks. In contrast, early concerns about the carcinogenic effects of TAM in the rat liver do not translate to the clinic, because there is no evidence from the Overview Analysis of an increase in either liver or colorectal cancer in patients who take TAM *(13)*.

BIOLOGICAL BASIS FOR TAM AS BC PREVENTIVE

Knowledge obtained over the past 25 yr converged to make the choice of testing TAM in well women a logical extension of clinical experience. TAM was selected for testing based on animal studies that demonstrated it could prevent carcinogenesis, an extensive clinical experience that showed few serious side effects, a beneficial profile of estrogen-like action in maintaining bone density, reducing circulating cholesterol. The fact that TAM was already known to reduce the incidence of contralateral BC made the drug the primary agent to test in high-risk women.

Animal Models

TAM prevents rat mammaty carcinogenesis induced by 1,2-dimethylbenz[a]anthracene (DMBA), N-methyl-N-nitrosourea (NMU), and ionizing radiation *(16,17,20,21)*, and long-term treatment prevents spontaneous carcinogenesis in C3WOUJ mice infected with mouse mammary tumor virus (22). The latter result is of interest, because TAM is classified as an estrogen in the uterus and vagina of the mouse *(23,24)*. This again illustrates the target-site specificity of TAM.

Bones

TAM maintains bone density in the ovariectomized rat *(25,26)*, and these observations have been translated to clinical trial. Sporadic reports *(27,28)* and placebo-controlled randomized trials *(29,30)* demonstrate that TAM can increase bone density, in the lumbar spine, forearm, and neck of the femur, by 1–2%. Although the increases are modest, compared to the results obtained with estrogen use or *bis*-phosphonates (≈ 5% increase in bone density), TAM produced a significant decrease in hip and wrist fractures as a secondary end point in the BC prevention trial *(31)*.

Lipids

TAM reduces circulating cholesterol *(32,33)*. Low-density lipoprotein (LDL) cholesterol is reduced by about 15%, but high-density lipoprotein (HDL) cholesterol is maintained. It is hypothesized that the magnitude of the decrease in circulating cholesterol is a good surrogate marker for protection from coronary heart disease (CHD) and atherosclerosis. In this regard, there is evidence that woman who have been treated with 5 yr of adjuvant TAM for BC have a reduced incidence of fatal myocardial infarction *(34,35)*. Additionally, longer treatment (5 yr) appears to be superior to shorter treatment (2 yr) in reducing the number of hospital admissions for any cardiac condition *(36)*. Conversely, a large study in the United States of 5 yr or more of TAM, for the adjuvant treatment of BC, found no statistically significant evidence for the protection of women from CHD *(37)*. Nevertheless, the incidence of CHD doubled, once TAM treatment was stopped, and there was no evidence for a detrimental effect of TAM, i.e., TAM did not increase the rate of CHD in pre- or postmenopausal women.

Uterus

It is well known that TAM produces a partial agonist action in the rat uterus *(23)*, but the histology is different than the epithelial hyperplasia noted with estradiol *(38)*. A variety of endometrial changes occur in unselected populations of woman *(39)*. The most significant finding is an increase in the stromal component, rather than endometrial hyperplasia *(40,41)*. Despite the fact that TAM has been used to treat endometrial cancer, the laboratory data suggesting that TAM has the potential to encourage the growth of pre-existing disease harbored in the uterus *(19–42)* provoked an intense investigation of the rates of detection of endometrial cancer in women using adjuvant TAM treatment for BC. These data have been reviewed *(44)*, and it is clear that TAM does not cause an excess of endometrial cancer in premenopausal women, but does increase risk by 3–4-fold in postmenopausal women. This is consistent with the fact that women harbor 4–5× the level of endometrial cancer than is detected clinically *(44)*. In other words, the increase in the detection of endometrial cancer from 1/1000 women per year to 3/1000 women per year is consistent with the known rate of occult disease. The stage and grade of endometrial cancer observed in women taking TAM is the same as the general population *(45)*.

PREVENTION OF BC WITH TAM

This subheading explores progress that has been achieved in the last decade to answer the question, Does TAM have worth in the prevention of BC in high-risk women? Two studies have addressed this question: The Royal Marsden Pilot Study and the National Surgical Adjuvant Breast and Bowel Project (NSABP) Protocol P-1. Additionally, an Italian report of the efficacy of TAM in a small number of low risk women (approx 5000) has been published. A comparison of patient characteristics in each trial is outlined in Table 4.

Royal Marsden Pilot Study

Powles et al. *(46)* recruited high-risk women aged 30–70 yr to a placebo-controlled trial using 20 mg TAM daily for up to 8 yr. Women were eligible if their risk of BC was increased because of family history (involving a first-degree relative). Women with a history of benign breast biopsy and an affected first-degree relative of any age were also eligible. A total of 2494 women consented to participate in the study, and 23 were excluded from final analysis, because of the presence of pre-existing ductal carcinoma *in situ* (DCIS) or invasive breast carcinoma *(47)*. The trial was undertaken to evaluate the problems of accrual, acute symptomatic toxicity, compliance, and safety as a basis for subsequent large national, multicenter trials designed to test whether TAM can prevent BC. However, the trial has also been analyzed for BC incidence *(47)*. The stated goal of this pilot study was to act as a vanguard for a 20,000-volunteer trial throughout the UK and Australia. The national study is still ongoing, but the recruitment goal has been cut to 12,000.

Table 4
Comparison of Patient Characteristics in TAM Prevention Trials

Characteristic	NSABP	Royal Marsden	Italian
Sample size	13,388	2471	5408
Women years of follow-up	46,858	12,355	5408
Patients <50 yr old	40%	62%	36%
First degree relative with BC	40%	62%	36%
Use of HRT	0%	42%	8%
Percent of women having bilateral oophorectomy	0%	0%	48%
BC events	368	62	41
BC incidence/1000			
Placebo	6.7	5.5	2.3
TAM	3.4	4.7	2.1

Acute symptomatic toxicity was low for participants on TAM or placebo in the vangard study, and compliance remained correspondingly high: 77% of women on TAM and 82% of women on placeco remained on medication at 5 yr. There was a significant increase in hot flashes (34 vs 20%), mostly in premenopausal women ($P < 0.005$); vaginal discharge (16 vs 4%; $P < 0.005$); and menstrual irregularities (14 vs. 9%; $P < 0.005$), respectively. At the most recent followup, 320 women had discontinued TAM and 176 had discontinued placebo prior to the study's completion ($P < 0.005$).

Until their report in 1994, (48), the Marsden group observed no thromboembolic episodes; at 70 mo, no significant difference in the incidence of deep vein thrombosis or pulmonary embolism was observed between groups. A significant fall in total plasma cholesterol occurred within 3 mo, and was sustained over 5 yr of treatment (49–51). The decrease affected LDLs, with no change in HDL cholesterol.

In contrast, TAM exerted estrogenic effects on bone density, depending on menopausal status. In premenopausal women, early findings demonstrated a small but significant ($P < 0.05$) loss of bone in both the lumbar spine and hip at 3 yr (49). In contrast, postmenopausal women had increased bone mineral density in the spine ($P < 0.005$) and hip ($P < 0.001$), compared to untreated women.

Finally, the Marsden group has made an extensive study of endometrial complications associated with TAM treatment in healthy women. Because uterine assessment by transvaginal ultrasound became available sometime after the trial's start, many subjects did not have a baseline evaluation. A careful examination of the uterus with transvaginal ultrasonography, using color Doppler imaging in women taking TAM, showed that the organ was usually larger; moreover, women with sonographic abnormalities had significantly thicker endometria (52). Recent observation (41) shows that 20 mg TAM daily caused a time-dependent proliferation of the endometrium in premenopausal and early postmenopausal women. This effect appeared to be mediated by the stromal component, since no cases of cancer, or even epithelial hyperplasia, were observed among the TAM-treated group in this Italian study with 33 women (41).

Although the Marsden study has provided invaluable information about the biological effects of TAM in healthy women, the trial was not designed to answer the question of whether TAM prevents BC. Despite this, an analysis of BC incidence was reported at a median follow-up of 70 mo, when 42% of the participants had completed therapy or withdrawn *(47)*. During the study, 336 women on TAM and 305 on placebo received hormone-replacement therapy (HRT), No difference in the incidence of BC was observed between the groups. There were 34 carcinomas in the TAM group and 36 in the placebo group, for a relative risk of 0.98. Of the 70 cancers, only eight were DCIS. An analysis of the subset of women on HRT did not demonstrate an interaction with TAM treatment.

NSABP/NCI Study

This study opened in the United States and Canada in May 1992 with an accrual goal of 16,000 women to be recruited at 100 North American sites. It closed after accruing 13,338 in 1997, because of the high-risk status of the participants. Those eligible for a entry included any woman over the age of 60 yr, or women between the ages of 35 and 59 yr, whose 5-yr risk of developing BC as predicted by the Gail model *(53)*, was equal to that of a 60-yr-old woman. Additionally, any woman over age 35 yr with a diagnosis of lobular carcinoma *in situ* (LCIS) treated by biopsy alone, was eligible for entry to the study. In the absence of LCIS, the risk factors necessary to enter the study varied with age, so that a 35-yr-old woman must have had a relative risk (RR) of 5.07; the required RR for a 45-yr-old woman was 1.79. Routine endometrial biopsies to evaluate the incidence of endometrial carcinoma in both arms of the study were also performed.

The BC risk of women enrolled in the study was extremely high, with no age group having an RR of less than 4, including the over-60-yr group. Recruitment was also balanced, with about one-third younger than 50-yr, one-third between 50 and 60 yr, and one-third older than 60 yr. Secondary end points of the study included the effect of TAM on the incidence of fractures and cardiovascular deaths. The study plans to provide the first prospective information about the role of genetic markers in the etiology of BC. It will also establish whether TAM has a role to play in the treatment of women who are found to carry somatic mutations in the *BRCA1* gene. Laboratory results are not yet available.

The first results of the NSABP study were reported m September 1998, after a mean follow-up of 47,7 mo *(31)*. There were a total of 368 invasive and noninvasive BCs in the participants: 124 in the TAM group and 224 in the placebo group. A 49% reduction in the risk of invasive BC was seen in the TAM group, and a 50% reduction in the risk of noninvasive BC was observed. A subset analysis of women, at risk because of a diagnosis of LCIS, demonstrated a 56% reduction in this group (Fig. 4) The most dramatic reduction was seen in women at risk because of atypical hyperplasia, in whom risk was reduced by 86% (Fig. 4).

The benefits of TAM were observed in all age groups, with a relative risk of BC ranging from 0.45 in women aged 60 yr and older to 0.49 for those in the 50–59 yr age group, and 0.56 for women aged 49 yr and younger (Fig. 5). A benefit for TAM was also observed for women with all levels of BC risk within the study, indicating that the benefits of TAM are not confined to a particular lower risk or higher risk subset (Fig. 6). Benefits were observed in women at risk on the basis of family history and in those whose risk resulted from other factors.

As expected, the effect of TAM was seen on the incidence of ER-positive tumors, which was reduced by 69%/yr. The rate of ER-negative tumors in the TAM group (1.46/1000 women) did not significantly differ from the placebo group (1.20/1000 women). TAM reduced the rate of invasive cancers of all sizes, but the greatest difference between the groups was in the incidence of tumors 2.0 cm in size or less. TAM also reduced the

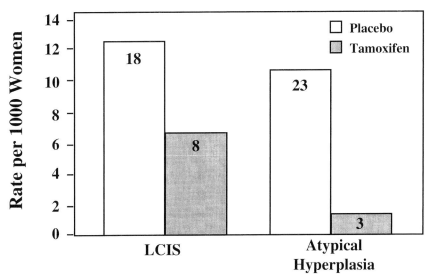

Fig. 4. Reduction in the incidence of BC of women with lobular carcinoma *in situ* (LCIS) and with prior diagnosis of atypical hyperplasia. Adapted with permission from ref. *31*.

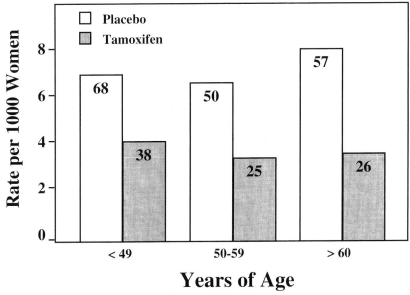

Years of Age

Fig. 5. Overall reduction in invasive BC observed in women at high risk for the disease, recruited to receive either TAM (20 mg daily) or placebo. For all women the number of BC was 175 women in the placebo group vs 89 women in the TAM group. The women were also subdivided into age groups and the same percentage reduction in the incidence of BC was observed. Adapted with permission from ref. *31*.

incidence of both node-positive and -negative BC. The beneficial effects of TAM were observed for each year of follow-up in the study. After yr 1, the risk was reduced by 33%, and, in yr 5, by 69%.

TAM also reduced the overall incidence of osteoporotic fractures of the hip, spine, and radius by 19%. However, the difference approached, but did not reach, statistical

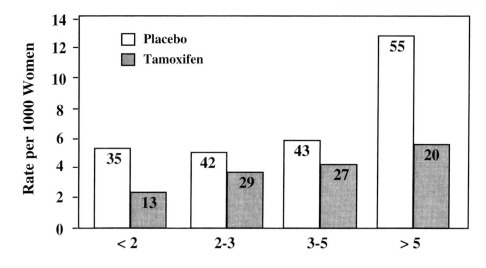

5 Year Predicted Breast Cancer Risk

Fig. 6. Reduction in the incidence of BC in the TAM prevention trial based on the calculated risk of developing the disease. Adapted with permission from ref. *31*.

significance. This reduction was greatest in women aged 50 yr and older at study entry. No difference in the risk of myocardial infarction, angina, coronary artery bypass grafting, or angioplasty was noted between groups.

This study confirmed the association between TAM and endometrial carcinoma. TAM-treated patients had a higher incidence of endometrial carcinoma, but this effect was seen mostly in the postmenopausal patients (Fig. 7). The relative risk of endometrial cancer in the TAM group was 2.5. The increased risk was seen in women aged 50 yr and older, whose relative risk was 4.01. All endometrial cancers in the TAM group were grade 1, and none of the women on TAM died of endometrial cancer. There was one endometrial cancer death in the placebo group. Although there is no doubt that TAM increases the risk of endometrial cancer, this increase translates to an incidence of 2.3/1000 women per year who develop endometrial carcinoma.

More women in the TAM group developed deep vein thrombosis (DVT) than in the placebo group. Again, this excess risk was confined to women aged 50 yr and older. The relative risk of DYT in the older age group was 1.71, (95% CI 0.85–3.58). An increase in pulmonary emboli was also seen in the older women taking TAM, with a relative risk of approx 3. Three deaths from pulmonary emboli occurred in the TAM arm, but all were in women with significant comorbidities. An increase incidence of stroke (RR 1.75) was also seen in the TAM group, but this did not reach statistical significance.

An assessment of quality of life showed no difference in depression scores between groups. Hot flashes were noted in 81% of the women on TAM compared to 69% of the placebo group, and the TAM-associated hot flashes appeared to be of no greater severity than those in the placebo group. Moderately bothersome or severe vaginal discharge was reported by 29% of the women in the TAM group and 13% in the placebo group.

Italian Study

The third TAM prevention study, performed in Italy, began in October 1992, and randomized 5408 women aged 35–70 yr to 20 mg TAM daily for 5 yr *(54)*. Women were

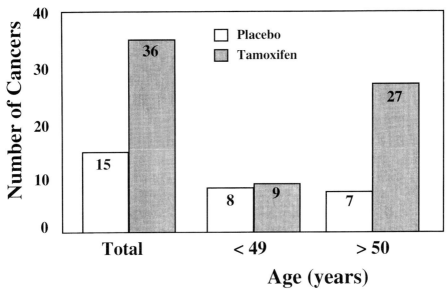

Fig. 7. The number of endometrial cancers in the TAM prevention trial. The increase in response to TAM incidence is seen in postmenopausal women, but not in premenopausal women. Adapted with permission from ref. *31*.

required to have had a hysterectomy for a nonneoplastic condition, to obviate concerns about an increased risk of endometrial carcinoma. There was no requirement that participants be at risk for BC development, and, in fact, whose who underwent premenopausal oophorectomy with hysterectomy actually had a slightly reduced risk of BC development. Women with endometriosis, cardiac disease, and OVT were excluded from the study. Although 5408 women were randomized into this study, 1422 withdrew and only 149 completed 5 yr of treatment.

The incidence of BC did not differ between groups, with 19 cases in the TAM group and 22 in the placebo group. Tumor characteristics, including size, grade, lymph node status, and receptor status, also did not differ between groups.

The incidence of thrombophlebitis was increased in the TAM group. A total of 64 events were reported: 38 in the TAM group and 18 in the placebo group ($P = 0.0053$). However, 42 of these were superficial phlebitis. No differences in the incidence of cerebrovascular ischemic events were observed.

Conclusions

Based on a single trial with a positive result and two with negative results, it may seem, at first glance, that the role of TAM in BC prevention remains unresolved. However, critical differences exist among these three studies (*see* characteristics in Table 5).

The negative finding in the Italian study *(54)* is readily explained by the relatively low risk of BC development in the study population, the high dropout rate, and the small number of participants who completed 5 yr of treatment. At present, the only conclusion that can be drawn from this study is that TAM's possible benefits are likely to be small in women with an average or decreased risk of BC.

The Royal Marsden study was initially described as a pilot study to examine toxicity and compliance *(46,48,51)*, which would serve as a feasibility assessment for a large trial

Table 5
Characteristics of Raloxifene

Decrease spine fractures, maintains bone density
Decreases LDL cholesterol
Decreased incidence of BC (preliminary results)
Less estrogenicity in the uterus than TAM

to determine if TAM prevents BC. Despite being designed as a pilot study, the trial is now said to have a 90% power to detect a 50% reduction in BC incidence, yet shows no effect *(47)*. The authors suggest that the positive results of the NSABP trial at 3.5 yr follow-up probably result from the treatment of clinically occult carcinoma, rather than the prevention of new BCs. However, of the 368 total cancers in the NSABP study *(31)*,104 (28%) were DCIS, compared to 11% of the 70 cancers in the Royal Marsden study. The higher percentage of DCIS in the NSABP trial indicates that the detection of subclinical cancers occurred, and that any treated occult cancer was not truly amenable to detection by currently available means. Whether occult carcinoma was treated, or whether true prevention occurred, a significantly greater number of women were spared surgery, irradiation, and chemotherapy.

Overall, the results of the NSABP trial *(31)*, with its large study population, clearly support the benefit of TAM for BC prevention in high-risk women. These findings are consistent with laboratory observations and with the contralateral BC risk reduction seen with TAM therapy. TAM was approved in 1998 for the reduction of risk in pre- and post-menopausal women with a high risk of BC. The results of the NSABP prevention trial have established TAM as the standard of care, but opened the door for the evaluation of other agents in clinical trial.

RALOXIFENE

Raloxifene (originally named keoxifene, or LY 156758 *[58]*) was discovered as part of the BC program at the laboratories of Eli Lilly in Indianapolis. The drug has a high binding affinity for ER *(55,56)*, primarily because it has strategically located phenolic groups. It is a member of the selective estrogen receptor modulator (SERM) group of antiestrogens, because it has been found to carry antiestrogenic activity in the breast and uterus and estrogenic action on the bones. Raloxifene's characteristics are listed in Table 5.

Antitumor Action

Raloxifene inhibits the growth of DMBA-induced rat mammary carcinomata *(57)*, but, dose for dose, TAM is more effective (Fig. 8). A small study of 18 ER-positive patients, with previously untreated metastatic disease, showed modest response rates of 30%, with a dose of 300 mg daily *(58)*. The key issue, which has not yet been addressed, is cross-resistance between raloxifene and TAM. More important, for the proposed evaluation as a preventative, raloxifene reduces the incidence of NMU-induced tumors *(59,60)*, if given after the carcinogen but before the appearance of palpable tumors (Fig. 8). However, as would be anticipated with a drug that has a short biological half-life, raloxifene is not superior to TAM at equivalent doses *(59)*. There is no doubt that raloxifene and its analogs are effective and potent inhibitors of the growth of BC cells in culture *(61,62)*, but

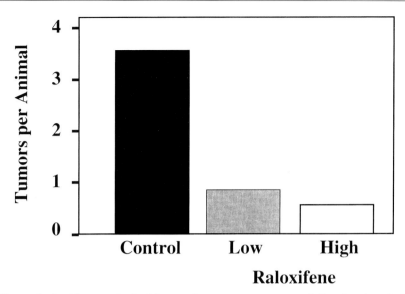

Fig. 8. Effects of raloxifene on the incidence of rat mammary tumors following the administration of NMU. Rats were treated with 100 and 500 μg raloxifene daily to prevent mammary carcinogenesis. Adapted with permission from ref. *59.*

the complication of first pass metabolism in vivo reduces potency. For this reason, doses above 60 mg raloxifene daily have been tested in clinical trial to prevent osteoporosis.

Based on the hypothesis that raloxifene could reduce the incidence of BC as a beneficial side effect of the prevention of osteoporosis *(63)*, the placebo-controlled trials with raloxifene have been monitored. There are two separate databases to test the hypothesis. First, an ongoing single trial entitled "Multiple Outcomes of Raloxifene Evaluation" has randomized 7704 postmenopausal women (mean age 66.5 yr), who had osteoporosis (hip or spine bone density at least 2.5 SD below normal mean, or had vertebrate fractures) and no history of BC or endometrial cancer, to placebo or to 60 or 120 mg raloxifene daily. Results at 2 yr, with a total of 32 cases of BC confirmed, indicate a 70% reduction in the risk of BC *(64)*. The second data base pools all placebo-controlled trials, and includes 10,553 women monitored for 3 yr. In this group, a 54% reduction in the incidence of BC in the raloxifene-treated patients is observed *(65,66)*. As was noted in the TAM study, raloxifene reduces the incidence of ER-positive BC, and has no effect on the incidence of ER-negative BC. It should be pointed out that the data from the raloxifine study actually represent three groups; one placebo control and two doses of raloxifene, 60 and 120 mg daily. Because the raloxifene data are pooled and represented in the abstracts as a percent of control, the events that can be calculated are artificially high. However, the result with raloxifene is strong preliminary data as a basis for the Study of Tamoxifen And Raloxifene (STAR), which is comparing TAM, the standard of care, with the test drug raloxifene in women with a high-risk for BC *(67)*.

Bones

Raloxifene can maintain bone density in ovariectomized rats *(25,67–73)*. Raloxifene increases bone density by 2.4 ± 0.4% in the lumber spine and 2.4 ± 0.4% for the total hip *(68)*. Although the percent increases in bone density are not as high as would be anticipated with estrogen or bisphosphonates, it is clear that raloxifene produces a 40% decrease in spine fractures. There are, however, no reports of a significant decrease in hip fractures with raloxifene. This contrasts with the 50% decrease noted with TAM in the prevention study *(31)*, and adds further support for the need to compare and contrast the clinical endocrinology of TAM and raloxifene in the STAR trial.

Lipids

Raloxifene produces a significant decrease in LDL cholesterol, but HDL cholesterol remains the same *(74,75)*. Additionally, triglycerides do not rise during raloxifene treatment. Laboratory data from the rabbit *(76)* strongly supports the value of raloxifene to prevent atherosclerosis. However, data from primates fed high cholesterol diets do not show a benefit for raloxifene *(76)*. These results have proved to be controversial *(77)*, because both HRT and TAM show positive results in the primate model. To address the issue directly, a prospective randomized clinical trial, Raloxifene Use for the Heart, is in place to address the question of whether raloxifene has merit for the reduction of risk for CHD in postmenopausal women with elevated risk factors.

Uterus

Raloxifene and its analogs have low estrogen-like actions in the rat uterus *(78,79)*. Indeed, the raloxifene analog, LY117018, is able to block (at high doses) the estrogen-like effect of TAM on the rat uterus *(80)*. However, raloxifene and its analogs cannot be classified as pure antiestrogens in these tests. There is not a complete lack of uterotropic properties *(81,82)*, and estrogen-regulated genes, such as the progesterone receptor, are partially activated *(83)*.

Raloxifene is receiving a rigorous evaluation in the human uterus. This is important, because the drug is used to treat and prevent osteoporosis. A current evaluation in women screened to ensure the absence of pre-existing endometrial abnormalities shows that raloxifene, unlike estrogen, does not increase endometrial thickness *(84)*. Raloxifene does have less estrogenicity in the uterus than TAM, and it only increases the growth of human endometrial carcinomas by about 50% of that noted with TAM *(85)*. This, coupled with the preliminary data with raloxifene as a potential preventive for BC in elderly women, is sufficient to propose testing against TAM as the current standard of care.

STUDY OF TAM AND RALOXIFENE (STAR)

The STAR trial is a Phase III, double-blind trial that will assign eligible postmenopausal women to either daily TAM (20 mg orally) or raloxifene (60 mg orally) therapy for 5 yr. Trial participants will also complete a minimum of an additional 2 yr follow-up after therapy is stopped.

The STAR trial's primary aim is to determine whether long-term therapy is effective in preventing the occurrence of invasive BC in postmenopausal women who are identified as being at high risk for the disease. Table 6 lists the eligibility criteria. The comparison will be made to the established drug, TAM. Its secondary aim is to establish the net effect of raloxifene therapy, by a comparsion of cardiovascular data, fracture data, and general toxicities, with TAM. It is clear that SERM is similar for TAM and ralaxifene, but the evaluation of the overall benefits of the agents will be an important new database on the new antiestrogen. The results from the STAR are anticipated by 2006.

Table 6
Eligibility Criteria for STAR Trial

1. Postmenopausal women over the age of 60 yr, regardless of their risk level for developing BC.
2. Postmenopausal women with a diagnosis of LCIS.
3. Postmenopausal women between the ages of 35 and 59 yr, who possess risk factors that place them at high risk for developing BC. Risk determination is based on a computerized calculation using the modified Gail model previously utilized in the P-1 trial. This group of women must have a combination of risk factors that increases the risk of developing BC.

These risk factors are based on:
- age
- number of first-degree relatives (mother, daughters, sisters) who have been diagnosed with BC
- whether a women had any children and her age at first delivery
- the number of times a woman has had breast lumps biopsied, especially if the tissue were shown to have atypical hyperplasia
- the woman's age at her first menstrual period

THE GOAL OF PREVENTION

The idea that BC could be prevented was first proposed by Lassagne *(1)* in 1936, and the concept of chemoprevention of cancer was proposed by Sporn in the mid-1970s *(86, 87)*. In 1998, two agents, TAM and raloxifene, which did or had the potential to reduce the risk of BC, were available to the medical community. Despite enormous progress through translational research, the prevention of BC is currently surrounded by controversy. The discussion is not whether the clinical trial data are valid, but rather what the results mean for women. At the heart of the debate lies the definition of prevention. The social issue has become whether a decrease in the incidence of BC within the time frame of a generation of clinical trials can be considered prevention.

TAM reduces the incidence of BC by 50% in high-risk women *(31)* in a single trial that was stopped at 4 yr. These early results have prompted the argument that this is not prevention, but the treatment of undetected disease. Indeed, the same argument was made before the prevention trial started in the United States *(88)*, so the debate is not new. The term "chemosuppression of BC" was proposed *(88)* to explain that the incidence would be suppressed only as long as the drug was administered. In fact, this is the definition of the prevention of osteoporosis with estrogen. However, this hypothesis may not be correct. TAM has an unique property of sustained biologic activity that should be studied further.

Data from the Overview Analysis *(13)* demonstrate a reduction in the incidence of contralateral BC, which continues for at least another 5 yr after TAM treatment is stopped. The pharmacologic effect of TAM to reduce the incidence of BC is clearly superior to the transient effect of estrogen to prevent osteoporosis. The challenge for future clinical investigations will be to determine how long will be long enough, i.e., extending the treatment duration for more that 5 yr, to determine the optimal protection from BC. Clearly, two competing issues will come into play, but cannot be predicted beforehand without further clinical trials. First, an optimal duration may be found that can prevent occult BC from growing, but this may be balanced out by the development of resistance to antiestrogen, resulting in the renewed growth of subclinical disease. It is unclear how soon antiestrogen resistance will appear, because the only model, thus far, has been adjuvant therapy to control the recurrence of genetically unstable micrometastatic disease. It may not be possible to use the model of adjuvant therapy to predict the optimal duration of antiestrogen use to hinder the development of primary disease. However, the issue will be critical over the next decade, because raloxifene is designed for indefinite use as a preventive for osteoporosis. It is only possible, at this point, to guess about the effectiveness of a long-term preventive strategy for postmenopausal women, because cardiovascular, bone, and cancer risks will all come into play for a woman's overall quality of life and, ultimately, longevity. Second, long durations of SERMs may be essential for true BC prevention during the promotion phase. The resolution of the competing effects of drug resistance and prevention can only be solved by large clinical trials or by an assessment of risk benefits of SERMs by a future generation of epidemiologists.

Despite the existing uncertainties, the successful translation of laboratory ideas to the clinic should not be dismissed. Two clinical strategies to reduce the incidence of BC are now available to women that were not available in 1997. Nevertheless, even though TAM has been evaluated clinically for two decades, there is still a need for the close monitoring of well women through their lives. Raloxifene, by contrast, has only been used for about 1 yr in the general population, and therefore requires very close monitoring for long-term toxicities. Only by testing raloxifene against TAM in the STAR trial can further advances in preventive therapeutics be established. The promising results with TAM and raloxifene should be viewed as a single step in the continuing process of BC research.

REFERENCES

1. Lacassagne A. Hormonal pathogenesis of adenocarcinoma of the breast. Am J Cancer 1936;27:211–225.
2. Jensen EV, Jacobson HI. Basic guides to the mechanism of estrogen action. Recent Prog Horm Res 1962;18:387–414.
3. Toft D, Gorski J. A receptor molecule for estrogen, isolation from rat uterus and preliminary characterization. Proc Natl Acad Sci USA 1996;55:1574–1581.
4. Toft D, Shyamala G, Gorski J. A receptor molecule for estrogens. Studies using a cell free system. Proc Natl Acad Sci USA 1967;57:1740–1743.
5. Jensen EV, Suzuki T, Kawashima T, Stumpf WE, Jungblut PW, DeSombre ER. A two-step mechanism for the interaction of estradiol with rat uterus. Proc Natl Acad Sci USA 1968;59:632–638.
6. Gorski J, Toft D, Shyamala G, Smith D, Notides A. Hormone receptors: studies on the interaction of estrogen with the uterus. Recent Prog Horm Res 1968;24:45–72.
7. Jensen EV, Block GE, Smith S, Kyser K, DeSombre ER. Estrogen receptors and breast cancer response to adrenalectomy: prediction of response in cancer therapy. Natl Cancer Inst Monogr 1971;34:55–70.
8. Jordan VC. Designer estrogens. Sci Am 1998;279:60–67.
9. Harper MJK, Walpole AL. A new derivative of triphenylethylene: effect on implantation and mode of action in rats. J Reprod Fertil 1967;13:101–119.
10. Harper MJK, Walpole AL. Mode of action of ICI 46,474 in preventing implantation in rats. J Endocrinol 1967;37:83–92.
11. Williamson JG, Ellis JD. The induction of ovulation by tamoxifen. J Obstet Gynaecol Br Comm 1973; 80:844–847.
12. Jordan VC. The development of tamoxifen for breast cancer: a tribute to the late Arthur L. Wadpole. Breast Cancer Res Treat 1988;11:197–209.
13. Early Breast Cancer Trialists' Collaborative Group. Tamoxifen for early breast cancer: an overview of the randomized trials. Lancet 1998;351:1451.
14. Jordan VC, Koerner S. Tamoxifen (ICI 46,474) and the human carcinoma 8S oestrogen receptor. Eur J Cancer 1975;11:205.
15. Jordan VC, Jaspan T. Tamoxifen as an antitumour agent: oestrogen binding as a predictive test for tumour response. J Endocrinol 1976;68:453.
16. Jordan VC. Antitumour activity of the antioestrogen ICI 46,474 (tamoxifen) in the dimethyl benzanthracene (DMBA)-induced rat mammary carcinoma model. J Steroid Biochem 1974;5:354.
17. Jordan VC. Effect of tamoxifen (ICI 46,474) on initiation and growth of DMBA-induced rat mammary carcinoma. Eur J Cancer 1976;12:419.

18. MacGregor JI, Jordan VC. Basic guide to the mechanisms of antiestrogen action. Pharm Rev 1998; 50:151.

19. Gottardis MM, Robinson SP, Satyaswaroo, PG, Jordan VC. Contrasting actions of tamoxifen on endometrial and breast tumor growth in the athymic mouse. Cancer Res 1988;48:812.

20. Jordan VC, Dix CJ, Alien KE. The effectiveness of long term tamoxifen treatment in a laboratory model for adjuvant hormone therapy of breast cancer. In: Salmon SE, Jones SE, eds. Adjuvant Therapy of Cancer II. Grune & Stratton, London, 1979, pp. 19–26.

21. Jordan VC, Allen KE. Evaluation of the antitumour activity of the nonsteroidal antioestrogen monohydroxytamoxifen in the DMBA-induced rat mammary carcinoma model. Eur J Cancer 1980;16:239.

22. Jordan VC, Lababidi MK, Langan-Fahey S. Suppression of mouse mammary tumorigenesis by longterm tamoxifen therapy. J Natl Cancer Inst 1991;83:492.

23. Harper MJK, Walpole AL. A new derivative of triphenylethylene: effect of on implantation and mode of action in rats. J Reprod Fertil 1967;13:101.

24. Terenius L. Structure-activity relationships of antioestrogens with regard to interaction with 17 β oestradiol in the mouse uterus and vagina. Acta Endocr 1971;66(Suppl):431.

25. Jordan VC, Phelps E, Lindgren JU. Effects of antiestrogens on bone in castrated and intact female rats. Breast Cancer Res Treat 1987;10:31.

26. Turner RT, Wakley GK, Hannon KS, Bell NH. Tamoxifen prevents the skeletal effects ovarian hormone deficiency in rats. J Bone Miner Res 1987;2:449.

27. Turken S, Siris E, Seldin D, Flaster E, Hyman G, Lindsay R. Effects of tamoxifen on spinal bone density in women with breast cancer. J Natl Cancer Inst 1989;81:1086.

28. Ward RL, Morgan G, Dalley D, Kelly PJ. Tamoxifen reduces bone turnover and prevents lumbar spine and proximal femoral bone loss in early postmenopausal women. Bone Miner 1993;22:87.

29. Love RR, Mazess RE, Barden HS, Epstein S, Newcomb PA, Jordan VC, Carbone PP, DeMets DL. Effects of tamoxifen on bone mineral density in postmenopausal women with breast cancer. N Engl J Med 1992;326:852.

30. Kristensen B, Ejlertsen B, Dolgard P, Larson L, Holmegaard SN, Transbol I, Mouridsen HT. Tamoxifen and bone metabolism in postmenopausal low risk breast cancer patients: a randomized study. J Clin Oncol 1994;12:992.

31. Fisher B, Costantino JP, Wickerham DL, Redmond C, Kovanah M, Cronin WM, et al. Tamoxifen for prevention of breast cancer: report of the National Surgical Adjuvant Breast and Bowel Project P-l Study. J Natl Cancer Inst 1998;90:1371.

32. Rossner S, Wallgren A. Serum lipoproteins and proteins after breast cancer surgery and effects of tamoxifen. Atherosclerosis 1984;52:339.

33. Love RR, Wiebe DA, Newcomb PA, Cameron L, Leventhal H, Jordan VC, Feyzi J, DeMets DL. Effects of tamoxifen on cardiovascular risk factors in postmenopausal women. Am Int Med 1991;115:860.

34. McDonald CC, Stewart HJ. Fatal myocardial infarction in the Scottish tamoxifen trial. Br Med J 1991; 303:435.

35. McDonald CC, Alexander FE, Wnyte BW, Forest AP, Steward HJ. Cardiac and vascular morbidity in women receiving adjuvant tamoxifen for breast cancer in a randomized trial. Br Med J 1995;311:977.

36. Rutquist LE, Matteson A. Cardiac and thromboembolic morbidity among postmenopausal women with early stage breast cancer in a randomized trial of tamoxifen: The Stockholm Breast Cancer Study Group. J Natl Cancer Inst 1993;85:1398.

37. Costantino JP, Kuller LH, Ives DG, Fisher B, Dignam J. Coronary heart disease mortality and adjuvant tamoxifen therapy. J Natl Cancer Inst 1997;89:776.

38. Jordan VC, Dix CJ. Effect of oestradiol benzoate, tamoxifen and monohydroxytamoxifen on immature rat uterine progesterone receptor synthesis and endometrial cell division. J Steriod Biochem 1979;11:285.

39. Assikis VJ, Jordan VC. Gynecological effects of tamoxifen and the association with endometrial cancer. Int J Gynecol Obstet 1995;49:241.

40. Goldstein SR. Unusual ultrasonographic appearance of the uterus in patients receiving tamoxifen. Am J Obstet Gynecol 1994;170:447.

41. Decensi A, Fontana V, Bruno S, Costa A. Effect of tamoxifen on endometrial proliferation. J Clin Oncol 1996;14:434.

42. Satyaswaroop PG, Zaino RJ, Mortel R. Estrogen-like effects of tamoxifen on endometrial carcinoma transplanted in nude mice. Cancer Res 1984;44:4006.

43. Assikis VJ, Neven P, Jordan VC, Vergote I. A realistic clinical perspective of tamoxifen and endometrial carcinogenesis. Eur J Cancer 1996;32A:1464.

44. Horwvitz RI, Feinstein AR, Horwitz SR. Necropsy diagnosis of endometrial cancer and detection-bias in case/control studies. Lancet 1981;ii:66.

45. Fisher B, Costantino JP, Redmond CK, Fisher ER, Wickerham DL, Cronin WM. Endometrial cancer in tamoxifen treated breast cancer patients. Findings from the National Surgical Adjuvant Breast and Bowel Project (NSABP). J Natl Cancer Inst 1994;86:527.

46. Powles TJ, Hardy JR, Ashley SE, Farrington GM, Cosgrove D, Dovey JB, et al. A pilot trial to evaluate the acute toxicity and feasibility of tamoxifen for prevention of breast cancer. Br J Cancer 1989;60:126.

47. Powles TJ, Eeles R, Ashley SE, Easton D, Chang J, Dowsett M, et al. Interim analysis of the incident breast cancer in the Royal Marsden Hospital tamoxifen randomized chemoprevention trial. Lancet 1998;362:98.

48. Powles TI, Jones AL, Ashley SE, O'Brien MER, Tidy VA, Treleavan J, et al. The Royal Marsden Hospital pilot tamoxifen chemoprevention trial. Breast Cancer Res Treat 1994;31:73.

49. Powles TJ, Hickish T, Kanis JA, Tidy VA, Ashley S. Effect of tamoxifen on bone mineral density measured by dual energy x-ray absorptiometry in healthy premenopausal and postmenopausal women. J Clin Oncol 1996;14:78.

50. Jones AL, Powles TJ, Treleaven J, Burman JF, Nicolson MC, Ching HI, Ashley SE. Haemostatic changes and thromboembolic risk during tamoxifen therapy in normal women. Br J Cancer 1992;66:744.

51. Powles TJ, Tillyer CP, Jones AL, Ashley SE, Treleaven J, Davey JB, McKinna JA. Prevention of breast cancer with tamoxifen: an update on the Royal Marsden pilot program. Eur J Cancer 1990;26:680.

52. Kedar RP, Bourne TH, Powles TJ. Effects of tamoxifen on uterus and ovaries of postmenopausal women in a randomizes breast cancer prevention trial. Lancet 1994;342:1318.

53. Call MH, Brinton LA, Byar DP. Projecting individualized probabilities of developing breast cancer for white females who are being examined annually. J Natl Cancer Inst 1989;81:1879.

54. Veronesi U. Maisonneuve P, Costa A. Prevention of breast cancer with tamoxifen: preliminary findings from the Italian randomized trial among hysterectomized women. Lancet 1998;362:93.

55. Black LJ, Jones CD, Clark JH, Clemens JA. LY156758: a unique antiestrogen displaying high afficity for estrogen receptors negligible estrogenic activity and nearly total estrogen antagonism in vivo. Breast Cancer Res Treat 1982;2:279.

56. Black LJ, Jones CD, Falcone JF. Antagonism of estrogen action with a new benzothiophene derived antiestrogen. Life Sci 1983;32:103.

57. Clemens JA, Bennett DR, Black LJ, Jones CD. Effects of new antiestrogen keoxifene LY156758 on growth of carcinogen-induced mammary tumors and on LH and prolactin levels. Life Sci 1983;32:2869.

58. Gradishar WJ, Glusman JE, Vogel CL, Mansi JL, Stuart NSA, Carmichael J, et al. Raloxifene HCl a new endocrine agent is active in estrogen receptor positive metastatic breast cancer. Breast Cancer Res Treat 1997;46:53(Abstract).

59. Gottardis MM, Jordan VC. The antitumor actions of keoxifene (raloxifene) and tamoxifen in the N-nitrosomethylurea-induced rat mammary carcinoma model. Cancer Res 1987;47:4020.

60. Anzano MA, Peer CW, Smith JM, Mullen LT, Shrader MW, Logsdon DL, et al. Chemoprevention of mammary carcinogenesis in the rat: combined use of raloxifene and 9-cis-retinoic acid. J Natl Cancer Inst 1996;88:123.

61. Poulin R, Merand Y, Poirier D, Levesque C, Dufor J-M, Labrie F. Antiestrogenic properties of keoxifene, trans 4-hydroxytamoxifen and ICI 164, 380, an new steroidal antiestrogen in ZR-75-1 human breast cancer cells. Breast Cancer Res Treat 1989;14:65.

62. Jiang SY, Parker CJ, Jordan VC. A model to describe how a point mutation of the estrogen receptor alters the structure function relationship of antiestrogens. Breast Cancer Res Treat 1993;26:139.

63. Lerner LJ, Jordan VC. Development of antiestrogens and their use in breast cancer. B.F. Cain Memorial Lecture. Cancer Res 1990;50:4177.

64. Cummings SR, Norton L, Eckert S, Grady D, Cauley J, Knickerbocker R, et al. for the MORE Investigators. Raloxifene reduces the risk of breast cancer and may decrease the risk of endometrial cancer in postmenopausal women. Two-year findings from the Multiple Outcomes of Raloxifene Evaluation (MORE) trial. Proc ASCO 1998;2a Abstract 3.

65. Jordan VC, Glusman JE, Eckert S, Lippman ME, Powles TJ, Costa A, Merrow M, Norton L. Incident primary breast cancers are reduced by raloxifene: integrated data from multicenter double blind, randomized trials in ~12,000 postmenopausal women. Proc ASCO 1998;122a Abstract 466.

66. Jordan VC, Glusman JE, Eckert S, Lippman ME, Powles TJ, Costa A, Merrow M, Norton L. Raloxifene reduces incident primary breast cancers. Integrated data from multicenter double blind, placebo controlled randomized trials in postmenopausal women. Breast Cancer Res Treat 1998;50;227(Abstract).

67. Black LJ, Sate M, Rowley ER, Magee DE, Bekele A, Williams DC, et al. Raloxifene (LY139 481 HC1) prevents bone loss and reduces serum cholesterol without causing uterine hypertrophy in ovariecto-mized rats. J Clin Invest 1994;93:63.

68. Frolick CA, Bryant HU, Black EC, Magee DE, Chandrasekhar S. Time-dependent changes in biochemi-cal bone markers and serum cholesterol in ovariectomized rats: effects of raloxifene HC1, tamoxifen, estrogen and alendronate. Bone 1996;18:621.

69. Sate M, McClintock C, Kim J, Turner CH, Bryant HU, Magee D, Slemenda CW. Dual-energy x-ray absorptiometry of raloxifene effects on the lumbar vertebrae and femora of ovariectomized rats. J Bone Miner Res 1994;9:715.

70. Sate M, Kim J, Short LL, Slemenda CW, Bryant HU. Longitudinal and cross sectional analysis of ral-oxifene effects on tibiae from ovariectomized aged rats. J Pharmacol Exp Ther 1995;272:1252.

71. Sate M, Bryant HU, Iverson P, Helterbrand J, Smietana F, Bemis K, et al. Advantage ofraloxifene over alendronate or estrogen on non-reproductive and reproductive tissues in the long term dosing of ovari-ectomized rats. J Pharmacol Exp Ther 1996;279:298.

72. Sate M, Rippy MK, Bryant HU. Raloxifene, tamoxifen, nafoxidine and estrogen effects on reproductive and non-reproductive tissues in ovariectomized rats. FASEB J 1996;10:905.

73. Turner CH, Sato M, Bryant HU. Raloxifene preserves bone strength and bone mass in ovariectomized rats. Endocrinology 1994;135:2001.

74. Draper MW, Flowers DE, Huster WJ, Neild JA. Effects of raloxifene (LY139,481 HC1) on biochemical markers of bone and lipid metabolism in healthy postmenopausal women. In: Christiansen C, Rii S, eds. Proceedings Fourth International Symposium on Osteoporosis and Consensus Development Confer-ence, Aalborg, Denmark, Handelstrykkeriet, Aalborg Ap. S. 1993, pp. 119.

75. Delmas PD, Bjarnason NH, Mitlak BH, Ravoux A-C, Shah AS, Huster WJ, Draper MW, Christiansen C. Effects of raloxifene on bone mineral density, serum cholesterol concentrations and uterine endo-metrium in postmenopausal women. N Engl J Med 1997;337:1641.

76. Clarkson TB, Anthony MS, Jerome CP. Lack of effect of raloxifene on coronary artery atherosclerosis of postmenopausal monkeys. J Clin Endocrinol Metab 1998;83:721.

77. Grese TA, Cho S, Finley DR, Godfrey AG, Jones CD, Lugar CW, et al. Structure-activity relationships of selective estrogen receptor modulators: modifications to the 2-arylbenzothiophene core of raloxifene. J Med Chem 1997;40:146.

78. Jones CD, Jevnikar MG, Pike AJ, Peters MK, Black LJ, Thompson AR, Falcone JF, Clemens JA. Anti-estrogens 2 structure-activity studies in a series of 3 aroyl-2-arylbenzo[b]thiophene derivatives leading to [6-hydroxy-2-(4-hydrotyphenyl) benzo[b] thiene-3-yl] [4-[2-(1 -piperidinyl) ethoxyl-phenyl] metha-none hydrochloride (LY156758), a remarkably effective estrogen antagonist with only minimal estro-genicity. J Med Chem 1984;27:1057.

79. Black LJ, Goode RL. Uterine bioassay of tamoxifen, trioxifene and a new estrogen antagonist (LY 117018) in rats and mice. Life Sci 1980;26:1453.

80. Jordan VC, Gosden B. Inhibition of the uterotropic activity of estrogens and antiestrogens by the short acting antiestrogen LY117018. Endocrinology 1983;113:463.

81. Grese TA, Sluka JP, Bryant HU, Cullinan GJ, Glasebrook AL, Jones CD, et al. Molecular determinants of tissue selectivity in estrogen receptor modulators. Proc Natl Acad Sci USA 1997;94:14,105.

82. Boss SM, Huster WJ, Neild JA, Giant MD, Eisenhut CC, Draper MW. Effect of raloxifene hydrochlo-ride on the endometrium of postmenopausal women. Am J Obstet Gynecol 1997;177:1458.

83. Levenson AS, Jordan VC. The key to the antiestrogenic mechanism of raloxifene is amino acid 351 (aspartate) in the estrogen receptor. Cancer Res 1998;58:1872.

84. Gottardis MM, Ricchio ME, Satyaswaroop PG, Jordan VC. Effect of steroidal and non steroidal anti-estrogens on the growth of a tamoxifen-stimulated human endometrial carcinoma (EnCa 101) in athymic mice. Cancer Res 1990;50:3189.

85. Sporn MB, Dunlop NM, Newton DL, Smith JM. Prevention of chemical carcinogenesis by vitamin A and its synthetic analogs (retinoids). Fed Proc 1976;35:1332.

86. Sporn MB. Approaches to prevention of epithelial cancer during the preneoplastic period. Cancer Res 1976;36:2699.

87. Jordan VC. Chemosuppression of breast cancer with tamoxifen: laboratory evidence and future clinical investigations. Cancer Invest 1988;6:589.

88. Fisher B, Dignam J, DeCillis A. Wickerham DL, Wolmark N, et al. Five years versus more than five years of tamoxifen therapy for breast cancer patients with negative lymph nodes and estrogen receptor-positive tumors. J Natl Cancer Inst 1996;88:1529.

7

Prolactin in Human Breast Cancer Development

Barbara K. Vonderhaar, PHD

CONTENTS

INTRODUCTION

In order to establish a role for a hormone in breast cancer (BC), three criteria must first be met: Specific receptors must be present in or on human BC cells, human BC cells must respond to the hormone as a mitogen, and a clinical response must be achieved when the hormone is prevented from binding to its receptors or following hormone ablation. In the case of estrogen, these three criteria have been met, and its role in human BC is widely accepted. However, the case for prolactin (PRL) has not been widely accepted, because the third criterion has been difficult to satisfy. Recent evidence from the author's and others' laboratories has presented a possible explanation that accounts for the difficulty in establishing the third criterion: Human BC cells synthesize and secrete their own biologically active PRL. This review examines the three criteria, in order to establish the validity of a potential role of PRL in human BC, and to explore possible implications in management of the disease.

CRITERION 1: PRL RECEPTORS

Receptor Forms

PRL receptors (PRLR) belong to the cytokine hematopoietic family of receptors *(1)*. The members of this superfamily are single-membrane-spanning receptors organized into three domains comprising an extracellular ligand-binding domain, a hydrophobic transmembrane domain, and an intracellular domain containing a proline-rich motif. Both normal and malignant mammary glands contain specific receptors for PRL.

From: *Contemporary Endocrinology: Endocrine Oncology*
Edited by: S. P. Ethier © Humana Press Inc., Totowa, NJ

Three different forms of the PRLR have been defined, which differ in their cytoplasmic domain. The long (90 kDa) and short (40 kDa) forms of the receptor differ only in the length of the cytoplasmic domain *(2)*. They are generated by differential splicing of a single gene. The intermediate form of the receptor lacks 198 amino acids in its cytoplasmic region, and is a deletion mutant of the long form. This form of the receptor is the predominant form in Nb2 rat lymphoma cells *(3)*. It is more sensitive to PRL, compared to the other forms, and may be present in some human BCs *(4)*. Both the long and the intermediate forms of the PRLR are able to induce differentiation, as measured by induction of milk protein gene expression *(5)*. The short form of the receptor acts as a negative regulator of PRL-induced differentiation *(6)*. All three forms induce mitogenesis *(7,8)*.

PRLRs in Human BC

By specific binding assays, PRLRs have been demonstrated in over 70% of breast biopsy samples *(9–12)*. Both normal and malignant mammary cells contain long and short forms of the receptor; the ratio of long and short forms is unknown. In human BC, there appears to be a correlation of disease parameters with binding to estrogen receptor (ER) and progesterone receptor (PR). However, no correlation with binding or presence of PRLR mRNA and disease parameters has been established. This may, in part, result from the multiple size and charged forms of the PRLR. Interaction of PRL with its receptor induces dimerization of the membrane-associated receptor *(13)*; a variety of dimeric combinations are possible. However, the physiological significance of homo- vs heterodimerization of the different-sized forms has not been explored.

More than 90% of BC surgical samples are positive for PRLR mRNA, but the amount varies considerably *(14,15)*. In the study by the author et al. *(15)*, receptor mRNA levels following *in situ* hybridization was regionally measured in areas corresponding to tumor cells and adipose cells in the same section. PRLR mRNA was found in normal breast, inflammatory lesions (mastitis), benign proliferative breast disease (fibroadenoma, papilloma, adenosis, epitheliosis), intraductal carcinoma or lobular carcinoma *in situ*, and invasive ductal, lobular, or medullary carcinoma. There was large individual variation, and no correlation with the level of PRLR mRNA was found with the histological type of lesion *(15)*. The expression of mRNA in malignant tissue was always greater than in adjacent uninvolved tissue, as determined by the polymerase chain reaction (PCR). Similarly, by immunohistochemistry, receptors were detected in some scattered stromal cells, but the staining intensity was always weaker than for the neoplastic epithelial cells (ECs). Using quantitative PCR and immunohistochemistry, Touraine et al. *(16)* made a similar observation in tissue from 29 patients.

In the author et al.'s study *(15)*, the expression of PRLR occurred regardless of the ER or PR status. In a similar study, Reynolds et al. *(14)* demonstrated by immunocytochemistry that >95% of BCs and >93% of normal breast tissues expressed the PRLR. There was no association between the expression of PRLR and ER or PR status. These observations are in contrast to the report from Ormandy et al. *(17)*, who found that the level of PRLR expression in BC cell lines was linearly related to that of the ER and PR.

PRL Mitogenic Signaling Pathways in Mammary Tissue

RECEPTOR-ASSOCIATED KINASES

The PRLR recruit kinases in order to transduce its mitogenic signals (Fig. 1). The receptor does not have intrinsic kinase activity. JAK2, a member of the Janus family of

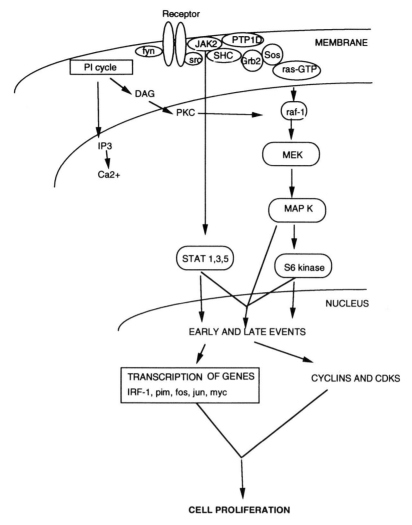

Fig 1. PRL signaling pathways. Reprinted with permission from ref. *53*.

kinases, is associated with the PRLR constitutively. JAK2 is phosphorylated on PRL binding in rat lymphoma *(18,19)*, mouse mammary explants *(20)*, and murine lymphoid BAF-3 cells *(21)*. JAK1 also is associated with the PRLR, and is phosphorylated on ligand binding in murine lymphoid BAF-3 cells transfected with the long form of the PRLR *(21)*. Phosphorylation of the JAK proteins may be one of the earliest cellular events in response to the hormone, which ultimately triggers a chain of events in the PRL signaling pathway. The PRLR is also phosphorylated in response to PRL within 1 min of hormone treatment both in vivo in rabbit mammary gland and in vitro in CHO cells transfected with the long form of PRLR cDNA *(22)*. PRLRs induce phosphorylation of cytoplasmic transcription factors signal transducer and activator of transcription 1 (STAT1), STAT3, and STAT5 *(23)*. STAT5 is activated during PRL-induced differentiation *(24)*. Recently, two different STAT5 proteins have been isolated from mouse mammary tissue (STAT5a and b). Both transcription factors recognize GAS sequences. Their expression is concurrent during mammary gland development, increasing from the virgin state, reaching a maximum at d 16 of pregnancy, and declining during lactation *(25)*.

STAT5a is essential for full lobuloalveolar development and lactation, as demonstrated by use of knockout mice (26). The phosphorylation of STAT proteins has also been reported in Nb2 cells (19) and in normal mouse mammary ECs (HC11) (24). The author et al. (27) have reported activation of STAT5 upon PRL treatment in T47D BC cells. DaSilva et al. (23) also reported the phosphorylation of STAT1, STAT3, and STAT5 in T47D cells upon PRL treatment. Activation of STAT proteins results in translocation of the transcription factors to the nucleus and activation of gene transcription (28).

PRL induces the association of PRLR with pp60 c-src and activation of its tyrosine kinase (TK) activity in hepatocytes of lactating rats (29), in which the short form of the receptor is predominant. PRL stimulation in rat lymphoma Nb2 cells induces the association and activation of src family protein TK p59 fyn (30), and also the guanine nucleotide-releasing factor (GNRF)-vav (31). Recently, a protein tyrosine phosphatase, PTP1D, was reported to be associated with the PRLR–JAK2 complex in Nb2 cells, which was essential for PRL signal transduction for induction of β-casein (32). In CHO cells transfected with the rabbit PRLR, two TK inhibitors, herbimysin A and tyrphostin, were able to decrease the expression of a β-lactoglobin promoter/catalase (CAT) construct by over 50%. Orthovanadate, an inhibitor of tyrosine phosphatase, was able to substitute for PRL in inducing CAT responses in these cells (33), which suggests an intricate role for both kinases and phosphatases in PRL signal transduction. Whether there is a difference in signaling for differentiation versus mitogenesis is unknown.

Ras-MAPK Pathway

A variety of growth factors and cytokines mediate proliferation by activating the ras-MAP kinase (MAPK) pathway of signal transduction. Activation of Ras p21 protein by PRL has been reported in a variety of cell systems by measuring the guanine nucleotides bound to the protein (34,35). Raf-1, MEK, and MAPK are downstream kinases in the ras-MAPK pathway, which are activated for mitosis induced by PRL. In Nb2 cells, PRL rapidly phosphorylates c-raf-1 (36). Raf-1 is closely associated with the PRLR in these cells. The author et al. have reported the rapid and transient activation of these enzymes in mammary cells in response to 5 min of PRL treatment. TK inhibitors block MAPK activity and PRL-induced growth in these mammary cells (27). Cells transfected with the long or short form of the PRLR cDNA also activate MAPK. There was rapid activation of MAPK reaching a peak within 5 min of PRL treatment in both of the transfectants (8), suggesting that both the long and short forms of the PRLR are able to induce mitosis through a common signaling pathway. Activation and nuclear translocation of protein kinase C (PKC) and MAPK have been reported during PRL-induced proliferation of Nb2 cells (37,38).

PKC Pathway

The phosphoinositide cycle plays a role in signal transduction for PRL, which then activates PKC. Endogenously added phospholipase C, an enzyme that hydrolyzes L-α-phosphoinositol 4,5-diphosphate to D-myo-inositol triphosphate and diacylglycerol (DAG), elicited PRL-like effects on ornithine decarboxylase activity and RNA synthesis in pregnant mouse mammary gland explants in culture (39). The author et al. have reported PRL-induced activation and translocation of PKC to the membranes in NOG-8 mammary cells within 5–10 min of exposure (40). Waters and Rillema (41), using explants from mouse mammary glands, showed translocation of PKC upon PRL treatment. The phosphorylation and activation of PI3-kinase for signal transduction of PRL in Nb2 cells has been reported (42).

SHC-Grb Pathway

Growth hormone receptor, which is a member of the same receptor family as the PRL receptor, activates the JAK–SHC pathway in 3T3-F442A cells *(43)*. In breast cells, both normal and malignant, the author et al. have shown that PRL can phosphorylate SHC proteins within 1 min of hormone treatment, followed by association with the Grb2–Sos complex. Also, JAK2 is phosphorylated and associated with SHC protein upon PRL activation in these mammary ECs *(44)*. Possible crosstalk between MAPK pathway and the JAK–STAT pathway has been suggested *(45)*.

Early-Response Genes

Modulation of early-response genes and late-response genes in the signaling pathways of a mitogen results in an increase in cell growth. PRL has been shown to induce transcription of early genes in a number of systems. PRL stimulates expression of *c-myc (46)* and rapidly induces expression of the proto-oncogenes c-*fos*, c-*jun*, and c-*src*, even in the presence of cyclohexamide *(29)*. This suggests that PRL stimulates the expression of genes with activating protein 1 (AP-1) or SRE sequences in their promoter regions. *Pim-1*, an early-response gene, is stimulated by PRL during mitogenesis *(47)*. Peak expression occurs at 2–4 h of PRL treatment, and is not affected by cyclohexamide. *Pim-1*, a proto-oncogene that encodes a conserved cytosolic serine/threonine protein kinase, is rapidly induced in hematopoietic cells, upon mitogen stimulation. Another early activation gene, induced over 20-fold in Nb2 cells by PRL, is interferon regulatory factor-1 (IRF-1). This gene is induced twice by PRL in a single cell cycle, first during G1 at 30–60 min, and again during early S-phase at 10–12 h of hormone treatment *(48)*. The second peak of IRF-1 mRNA expression in early S-phase is dependent on the continuous presence of PRL throughout G1, and is correlated tightly with DNA synthesis and subsequent cell proliferation. The GAS site in the IRF-1 promoter is thought to act as a PRL-responsive element that responds to the mitogenic signal of PRL in T-cells. Its activation in breast cells has not been established.

Late-Response Genes

Cyclins play an important role in the progression of the cell cycle *(49)*. Several cyclins are amplified in malignant cells, compared to their normal counterpart. Cyclin D1 is among the most commonly overexpressed oncogenes in BC. Cyclin D1 knockout mice have abnormal mammary gland development, and they are devoid of PRL-dependent lobuloalveolar structures in the mature gland *(50)*. In addition, following PRL stimulation of quiescent Nb2 cells, cyclin D2 mRNA level increase in mid-G1-phase and decrease sharply before S-phase. Cyclin D3 level increased in late G1–early S-phase, and gradually decreases during S-phase *(51)*. Further elucidation of the activation of specific late-response genes should help clarify the distinguishing events in PRL-induced mitogenesis vs differentiation.

CRITERION 2: BIOLOGICAL RESPONSE

PRL as Mitogen

In the mammary gland, PRL is both a differentiating agent and a mitogen. It is well established that terminal differentiation, as defined by the induction of milk protein synthesis, is dependent on PRL both in vivo and in vitro *(52)*. Less well-recognized is the mitogenic action of PRL *(53)*. Although the ovarian steroids, estrogen and progesterone, are involved in mammary ductal growth and branching, strong evidence suggests that lobuloalveolar development and extensive growth of the alveolar cells require PRL *(52,54)*. The development of PRL knockout mice has underscored the role of PRL. Although a ductal tree develops in these mice, it is devoid of alveolar buds and is unable to undergo full lobuloalveolar development *(55)*. Progesterone acts synergistically with PRL to induce mitogenesis throughout mammary gland development, possibly by increasing the PRLR levels in these glands *(56)*. On the other hand, PRL has been implicated in regulation of ER in the mammary gland *(57,58)*.

Rodent Mammary Cancer

The same hormones that are important for normal growth are also involved to varying degrees in the development of BC. PRL's role in rodent mammary cancer is well established *(59)*. Multiple pituitary isografts in mice result in large amounts of PRL secreted into the circulation. Subsequently, there is a significant increase in the incidence of spontaneous mammary tumors *(60)*. There is a direct correlation between serum PRL levels and susceptibility of various rat strains to induction of tumors by chemical carcinogens *(61)*. Both N-methyl(-N-nitrosourea-) and 1,2-dimethylbenz(a)anthracene-induced tumors in rats are dependent on PRL for sustained growth *(62)*. There is a direct correlation between drug-induced hyperprolactinemia and increased tumor growth and hypo-prolactinemia and retarded tumor growth in rodents *(63,64)*.

Human BC

SERUM PRL LEVELS

The function of PRL in the etiology and progression of human BC, in contrast to its function in rodent model systems, is not well established. Significant contradictory evidence has clouded the literature for several years. However, recent studies suggest that a re-examination of the role of PRL in human BC is in order. As many as 44% of patients with metastatic breast disease have been reported to have hyperprolactinemia during the course of the disease *(65)*. Several cases of breast carcinoma in association with prolactinoma have been reported *(66)*. More than 70% of human breast biopsies are positive for PRLRs *(9–12)*. Approximately 80% of BC cells in culture respond to PRL's mitogenic signal, when proper conditions of reduced serum or serum-free conditions are employed *(67)*. Basal serum PRL levels are significantly elevated in a subset of women at risk for familial BC *(68,69)*. In addition, the circadian rhythm of PRL secretion from the pituitary differs between groups at high vs low risk of BC *(70)* with no seasonal variations *(71)*. In one study of node-positive BC patients, both when evaluated singly and in conjunction with steroid receptor status, hyperprolactinemia was found to be an important indicator of unfavorable prognosis *(72)*. In another study *(73)*, aggressiveness of the tumor, early disease relapse or metastases, and poor overall survival in patients with node-negative BC were associated with hyperprolactinemia and/or alterations in levels of p53. In contrast, a surgery-induced rise in PRL was paradoxically associated with a longer disease-free survival in operable breast carcinoma in patients both with or without axillary node involvement, despite the potential stimulation of cancer cell growth by the hormone *(74)*. However, surgery-induced hyperprolactinemia was associated with a significant decline in the serum level of insulin-like growth factor I (IGF-I) *(75)*, suggesting that the balance of specific hormones and growth factors may be a key etiological factor.

BIOLOGICAL RESPONSES TO PRL IN VIVO

Immunologically detectable PRL appears in 60–85% of human BC biopsies *(76,77)*; specific PRLRs have been demonstrated in more than 70% of biopsy samples *(9–12)*. However, there is no clear correlation between circulating PRL levels and the etiology or prognosis of the BC *(69,78,79)*. When patients were treated with PRL-inhibiting ergot drugs, which significantly diminish circulating pituitary PRL, no change in disease state was observed *(80,81)*. Operating on the assumption that the lack of effect may have been caused by the presence of human growth hormone (hGH), which is also a lactogen, Manni et al. *(82)* administered a combination therapy of bromocriptine and a somatostatin analog to a group of women with advanced BC. Circulating levels of PRL, detected by a single assay, were abolished nearly completely in 8/9 patients; hGH levels were suppressed in 7/9 patients during treatment. Although overall antitumor effects could not be assessed reliably, because the patients entering the study had been pretreated heavily with chemotherapeutic agents, only one patient experienced disease stabilization. In a similar study, Anderson et al. *(83)* treated patients long-term with bromocriptine and the long-acting, superpotent somatostatin analog, octretide, and found that there was no evidence of disease progression for periods up to 6 mo in 4/6 patients with advanced BC, who had failed first- and second-line endocrine therapies. Although immunoreactive PRL, GH, and IGF-I, in 24 h profiles of serum, were greatly reduced by these treatments, diurnal peaks of bioreactive lactogenic hormone, as well as GH levels, were still apparent, although much reduced.

BIOLOGICAL RESPONSES TO PRL IN VITRO

In contrast to the lack of convincing data in vivo, investigations in vitro using human breast tumor tissue and cells, show clear responses to PRL. These responses include increased DNA *(84–87)*, protein *(88)*, and α-lactalbumin *(89)* synthesis; colony formation *(90,91)*; and changes in shape, adhesion, lipid accumulation *(92)* and ER content *(93)*. Primary breast biopsy samples grown in nude mice respond to lactogenic hormones with increased growth *(94)*. Malarkey et al. *(90)* found that physiological levels of human PRL (hPRL) and hGH increased the population doubling of primary breast tumor cultures. The author et al. have shown that the majority of human BC cell lines, ER-positive and -negative, express PRL receptors, and that more than 80% of human BC cell lines tested respond to PRL's mitogenic signal *(67,95)*. Direct effects of PRL on growth of the ER-positive cell lines, MCF-7, T47D, and ZR75.1, can be demonstrated only under proper growth conditions in the presence of charcoal-stripped serum (CSS). PRL-stimulated growth of MCF-7 cells was greater in the presence of 1% CSS, compared to 10% serum containing medum *(67)*. Growth effects were seen at concentrations as low as 25 ng/mL; the maximal effect was observed at 100–250 ng/mL hPRL. Growth was also stimulated by hGH, human placental lactogen, and ovine PRL, but required higher concentrations to achieve the same effect. Thus, MCF-7 cells were more sensitive to the mitogenic effect of hPRL than to other lactogens. Bovine PRL had no effect on the growth of these human BC cells. The ER-negative cell line, T47Dco, also responds to PRL as a mitogen in the presence of CSS *(96)*. PRL acts as a mitogen in MCF-7 and ZR75.1 grown in serum-free media *(97)*.

Effects of PRL on the growth of BC cells are modulated by the presence of other growth factors and hormones. Melatonin, the primary hormone from the pineal gland, completely blocks hPRL-induced growth of MCF-7 and ZR75.1 (97). Bovine PRL, when added simultaneously with hPRL, blocked the effect of hPRL on the growth of MCF-7 cells (67). As little as 50–100 ng/mL bovine PRL was able to block the hPRL-induced growth of these cells. In contrast, bovine PRL is an effective mitogen in normal mouse mammary cell lines. The ability of bovine PRL to act as an antagonist of hPRL may be unique to the mitogenic action of PRL in human BC cells.

CRITERION 3: RESPONSE TO HORMONE ABLATION

PRL Synthesis by Mammary Cells

EXTRAPITUITARY PRL

In human BC, the lack of correlation between clinical data and in vitro responses to PRL may be explained, in part, by the observation that BC cells themselves synthesize and secrete this hormone. Although hPRL was first characterized as a 22–25-kDa pituitary (pit) hormone, in recent years, synthesis of PRL and PRL-like molecules by a variety of tissues other than the pit has been reported (98). In humans, circulating levels of all pit hormones, except for PRL, become undetectable following surgical removal of the pituitary. Circulating levels of PRL remained at 30–80% of the presurgical levels for as long as 10 mo in BC patients who received a total hypophysectomy (99). Patients given bromocriptine plus somatostatin persistently maintained low levels of circulating bioactive PRL (83). These data could result from other PRL-like molecules circulating in the blood, but it was also possible that PRL itself was produced by peripheral tissues. Both normal tissue and tumors appear to generate this hormone. Placenta is the richest extrapituitary source (100). It is now well established that the high concentrations of PRL in human amniotic fluid result from the decidua. PRL is also produced by the brain, uterus, prostate, dermal fibroblasts, and the immune system (100–105).

MAMMARY PRL

Several laboratories, including the author's, have shown that PRL is produced by both normal and malignant mammary ECs, and thus may be an autocrine/paracrine factor for this tissue (Fig. 2). By in situ hybridization, Steinmetz et al. (106) showed that PRL gene transcripts are present in secretory mammary ECs from pregnant rats. PRL mRNA has also been demonstrated by both Northern analysis and reverse transcriptase (RT)-PCR in mammary glands from lactating rats (107), and goats (108), suggesting local synthesis of PRL by this gland. More recently, the presence of PRL mRNA has been demonstrated in human BC cells line in this laboratory (109), and in some primary human breast carcinomas (4).

In addition to the mRNA for the hormone, the author determined that bioactive PRL is synthesized by human BC cells and acts in an autocrine manner to stimulate cell proliferation. Growth of both T47Dco and MCF-7 human BC cell lines was inhibited by 20–90% when cells were treated with monoclonal antibodies (mAbs) raised against human pit PRL (109). In addition, when T47Dco cells were treated with antisense RNA directed against the gene encoding for pit PRL, significant growth inhibition (>50%) was obtained (110). In parallel cultures treated with a randomized antisense RNA sequence, the cells

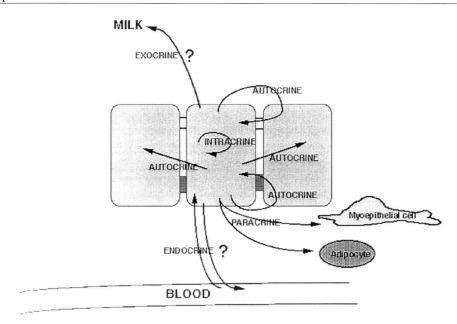

Fig 2. Autocrine/paracrine action of PRL in the mammary gland. Reprinted with permission from ref. *104*.

grew at the same rate as untreated controls. RT-PCR, followed by Southern analysis using pit hPRL cDNA as the probe, confirmed the presence of the mRNA in T47Dco and MCF-7 cells *(109)*. In addition, 82% of all BC cell lines tested contained mRNA for PRL *(110)*.

That the protein is actually synthesized and secreted by the cells in culture was confirmed by metabolically labeling T47Dco cells with ^{35}S-cysteine. Conditioned media and cell extracts both contain a 22-kDa protein precipitated by anti-hPRL mAb. Conditioned media prepared from T47Dco cells stimulated the PRL-responsive Nb2 rat lymphoma cells to grow in a concentration-dependent manner. These cells respond to picogram quantities of lactogens. The level of biological activity in the conditioned media is equivalent to 0.7 mg/mL (14.5 pg PRL/cell) of pit PRL, as measured by the Nb2 assay, and is approx 30% of the amount normally produced by the rat pit cell line, GH3 *(111,112)*. By using a specific RIA for human pit PRL, 0.35 mg /mL of PRL protein was detected. The activity in the conditioned media, like that of the human pit PRL, was abolished when the media were pretreated with antipit PRL Ab *(109)*.

More than 80% of all BC cell lines tested contain mRNA for PRL *(95)*. In this sample of cell lines, there is no correlation of ER status with PRLR or with the ability to synthesize PRL. When human BC cells were grown as solid tumors in nude mice, the resulting tumors contained PRL gene transcripts *(110)*. Immunologically detectable PRL was present in 60–85% of human BC biopsies *(76,77)*. In addition, the author found that more than 75% of primary BC surgical samples also contained mRNA for PRL. In the majority of cases, the amount of mRNA for PRL and its receptors is significantly elevated in cancerous vs adjacent, noninvolved tissue from the same patient. Similar results were reported by Touraine et al. *(16)*, who found PRL mRNA in all breast samples tested from 29 patients.

Posttranslational Modifications of PRL

Although alternate splicing of the PRL mRNA from rat brain has been reported, which results in a variant lacking exon 4 *(113)*, sequence analysis of the cDNA for PRL synthesized by late pregnant and lactating sheep and goat mammary glands differed from pit transcripts by only three mutations, two of which were silent *(108)*. Recent (unpublished) data by the author et al. suggest at least 90% sequence identity between the mRNA from the pit and BC cells. This agrees with the observation of Shaw-Bruha et al. *(114)* in a variety of human BC cell lines and neoplastic breast tissue samples. Hence, posttranslational modifications of the hormone may play a key role in its action. There is significant evidence that many diverse activities of PRL are modulated by different posttranslational modifications. The immunoreactivity and biological activity of pit PRL are modified by glycosylation and phosphorylation *(115,116)*. Phosphorylated forms of PRL are present in murine, bovine, and avian species *(117)*; phosphorylated PRL has less activity, compared to the nonphosphorylated form *(118)*. Because of conformational change in the hormone, the phosphorylated form of PRL is unable to bind to the receptor; dephosphorylation of PRL restores its biological activity. The biological activity of glycosylated PRL in mammary casein synthesis, and in the Nb2 proliferation assay, is similar to, or lower than, that of the nonglycosylated PRL *(119,120)*. However, receptor-binding activity and immunological crossreactivity are greatly reduced as a result of glycosylation. Hoffman et al. *(121)* suggested that glycosylation may selectively downregulate PRL action in target tissues. Recombinant human PRL, both glycosylated and nonglycosylated forms, was purified from the murine C127 cell expression system. The 23-kDa nonglycosylated form of the PRL was 3–4× more active in the Nb2 mitogenesis bioassay, compared to the 25-kDa glycosylated form *(122)*. The physiologically diverse effects of PRL on target tissues may be caused by changes in the ratio of glycosylated and nonglycosylated forms of PRL *(123)*.

The nature of the posttranslational alterations of PRL synthesized by the mammary gland and BC cells is unknown. Observations *(109)* that a panel of mAbs directed against pit PRL vary in their ability to recognize the PRL produced by BC cells suggest that there are marked differences in posttranslational modifications between the pit and the mammary gland.

Regulation of Expression of PRL

The hormones and growth factors that regulate expression of PRL by human BC cells in vivo and in vitro are currently unknown. In the normal sheep and goat mammary gland, the PRL gene appears to be transcribed from the same promoter as in the pit *(108)*. However, recent studies *(114)* suggest that PRL synthesis is regulated in T47D cells by the distal promoter used by decidua and lymphocytes, rather than the proximal promoter used by the pit. The author et al.'s data (unpublished) show that one of the most effective regulators of mammary PRL synthesis is the hormone itself, suggesting an autoregulatory feedback mechanism. Such a mechanism may explain the observation that treatment of lactating rats with bromocriptine results in a decrease in PRL localization to the endocytic organelles, and an increase in localization to the organelles associated with synthesis and exocytosis *(124)*.

Cleaved PRL and Tumor Angiogenesis

The ability of the mammary gland to cleave PRL has been known for some time *(125)*. In rat mammary tissue, three PRL species (25-, 23-, and 14-kDa) have been detected immunologically *(124)*. Extracts of normal mouse mammary tissue cleaved PRL to yield two fragments; extracts from a transplantable rat tumor were unable to cleave PRL *(126)*. The larger fragment of cleaved PRL, either 14-kDa or 16-kDa, has been shown to have antiangiogenic activity and inhibits vascular endothelial growth factor (VEGF)-induced growth of capillary endothelial cells *(127,128)*. VEGF is essential for initial, but not continued, in vivo growth of human breast carcinoma cells *(129)*.

INHIBITION OF PRL ACTION

Hormone Antagonists

The fact that the mammary gland can make its own PRL, and the majority of human breast tumors contain PRL receptors, suggests that manipulation of pituitary PRL is not a valid approach to therapy for this disease, and that new approaches based on the concept of an autocrine/paracrine PRL may be necessary. The use of specific drugs acting as antilactogens (i.e., anti-PRLs) *(96)* or analogs of the hormone, which act directly at the receptor level, may present an alternate clinical approach to controling this disease in PRL-responsive tumors. Included among these are mutants of hGH and hPRL, some of which have been shown to have antilactogenic activity in vitro under defined-growth conditions *(13,130–135)*. These mutants usually involve that portion of the hormone identified as site 2 (Fig. 3), where amino acids with small side-chain residues are replaced with amino acids carrying large side chains. Steric hindrance prevents binding of the mutant to the second receptor in the dimer, and hence they act as hormone antagonists *(13)*.

Antilactogen Binding Site

Tamoxifen (TAM), the first line of therapy in pre- and postmenopausal, ER-positive BC patients, is also an antilactogen (Fig. 3; *136*). TAM therapy has been shown to be effective in 14–30% of ER-negative BC patients *(137–139)*. Frequently, inhibition of cell proliferation in vitro, with lower concentrations of TAM, can be reversed by estrogens. However, the growth rates cannot be restored by estradiol in the presence of higher concentrations of the antiestrogen *(140)*. Micromolar concentrations of TAM inhibit the growth of several ER-negative human BC cell lines *(96,141,142)*. Besides the ER, there are several other cellular proteins that may be directly affected by TAM *(136)*. Pollak et al. *(143)* have suggested that during TAM therapy, there is a decrease in circulating IGF-I, which could account for the estrogen-independent response in some patients. Others have suggested that direct interaction of TAM with PKC may be responsible *(144)*. The author et al. have shown that the antilactogenic activity of TAM results from interaction with the antilactogen binding site (ALBS) *(145)*, which is located on the PRLR (Fig. 3).

The ALBS is a member of the family of high-affinity membrane-associated binding sites called antiestrogen binding sites (AEBS) *(146,147)*, which have been identified in a variety of tissues *(148,149)*. The TAM-resistant clone of MCF-7 cells, RTx6, differs from the parent MCF-7 cells in having no AEBS, but is identical to the parent cells with respect to the ER content and hormone affinity *(150)*. These cells cannot be inhibited by TAM, as MCF-7 cells are. Antiestrogens, acting through the ALBS, inhibit the growth of PRL-responsive cells, even in the absence of ER *(151)*. The ALBS, located on cellular membranes, binds TAM and related nonsteroidal antiestrogens with high affinity, but does not bind estrogens (Fig. 4; *136,152*). It is through the ALBS that TAM inhibits PRL-induced growth of ER-negative, Nb2 rat lymphoma cells *(153)*: these effects are not

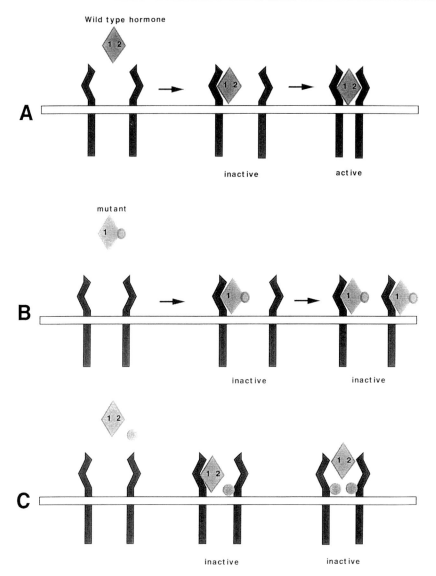

Fig 3. Inhibition of ligand-induced receptor dimerization. (**A**) Sequential hormone binding, first, through binding site 1, forming an inactive complex. The hormone then binds to a second receptor through site 2, which leads to dimerization and formation of an active complex. (**B**) Site 2 mutants prevent formation of active dimers. (**C**) Inhibitors, such as TAM, interfere with the ability of the hormone to bind to the receptor. Reprinted with permission from ref. *154.*

reversed by estradiol. The order of affinities of various nonsteroidal antiestrogens for the ALBS parallels the order of their potencies as growth and PRL-binding inhibitors. Binding of lactogenic hormones to particulate and solubilized microsomal membranes, isolated from normal mammary glands of lactating mice, was inhibited by direct addition of 10^{-10} *M* or greater concentrations of TAM to the binding assays *(152)*. Estradiol did not have this effect. Maximal inhibition of PRL binding by TAM was observed in the light microsomes that contain the plasma membranes.

TAM acts by inhibiting the binding of PRL to its receptor, rather than promoting dissociation of the hormone-receptor complex (Fig. 3; *145*). Both the ER-positive T47D

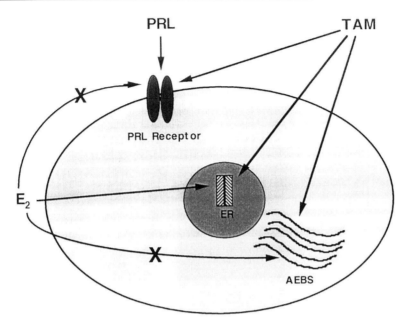

Fig. 4. Interactions at the antilactogen binding site (ALBS) on the PRL receptor. Reprinted with permission from ref. *154.*

and the ER-negative T47Dco cell lines bind lactogenic hormones specifically, and this binding was inhibited by 70–90% when $10^{-9}\,M$ TAM was added directly to the T47D whole-cell binding reaction *(96)*. A similar inhibition of PRL binding was achieved in the ER negative mouse mammary EC line, NOG-8 *(151)*. Subsequently, TAM, at concentrations as low as $10^{-9}\,M$, rapidly inhibited PRL signal transduction in these cells. This, in turn, led to an inhibition of PRL-induced growth. Thus, it appears that TAM acts primarily by inhibiting PRL's binding to its receptor and, subsequently, by blocking the hormone's signal transduction pathways. TAM acts by decreasing the number of binding sites without changing the receptor's affinity for PRL. The ALBS and PRL receptor co-purify on either PRL-Sepharose or TAM-Sepharose affinity columns, and both are recognized by the anti-PRLR mAb, B6.2 *(145)*. Taken together, these data suggest that the ALBS is on the PRLR, and that TAM, and other related, nonsteroidal, triphenylethylene antiestrogens, can inhibit growth of ER-negative human BC cells through this mechanism.

CONCLUSION

The role of PRL in human BC is still mostly undefined. The ability of this hormone to stimulate growth of human BC cells in culture, coupled with the presence of active receptors for PRL on the majority of breast carcinomas, suggests that this peptide hormone is an active player in this disease. Understanding its role is complicated by the fact that human BC cells synthesize and secrete significant amounts of biologically active PRL. These data suggest that clinically useful reagents should be sought that act at the level of the target tissue. The drug, TAM, in addition to its action as an antiestrogen, is also an antilactogen, and hence may have clinical usefulness in patients whose tumors are PRLR-positive, even if they are ER-negative.

REFERENCES

1. Kelly PA, Djiane J, Postel-Vinay MC, Edery M. The prolactin/growth hormone receptor family. Endocrine Rev 1991;12:235–251.
2. Kelly PA, Ali S, Rozakis M, Goujon L, Nagano M, Pellegrini I, et al. The growth hormone/prolactin receptor family. Rec Prog Hormone Res 1993;48:123–164.
3. Ali S, Edery M, Pellegrini I, Lesueur L, Paly J, Djiane J, Kelly PA. The Nb2 form of prolactin receptor is able to activate a milk protein gene promoter. Mol Endocrinol 1992;6:1242–1248.
4. Clevenger CV, Chang WP, Ngo W, Pasha TLM, Montone KT, Tomaszewski JE. Expression of prolactin and prolactin receptor in human breast carcinoma. Am J Pathol 1995;146:695–705.
5. Lesueur L, Edery M, Ali S, Paly J, Kelly PA, Djiane J. Comparison of long and short forms of the prolactin receptor on prolactin-induced milk protein gene transcription. Proc Natl Acad Sci USA 1991;88:482–828.
6. Berlanga JJ, Garcia-Ruiz JP, Perrot-Applanat M, Kelly PA, Edery M. The short form of the prolactin (PRL) receptor silences PRL induction of the β-casein gene promoter. Mol Endocrinol 1997;11:1449–1457.
7. O'Neal KD, Yu Lee L. Differential signal transduction of the short, Nb2, and long prolactin receptors. J Biol Chem 1994;269:26,076–26,082.
8. Das R, Vonderhaar BK. Transduction of prolactin's growth signal through both the long and short forms of the prolactin receptor. Mol Endocrinol 1995;9:1750–1759.
9. Codegone ML, DiCarlo R, Muccioli G, Bussolati G. Histology and cytometrics in human breast cancers assayed for the presence of prolactin receptors. Tumori 1981;67:549–552.
10. Peyrat JP, DeWailly D, Djiane J, Kelly PA, Vandewalle B, Bonneterre J, LeFebvre J. Total prolactin binding sites in human breast cancer biopsies. Breast Cancer Res Treat 1981;1:369–373.
11. Bonneterre J, Peyrat JP, Vandewalle B, Beuscart R, Vie MC, Cappelaere P. Prolactin receptors in human breast cancer. Eur J Cancer Clin Oncol 1982;18:1157–1162.
12. L'Hermite-Baleriaux M, Casteels S, Vokaer A, Loriaus C, Noel G, L'Hermite M. Prolactin and prolactin receptors in human breast disease. Prog Cancer Res Ther 1984;31:325–334.
13. Goffin V, Kelly PA. The prolactin/growth hormone receptor family: structure/function relations. J Mammary Gland Biol Neoplasia 1997;2:7–17.
14. Reynolds C, Montone KT, Powell CM, Tomaszewski JE, Clevenger CV. Expression of prolactin and its receptor in human breast carcinoma. Endocrinology 1997;138:5555–5560.
15. Mertani HC, Garcia-Caballero T, Lambert A, Gerard F, Palayer C, Boutin JM, et al. Cellular expression of growth hormone and prolactin receptors in human breast disorders. Int J Cancer 1998;79:201–211.
16. Touraine P, Martini JF, Zafrani B, Durand JC, Labaille F, Malet C, et al. Increased expression of prolactin receptor gene assessed by quantitative polymerase chain reaction in human breast tumors versus normal breast tissue. J Clin Endocrinol Metab 1998;83:667–674.
17. Ormandy CJ, Hall RE, Manning DL, Robertson JFR, Blamey RW, Kelly PA, Nicholson RI, Sutherland RL. Coexpression and cross-regulation of the prolactin receptor and sex steroid hormone receptors in breast cancer. J Clin Endocrinol Metab 1997;82:3692–3699.
18. Rui H, Kirken RA, Farrar WL. Activation of receptor-associated tyrosine kinase JAK2 by prolactin. J Biol Chem 1994;269:5364–5368.
19. David M, Petricoin EF, Igarashi KI, Feldman GM, Finbloom DS, Larner AC. Prolactin activates the interferon-regulated p91 transcription factor and the JAK2 kinase by tyrosine phosphorylation. Proc Natl Acad Sci USA 1994;91:7174–7178.
20. Campbell GS, Argetsinger LS, Ihle JN, Kelly PA, Rillema JA, Carter-Su C. Activation of JAK (JAK2) tyrosine kinase by prolactin receptors in NB (NB2) cells and mouse mammary gland explants. Proc Natl Acad Sci USA 1994;91:5232–5236.
21. Dusanter-Fourt I, Muller O, Ziemiecki A, Mayeux P, Drucker B, Djiane J, et al. Identification of JAK protein tyrosine kinases as signaling molecules for prolactin. Functional analysis of prolactin receptor and prolactin-erythropoietin receptor chimera expressed in lymphoid cells. EMBO J 1994;13:2538–2591.
22. Waters MJ, Daniel N, Bignon C, Djiane J. The rabbit mammary gland prolactin receptor is tyrosine phosphorylated in response to prolactin in vivo and in vitro. J Biol Chem 1995;270:5136–5143.
23. DaSilva L, Rui H, Erwin RA, Howard OMZ, Kirken RA, Malabarba MG, et al. Prolactin recruits STAT1, STAT3 and STAT5 independent of conserved receptor tyrosine TYR402, TYR479, TYR515 and TYR580. Mol Cell Endocrinol 1996;117:131–140.

24. Wakao H, Gouilleux F, Groner B. Mammary gland factor (MGF) is a novel member of the cytokine regulated transcription factor gene family and confers the prolactin response. EMBO J 1994;13:2182–2191.

25. Liu X, Robinson GW, Gouilleux F, Groner B, Hennighausen L. Cloning and expression of Stat5 and an additional homologue (Stat5b) involved in prolactin signal transduction in mouse mammary tissue. Proc Natl Acad Sci USA 1995;92:8831–8835.

26. Liu X, Robinson GW, Wagner KU, Garrett L, Wynshaw-Boris A, Hennighausen L. Stat5a is mandatory for adult mammary gland development and lactogenesis. Genes Dev 1996;11:179–186.

27. Das R, Vonderhaar BK. Activation of raf-1, MEK and MAP kinase in prolactin responsive mammary cells. Breast Cancer Res Treat 1996;40:141–149.

28. Darnell JE Jr, Kerr IM, Stark GR. Jak-STAT pathways and transcriptional activation in response to IFNs and other extracellular signaling proteins. Science 1994;264:1415–1421.

29. Berlanga JJ, Vara JAF, Martin-Perez J, Garcia-Ruiz JP. Prolactin receptor is associated with c-src kinase in rat liver. Mol Endocrinol 1995;9:1461–1467.

30. Clevenger CV, Medaglia MV. The protein tyrosine kinase p59fyn is associated with prolactin (PRL) receptor and is activated by PRL stimulation of T-lymphocytes. Mol Endocrinol 1994;8:674–681.

31. Clevenger CV, Ngo W, Sokol DL, Luger SM, Gewirtz AM. Vav is necessary for prolactin-stimulated proliferation and is translocated into the nucleus of a T-cell line. J Biol Chem 1995;270:13,246–13,253.

32. Ali S, Chen Z, Lebrun J-J, Vogel W, Kharitonenkov A, Kelly P, Ullrich A. PTP1D is a positive regulator of the prolactin signal leading to β-casein promoter activation. EMBO J 1996;15:135–142.

33. Daniel N, Waters MJ, Bignon C, Djiane J. Involvement of a subset of tyrosine kinases and phosphatases in regulation of the β-lactoglobulin gene promoter by prolactin. Mol Cell Endocrinol 1996;118:25–35.

34. Erwin RA, Kirken RA, Malabarba MG, Farrar WL, Rui H. Prolactin activates Ras via signaling proteins SHC, growth factor receptor bound 2 and son of sevenless. Endocrinology 1995;136:3512–3518.

35. Elberg G, Rapoport MJ, Vashdi-Elberg D, Gertler A, Scechter Y. Lactogenic hormones rapidly activate p21 ras/mitogen-activated protein kinase in Nb2-11C rat lymphoma cells. Endocrine 1996;4:65–71.

36. Clevenger CV, Torigoe T, Reed JC. Prolactin induces rapid phosphorylation and activation of prolactin receptor-associated RAF-1 kinase in a T-cell line. J Biol Chem 1994;269:5559–5565.

37. Buckley AR, Rao YP, Buckley DJ, Gout PW. Prolactin-induced phosphorylation and nuclear translocation of MAP kinase in Nb2 lymphoma cells. Biochem Biophys Res Commun 1994;204:1158–1164.

38. Ganguli S, Hu L, Menke P, Collier RJ, Gertler A. Nuclear accumulation of multiple protein kinases during prolactin-induced proliferation of Nb2 rat lymphoma cells. J Cell Physiol 1996;167:251–260.

39. Rillema JA, Wing LY, Foley KA. Effects of phospholipases on ornithine decarboxylase activity in mammary gland explants from midpregnancy mice. Endocrinology 1983;113:2024–2028.

40. Banerjee R, Vonderhaar BK. Prolactin induced protein kinase C activity in a mouse mammary epithelial cell line NOG-8. Mol Cell Endocrinol 1992;90:61–67.

41. Waters SB, Rillema JA. Role of protein kinase C in the prolactin-induced responses in mouse mammary gland explants. Mol Cell Endocrinol 1989;63:159–166.

42. Alsakkaf KA, Dobson PRM, Brown BL. Activation of phosphatidylinositol 3-kinase by prolactin in Nb2 cells. Biochem Biophys Res Commun 1996;221:779–784.

43. VanderKuur J, Allevato G, Billestrup N, Norstedt G, Carter-Su C. Growth hormone-promoted tyrosyl phosphorylation of SHC proteins and SHC association with Grb2. J Biol Chem 1995;270:7587–7593.

44. Das R, Vonderhaar BK. Involvement of SHC, Grb2, Sos and ras in prolactin signal transduction in mammary cells. Oncogene 1996;13:1139–1145.

45. David M, Petricoin E III, Benjamin C, Pine R, Weber MJ, Larner AC. Requirement for MAP Kinase (ERK2) activity in interferon α- and interferon β-stimulated gene expression through STAT proteins. Science 1995;269:1721–1723.

46. Zabala MT, Garcia-Ruiz JP. Regulation of expression of the messenger ribonucleic acid encoding the cytosolic form of phosphoenolpyruvate carboxykinase in liver and small intestine of lactating rats. Endocrinology 1989;125:2587–2593.

47. Buckley AR, Buckley DJ, Leff MA, Hoover DS, Magnuson NS. Rapid induction of pim-1 expression by prolactin and interleukin-2 in rat Nb2 lymphoma cells. Endocrinology 1995;136:5252–5259.

48. Stevens AN, Wang Y, Sieger KA, Lu H-F, Yu-Lee LY. Biphasic transcription regulation of the interferon regulatory factor-1 gene by prolactin: involvement of γ-interferon-activated sequence and stat-related proteins. Mol Endocrinol 1995;9:513–525.

49. Musgrove EA, Hui R, Sweeney KJE, Watts CKW, Sutherland RL. Cyclins and breast cancer. J Mammary Gland Biol Neoplasia 1996;1:153–162.

50. Sicinski P, Donaher JL, Parker SB, Li T, Fazeli A, Gardner H, et al. Cyclin D1 provides a link between development and oncogenesis in the retina and breast. Cell 1995;82:621–630.
51. Hosokawa Y, Onga T, Nakashima K. Induction of D2 and D3 cyclin-encoding genes during promotion of the G1/S transition by prolactin in rat Nb2 cells. Gene 1994;147:249–252.
52. Vonderhaar BK. Prolactin: transport function and receptors in mammary gland development and differentiation. In: Neville MC, Daniel CW, ed. The Mammary Gland. Plenum, New York, 1987, pp. 383–438.
53. Das R, Vonderhaar BK. Prolactin as a mitogen in mammary cells. J Mammary Gland Biol Neoplasia 1997;2:29–39.
54. Vonderhaar BK. Hormones and growth factors in mammary gland development. In: Veneziale CM, ed. Control of Cell Growth and Proliferation. Van Nostrand, New York, 1984, pp. 11–33.
55. Horseman ND, Zhao W, Montecino-Rodriguez E, Tanaka M, Nakashima K, Engle SJ, et al. Defective mammopoiesis, but normal hematopoiesis, in mice with a targeted disruption of the prolactin gene. EMBO J 1997;16:6926–6935.
56. Nagasawa H, Miur K, Niki K, Namiki H. Interrelationship between prolactin and progesterone in normal mammary gland growth in SHN virgin mice. Exp Clin Endocrinol 1985;86:357–360.
57. Muldoon TG. Interplay between estradiol and prolactin in the regulation of steroid hormone receptor levels, nature, and functionality in normal mouse mammary tissue. Endocrinology 1981;109:1339–1346.
58. Muldoon TG. Prolactin mediation of estrogen-induced changes in mammary tissue estrogen and progesterone receptors. Endocrinology 1987;121:141–149.
59. Vonderhaar BK, Bhattacharjee M. The mammary gland: a model for hormonal control of differentiation and preneoplasia. In: Mihich E, ed. Biological Responses in Cancer, vol. 4. Plenum, New York, 1985, pp. 125–159.
60. Muhlbock O, Boot LM. Induction of mammary cancer in mice without the mammary tumor agent by isografts of hypophyses. Cancer Res 1959;19:402–412.
61. Boyns AR, Buchan R, Cole EN, Forrest APM, Griffiths K. Basal prolactin blood levels in three strains of rat with differing incidence of 7,12–dimethylbenzanthracene-induced mammary tumors in rats. Eur J Cancer 1973;9:169–171.
62. Mershon J, Sall W, Mitchner N, Ben-Jonathan N. Prolactin is a local growth factor in rat mammary tumors. Endocrinology 1995;136:3619–3623.
63. Welsch CW, Gribler C. Prophylaxis of spontaneously developing mammary carcinoma in C3H/HeJ female mice by suppression of prolactin. Cancer Res 1973;33:2939–2946.
64. Welsch CW, Nagasawa H. Prolactin and murine mammary tumorigenesis: a review. Cancer Res 1977; 37:951–963.
65. Holtkamp W, Nagel GA, Wander HE, Rauschecker HF, VonHeyden D. Hyperprolactenemia is an indicator of progressive disease and poor prognosis in advanced breast cancer. Int J Cancer 1984;34:323–328.
66. Strungs I, Gray RA, Rigby HB, Strutton G. Two case reports of breast carcinoma associated with prolactinoma. Pathology 1997;29:320–323.
67. Biswas R, Vonderhaar BK. Role of serum in prolactin responsiveness of MCF-7 human breast cancer cells in long term tissue culture. Cancer Res 1987;47:3509–3514.
68. Love RR, Rose DP. Elevated bioactive prolactin in women at risk for familial breast cancer. Eur J Cancer Clin Oncol 1985;21:1553,1554.
69. Love RR, Rose DR, Surawicz TS, Newcomb PA. Prolactin and growth hormone levels in premenopausal women with breast cancer and healthy women with a strong family history of breast cancer. Cancer 1991;68:1401–1405.
70. Haus E, Lakatua DJ, Halberg F, Halberg E, Cornelissen G, Sackett LL, et al. Chronobiological studies of plasma prolactin in women in Kyushu, Japan and Minnesota, USA. J Clin Endocrinol Metab 1980; 51:632–640.
71. Holdaway IM, Mason BH, Gibbs EE, Rajasoorya C, Lethaby A, Hopkins KD, et al. Seasonal variation in the secretion of mammotrophic hormones in normal women and women with previous breast cancer. Breast Cancer Res Treat 1997;42:15–22.
72. Bhatavdekar JM, Patel DD, Vora HH, Ghosh N, Shah NG, Karelia NH, et al. Node-positive breast cancer: prognostic significance of the plasma prolactin compared with steroid receptors and clinicopathological features. Oncol Rep 1994;1:841–845.
73. Patel DD, Bhatavdekar JM, Chikhlikar PR, Ghosh N, Suthar TP, Shah NG, Mehta RH, Balar DB. Node negative breast carcinoma: hyperprolactinemia and/or overexpression of p53 as an independent predictor of poor prognosis compared to newer and established prognosticators. J Surg Oncol 1996;62:86–92.

74. Lissoni P, Barni S, Cazzaniga M, Ardizzoia A, Rovelli F, Tancici G, Brivio F, Frigerio F. Prediction of recurrence in operable breast cancer by postoperative changes in prolactin secretion. Oncology 1995;52:439–442.

75. Barni S, Lissoni P, Brivio F, Fumagalli L, Merlini D, Cataldo M, Rovelli F, Tancini G. Serum levels of insulin-like growth factor-I in operable breast cancer in relation to the main prognostic variables and their perioperative changes in relation to those of prolactin. Tumori 1994;80:212–215.

76. Purnell DM, Hillman EA, Heatfield BM, Trump BF. Immunoreactive prolactin in epithelial cells of normal and cancerous human breast and prostate detected by the unlabeled antibody peroxidase-anti-peroxidase method. Cancer Res 1982;42:2317–2324.

77. Agarwal PK, Tandon S, Agarwal AK, Kumar S. Highly specific sites of prolactin binding in benign and malignant breast disease. Indian J Exper Biol 1989;27:1035–1038.

78. Wang DY, Hampson S, Kwa HG, Moore JW, Bulbrook RD, Fentiman IS, et al. Serum prolactin levels in women with breast cancer and their relationship to survival. Eur J Cancer Clin Oncol 1986;22:487–492.

79. Ingram DM, Nottage EM, Roberts AN. Prolactin and breast cancer risk. Med J Aust 1990;153:469–473.

80. Henson JC, Coune A, Staquet M. Clinical trial of 2-Br-α-ergocryptine (CB154) in advanced breast cancer. Eur J Cancer 1972;8:155,156.

81. Pearson OH, Manni A. Hormonal control of breast cancer growth in women and rats. In: Martini L, James VHT, ed. Current Topics in Experimental Endocrinology. Academic, New York, 1978, pp. 75–92.

82. Manni A, Boucher AE, Demers LM, Harvey HA, Lipton A, Simmonds MA, Bartholomew M. Endocrine effects of combined somatostatin analog and bromocriptine therapy in women with advanced breast cancer. Breast Cancer Res Treat 1989;14:289–298.

83. Anderson E, Ferguson JE, Morten H, Shalet SM, Robinson EL, Howell A. Serum immunoreactive and bioactive lactogenic hormones in advanced breast cancer patients treated with bromocriptine and octeotide. Eur J Cancer 1993;29A:209–217.

84. Salih H, Brander W, Flax H, Hobbs JR. Prolactin dependence in human breast cancers. Lancet 1972;2:1103–1105.

85. Welsch CW, Iturri GC, Brennan MJ. DNA synthesis of human, mouse, and rat mammary carcinomas in vitro: influence of insulin and prolactin. Cancer 1976;38:1272–1281.

86. Peyrat JP, Djiane J, Bonneterre J, Vandewalle B, Vennin P, Delobelle A, Depadt G, Lefebvre J. Stimulation of DNA synthesis by prolactin in human breast tumor explants. Relation to prolactin receptors. Anticancer Res 1984;4:257–261.

87. Calaf G, Garrido F, Moyano C, Rodriguez R. Influence of hormones on DNA synthesis of breast tumors in culture. Breast Cancer Res Treat 1986;8:223–232.

88. Burke RE, Gaffney EV. Prolactin can stimulate general protein synthesis in human breast cancer cells (MCF-7) in long-term culture. Life Sci 1978;23:901–906.

89. Wilson GD, Woods KL, Walker RA, Howell A. Effect of prolactin on lactalbumin production by normal and malignant breast tissue in organ culture. Cancer Res 1980;40:486–489.

90. Malarkey WB, Kennedy M, Allred LE, Milo G. Physiological concentrations of prolactin can promote the growth of human breast tumor cells in culture. J Clin Endocrinol Metab 1983;56:673–677.

91. Manni A, Wright C, Davis G, Glenn J, Joehl R, Feil P. Promotion by prolactin of the growth of human breast neoplasms cultured in vitro in the soft agar clonogenic assay. Cancer Res 1986;46:1669–1672.

92. Shiu RP, Paterson JA. Alterations of cell shape, adhesion, and lipid accumulation in human breast cancer cells (T-47D) by human prolactin and growth hormone. Cancer Res 1984;44:1178–1186.

93. Shafie SM, Grantham FH. Role of hormones in the growth and regression of human breast cancer cells (MCF-7) transplanted into athymic nude mice. J Natl Cancer Inst 1981;67:51–56.

94. McManus MJ, Welsch CW. The effect of estrogen, progesterone, thyroxine, and human placental lactogen on DNA synthesis of human breast ductal epithelium maintained in athymic nude mice. Cancer 1984;54:1920–1927.

95. Vonderhaar BK. Prolactin: the forgotten hormone of human breast cancer. Pharmacol Ther 1998;79:169–178.

96. Das R, Ginsburg E, Vonderhaar BK. Tamoxifen as an antilactogen in human breast cancer cells, In: Rao RS, Deo MG, Sanghvi LD, Mittra I, ed. Proceedings of the International Cancer Congress. Monduzzi Editore, Bologna, 1994, pp. 1487–1491.

97. Lemus-Wilson A, Kelly PA, Blask DE. Melatonin blocks the stimulatory effects of prolactin on human breast cancer cell growth in culture. Br J Cancer 1995;72:1435–1440.

98. Ben-Jonathan N, Mershon JL, Allen DL, Steinmetz RW. Extrapituitary prolactin: distribution, regulation, functions, and clinical aspects. Endocr Rev 1996;17:639–669.

99. Lachelin GCL, Yen SSC, Alksne JF. Hormonal changes following hypophysectomy in humans. Obstet Gynecol 1977;50:333–339.

100. Sinha YN. Structural variants of prolactin: occurrence and physiological significance. Endocr Rev 1995;16:354–369.

101. Clevenger CV, Russell DH, Appasamy PM, Prystowsky MB. Regulation of IL-2-driven T-lymphocyte proliferation by prolactin. Proc Natl Acad Sci USA 1990;87:6460–6464.

102. Gellerson B, Kempf R, Teglmann R, DiMattia GE. Nonpituitary human prolactin gene transcription is independent of pit-1 and differentially controlled in lymphocytes and in endometrial stroma. Mol Endocrinol 1994;8:356–373.

103. Richards RG, Hartman SM. Human dermal fibroblast cells express prolactin in vitro. J Invest Dermatol 1996;106:1250–1255.

104. Vonderhaar BK. Prolactin in development of the mammary gland and reproductive tract. In: Dickson RB, Salomon DS, ed. Hormones and Growth Factors in Development and Neoplasia. Wiley-Liss, New York, 1998, pp. 193–206.

105. Nevalainen MJ, Valve EM, Ingleton PM, Nurmi M, Martikainen PM, Harkonen PL. Prolactin and prolactin receptors are expressed and functioning in human prostate. J Clin Invest 1997;99:618–627.

106. Steinmetz RW, Grant AL, Malven PV. Transcription of prolactin gene in milk secretory cells of the rat mammary gland. J Endocrinol 1993;36:271–276.

107. Kurtz A, Bristol LA, Toth BE, Lazar-Wesley E, Takacs L, Kacsoh B. Mammary epithelial cells of lactating rats express prolactin messenger ribonucleic acid. Biol Reproduction 1993;48:1095–1103.

108. LeProvost F, Leroux C, Martin P, Gaye P, Djiane J. Prolactin gene expression in ovine and caprine mammary gland. Neuroendocrinology 1994;60:305–313.

109. Ginsburg E, Vonderhaar BK. Prolactin synthesis and secretion by human breast cancer cells. Cancer Res 1995;55:2591–2595.

110. Ginsburg E, Das R, Vonderhaar BK. Prolactin: an autocrine growth factor in the mammary gland. In: Wilde CJ, Peaker M, Taylor E, eds. Biological Signalling in the Mammary Gland. Hannah Institute, Ayr, Scotland, 1997, pp. 47–58.

111. Bancroft FC, Tashjian AH. Growth in suspension culture of rat pituitary cells which produce growth hormone and prolactin. Exp Cell Res 1971;64:125–128.

112. Tanaka T, Shiu RPC, Gout PW, Beer CT, Noble RL, Friesen HG. New sensitive and specific bioassay for lactogenic hormones: measurement of prolactin and growth hormone in human serum. J Clin Endocrinol Metab 1980;51:1058–1063.

113. Emanuele NV, Jurgens JK, Halloran MM, Tentler JJ, Lawerence AM, Kelley MR. The rat prolactin gene is expressed in brain tissue: detection of normal and alternatively spliced prolactin messenger RNA. Mol Endocrinol 1992;6:35–42.

114. Shaw-Bruha CM, Pirrucello SJ, Shull JD. Expression of the prolactin gene in normal and neoplastic human breast tissues and human mammary cell lines: promoter usage and alternative mRNA splicing. Breast Cancer Res Treat 1997;4:243–253.

115. Markoff E, Sigel MB, Lacour N, Seavey BK, Friesen HG, Lewis UJ. Glycosylation selectively alters the biological activity of prolactin. Endocrinology 1988;123:1303–1306.

116. Lewis UL, Singh RNP, Lewis LJ. Two forms of glycosylated prolactin have different pigeon crop sac-stimulating activities. Endocrinology 1989;124:1558–1563.

117. Walker AM. Phosphorylated and nonphosphorylated prolactin isoforms. Trends Endocrinol Metab 1994;5:195–200.

118. Wicks JR, Brooks CL. Biological activity of phosphorylated and dephosphorylated bovine prolactin. Mol Cell Endocrinol 1995;112:223–229.

119. Pellegrini I, Lebrun JJ, Ali S, Kelly PA. Expression of prolactin and its receptors in human lymphoid cells. Mol Endocrinol 1992;6:1023–1031.

120. Sinha YN, DePaolo LV, Haro LS, Singh RNP, Jacobsen BP, Scott KE, Lewis UJ. Isolation and biochemical properties of four forms of glycosylated porcine prolactin. Mol Cell Endocrinol 1991;80: 203–213.

121. Hoffman T, Penel C, Ronin C. Glycosylation of human prolactin regulates hormone bioactivity and metabolic clearance. J Endocrinol Invest 1993;16:807–816.

122. Price AE, Loginenko KB, Higgins EA, Cole ES, Richards S. Studies on the microheterogeneity and in vitro activity of glycosylated and nonglycosylated recombinant human prolactin separated using a novel purification process. Endocrinology 1995;136:4827–4833.

123. Young KH, Buhi WC, Horseman N, Davis J, Kraeling R, Linzer D, Bozer FW. Biological activities of glycosylated and nonglycosylated porcine prolactin. Mol Cell Endocrinol 1990;71:155–162.

124. Lkhider M, Delpal S, Olivier-Bousquet M. Rat prolactin in serum, milk and mammary tissue: characterization and intracellular localization. Endocrinology 1996;137:4969–4979.

125. Wong VLY, Compton MM, Witorsch RJ. Proteolytic modification of rat prolactin by subcellular fractions of the lactating rat mammary gland. Biochim Biophys Acta 1986;881:167–175.

126. Baldocchi RA, Tan L, Hom YK, Nicoll CS. Comparison of the ability of normal mouse mammary tissues and mammary adenocarcinoma to cleave rat prolactin. Proc Soc Exp Biol Med 1995;208: 283–287.

127. Ferrara N, Clapp C, Weiner R. The 16K fragment of prolactin specifically inhibits basal and fibroblast growth factor stimulated growth of capillary endothelial cells. Endocrinology 1991;129:896–900.

128. D'Angelo G, Struman I, Martial J, Weiner RI. Activation of mitogen-activated protein kinases by vascular endothelial growth factor and basic fibroblast growth factor in capillary endothelial cells is inhibited by the antiangiogenic factor 16-kDa N-terminal fragment of prolactin. Proc Natl Acad Sci USA 1995;92:6374–6378.

129. Yoshiji H, Harris SR, Thorgeirsson UP. Vascular endothelial growth factor is essential for initial but not continued in vivo growth of human breast carcinoma cells. Cancer Res 1997;57:3924–3928.

130. Fan G, Rillema JA. Prolactin stimulation of protein kinase C in isolated mouse mammary gland nuclei. Horm Metab Res 1993;25:564–568.

131. Fuh G, Cunningham BCRF, Nagata S, Goeddel DV, Wells JA. Rational design of potent antagonists to the human growth hormone receptor. Science 1992;256:1677–1679.

132. Fuh G, Colosi P, Wood WI, Wells JA. Mechanism-based design of prolactin receptor antagonists. J Biol Chem 1993;268:5376–5381.

133. Fuh G, Wells JA. Prolactin receptor antagonists that inhibit the growth of breast cancer cell lines. J Biol Chem 1995;270:13,133–13,137.

134. Dattani MT, Hindmarsh PC, Brook GD, Robinson ICAF, Kopchick JJ, Marshall NJ. G120R, a human growth hormone antagonist, shows zinc-dependent agonist and antagonist activity on Nb2 cells. J Biol Chem 1995;270:9222–9226.

135. Mode A, Tollet P, Wells T, Carmignac DF, Clark RG, Chen WY, Kopchick JJ, Robinson ICAF. The human growth hormone (hGH) antagonist G120RhGH does not antagonize GH in the rat but has paradoxical agonist activity, probably via the prolactin receptor. Endocrinology 1996;137:447–454.

136. Vonderhaar BK, Banerjee R. Is tamoxifen also an antilactogen? Mol Cell Endocr 1991;79:C159–C163.

137. Hawkins RA, Roberts MM, Forest APM. Estrogen receptors and breast cancer: current status. Br J Surg 1980;67:153–169.

138. Furr BJA, Jordan VC. The pharmacology and clinical uses of tamoxifen. Pharmac Ther 1984;25:127–205.

139. Nolvadex Adjuvant Trial Organization. Controlled trial of tamoxifen as single adjuvant agent in management of early breast cancer. Lancet 1985;i:836–839.

140. Sutherland RL, Watts CKW, Hall RE, Ruenitz PC. Mechanism of growth inhibition by nonsteroidal antioestrogens in human breast cancer cells. J Steroid Biochem 1987;27:891–897.

141. Green MD, Whybourne AM, Taylor IW, Sutherland RL. Effects of antioestrogens on the growth and cell cycle kinetics of cultured human mammary carcinoma cells. In: Sutherland RL, Jordan VC, ed. Non-Steroidal Antiestrogens: Molecular Pharmacology and Antitumor Actions. Academic, New York, 1981, pp. 397–412.

142. Chouvet C, Vicard E, Frappart L, Falette N, Lefebvre MF, Saez S. Growth inhibitory effect of 4-hydroxy-tamoxifen on the BT-20 mammary cancer cell line. J Steroid Biochem 1988;31:655–663.

143. Pollak M, Constantino J, Polychronakas C, Blauer HG, Guyda H, Redmond C, Fisher B, Margolese R. Effect of tamoxifen on serum insulin-like growth factor I levels of stage I breast cancer patients. J Natl Cancer Inst 1990;82:1693–1697.

144. O'Brian CA, Liskamp RM, Solomon DH, Weinstein IB. Inhibition of protein kinase C by tamoxifen. Cancer Res 1985;45:2462–2465.

145. Das R, Biswas R, Vonderhaar BK. Characteristics of the antilactogen binding site in mammary gland membranes. Mol Cell Endocrinol 1993;98:1–8.

146. Sutherland RL, Foo MS. Differential binding of antiestrogen by rat uterine and chick oviduct cytosol. Biochem Biophys Res Commun 1979;91:183–191.

147. Sutherland RL, Murphy LC, Foo MS, Green MD, Whybourne AM, Krozowski ZS. High-affinity antioestrogen binding sites distinct from the oestrogen receptor. Nature 1980;288:273–275.

148. Gulino A, Pasqualini JR. Heterogeneity of binding sites for tamoxifen and tamoxifen derivatives in estrogen target and non-target fetal organs of guinea pig. Cancer Res 1982;42:1913–1921.

149. Mehta RG, Cerny WL, Moon RC. Distribution of antiestrogen-specific binding sites in normal and neoplastic mammary gland. Oncology 1984;41:387–392.

150. Faye JC, Fargin A, Valette A, Bayard F. Antiestrogens, different sites of action than the estrogen receptor? Hormone Res 1987;28:202–211.

151. Das R, Vonderhaar BK. Tamoxifen inhibits prolactin signal transduction in estrogen receptor negative NOG-8 mammary epithelial cells. Cancer Lett 1997;116:41–46.

152. Biswas R, Vonderhaar BK. Tamoxifen inhibition of prolactin action in the mouse mammary gland. Endocrinology 1991;128:532–538.

153. Biswas R, Vonderhaar BK. Antiestrogen inhibition of prolactin induced growth of the Nb2 rat lymphoma cell line. Cancer Res 1989;49:6295–6299.

154. Vonderhaar BK. Prolactin and breast cancer: the new chapter. Women Cancer 1999;1:7–20.

8

Human Chorionic Gonadotropin in Breast Cancer Prevention

Jose Russo, MD *and I. H. Russo,* MD

CONTENTS

INTRODUCTION

Breast cancer (BC) is the most common cancer diagnosed in American and Northern European women, and the number one cause of cancer-related death in nonsmokers *(1,2)*. Although a reduction in the mortality caused by this disease has been observed in the United States during the past few years, the incidence of BC is progressively and steadily increasing in most Western countries, and in societies that are becoming westernized *(3–5)*. Although the reasons for this increase are uncertain, epidemiological and clinical evidence indicates that endocrinological and reproductive influences play major roles in this phenomenon. It has long been known that the incidence of BC is greater in nulliparous than in parous women *(5–7)*. Changes in lifestyle, which in turn influence the endocrinology of women, have been observed during recent decades in American women, namely, a progressive decrease in the age of menarche *(5)* and a progressive increase in the age at which a woman bears her first child *(6)*.

The significance of these changes is highlighted by the reduction in BC risk associated with late menarche and the completion of a full term pregnancy before age 24 yr, with

From: *Contemporary Endocrinology: Endocrine Oncology*
Edited by: S. P. Ethier © Humana Press Inc., Totowa, NJ

further reduction in the lifetime BC risk as the number of pregnancies increases *(5–7)*. Women who undergo their first full-term pregnancy after age 30 yr, on the other hand, appear to be at higher risk of BC development than nulliparous women, suggesting that parity-induced protection against BC is related to the timing of a first full-term pregnancy. Although pregnancy appears to have a dual effect on BC risk, a transient increase (relative to nulliparous women), lasting 10–15 yr, followed thereafter by a decreased risk, the protection conferred lasts a lifetime *(6)*. Women from different countries and ethnic groups exhibit a similar degree of parity-induced protection from BC, regardless of the endogenous incidence of this malignancy *(8,9)*. This observation suggests that the reduction in BC risk associated with early first full-term pregnancy does not result from factors specific to a particular environmental, genetic, or socioeconomic setting, but rather from an intrinsic effect of parity on the biology of the breast (which nevertheless may be modified by environmental, genetic, or other factors) *(4–11)*.

These observations indicate that an early first full-term pregnancy modifies, through mechanisms still poorly understood, specific biological characteristics of the breast, which result in a lifetime decreased risk of cancer development. This protection has been attributed, in great part, to the induction of terminal differentiation of the mammary gland, a mechanism that has been found to reduce the susceptibility of the mammary epithelium to carcinogenesis *(7,8,12–18)*. These observations indicate that the terminally differentiated state of lactation should be reached for attaining protection, although other mechanisms have been proposed for the protective effect of early first full-term pregnancy, including the occurrence of sustained changes in the level or regulation of hormones that affect the breast *(19,20)*. Regardless of the intervening mechanism, the end result of the first pregnancy is a dramatic modification of the architecture of the breast *(16–18)*.

NORMAL BREAST DEVELOPMENT

The development of the breast is the result of a combined process of growth of the mammary parenchyma and stromal changes. This process, which is initiated at childhood, is manifested as the elongation and branching of ducts: It proceeds during puberty through sprouting of lobular structures, which evolve from the undifferentiated lobule type 1 (Lob 1) to the more differentiated Lob 2 and Lob 3, which originate under the cyclic hormonal stimulation of the ovaries. Full differentiation to Lob 4 is achieved by the end of pregnancy and during lactation *(16,17)*. Lob 1, which are more frequently found in the breast of young nulliparous women, have a high rate of cell proliferation and a high content of estrogen (ER) and progesterone (PR) receptors. Both the rate of epithelial cell (EC) proliferation and the content of steroid hormone receptors decrease progressively in the more differentiated Lob 2 and Lob 3, reaching their lowest values in the fully differentiated secretory Lob 4 *(21–23)*. The more differentiated lobules express, instead, specific markers associated with cell differentiation, such as inhibin *(24–26)* and mammary-derived growth inhibitor *(27)*.

EFFECT OF HUMAN CHORIONIC GONADOTROPIN TREATMENT ON MAMMARY GLAND DEVELOPMENT AND CARCINOGENESIS

The direct association of BC risk with nulliparity, as well as the protection afforded by early first full-term pregnancy, have been in great part explained by experimental studies. This and other laboratories have demonstrated that mammary cancer in rodents can be induced with chemical carcinogens, such as dimethylbenz[a]anthracene (DMBA) or N-methyl-N-nitrosourea only in the young nulliparous females; completion of pregnancy prior to carcinogen exposure prevents carcinoma development *(7,12–15,19,20, 28,29)*. This preventive effect has been attributed to the differentiation of the mammary gland induced by pregnancy. In the DMBA model, the authors have successfully reproduced this effect by treating virgin rats with human chorionic gonadotropin (hCG) *(28–32)*.

Mechanism of Action of hCG

Chorionic gonadotropin (CG) is a glycoprotein hormone first secreted by the fertilized egg, and later by the placenta *(33)*. The detection of hCG in the maternal circulation is the only established way of determining the presence of pregnancy *(33)*. The best known function of hCG in the female is the maintenance of the corpus luteum, through its interaction with a receptor shared with pituitary (pit) luteinizing hormone (LH), and the lutropin-choriogonadotropin-receptor (LH-CG-R) present in the granulosa and luteal cells of the ovary *(34)*. Upon interaction with its receptor, CG increases adenylyl cyclase activity, an effect mediated by intracellular-membrane-associated G proteins. This, in turn, results in cAMP increases, leading to steroid and polypeptide hormone synthesis, with resulting increases in serum levels of estrogen and progesterone in most species. Inhibin has been also found to be elevated in hCG-treated women *(33–36)*.

Mammary Gland Development Under Influence of hCG

The study of mammary gland development in the rat requires an evaluation of changes in the parenchyma of the gland, because, unlike in women, no significant external changes occur in this organ after puberty *(13,26,37)*. The six pairs of mammary glands of the young virgin rat are composed of ducts ending in club-shaped terminal end buds (TEBs), which are multilayered structures measuring 100–140 µm in diameter. They are lined by a 3–10-layer thick cuboidal epithelium that rests on a discontinuous layer of myo-ECs *(37)*. After the beginning of ovarian function, the mammary ducts undergo further longitudinal lengthening and branching with sprouting of a few alveolar buds, which progressively evolve to lobular structures. The lobules found in the rat mammary gland can be classified according to their degree of development as Lob 1, which consists of clusters of approx 10 ± 4 ductules per unit. Individual ductules are lined by a single layer of cuboidal ECs and few myo-ECs. With further growth, Lob 1 evolves to Lob 2, which is larger, and composed of approx 40 ± 7 ductules; these progress to Lob 3, which contain approx 60 ± 12 ductules or alveoli per lobule *(32)*.

The administration of 100 IU/hCG/d for 40 d, to young virgin rats, dramatically affects the development of the mammary gland, modifying profoundly the relative proportions of Lob 1, Lob 2, and Lob 3. Although the concentration of Lob 1 in the mammary gland of untreated or saline-injected control virgin rats decreases slightly as a consequence of aging, in hCG-treated animals, the number of Lob 1 begins to decrease by d 10 of hormonal treatment, and decreases further between d 20 and 40 (Fig. 1). After cessation of treatment, their number increases sharply, reaching the same values found in control animals. Lob 2 are practically nonexistent in the 45-d-old animals; they first become evident when the animals reach the age of 75 d, and their percentage increases even further in the next 10 d, reaching its peak in 85-d-old animals, remaining unchanged thereafter (Fig. 1). Under hCG treatment, the Lob 2 develop in a biphasic pattern. Their concentration increases progressively from 70 to 85 d of age, decrease significantly by

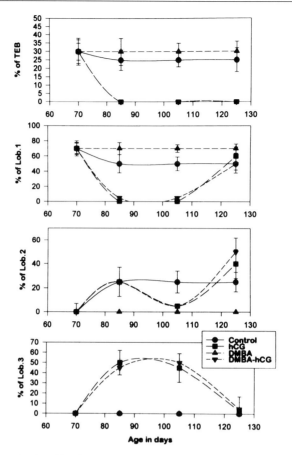

Fig. 1. Percenteage of terminal end buds (TEB), lobules type 1 (Lob 1), lobules type 2 (Lob 2), and lobules type 3 (Lob 3) in control; hCG, animals injected daily with 100 IU hCG from 65 to 105 d of age; DMBA, rats treated with DMBA when they were 45 d old, followed by a daily ip saline injection, and DMBA + hCG, animals treated with DMBA at the age of 45 d, and daily with hCG from 65 to 105 d of age. Five animals per group were sacrificed at each one of the age periods indicated.

the time the animals reach the age of 105 d, and increase again after cessation of treatment (Fig. 1). Lob 3 formation, on the other hand, starts at d 10 of treatment, increases progressively between d 20 and 40, and decreases only after cessation of the hormonal treatment, because of their regression to Lob 2. The resulting recovery of this type of lobule is absent in control animals (Fig. 1).

Hormonal Profile Induced by hCG

The evaluation of the effect of hCG on the development of the mammary gland requires one to assess the effect of this hormone on two important endocrine organs: the ovary and the pituitary gland. Evaluation of the hormonal profile at various times during and after hCG treatment requires determination of serum levels of the β-subunit of the injected hCG, as well as determination of the levels of the ovarian hormones, estrogen, P, and inhibin, and the pituitary hormones, prolactin (PRL), follicle-stimulating hormone (FSH), and LH *(38,39)*.

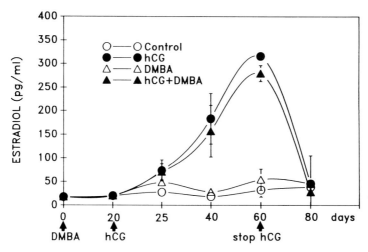

Fig. 2. Estrogen serum levels. Mean ± SD of 5–10 animals/group. Groups as in Fig. 1. Abscissa: days after DMBA treatment.

Serum Levels of β-hCG

The determination of the serum levels of the β-subunit of hCG by radioimmunoassay revealed that this hormone was completely absent at the beginning of treatment and in control animals. By the fifth day of treatment, it had reached a level of 2,845±575 mIU/mL. The levels remained elevated until d 20, declining rapidly thereafter, despite continuous administration of the hormone for an additional 20 d. The progressive increase in hCG serum levels paralleled the increase in ovarian size, which occurred because of the increased number and size of corpora lutea. Ovarian-size returned to normal after cessation of the hormonal treatment *(38)*.

Serum Levels of Ovarian Hormones

In control animals, serum estradiol levels ranged from 32.4 to 50.2 pg/mL, with no significant variations observed in association with aging. Serum estradiol levels were elevated in hCG-treated animals. Maximal values were observed between d 20 and 40 of hormonal treatment (Fig. 2). The levels of estradiol decreased below those of the controls in the hCG-treated group after the fortieth injection, and even further 20 d later *(39)*.

P levels were significantly elevated in hCG-treated groups in comparison to control animals (Fig. 3). The serum levels of P peaked between d 20 and 40 of hormonal treatment. In the hCG group, the serum levels dropped to the levels observed in the controls by the time of the fortieth injection, and they remained low by 20 d after cessation of treatment *(39)*.

Serum Levels of Pituitary Hormones

Serum levels of the pituitary hormone, LH, were similar in all groups of animals studied, ranging from 3.2 to 8.5 ng/mL. It became evident that hCG treatment had no significant effect on the synthesis and/or secretion of LH, because the levels of LH measured in the serum of saline-treated rats were not significantly different from the levels in the hCG-treated groups *(39)*. Serum FSH levels of female rats were not modified by treatment with hCG. All groups of animals had similar FSH levels, and no changes in serum levels were

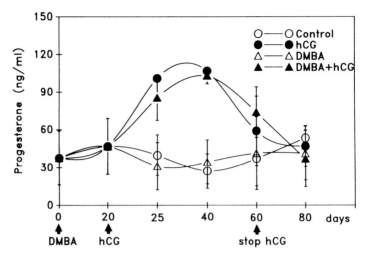

Fig. 3. Progesterone serum levels. Mean ± SD of 5–10 animals/group. Abbreviations as in Fig. 1. Abscissa: days after DMBA treatment.

observed with aging. The daily injections of hCG neither stimulated nor inhibited its production *(39)*. The serum levels of PRL were not modified by aging. The hormonal treatment moderately affected PRL levels, since an elevation in serum levels was observed in hCG-treated groups, but the differences with controls were not significant *(39)*.

Administration of hCG to young virgin rats raised the serum levels of estrogen and progesterone, but the levels of PRL, FSH, LH, and inhibin were not modified significantly by the hormonal treatment *(38,39)*. The increment in estrogen and P levels induced by hCG was accompanied by an increase in the size of the ovaries, which was mostly caused by the enlargement of the corpora lutea. These effects were transient, because ovarian size regressed to normal values as early as 5 d after cessation of the hormonal treatment. The effect of hCG treatment on the mammary gland, however, persisted even after the cessation of treatment, indicating that the hormonal milieu induced by hCG sufficed for differentiating the mammary epithelium.

ROLE OF PREGNANCY AND hCG
IN MAMMARY CANCER INHIBITION

The direct association of BC risk with the prolongation in the period encompassed between menarche and the first full-term pregnancy, as well as the protection afforded by pregnancy, have been partially explained by experimental studies performed in this laboratory *(7,12,28–32)*. The authors have demonstrated that mammary cancer in rodents can be induced with the polycyclic hydrocarbon, DMBA, preferentially when the carcinogen is administered to young nulliparous females *(40)*. Those females that have completed a full-term pregnancy prior to carcinogen exposure fail to develop carcinomas *(7,12–15)*. The authors have demonstrated that the inhibitory effect of pregnancy on mammary cancer initiation is mediated by hCG, because virgin rats, treated for 21 d with a daily intraperitoneal injection of this hormone prior to carcinogen administration, exhibit a dose-related reduction in tumor incidence and multiplicity *(26,28–32)*. This phenomenon is in great part mediated by the induction of mammary gland differentiation, inhibition of cell proliferation, increase in the DNA repair capabilities of the mammary epithelium, decreased binding of the carcinogen to the DNA, and activation of genes controling programmed cell death (PCD) *(12,28–32,41–43)*. The activation of these genes by hCG is of great relevance, because PCD is a physiological and phylogenetically conserved form of active cell death (or apoptosis), which has been associated with specific phases of development that control cell proliferation and differentiation *(41–43)*.

ROLE OF hCG IN BC PROGRESSION

The authors' studies of the protective effect of hCG-induced differentiation on experimental mammary carcinogenesis led to postulation of the possibility that hCG may be useful in preventing the development of BC in women. The fact that the time of initiation of BC in the female population is not known represented a major drawback for accomplishing the goal of instituting a truly preventative hormonal treatment. Thus, it has to be assumed that all women are at risk of being carriers of initiated lesions. This assumption requires that, before hormonal treatment is undertaken, it has to be proven that it either inhibits the progression of initiated cells, or at least does not cause tumor progression. Based on previous observations that the chemical carcinogen, DMBA, induces neoplastic transformation in the mammary gland by acting on the highly proliferating TEBs of the virgin animal *(7,12,37)*, and that, once initiated, these structures progress to intraductal proliferations (IDPs) within 3 wk of exposure to the carcinogen *(7,37)*, the authors tested the effect of hCG on tumor progression by administering 8 mg DMBA/100 g body wt to 45-d-old virgin Sprague-Dawley rats. Twenty d later, when IDPs were already evident, the animals were treated with 100 IU/hCG/d for 40 d (DMBA + hCG group). Age-matched, untreated, hCG–, and DMBA + saline-treated rats were used as controls. Tissues were collected at the time of DMBA administration, and at 5, 10, 20, and 40 d of hCG injection, and 20 d postcessation of treatment *(43)*.

Effect of hCG on TEBs, Intraductal Proliferations, and Ductal Carcinomas In Situ

The mammary gland of 45-d-old virgin rats contains the highest number of TEBs. In animals of the saline control group, the number of TEBs decreased slightly as a function of age, as has been previously described *(23)*; in the DMBA group, their number remained constant. In both hCG-treated groups, a diminution in the relative percentage of TEBs was observed as early as 5 d after the initiation of treatment, and more sharply between d 10 and d 20 before reaching a plateau. The percentage of TEBs in these two groups of animals was significantly lower than the values found in the saline control and DMBA groups ($P < 0.01$) (Fig. 4). A more noticeable effect of the hormonal treatment occurred at the level of IDPs and ductal carcinomas *in situ* (DCIS) (Fig. 4). In DMBA-treated animals there were 5.80 IDPs/gland when they reached the age of 105 d, which is, 25-fold higher than the values observed in the hCG-treated animals, in which there were 0.23 IDP/gland. These differences were still significant in the 125-d-old animals.

The number of DCIS was also higher in the DMBA-treated group, and their number was decreased 13-fold by hCG treatment. The number of DCIS increased slightly when the animals reached the age of 125 d, averaging 1.76 DCIS/gland; however, this was still significantly lower than that observed in the DMBA group of animals, which contained 23 DCIS/gland (Fig. 4). Occasional lactating adenomas were observed in both hCG and DMBA + hCG-treated animals *(43)*.

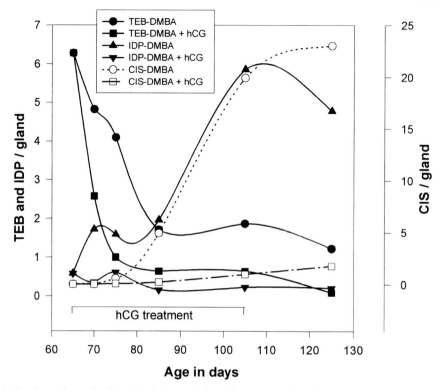

Fig. 4. Number of terminal end buds (TEB), intraductal proliferations (IDP) (lefthand side ordinate), and carcinoma in situ (CIS) (righthand side ordinate) in animals treated with DMBA when they were 45 d old, followed by a daily ip saline injection (DMBA) or hCG from 65 to 105 d of age (DMBA + hCG).

Effect of hCG Treatment on DMBA-Induced Tumor Progression

Although mammary tumors were palpated as early as 25 and 30 d postcarcinogen administration in the DMBA + hCG and DMBA groups, respectively, none of the animals in the saline control or the hCG-treated groups developed tumors. In the group of animals treated with DMBA, the number of palpable tumors continued increasing until the end of the experiment. In the DMBA + hCG group, the number of palpable tumors reached a plateau when the animals were 105 d old, and no additional tumors were detected in the 125-d-old animals. The highest total number of tumors and number of tumors per animal were observed in the DMBA group; the DMBA + hCG group showed a reduction in the total number of palpable tumors and number of tumors per animal at all time-points studied. The histopathological analysis of both palpable tumors and microscopic lesions revealed that most of them were adenocarcinomas with papillary, cribriform, or comedo features. Only three fibroadenomas developed in the DMBA and two in the DMBA + hCG groups, respectively. The hormonal treatment more noticeably reduced the incidence of adenocarcinomas, from 8.3 in the DMBA to 1.8 adenocarcinomas per animal in the DMBA + hCG group (Fig. 5; *43*).

hCG treatment inhibited the progression of mammary carcinomas by stopping the development of early lesions, i.e., IDPs and carcinomas *in situ* (CIS). These findings indicated that hCG has a significant potential as a chemopreventive agent, not only before

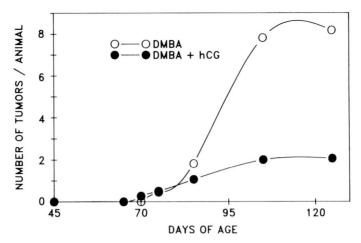

Fig. 5. Number of palpable tumors per animal in rats treated with DMBA when they were 45 d old, followed by a daily ip saline injection (DMBA) or hCG from 65 to 105 d of age (DMBA + hCG).

the cell is initiated, but after the carcinogenic process has been initiated, and is vigorously progressing. The authors' report was the first to indicate that a hormone preventive agent, such as hCG, is able to stop initiated cells by inhibiting the formation of the intermediate step, represented by the CIS *(38–43)*.

EFFECT OF hCG ON INHIBIN EXPRESSION AND ITS RELATION TO ACTIVATION OF EARLY-RESPONSE GENES

The authors' observations that the hCG-induced differentiation of the mammary gland is associated with the synthesis of inhibin, a heterodimeric protein that is structurally related to the transforming growth factor-β (TGF-β) family *(24,25,35,36,44)*, led to test of whether inhibin was also involved in the regression of DMBA-induced rat mammary carcinomas. For these purposes, virgin rats that received 8 mg DMBA/100 g body wt, when they were 45 d old, were injected 20 d later with 100 IU/hCG/d for 40 d, as described above. Corresponding age-matched controls received saline, hCG-, or DMBA + saline treatments. Mammary glands and ovaries were collected at the time of DMBA administration, and at 5, 10, 20, and 40 d of hCG injection, and 20 d postcessation of treatment *(43)*. Total and polyadenylated RNAs were probed for inhibin A, B, c-myc, c-fos, and c-jun. The mammary glands of hCG-treated animals exhibited elevated expression of inhibin A (1.5–4-fold) and inhibin B (1.5–3-fold), from d 5 of hCG treatment to 20 d posttreatment. The expression of these genes was also enhanced by hCG in the DMBA-treated group; no changes occurred in the animals treated with DMBA alone. The hormonal treatment markedly increased the expression of c-myc and c-jun by 4–7-fold and 2–3-fold, respectively. No significant changes were found in the levels of c-fos expression, and DMBA treatment alone did not modify the expression of these genes. Immunohistochemical staining showed a strong immunoreactivity for inhibin α- and β-subunits in the lobular epithelium. Inhibin expression became evident by d 10 of treatment, reaching a peak of expression by d 20. A similar pattern of reactivity was observed in animals treated with hCG alone, or after DMBA. The expression of both inhibin subunits remained elevated until 20 d posthormone withdrawal, even though the lobular structures had

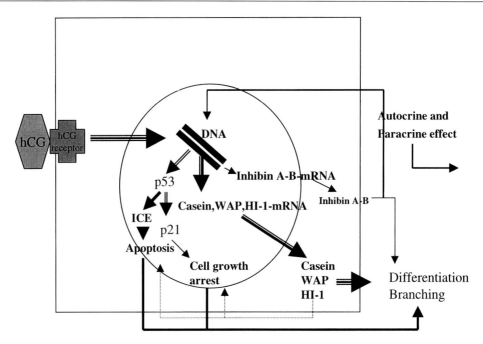

Fig. 6. Postulated mechanism of action of hCG. The hormone binds to a specific membrane receptor, activating genes identified to be specific for pregnancy- or hCG-induced differentiation, and that have been found to be correlated with the lobular development of the mammary tissue. Thus, a pathway of activation of p53 and ICE may lead to apoptosis, or through p21 to cell growth arrest. Activation of inhibin α and β, and of the milk proteins, casein, whey acidic protein (WAP), and HI-1, may lead to differentiation through autocrine or paracrine mechanisms.

involuted from the well-developed secretory Lob 3 and Lob 4 to Lob 2 and Lob 1. The finding that c-*myc* and c-*jun* were also elevated at the time of maximal inhibin synthesis indicated that early-response genes could be involved in the pathway of hCG-inhibin-induced synthesis (Fig. 6; *46–48*).

The expression of both inhibin α and β was increased in the mammary gland of rats treated with hCG, either alone or after DMBA, but it was absent in the mammary gland of the saline control and DMBA groups. The inhibin mRNA levels were maximal by d 20 of treatment, but they remained elevated, even after hormone withdrawal. The changes observed at the mRNA level were confirmed at protein level, since immunocytochemical stains revealed increased expression of inhibin α- and β-subunits in the cytoplasm of lobular ECs. Inhibin was immunocytochemically detected, even in the lobules that had regressed after hormone withdrawal. There were differences, however, in the pattern of inhibin distribution between those animals treated with hCG alone and those that received DMBA before the hCG. In the former, both inhibin subunits were diffusely distributed in the cytoplasm of the lobular ECs; in the DMBA + hCG group, inhibin tended to form clumps in localized areas of the cytoplasm. The effect of hCG was accompanied by a significant activation of c-*myc* and c-*jun*, while c-*fos* was not modified by the treatment. These early genes remained activated, even after the cessation of hCG treatment, an indication that their expression was regulated by the hCG treatment in a fashion similar to that described for inhibin. Even though inhibin belongs to the TGF-β family, hCG treatment did not affect the level of expression of TGF-β, or of other members of this family. The authors' results clearly support the concept that hCG acts as an inducer of inhibin, and early-response gene expression, even in the mammary gland affected by a chemical carcinogen. Although more work needs to be done to understand the mechanisms mediating hCG's effect on gene activation, our results indicate that both inhibin subunits can be used as intermediate surrogate markers for evaluating the effect of hCG in the mammary gland.

EFFECT OF hCG ON PCD GENE EXPRESSION

The mammary glands of hCG– and DMBA + hCG groups of animals showed elevated expression of testosterone repressed prostate message 2 (TRPM2) and interleukin-1β-converting enzyme (ICE) transcripts as early as 5 d after initiation of treatment (70-d-old groups): Their values remained elevated at all subsequent time-points tested, and up to 20 d posttreatment (125-d-old groups) *(43)*. The hormonal treatment induced an increase of 2.5–5-fold and 1.5–5-fold in the expression of TRPM2 and ICE transcripts, respectively. Maximal induction was observed in the animals sacrificed at the ages of 85 and 105 d. DMBA treatment alone, on the other hand, did not modify, or even slightly reduce, the expression of TRPM2 and ICE transcripts, since the values found were similar to those of the respective control groups. The product of the proto-oncogene, *bcl2* and one of its family members, *bcl*-XL, are known to play a role in promoting cell survival and inhibiting apoptosis, and expression of *bcl*-XS is associated with the induction of apoptosis. The authors examined, by Northern blot analysis, the effects of hCG treatment on the mRNA expression of *bcl2*, *bcl*-XL and *bcl*-XS. Results demonstrated that neither DMBA nor hCG treatments had an effect on the expression of *bcl2* and *bcl*-XL at any of the time periods tested. Treatment with hCG, either alone or after DMBA, on the other hand, induced the expression of *bcl*-XS, an effect that was not observed in the DMBA-treated group *(43)*.

In order to determine whether the activation of PCD genes by hCG was dependent on *p53* and *c-myc*, the authors studied their expression at different time periods after the initiation of the hormonal treatment. hCG treatment induced an increase in the expression of *p53* (3–5-fold) and *c-myc* (2–4-fold) in the mammary gland. This increased expression was maintained from d 5 of treatment (70-d-old animals) until 20 d posttreatment (125-d-old animals). DMBA treatment did not modify the expression of these genes, but, in the DMBA + hCG group, a dramatic increase in the expression of p53 (10–14-fold increase) and *c-myc* (sevenfold increase) was noted in the groups of animals sacrificed at the ages of 85 and 105 d. These findings indicated that the induction of PCD observed in the mammary gland of hCG-treated animals, was dependent on both p53 and *c-myc* (Fig. 6). TGF-α and TGF-β genes were normally expressed in the mammary glands of control animals. Administration of hCG, either alone or after DMBA treatment, had little or no effect on the expression of TGF genes *(43)*.

Effect of hCG Treatment on the Expression of Apoptotic Genes in DMBA-Induced Mammary Carcinomas

Mammary adenocarcinomas that reached 1.5 cm in diameter, from the DMBA– and the DMBA + hCG groups, were tested for the expression of the same genes described above. In the nontumoral mammary glands and in the adenocarcinomas developed in those animals treated with DMBA alone, the expression of *p53*, *c-myc*, ICE, *bcl2*, and

TGF-β was not modified in any of the groups studied; in those animals that received hCG after carcinogen treatment, the levels of *p53*, *c-myc*, and ICE were significantly elevated *(43)*. The elevation was more marked in the nontumoral mammary gland than in the tumors, but the differences from the levels observed in adenocarcinomas developed by the animals treated with DMBA alone were significant. The expression of TRPM2 was significantly elevated in the nontumoral mammary glands of DMBA + hCG-treated animals, but it was not modified in any of the tumors. Neither the nontumoral mammary glands nor the tumors exhibited changes in the expression of *bcl*2 and TGF-β, or TGF-α, as a consequence of the hCG or DMBA treatments. These observations indicated that, even though in certain animals treated with hCG, tumors developed, the hormone was still capable of inducing a certain degree of activation of the apoptotic genes, which may account for the lower overall tumorigenic response in hCG-treated animals *(42,43)*.

Effect of hCG Treatment on the Expression of Apoptotic Genes in the Ovary

The specificity of the effect of hCG on the expression of apoptotic genes in the mammary gland was verified by a comparison with the expression of these genes in the ovaries of the same animals. Northern blot analysis revealed that the ovaries of control animals had detectable basal levels of all the apoptotic transcripts tested in the mammary glands, as well as of TGF-α and TGF-β. No significant alterations in mRNA expression in any of the genes studied were observed to be induced by either hCG or DMBA treatments, at any of the time periods tested. These results indicated that the induction of PCD expression by hCG occurred specifically in the mammary gland, but did not modify these parameters in the ovary, despite it being the target organ of hCG action.

Effect of hCG Treatment on Apoptosis

Apoptosis was detected in 4-μm sections of formalin-fixed, paraffin-embedded tissue sections of nontumoral mammary glands of control, hCG, DMBA and DMBA + hCG-treated animals, and in DMBA-induced mammary carcinomas in the two latter groups of animals. Apoptotic cell nuclei were identified using the ApopTag kit (Oncor, Gaithersburg, MD), utilizing standard procedures *(43)*. The number of cells containing apoptotic nuclei was counted in ducts and lobules of nontumoral mammary glands of animals of the four groups under study, and in three DMBA-induced tumors developed in the DMBA and three in the DMBA + hCG groups of animals.

The percentage of positive cells over the total number of cells counted in each specific structure represented the apoptotic index. In the nontumoral mammary gland, the lowest apoptotic index was observed in control animals, and this parameter was not modified by aging. The second lowest index was observed in the DMBA group of animals. Treatment with hCG induced an increase in the apoptotic index, which reached its maximum when the animals were 85 d old, and it remained elevated at the same level, even after cessation of the hormonal treatment. Administration of hCG after DMBA induced a steady increase in the apoptotic index which reached a peak by the time the animals were 105 d old, but its value decreased sharply after the discontinuation of the hormonal treatment *(43)*. The apoptotic index of DMBA-induced mammary carcinomas was markedly lower than that of the nontumoral mammary gland of the animals in the same group. hCG treatment resulted in a marked increase in the apoptotic index of mammary adenocarcinomas, with respect to the values found in the tumors of the DMBA group, and were also higher than in the nontumoral mammary glands of the same group of animals (Fig. 6).

ISOLATION AND CHARACTERIZATION OF NEW GENES INDUCED BY hCG TREATMENT IN THE RAT MAMMARY GLAND

The authors tested the dual hypotheses that the inhibitory effect of hCG mammary carcinogenesis was mediated by activation or downregulation of specific genes, and that the changes induced in gene expression would be practically permanent, and not only limited to the period of hormone administration. For this purpose, the authors analyzed, by differential display, RNA from mammary glands obtained from four groups of animals: 15 d-pregnant rats; parous rats sacrificed 21 d postweaning; virgin rats treated with a daily injection of 100 IU hCG, administered for 15 d, and sacrificed on the day of the last injection; and virgin rats treated with a daily injection of 100 IU hCG, administered for 15 d, and sacrificed 48 d after the last injection. Untreated, age-matched virgin rats were used as controls for every group. Mammary gland RNA was isolated and reverse-transcribed, and cDNAs were amplified using four different sets of arbitrary primers. Selected fragments were cloned, sequenced, and used as probes in Northern blot analysis.

Three cDNA fragments were isolated. Two of the cDNA bands, which were called R3A7 and R5C9, were found to be differentially expressed in differential display gels in pregnant, and hCG-treated animals, but they were absent in the virgin rat mammary gland. Differential expression was confirmed by Northern Blot for the two bands, after ^{32}P-labeling of their cloned cDNA fragments. Both R3A7 and R5C9 were found to be overexpressed in both hCG-treated groups, as well as in the pregnant group. These genes were found to be upregulated during the hormonal treatment and during pregnancy, and they remained activated, even after hormone withdrawal and after weaning of the pups. The isolated and differentially expressed bands, R5C9 and R3A7, were 625 and 480 bp in length, respectively, and showed 97% homology to the rat β-casein mRNA (R5C9) and 98% homology to the rat whey acidic protein mRNA (R3A7). The third cDNA fragment, HI-I, was found differentially displayed in another gel, in the lanes containing polymerase chain reaction products from hCG and pregnant animals, but it was absent in the virgin rat mammary gland lane. The differential expression was confirmed in the same Northern blots used for the other two isolated fragments. No sequence homology match in the gene bank was found for the third cloned fragment HI-1, indicating that this may represent a novel gene (Fig. 6; *45*).

SUMMARY AND CONCLUSIONS

The novel finding that hCG treatment inhibits the progression of DMBA-induced mammary tumors led the authors to capitalize on knowledge of the pathogenesis of mammary cancer, for testing the effect of this hormone on the early phases of tumor progression, namely, from TEBs damaged by DMBA to IDPs, *in situ* carcinomas, and invasive carcinomas. The authors observed that treatment of young virgin rats with hCG induced a profuse lobular development of the mammary gland, practically eliminating the highly proliferating TEBs, with overall reduction in the proliferative activity of the mammary epithelium, and induction of the synthesis of inhibin, a secreted protein with tumor-suppressor activity. The hormonal treatment induced differentiation of the mammary gland, which was manifested at morphological, cell-kinetic, and functional levels. The morphological changes consisted of progressive branching of the mammary parenchyma and lobule formation, which was accompanied by a reduction in the rate of cell proliferation. The functional changes included increased synthesis of inhibin, β-casein, and other milk-related bioactive peptides. In addition, hCG also increased the expression of the PCD gene, TRPM2, ICE, p53, c-myc, and *bcl-XS*. The authors found that PCD genes were activated through a p53-dependent process, modulated by c-myc, and with partial dependence on the *bcl-2* family-related genes. Lobular development, which reached its maximal expression after d 15 of hCG treatment, regressing after hormone withdrawal, was preceded by activation of genes associated with the expression of PCD, and, furthermore, the expression of these genes, including the newly identified gene, HI-1, was still elevated 20 d postcessation of treatment. Although lobular development regressed after the cessation of hormone administration, PCD genes remained activated. The authors postulate that this mechanism plays a major role in the longlasting protection exerted by hCG from chemically induced carcinogenesis (Fig. 6), and may be even involved in the lifetime reduction in BC risk induced in women by full-term and multiple pregnancies. The implications of these observations are twofold: First, they indicate that hCG, as in pregnancy, may induce early genomic changes that control the progression of the differentiation pathway, and second, they show that these changes are permanently imprinted in the genome, regulating the longlasting refractoriness to carcinogenesis. The permanence of these changes, in turn, makes them ideal surrogate markers of the hCG effect in the evaluation of this hormone as a BC preventive agent.

ACKNOWLEDGMENTS

This work was supported by grant RO1 CA64896 from National Institutes of Health, National Cancer Institute, Department of Health and Human Services, and Development Command Grant DAMD-J-94-2463.

REFERENCES

1. Parker SL, Tong T, Bolden S, Wingo PA. Cancer statistics, 1997. CA Cancer J Clin 1997;47:5–27.
2. Landis SH, Murray T, Bolden S, Wingo PA. Cancer statistics, 1998. CA Cancer J Clin 1998;48:6–29.
3. King SE, Schottenfeld D. The epidemic of breast cancer in the U. S.—determining the factors. Oncology 1996;10:453–462.
4. Gaudette LA, Silberberg C, Altmayer CA, Gao RN. Trends in breast cancer incidence and mortality. Health Rep 1996;8:29–40.
5. Kelsey JL, Horn-Ross PL. Breast cancer: magnitude of the problem and descriptive epidemiology. Epidemiol Rev 1993;15:7–16.
6. Lambe M, Hsieh C-C, Chan H-W, Ekbom A, Trichopoulos D, Adami HO. Parity, age at first and last birth, and risk of breast cancer: a population-based study in Sweden. Breast Cancer Res Treat 1996;38: 305–311.
7. Russo J, Tay LK, Russo IH. Differentiation of the mammary gland and susceptibility to carcinogenesis. Breast Cancer Res Treat 1982;2:5–37.
8. Rao DN, Ganesh B, Desai PB. Role of reproductive factors in breast cancer in a low-risk area: a case-control study. Br J Cancer 1994;70:129–152.
9. Coe K. Breast cancer in Hispanic women. Women Cancer 1998;1(Suppl):38–43.
10. Apter D. Hormonal events during female puberty in relation to breast cancer risk. Eur J Cancer Prev 1996;5:476–482.
11. Shivvers SA, Miller DS. Preinvasive and invasive breast and cervical cancer prior to or during pregnancy. Clin Perinatol 1997;24:369–389.
12. Russo J, Wilgus G, Russo IH. Susceptibility of the mammary gland to carcinogenesis. I. Differentiation of the mammary gland as determinant of tumor incidence and type of lesion. Am J Pathol 1979;96:721–734.
13. Russo J, Russo IH. Influence of differentiation and cell kinetics on the susceptibility of the mammary gland to carcinogenesis. Cancer Res 1980;40:2677–2687.
14. Russo J, Russo IH. Susceptibility of the mammary gland to carcinogenesis. II. Pregnancy interruption as a risk factor in tumor incidence. Am J Pathol 1980;100:497–512.

15. Russo J, Russo IH. Toward a physiological approach to breast cancer prevention. Cancer Epidemiol. Biomarkers Prev 1994;3:353–364.
16. Russo J, Rivera R, Russo IH. Influence of age and parity on the development of the human breast. Breast Cancer Res Treat 1992;23:211–218.
17. Russo J, Russo IH. Developmental pattern of the human breast and susceptibility to carcinogenesis. Eur J Cancer Prev 1993;2:85–100.
18. Magnusson C. Breast cancer epidemiology-Influence of hormone-related factors. *Duvbo tryckeri ab*, Stockholm, 1998.
19. Nandi S, Guzman RC, Yang J. Hormones and mammary carcinogenesis in mice, rats and humans: a unifying hypothesis. Proc Natl Acad Sci USA 1995;92:3650–3657.
20. Sinha DK, Patzik JE, Dao TL. Progression of rat mammary development with age and its relationship to carcinogenesis by a chemical carcinogen. Int J Cancer 1983;31:321–327.
21. Russo IH, Russo J. Role of hormones in cancer initiation and progression. J Mammary Gland Biol Neoplasia 1998;3:49–61.
22. Russo IH, Russo J. Role of pregnancy and chorionic gonadotropin in breast cancer prevention. In: Birkhauser MH, Rozenbaum H, eds. Proc. IV. European Congress on Menopause. Editions ESKA, Paris, 1998, pp. 133–142.
23. Russo J, Ao X, Grill C, Russo IH. Pattern of distribution of cells positive for estrogen receptor α and progesterone receptor in relation to proliferating cells in the mammary gland. Breast Cancer Res Treat, 1999;53:217–227.
24. Alvarado ME, Alvarado NE, Russo J, Russo IH. Human chorionic gonadotropin inhibits proliferation and induces expression of inhibin in human breast epithelial cells in vitro. In Vitro 1994;30A:4–8.
25. Alvarado MV, Russo J, Russo IH. Immunolocalization of inhibin in the mammary gland of rats treated with hCG. J Histochem Cytochem 1993;41:29–34.
26. Russo IH, Russo J. Role of hCG and inhibin in breast cancer. Int J Oncol 1994;4:297–306.
27. Hu YF, Russo IH, Ao X, Russo J. Mammary derived growth inhibitor (MDGI) cloned from human breast epithelial cells is expressed in fully differentiated lobular structures. Int J Oncol 1997;11:5–11.
28. Russo IH, Koszalka M, Russo J. Comparative study of the influence of pregnancy and hormonal treatment on mammary carcinogenesis. Br J Cancer 1991;64:481–484.
29. Russo IH, Koszalka M, Russo J. Protective effect of chorionic gonadotropin on DMBA-induced mammary carcinogenesis. Br J Cancer 1990;62:243–247.
30. Russo IH, Russo J. Chorionic gonadotropin: a tumoristatic and preventive agent in breast cancer. In: Teicher BA, ed. Drug Resistance in Oncology. Marcel Dekker, New York, 1993, pp. 537–560.
31. Russo IH, Koszalka M, Russo J. Human chorionic gonadotropin and rat mammary cancer prevention. J Natl Cancer Inst 1990;82:1286–1289.
32. Russo IH, Koszalka M, Russo J. Effect of human chorionic gonadotropin on mammary gland differentiation and carcinogenesis. Carcinogenesis 1990;11:1849–1855.
33. Chen C, Jones WR, Fern B, Forde C. Monitoring embryos after in vitro fertilization using early pregnancy factor. In: Seppälä M, Edwards RG, eds. In Vitro Fertilization and Embryo Transfer. Ann NY Acad Sci 1985, pp. 420–428.
34. Hamberger L, Hahlin M, Hillensjö T, Johanson C, Sjögren A. Luteotropic and luteolytic factors regulating human corpus luteum function. In: Jones HW Jr, Schrader C, eds. In Vitro Fertilization and Other Assisted Reproduction. Ann NY Acad Sci 1988;541:485–497.
35. Woodruff TK, Mayo KE. Regulation of inhibin synthesis in the rat ovary. Annu Rev Physiol 1990; 52:807–827.
36. Meunier H, Rivier C, Evans R, Vale W. Gonadal and extragonadal expression of inhibin α-, βA-, and βB-subunits in various tissues predicts diverse functions. Proc Natl Acad Sci USA 1988;85:247–251.
37. Russo IH, Russo J. Mammary gland neoplasia in long-term rodent studies. Environ Health Perspec 1996;104:938–967.
38. Mgbonyebi OP, Tahin Q, Russo J, Russo IH. Serum levels of chorionic gonadotropin in treated female rats during the progression of DMBA-induced tumorigenesis. Proc Am Assoc Cancer Res 1996;37: 1564a.
39. Tahin Q, Mgbonyebi OP, Russo J, Russo IH. Influence of hormonal changes induced by the placental hormone chorionic gonadotropin on the progression of mammary tumorigenesis. Proc Am Assoc Cancer Res 1996;37:1622a.
40. Russo J, Saby J, Isenberg W, Russo IH. Pathogenesis of mammary carcinoma induced in rats by 7,12-dimethylbenz(a)anthracene. J Natl Cancer Inst 1977;59:435–445.

41. Russo J, Russo IH. Toward a unified concept of mammary carcinogenesis. In: Aldaz MC, Gould MN, McLachlan J, Slaga TJ, eds. Progress in Clinical and Biological Research, vol. 396, Etiology of Breast and Gynecological Cancers. Wiley-Liss, New York, 1997, pp. 1–16.
42. Russo IH, Srivastava P, Mgbonyebi OP, Russo J. Activation of programmed cell death by human chorionic gonadotropin in breast cancer therapy. Acta Haematol 1997;98(Suppl):16.
43. Srivastava P, Russo J, Russo IH. Chorionic gonadotropin inhibits rat mammary carcinogenesis through activation of programmed cell death. Carcinogenesis 1998;18:1799–1808.
44. Matzuk MM, Finegold MJ, Su J-G, Hsueh AJW, Bradley E. β-Inhibin is a tumour-suppressor gene with gonadal specificity in mice. Nature 1992;360:313–319.
45. Silva IDCG, Srivastava P, Russo J, Russo IH. Gene expression during differentiation of the rat mammary gland induced by pregnancy and human chorionic gonadotropin. Proc Am Assoc Cancer Res 1998;39:776a.

9

Epidermal Growth Factor-Related Peptides in Endocrine Neoplasias

David S. Salomon, PHD,
Caterina Bianco, MD, PHD,
Marta De Santis, PHD,
Isabel Martinez-Lacaci, PHD,
Christian Wechselberger, PHD,
and Andreas D. Ebert, MD, PHD

INTRODUCTION

The development of cancer results from the cumulative acquisition of somatic and/or germline mutations in regulatory genes that control various aspects of cellular proliferation, differentiation, apoptosis, and DNA repair *(1–6)*. Gain or loss of function in proto-oncogenes or tumor suppressor genes accounts for the majority of these genetic defects *(6–8)*. Generally, gain of function is observed in dominantly transforming oncogenes, which can occur by point mutations, gene amplification, chromosomal translocation, or insertional mutagenesis *(6,9,10)*. Conversely, loss of function, because of the inactivation of tumor suppressor genes, can occur by point mutations or a loss of heterozygosity (LOH) in one allele *(11,12)*. Changes in the expression of these genes can also contribute to the pathogenesis of cancer, and may be caused by environmental stimuli such as viruses, radiation, carcinogens, hormones, and growth factors (GFs) *(6–10)*.

From: *Contemporary Endocrinology: Endocrine Oncology*
Edited by: S. P. Ethier © Humana Press Inc., Totowa, NJ

GFs and growth inhibitors are locally acting peptides that are normally involved in regulating cellular proliferation, survival, and differentiation *(13–16)*. The expression of GFs in different tissues is tightly regulated by various systemic hormones and cytokines *(16)*. However, in carcinoma cells, in which proliferation becomes accelerated, there can be a reduction in the requirement for exogenously supplied GFs, compared to their non-transformed counterparts, which may contribute to this phenotype *(14)*. This relaxation in GF dependency may result in part, from the ability of tumor cells to synthesize and respond to endogenously produced GFs *(15)*. Tumor-derived GFs are known to function through intracrine, juxtacrine, autocrine, or paracrine mechanisms, to regulate cellular proliferation and survival in an autonomous manner, in cells that are also expressing cognate receptors for these peptides *(15,16)*. Additionally, overexpression of GF receptors can hypersensitize carcinoma cells to low concentrations of host- or tumor-derived GFs. These effects may result from the activation of oncogenes, which have the capacity to indirectly regulate the expression of, or encode directly for, proteins that are GFs, GF receptors, or intracellular proteins that are situated within GF-activated signal transduction pathways *(8–16)*.

The complexion of cancer therapy will drastically change in the 21st century. Conventional chemotherapy (Chemo) regimes will ultimately be wedded to more rational and biologically oriented therapies. One important target for these novel therapeutic approaches in solid tumors will be the epidermal growth factors (EGF)-related GFs and their receptors.

THE EGF FAMILY

The EGF-related peptide GF family constitutes one of the larger families of GFs, which have been demonstrated to be important in regulating various aspects of carcinoma development and growth *(17)*. In fact, peptide GFs in this family are part of a larger superfamily of proteins of diverse function, which are related by possessing singular or multiple copies of a common motif, the EGF-like module (Table 1; *18*). Proteins in this superfamily perform an important role during early embryonic development, by specifying and determining body axis and cell fate in *Caenorhabditis elegans* and *Drosophila*, and in mammals, and in regulating the renewal of stem cells in adult tissues *(18–20)*. These proteins can be either secreted or membrane-bound, and can function as GFs, morphogens, proteases, adhesion molecules, receptors, or extracellular matrix-associated molecules. The EGF-like domain, which is central to the biological activity of the GFs in this family, and which is also involved in mediating interactions with other proteins in this superfamily, consists of a stretch of six conserved cysteine residues spaced at defined intervals within a region of approx 40 amino acids (Fig. 1; *18*). The cysteine residues within this region are capable of forming three intramolecular disulfide bonds, which restrain the molecule in this domain in a three-loop secondary structure (Fig. 2; *21*). The peptide GFs that are members of this family of proteins include EGF, transforming growth factor-α (TGF-α), heparin-binding EGF (HB-EGF), amphiregulin (AR), beta-cellulin (BTC), epiregulin (EPR), and the neuregulin (NRG) and EGF-CFC (cripto) subfamilies. The NRG subfamily includes α and β heregulins (HRG), glial growth factors, sensory motor neuron-derived growth factor, and acetylcholine receptor-inducing activity (Table 2; *22–41*). There are at least 45 known structural variants in this subfamily, which are derived from three distinct HRG genes by alternative mRNA splicing *(22,34, 35)*. Unlike other members in the EGF family, which are expressed predominantly in epithelial cells (ECs), NRGs are expressed in mesenchymal and neuronal tissues *(33–35)*.

Table 1
EGF Superfamily and EGFR (*erb*B) Family

Protein	Function
EGF	GF
Heparin-binding EGF (HB-EGF)	GF
Transforming growth factor α (TGF-α)	GF
Amphiregulin (AR)	GF
Betacellulin (BTC)	GF
Epiregulin (EPR)	GF
Neuregulin α and β (HRG)-1	GF
Neuregulin-2	GF
Neuregulin-3	GF
Cripto-1 (CR-1)	GF/Morphogen
Cryptic (mouse)	Morphogen
One-eyed pinhead (oep/Zebrafish)	Morphogen
FRL-1 (*Xenopus laeavis*)	Morphogen
Vaccina virus growth facator (VGF)	GF
Shopes fibroma virus growth factor (SFGF)	GF
Myxoma virus growth factor (MGF)	GF
pfs (*Plasmodium falciparum*)	
Notch (*Drosophilia*)	Adhesion/neurogenesis
Delta (*Drosophilia*)	Adhesion/neurogenesis
Serrate (*Drosophilia*)	Adhesion/neurogenesis
Crumbs (*Drosophilia*)	Cell polarity
Slit (*Drosophilia*)	Adhesion
Gurken (*Drosophilia*)	GF
Spitz (*Drosophilia*)	GF
Vein (*Drosophilia*)	GF
Argos (*Drosophilia*)	GF antagonist
lin-3 (*C. elegans*)	GF
glp-1 (*C. elegans*)	Adhesion
uEGF1 (sea urchin *S. purpuratus*)	Exogastrulation(?)
SpEGF2 (sea urchin *S. purpuratus*)	Exogastrulation(?)
Pref-1 (mouse)	Adhesion
Ascites sialoglycoprotein-2 (rat)	GF (?)
Urokinase	Serine protease
Tissue plasminogen activator (tPA)	Serine protease
Clotting factors (VII, IX, X, XII)	
LDL receptor	LDL uptake
Laminin β1 chain	ECM protein
Thrombospondin	ECM protein
Tenascin (Cytotactoin)	ECM protein
Nidogen	ECM protein
Human proteoglycan core protein	ECM protein
Type I EGFR family of cell surface TKs	
*c-erb*B/DER/*let-23*	p170-EGFR
*c-erb*B-2 (HER-2/*c-neu*)	p185
*c-erb*B-3 (HER-3)	p180
*c-erb*B-4 (HER-4)	p180

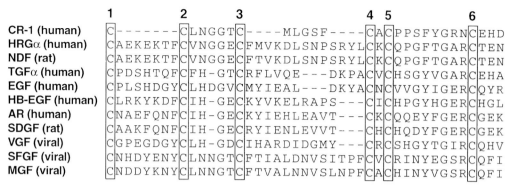

Fig. 1. Alignment of amino acid residues in EGF-like domains of GFs with six conserved cysteine residues (yellow).

The EGF-CFC subfamily includes human cripto-1 (CR-1)/teratocarcinoma-derived growth factor 1, mouse cripto-1, mouse cryptic, Zebrafish one-eyed pinhead, *Xenopus* FRL-1 *(37–41)*. Cripto-related proteins possess a modified EGF-like motif that lacks an A loop, but possesses a truncated B loop and has a complete C loop. This structure differentiates the EGF-CFC subfamily from other members within the EGF family of peptides. In addition to these vertebrate GFs, there are peptides in *Drosophilia*, such as *spitz*, *gurken*, *vein*, and *argos* or in *C. elegans*, such as *lin-3*, which can function as EGF-like GFs or GF antagonists by binding to the *Drosophilia* EGF receptor or to the *C. elegans* EGF receptor, *let-23 (18–21)*. Finally, there is a series of DNA pox virus-derived peptides, including vaccinia virus growth factor (VGF), Shope fibroma growth factor, and myxoma virus growth factor, which possess an EGF motif, and which can bind to the mammalian EGF receptor (EGFR) *(21)*. EGF, HB-EGF, BTC, TGF-α, AR, EPR, VGF, and some of the isoforms of NRG, are synthesized as glycosylated membrane-associated precursors that are biologically active, and that can function as such through a cell–cell, juxtacrine-mediated pathway (Fig. 3; *26*). Some of these cell-associated molecules can also serve as cell–cell adhesion molecules, which suggests that they may be important in regulating chemotactic migration, and in controlling the colonization of specific organs during metastasis *(18,26)*. Selective and tissue-specific processing of the larger cell-associated forms of these GFs can lead to cleavage at residues that flank the EGF domain, and which leads to the production of soluble, smaller peptides. This processing occurs under the action of a specific group of serine proteases and elastase-like enzymes, which may limit the diffusion and range of activity of these peptides *(26,28,35)*. In addition to the conserved, extracellular, juxtamembrane EGF domain in these GFs, the NRG subfamily contains immunoglobulin (IgG) and kringle-like motifs that may serve other functions (Fig. 3).

*erb*B-RELATED TYPE 1 TYROSINE KINASE FAMILY OF RECEPTORS

There are four distinct members of the *erb*B type 1 GF receptor tyrosine kinase (TK) family, which includes the EGFR/*erb*B, c-*erb*B-2 (HER-2), c-*erb*B-3 (HER-3), and c-*erb*B-4 (HER-4) *(42–48)*. The EGFR exhibits considerable homology to the avian erythroblastosis virus transforming protein, v-*erb*B. This family of receptors is of particular interest because of their frequent involvement in several types of human cancer *(17,42, 43)*. For example, amplification of the EGFR and *erb*B-2 genes has been detected in

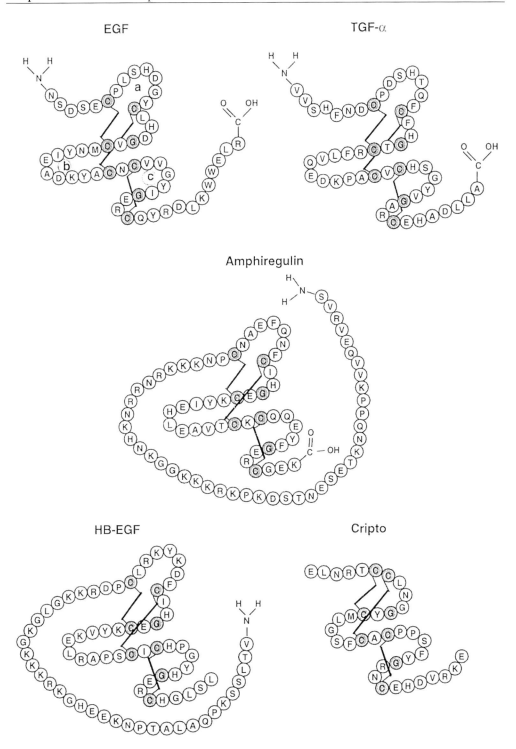

Fig. 2. Proposed tertiary structure of EGF-like domains demonstrating three intramolecular disulfide bridges, which can restrain the EGF-like motif in a structure that can form three intramolecular disulfide-bonded loops, designated a, b, and c. Yellow amino acid residues represent basic amino acid residues that could potentially function as nuclear localization sequences in AR and HB-EGF.

Table 2
EGF-Related GF Family and Their Receptors

Ligand	Receptor
Epidermal growth factor (EGF)	EGF Receptor (EGFR/*erb*B)
Transforming growth factor α (TGF-α)	
Amphiregulin (AR)	
Epiregulin (EPP)	EGFR and *erb*B-4
Heparin-binding EGF (HB-EGF)	EGFR and *erb*B-4
Betacellulin (BTC)	EGFR< *erb*B-3 and *erb*B-4
?	*erb*B-2
Neuregulins	*erb*B-3 and *erb*B-4
Heregulin (HRGα and β)-1	
Glial cell growth factor (GGF)	
Sensory motor neuron-derived growth factor (SMDGF)	
Acetylcholine receptor-inducing activity (ARIA)	*erb*B-4 > *erb*B-3
Heregulin-2	
Heregulin-3 (DON)	
Cripto-1 (CR-1)	?
Cryptic	
FRL-1	
oep	

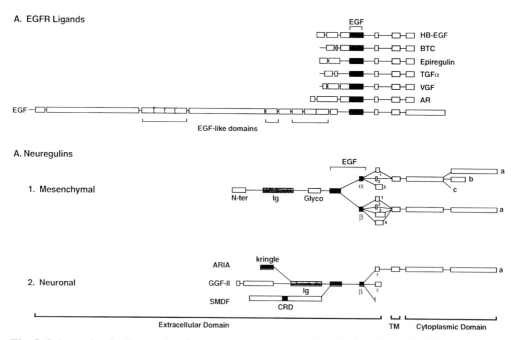

Fig. 3. Schematic of cell-associated precursor structures for EGF-related peptide GFs. Conserved extracellular EGF-like motif (EGF in purple) and transmembrane domains (TM) in pink.

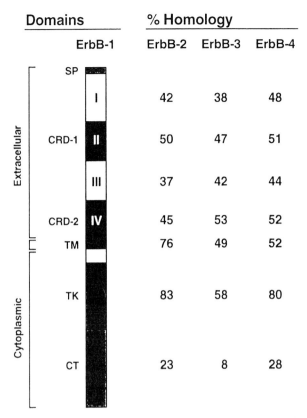

Fig. 4. Schematic of type 1 *erb*B receptor structure. Amino acid sequence homology of different domains between EGFR (*erb*B-1) and the three other *erb*B TK receptors. SP, signal peptide; CRD, cysteine-rich domain; TM, transmembrane domain; TK, tyrosine kinase domain; and CT, cytoplasmic tail.

several types of human malignancies; deletions or truncations of the EGFR, which constitutively activate the receptor in the absence of ligand binding, are also frequently observed *(17,43)*. All of these receptors were identified by low-stringency screening of human cDNA libraries with a v-erbB probe or degenerate oligonucleotides to the conserved TK domain regions in these receptors. Receptor proteins in this family are glycosylated, and share a similar structure, consisting of an extracellular, ligand-binding domain (ECD), which has two cysteine-rich regions, a short juxtamembrane sequence, a hydrophobic transmembrane region, and an intracellular domain that contains a TK domain that is adjacent to a hydrophilic carboxyl tail (Fig. 4). The carboxyl tail displays sequence heterogeneity and carries several tyrosine autophosphorylation sites *(42)*, which serve as docking sites for various cytoplasmic signaling proteins that share a *src* homology 2 (SH2)-domain. Signal transduction by type 1 receptor TKs is initiated by ligand-induced dimerization, which is followed by receptor autophosphorylation and recruitment, and binding of specific SH2-domain-containing signaling proteins *(17,42,43)*. Besides differences in docking sites for different SH2-containing proteins, the intrinsic catalytical activities of each *Erb*B protein differ, in that *Erb*B-2 is characterized by a constitutively active, TK, whereas *Erb*B-3 possesses an impaired TK *(23,46)*. In addition, ligand-induced downregulation, resulting from internalization and degradation, occurs only for the EGFR, demonstrating that endocytosis of the other *erb*B receptors is impaired *(49)*. Ligands that bind exclusively to the EGFR include EGF, TGF-α, and AR (Table 2; Fig. 5).

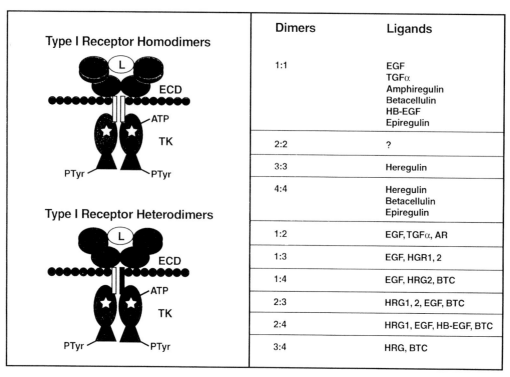

Fig. 5. Homodimerization and heterodimerization between the *erb*B type 1 receptors. Ten possible dimeric combinations are presented with known ligand (L) binding preferences. ECD, extracellular domain; TK, tyrosine kinase.

EPR, HB-EGF, and BTC are more promiscuous, because these peptides can also bind to *erb*B-3 and *erb*B-4 *(23,50–52)*. In contrast, the NRGs bind to only *erb*B-3 or *erb*B-4. Therefore, a single EGF-like peptide may bind to multiple *erb*B receptors, and, recipro-cally, a single *erb*B receptor may accommodate multiple EGF-like ligands, suggesting that signaling via this family of GFs may be quite complex *(23)*. There is no known ligand that directly binds to and activates *erb*B-2. Finally, the EGF-CFC subfamily of peptides does not directly bind to any of the known *erb*B receptors, and its receptor has not yet been identified *(53)*.

A common and important feature of the *erb*B receptor family is their ability to hetero-dimerize after ligand binding *(54–57)*. Heterodimerization after ligand binding and activa-tion, which can lead to tyrosine phosphorylation *in trans* between two different receptors, increases signal diversification and the spectrum of biological responses, by recruiting different SH2-containing proteins to these receptor complexes *(22,23,56*; Fig. 6). In this context, *erb*B-2 functions as a co-receptor for the other three *erb*B receptors, and is the preferred heterodimerization partner *(54,55)*. In fact, there may be a hierarchy between different receptor heterodimers, depending on the type and stoichiometry of *erb*B recep-tors that are expressed on a target cell and the nature of the activating ligand *(50,54)*. Ligand activation of heterodimers containing *erb*B-2 as a partner leads to a more sus-tained intracellular signal than homodimer activation, probably because of the impaired internalization of *erb*B-2 *(23,49)*. Another important consequence of heterodimerization with *erb*B-2 is to increase the affinity of respective ligand binding to the EGFR, *erb*B-3 or *erb*B-4 *(22,23,55)*. However, this may be mutually exclusive, since binding of HRG

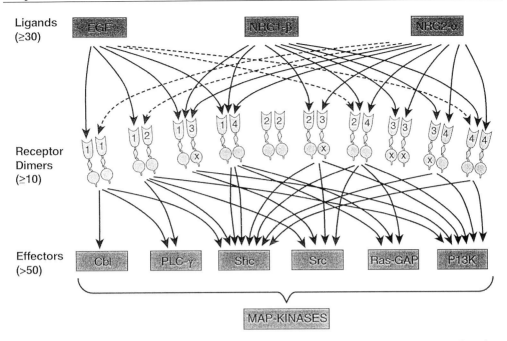

Fig. 6. Intracellular signal diversification resulting from ligand-induced type 1 receptor dimerization. Reproduced with permision from ref. *35.*

to *erb*B-3, or *erb*B-4 in some types of tumor cells can indirectly inhibit EGF binding to the EGFR *(22).* In addition to modulating affinity, heterodimers may also generate novel, or expose previously cryptic, ligand binding sites that are not normally utilized in homodimeric pairs. For example, *erb*B-2 overexpression in the context of *erb*B-4 or *erb*B-3 can lead to EGF or TGF-α binding to *erb*B-3 or *erb*B-4 *(52,57),*which suggests that EGF-like ligands are bivalent in their binding capacity, with a high-affinity NH_2 terminal site and a low-affinity COOH-terminal site in the molecule *(58).* There is also evidence that secondary dimerization between *erb*B receptors can occur *(59).* In this case, GF-induced dimerization and receptor transphosphorylation results in the dissociation of the original receptor dimer. Each phosphorylated monomer then interacts with a new receptor partner to form a secondary dimer. This second wave of signals might elongate or terminate the effects induced by the first wave, thereby providing a means for control and fine-tuning of the primary signal. Finally, autoinduction and crossinduction within the EGF-related GF family has been identified in several different types of ECs *(60).* All this evidence implies that a very complex network of interligand and *erb*B crosstalk exists, leading to signal diversification *(22,23).* It also suggests that activation of multiple *erb*B receptors in tumors may contribute to synergistic or novel sets of biological responses to different endogenously produced EGF-like ligands *(51).*

BREAST CANCER

Breast cancer (BC) afflicts nearly 180,000 women each year, or 1/9 women in the United States, and accounts for approx 48,000 deaths/year. BC is the leading cause of cancer deaths in women. Therefore, a large investment has been made in attempting to identify genetic and epigenetic factors that can regulate the normal and abnormal growth and development of the mammary gland, because these facts may provide important clues to the pathogenesis of BC and information for improving prevention, diagnosis, and therapy *(61)*. Approximately 60% of BCs are initially estrogen-dependent at the time of diagnosis, possess functional estrogen receptors (ER), and respond to some sort of anti-estrogen therapy *(62)*. It is conceivable that estrogens may indirectly function as mitogens or morphogens for mammary ECs, by their ability to regulate the local synthesis, processing, and/or secretion of a spectrum of different endogenous peptide GFs or growth inhibitors, or their ability to modulate the expression of specific GF receptors *(62–65)*. Alterations in GF signaling pathways is therefore also one factor that is likely to contribute to the etiology and progression of BC *(62–67)*.

GFs in Rodent Mammary Gland Development and Carcinogenesis

The mouse has been an important model for studying the genetics and development of human diseases. In this context, mammary gland growth and development has been extensively studied in this species *(68)*. Ductal growth and branching in the virgin mouse and lobuloalveolar development in the parous animal are tightly regulated and orchestrated by a complex interplay of systemic ovarian and pituitary (pit) hormones, such as estrogen, progesterone (P), and prolactin. Hormonal responsiveness in the rodent mammary gland is in turn regulated by stromal–epithelial interactions that are mediated by components of the ECM and by various locally derived GFs *(62–67,69)*.

GFs in Mammary Gland Development

Several different types of GFs are expressed either in the mammary stroma as paracrine effectors or in the ductal or secretory epithelium as autocrine factors, at defined periods during mammary gland development in the mouse *(70–72)*. In this context, EGF, TGF-α, AR, and HRGα have been shown to be involved in various aspects of mammary gland development *(73–85)*. EGF, AR, and TGF-α are expressed in the virgin mouse mammary gland, in either ductal ECs (EGF and AR) or in the cap stem cells (TGF-α) within the growing terminal end buds (TEBs); HRGα expression is generally restricted to a subpopulation of mesenchymal cells *(74,75,77,84)*. More recently, HB-EGF, BTC, and EPR have been detected in the virgin and/or pregnant mammary gland *(78)*. Expression of EGF is under the control of estrogen in the pubertal mammary gland, and lactational hormones may regulate TGF-α and HRGα expression during pregnancy and lactation *(76,79, 77)*. All four *erb*B receptors are expressed in the epithelium during pregnancy and lactation, but only the EGFR and *erb*B-2 are expressed in the virgin mouse mammary gland *(78)*. When implanted in Elvax pellets in vivo, EGF, TGF-α , HRGα, HRGβ, CR-1, and, to a lesser extent AR, can induce, to different degrees, longitudinal ductal growth, ductal branching, and TEB development in the mammary gland of ovariectomized virgin mice *(79–85)*. Conversely, targeted expression of a dominant-negative EGFR to the mammary gland in virgin transgenic mice produces an inhibition of mammary ductal development in which TEBs are smaller and less frequent, and in which lateral and terminal ductal branching are severely impaired *(86)*. These peptides can also influence biochemical differentiation in the mammary gland. For example, EGF, TGF-α, CR-1, or various HRGβ isoforms can either stimulate or inhibit the transcriptional expression of milk proteins, such as β-casein and whey acidic protein, depending on the presence or absence of prolactin, and depending on whether the mammary epithelial primary cultures or explants were initiated from mammary glands obtained from virgin or pregnant mice *(77,83,87–89)*.

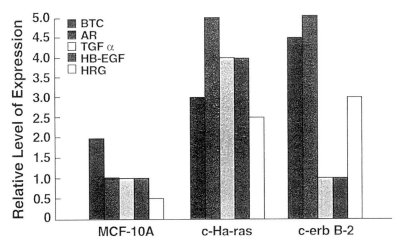

Fig. 7. Coexpression of multiple EGF-related peptide GFs in nontransformed and c-Ha-*ras* and c-*erb*B-2 transformed human mammary MCF-10A ECs.

Carcinogen-induced rat mammary tumors, spontaneous mouse mammary tumors, and tumors in transgenic mice, which overexpress oncogenes in the mammary gland, also exhibit elevated expression of EGF, TGF-α, AR, CR-1, and/or HRG, which can potentially function as autocrine GFs in some of these cases *(90–92)*. Overexpression of TGF-α, HRGβ2, CR-1, or c-*erb*B-2 has been formally demonstrated to contribute to the malignant transformation of mouse, rat, or human mammary ECs in vitro and/or in vivo in transgenic mice or rats, utilizing mammary-directed promoters such as WAP, or mouse mammary tumor virus promoters to drive expression of the transgene *(93–102)*. In fact, TGF-α and HRGβ$_2$ overexpression in transgenic mice or rats leads to the persistence of TEBs, the appearance of hyperplastic alveolar nodules, and to a retardation in apoptosis in secretory alveolar ECs during involution *(96,97,100)*. These events may collectively contribute to subsequent mammary tumor development in multiparous rodents, by facilitating the survival of a potential stem cell population that normally would regress during involution, and that may persist and be susceptible to genetic or hormonal insult *(97)*. There is also a synergistic enhancement in the acceleration of mammary tumor formation and number in bitransgenic mice that overexpress c-*myc* or *erb*B-2 in combination with TGF-α *(103–105)*.

In addition to contributing directly to mammary EC transformation, some of these GFs, such as TGF-α, AR, HB-EGF, and HRG, may also indirectly mediate the transforming activity of different oncogenes, such as c-H-*ras* and c-*erb*B-2, since these GFs can be differentially upregulated in oncogene-transformed mammary ECs, and since blockade of their action can significantly inhibit the growth of these transformed cells (Fig. 7; *92–94,106–109*). Estrogen and antiestrogens can also regulate the expression of TGF-α and AR in ER-positive human BC cell lines *(110–114)*. In this respect, physiological, growth-promoting concentrations of 17β-estradiol (E$_2$) can induce a 2–10-fold increase of TGF-α and AR mRNA and protein expression in ER-positive BC cells *(110,111)*. The estrogen-induced increase in TGF-α and AR expression in vitro is an ER-mediated response that can be blocked by treatment with the antiestrogens, tamoxifen, (TAM), or droloxifene *(111,112)*. Blocking expression of TGF-α or impairing the activity of the EGFR, can significantly mute the growth-promoting effects of estrogen or P, suggesting that TGF-α may function as a mediator of estrogen and/or P action *(66,115,116)*. Basal

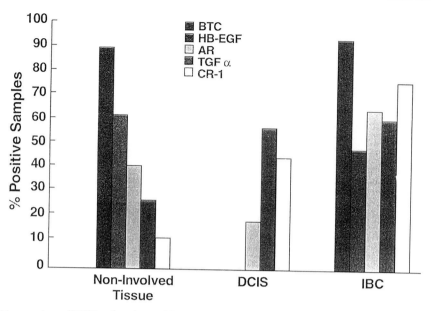

Fig. 8. Expression of EGF-related peptide GFs in invasive human BC (IBC), ductal carcinoma *in situ* (DCIS), and noninvolved, adjacent breast tissue.

levels of TGF-α are generally higher in ER-negative, estrogen-nonresponsive BC cell lines than in ER-positive, estrogen-responsive cell lines; the reciprocal is observed for AR mRNA expression *(111,120)*. Some human BC cell lines also express EGF mRNA *(112,117,118)*. Specifically, the ER-positive BC cell lines, T47-D and ZR-75-1, exhibit high levels of EGF mRNA expression. Progestins can increase the levels of EGF mRNA in T47-D cells; E_2 has no effect on EGF mRNA levels in these cells *(118,119)*. In addition to TGF-α, EGF, and AR, human BC cell lines can also express HB-EGF, BTC, HRG, and CR-1 *(119,120)*. In fact, co-expression of several of these GFs is a frequent observation in human breast carcinoma cell lines *(119–121)*. In BC cells that express sufficiently high levels of *erb*B-2, endogenous HRG may not only function as an EGF-like GF, but also as a surrogate insulin-like growth factor-I (IGF-I), especially in cells that are autonomous for several exogenous GFs, such as EGF and IGF-I *(122,123)*.

EGF-like Ligands in Primary Human Breast Tumors

Cumulative data obtained from multiple studies, representing nearly 1000 invasive breast tumors, have demonstrated expression of HB-EGF and BTC, and overexpression (and, in a majority of cases, co-expression) of TGF-α, AR, and/or CR-1 in breast tumors, relative to the level of expression in adjacent noninvolved breast tissue (Fig. 8; *124*). In addition, overexpression of some of these GFs, such as TGF-α and CR-1, can first be detected in ductal carcinomas *in situ* (DCIS) *(124)*. EGF mRNA has been detected in 83% of human BC biopsy samples *(125)*. In this subset of tumors, a higher proportion of ER- and progesterone receptor (PR)-positive tumor biopsies had detectable EGF mRNA levels, compared to tumors that were negative for ER or PR mRNA *(125)*. Mizukami et al. *(126)* found an inverse correlation between ER status and EGF protein expression in breast carcinomas. They also found that EGF expression was correlated with poor prognosis in BC patients, but no correlations between EGF expression and tumor size, degree of differentiation, or metastatic progression were observed. In contrast, Pirinen et al.

(127) has found, in 198 human breast carcinomas, expression of immunoreactive EGF protein in 34% of the breast tumor specimens, with no association with steroid receptor status or with overall survival.

Examination of TGF-α expression in breast tumor specimens has been more thoroughly investigated. TGF-α-specific mRNA has been found in 40–70% of primary and metastatic human breast tumors *(111,128–133)*. *In situ* hybridization has shown that TGF-α mRNA is expressed in breast tumor cells, and not in the surrounding stromal cells or in infiltrating lymphoid cells *(129)*. Most studies have found no significant correlation between TGF-α mRNA expression and steroid receptor status, axillary lymph node involvement, or patient relapse and survival *(128–131,136,137)*. However, one study *(133)* has shown significantly higher levels of TGF-α and EGF in ER-positive human breast tumors than in ER-negative tumors. There is no evidence for rearrangements or amplifications of the TGF-α gene in human breast tumors that could account for elevated expression *(129)*. Immunoreactive and bioactive TGF-α protein have also been detected in premalignant atypical ductal hyperplasias, ductal hyperplasias, DCIS, and in 30–50% of primary and metastatic human breast carcinomas, at levels that generally are 2–3-fold higher than TGF-α levels found in benign breast lesions or in normal mammary tissues *(126, 134,135,137–141)*. The majority of BCs that express high levels of TGF-α co-express EGFR, suggesting that an autocrine loop may exist in vivo *(132,133,135,136,138,142)*. TAM can reduce the production of immunoreactive TGF-α by 30–70% in primary human breast tumors that are ER positive and PR-positive *(143)*. In addition, in one study, TAM treatment of BC patients resulted in a 10-fold reduction in tumor-associated TGF-α *(144)*. Bioactive and immunoreactive TGF-α has also been found in pleural effusions and in urine from metastatic BC patients *(129,145)*. High levels of TGF-α in pleural effusions correlate with a poor prognosis and performance status, and with tumor burden.

Normal human mammary EC strains and nontransformed human mammary EC lines express AR mRNA and protein *(146–148)*. AR can function as an autocrine GF in these cells *(119,146–148)*. AR protein is expressed in approx 80% of human primary breast carcinomas, as detected by immunocytochemistry *(137)*. Immunoreactive AR was also found in 43% of the adjacent noninvolved mammary EC specimens, but generally at lower levels, compared to the carcinomas *(137)*. The pattern of staining was mostly cytoplasmic, but nuclear staining was also observed. A similar nuclear localization has been noted for HRG in *erb*B-2-overexpressing breast carcinoma cells, which may relate to the presence of nuclear localization sequences in both AR and HRG *(119,149)*. AR expression is statistically associated with tumor histology, because a significantly higher percentage of tumor cells in infiltrating lobular carcinomas were found to express AR, compared to infiltrating ductal carcinomas *(137)*. An inverse relationship between AR expression and the presence of a point-mutated *p53* gene has also been observed. No correlation between AR expression, ER status, axillary lymph node involvement, histologic grade, tumor size, proliferative index or LOH on chromosome 17p was found in this study *(137)*. However, a strong correlation between AR and ER expression was found in a different subset of human primary breast carcinomas that were examined for AR mRNA expression by Northern blot analysis. AR mRNA expression was found in approx 60% of these tumors, and all the tumors that were positive for AR expression were also found to be ER-positive *(121)*. LeJeune et al. *(150)* reported AR expression in only 37% of human primary breast carcinomas, as assessed by immunocytochemistry and by RNA dot blot analysis. LeJeune et al. also found that expression of AR was more common in lymph-node-positive cases than in lymph-node-negative cases, and no correlation between AR expression and tumor histology or p53 expression was observed. Finally, Visscher et al. *(151)* found that AR is expressed in 71% of breast tumors and in 59% of surrounding host stromal cells.

HRGα mRNA has been detected in both normal and malignant breast tissues *(151–155)*. Visscher et al. *(151)* showed that immunoreactive HRG could be detected in 38% of the tumors, and in the stroma in 50% of the cases. Peritumoral host stromal AR and HRG staining was significantly correlated with tumor recurrence. In this study, medullary carcinomas were found to express HRG at a higher frequency than infiltrating ductal carcinomas *(151)*. HRG may regulate estrogen-responsiveness. In this respect, HRG-transfected MCF-7 cells become estrogen-independent and develop resistance to antiestrogens *(157)*. This phenotype may result from the ability of HRG to downregulate ER expression *(158)*. A similar phenotype is observed after transfection and overexpression of c-*erb*B-2 in MCF-7 BC cells *(159,160)*. Finally, HRGβ3 can induce apoptosis in BC cells that are overexpressing *erb*B-2 *(161)*.

Immunohistochemical (IHC) detection of CR-1 has been observed in approx 80% of human primary infiltrating breast carcinomas, in approx 47% of DCIS, and in only 13% of noninvolved breast tissue samples *(124,137,156,162,163)*. Since TGF-α and AR are expressed in 29 and 43% of noninvolved, adjacent breast tissues, respectively, this suggests that the differential expression of CR-1 in malignant mammary ECs may serve as a more useful tumor marker than expression of other GFs for the early detection of BC *(137,162,163)*. Nonetheless, no significant correlations were found between the percentage of carcinoma cells that were positive for CR-1 and ER status, axillary lymph node involvement, histologic grade, tumor size, proliferative index, LOH on chromosome 17p, or overall patient survival *(137,162,163)*.

erbB Receptors in Primary Human Breast Tumors

Expression of the EGFR was the first *erb*B TK to be detected in both lobular and ductal human breast carcinomas *(164)*. EGFR expression is generally associated with an estrogen-independent phenotype *(164)*. ER-negative BC cell lines usually express higher numbers of EGFRs than ER-positive cell lines, and estrogen and P treatment upregulates expression of EGFR in ER-positive BC cells *(165)*. However, overexpression of the EGFR alone is not sufficient to induce ER downregulation, and the appearance of a hormone-independent phenotype in vitro, in human BC cells *(166)*. Several groups have reported EGFR expression in human breast carcinomas, with an incidence ranging from 14 to 91% and a median value of 48% *(164,167)*. Increased levels of EGFR expression that are observed in primary breast tumors, or in BC cell lines, are not the result of gene amplification, but generally result from an increased level of EGFR mRNA and protein expression *(168)*. Although activating mutations within the EGFR gene are rare, at least in BC, one study *(169)* has demonstrated in a subset of BC patients the existence of type VIII mutations in the EGFR, in which regions of the ECD are deleted. Several studies have correlated high expression of EGFR in breast tumors that have higher proliferative rates and axillary lymph node involvement *(167)*. Studies following patients for longer than 5 yr generally do not show a significant relationship between EGFR expression and relapse-free survival or overall survival; studies analyzing patients after 1–2 yr have found this association *(167)*. These results indicate that EGFR status may define a subset of early-relapsing, poor-prognosis patients. It has been demonstrated that EGFR expression is second only to lymph node involvement as a prognostic marker in lymph-node-positive patients, and is the only predictive marker for recurrence and overall survival in node-negative patients during short-term follow-up *(170,171)*. These results have been recently confirmed by a prospective study demonstrating that EGFR expression is indicative of poor prognosis in BC patients *(172)*. A statistically significant inverse relationship between EGFR and ER expression in human primary BC has also been found in several studies *(167)*. The relapse-free survival and the overall survival for ER-negative, EGFR-positive patients has been demonstrated to be significantly worse than for double-negative patients *(170,173)*. Thus, EGFR status stratifies the ER-negative population into good and poor prognosis subgroups. Expression of EGFR in breast tumors of patients treated with primary endocrine therapy has also been correlated with accelerated disease progression and with a poor response to antiestrogen treatment *(174,175)*. In addition, EGFR expression is also associated with a lack of response to endocrine therapy in patients with BC relapse after surgical treatment, compared to EGFR-negative tumors in antiestrogen-treated patients *(174–176)*.

The c-*erb*B-2 protein is expressed at generally low levels in normal breast ECs and myo-ECs *(177)*. Oncogenic activation of the c-*erb*B-2 protein may occur both by point-mutation in the transmembrane region or by overexpression of the wild-type protein *(178–181)*. Although no activating transmembrane mutations have been detected in the c-*erb*B-2 proto-oncogene in primary human primary breast carcinomas, c-*erb*B-2 proto-oncogene amplification and/or erbB-2 protein overexpression has been detected in several human BC cell lines, and in approx 15–30% of primary human breast tumors *(43,177,182,183)*. More recently, tyrosine phosphorylated *erb*B-2, which is indicative of the presence of an activated receptor, has been found in 35% of the *erb*B-2-positive cases *(184,185)*. Overexpression of *erb*B-2 mRNA and protein can occur both in the presence or absence of gene amplification *(186)*. Overexpression of *erb*B-2 is associated with resistance to TAM and other drugs, suggesting that patients presenting with breast tumors that overexpress *erb*B-2 may derive the best benefits from high-dose Chemo *(43,183, 187,188)*. In benign tumors, overexpression of *erb*B-2 is relatively rare, although expression of low levels of p185^{erbB-2} protein frequently occurs *(189,190)*. In comedo types of DCIS, over 90% of these lesions overexpress c-*erb*B-2, but other DCIS subtypes are negative *(191)*. In addition, c-*erb*B-2 overexpression in comedo DCIS is associated with tumors with a greater invasive potential *(183,192)*. Overexpression of c-*erb*B-2 in invasive breast tumors is essentially confined to ductal carcinomas, and is more frequent in inflammatory ductal carcinomas than in noninflammatory tumors *(193,194)*. There is no association of elevated c-*erb*B-2 expression with age, grade, size, or nodal involvement; there is a significant inverse association with steroid hormone receptor status, similar to expression of the EGFR *(177,183)*. This may be mechanistically significant, since it has recently been demonstrated that E_2 can induce a dose-dependent decrease in c-*erb*B-2 expression in estrogen-responsive human BC cells *(187,195)*. In contrast, an increase in c-*erb*B-2 expression is observed in TAM-treated BC patients, suggesting that antiestrogen therapy may be contraindicated in *erb*B-2-positive tumors *(187)*. *erb*B-2 overexpression in lymph-node-positive patients is predictive of a poor outcome, independent of other prognostic indicators *(183)*. More controversial is the role of c-*erb*B-2 status as a prognostic indicator in node-negative patients. However, some recently published studies have reported a prognostic role for c-*erb*B-2 that is independent of stage and nodal status of patients *(183,196)*. *erb*B-2 overexpression is a reasonable indicator of poor survival in node-negative patients with breast tumors that possess low nuclear grade, and who normally represent a low-risk group *(197)*. Co-overexpression of c-*erb*B-2 and EGFR in the same tumor is associated with a poorer prognosis than overexpression of either oncogene alone *(183,198,199)*. This may be functionally significant, because the EGFR can form heterodimers with p185[erbB-2], can transphosphorylate p185 [erbB-2] in response to ligand binding, and can synergistically enhance cellular transformation in vitro with c-*erb*B-2 *(23,43)*.

c-*erb*B-3 is expressed in both luminal ECs and myo-ECs of the adult mammary gland *(200)*. Overexpression of c-*erb*B-3 has been found in several human BC cell lines in the absence of either gene rearrangement or amplification *(201)*. *erb*B-3 shows a wide range of expression in primary breast carcinomas. It is expressed in 60–90% of primary human breast tumors, and is overexpressed when compared to the adjacent noninvolved mucosa in approx 15–30% of the tumors *(202–205)*. Overexpression of c-*erb*B-3 is caused by an increase in gene transcription, since no evidence of gene amplification has been found *(202)*. High expression of c-*erb*B-3 is also positively associated with the presence of lymph node metastases, but not with patient survival *(202)*. c-*erb*B-4 is expressed in several human BC cell lines *(155,203)*. In addition, approx 50–70% of primary human breast tumors express *erb*B-4 in which *erb*B-4 expression correlates with ER and PR expression *(155)*. In a more recent study *(204)*, *erb*B-4 expression in a small panel of breast tumors was found to be elevated in approx 20% of primary breast tumors, compared to adjacent noninvolved breast tissue.

PROSTATE CANCER

Prostate cancer (PC) is the most common cancer in men. There are approx 190,000 new cases per year, of which there are nearly 38,000 deaths per year from this disease *(205)*. The incidence of PC increases significantly with age. Less than 1% of PCs are diagnosed in men under 50 yr of age; 10% of men in the age range of 50–60 yr and 50% of men in the 70–80-yr range have histological foci of cancer within their prostate glands *(203–207)*. This may relate to the fact that nearly 80% of men over 70 yr of age have some degree of benign prostatic hypertrophy (BPH). Similar to BC, PC begins as a hormone-dependent disease with tumors that are androgen-receptor-positive and androgen-dependent, and eventually progress to a more aggressive, androgen-independent phenotype. In addition, as in BC, it is unclear whether androgens have a direct mitogenic effect on prostate ECs or function to enhance the expression of autocrine or paracrine factors in the prostate stroma that mediate this effect *(205,208–210)*.

EGF and TGF-α can function as mitogenic and survival factors in both normal and malignant prostate ECs *(209–213)*. EGF has been detected in the ECs of the prostate gland of rodents; TGF-α is expressed both in the epithelium and in the stroma *(211, 214,215)*. EGF is mitogenic for normal rat and human prostate cells *(211,216,217)*, as well as for rat and human prostate carcinoma cells *(211,215,216,218)*. EGF, AR, and TGF-α expression in the rodent prostate, and in some human prostate carcinoma cell lines, are inducible by androgens *(219–222)*. Some human prostate carcinoma cell lines contain high levels of TGF-α mRNA and exhibit an increased proliferation in response to TGF-α *(223)*. The androgen-independent prostate carcinoma cell line, PC-3, exhibits a reduced requirement for exogenous GFs. This results, in part, from the secretion of TGF-α into the medium. and from the expression of EGFR on these cells *(224)*. Pretreatment of

PC-3, DU-145, or ALVA101 prostate carcinoma cells with a humanized EGFR-blocking monoclonal antibody (mAb) or TGF-α-neutralizing Ab is able to block the growth stimulatory effects of TGF-α in vitro, and to significantly inhibit the growth of PC-3, DU-145, and ALVA101 tumor xenografts *(221,224)*. Likewise, growth of PC-3 tumor xenografts in nude mice can be significantly retarded by the intratumoral injection of TGF-α or EGFR antisense oligodeoxynucleotides *(225)*. LNCaP cells can be stimulated to proliferate with either EGF or TGF-α *(226)*. The synthetic androgen, R1881, can stimulate the growth and increase the number of EGF receptors in these cells, suggesting that the increased growth rate of LNCaP cells is related in part to the increase in EGFR expression, thereby hypersensitizing these cells to endogenously produced TGF-α *(226)*. In contrast to EGF or TGF-α, HRG was found to inhibit LNCaP growth, and to induce a more differentiated phenotype *(227)*. Treatment of DU-145 cells, an androgen-independent human prostate carcinoma cell line, with suramin (a trypanocidal drug that can inhibit the binding of various GFs to their receptors), specifically reduced the binding of TGF-α to DU-145 cells and EGF to LNCaP cells *(228,229)*. This effect was substantially reversed by culturing the cells in the presence of an excess of TGF-α *(229)*.

TGF-α and EGF expression in prostate carcinomas is generally elevated, relative to BPH or prostatic intraepithelial neoplasia (PIN) *(230,231)*. In the normal human prostate, TGF-α may function as a paracrine effector, because it is expressed in the stroma; in prostate carcinoma cells, this GF probably becomes a predominantly autocrine growth regulator *(208,210,231)*. The most intensive staining for TGF-α has been demonstrated in less-differentiated prostate tumors. TGF-α expression has been shown to be significantly correlated with the histopathological grade of the tumors, but not with the expression of proliferation markers, such as Ki-67 *(231)*. More recently, immunoreactive HRGα has been demonstrated to be expressed in nearly 70% of prostate carcinomas; its receptor, *erb*B-3, is expressed in 54% of the cases in the tumor ECs *(232)*. Increased expression of *erb*B-3 can be detected in PINs and prostate carcinoma, compared to nondysplastic normal secretory prostate epithelium *(233)*. In a second study, 95% of prostate carcinomas were found to express *erb*B-3 and only 23% *erb*B-4 *(234)*. In contrast, HRG expression was found to be restricted to the stroma of normal and benign prostate lesions *(234)*.

In contrast to TGF-α and HRGα, which are expressed in the normal prostate stroma, EGFR, *erb*B-2, *erb*B-3, and *erb*B-4 expression is restricted to the epithelial compartment, where expression of the EGFR is elevated in human prostate carcinomas, compared to normal or benign human prostate tissues *(222,232–235)*. EGFR expression is negatively regulated by androgens, and is correlated with high-grade tumors and with less-differentiated tumors *(222,236,237)*. More recently, it has been demonstrated that expression of EGFR is highest in BPH, compared to PIN or prostate carcinoma *(238)*. These data are at variance with other data, which demonstrate higher levels of EGFR expression in PC tissue, compared to BPH *(222,236)*.

There are conflicting data on the relative levels of expression of c-*erb*B-2 in BPH or prostate carcinomas, since expression levels range from 30 to 86% in prostate tumor samples and from 0 to 62% in BPH samples. For example, no staining was found in 23 PCs or in 10 BPH specimens, using an anti-*erb*B-2 Ab *(239)*. In contrast, another study *(240)* found that 86% of 19 primary prostate tumors were moderately to strongly stained. Similar to EGFR expression, expression of *erb*B-2 mRNA is enhanced by androgens *(241)*. More recently, 53 prostate carcinomas and 9 cases of BPH were examined for c-*erb*B-2 gene amplification and *erb*B-2 overexpression *(242,243)*. Enhanced staining

Table 3
Novel Therapeutic Targets

Growth factors
    Neutralizing antibodies
    Antagonists
    Sequestration drugs (Suramin/PPS)
    Antisense ODNs
Growth factor receptors
    Immunotherapy and blocking antibodies
    Ligand-based toxins
    Protein kinase inhibitors
    Antisense ODNs
    Vaccines
Intracellular signal transduction components
    Peptide antagonists for SH2/PID
    Farnesylation inhibitors
    PI-3-Kinase inhibitors
    MAPK inhibitors

was detected in 34% of the carcinomas and in none of the BPH samples *(243)*. Over-expression of c-*erb*B-2 results fromenhanced levels of transcription, but also amplification has been detected by fluorescence *in situ* hybridization analysis and found to correlate with Gleason score in approx 40% of prostate tumors that are generally nondiploid *(244,245)*. Similar to EGFR expression, enhanced staining for *erb*B-2 was more prevalent in poorly differentiated carcinomas than in well-differentiated prostate tumors.

DIAGNOSTIC, PROGNOSTIC, AND THERAPEUTIC APPLICATIONS

Differential overexpression of the EGFR or *erb*B-2 in breast, ovarian, and endometrial carcinomas has already proven to be efficacious in stratifying patients with respect to subsequent Chemo, and in prediction of shorter disease-free survival or overall survival. This suggests that these receptors, or the GFs or signaling proteins that function either upstream or downstream from these receptors, may represent novel targets for selective therapy (Table 3; *246–255*). In addition, the detection of elevated levels of GFs in the urine and in the serous effusions of BC patients or the shed ECD of GF receptors, such as the ECD of c-*erb*B-2, in the serum of BC or PC patients, suggests that these proteins may have some utility in the early diagnosis of BC. Detection of these peptides could also be useful in the prognosis of BC, PC, or ovarian cancer (OC), particularly for following the response to therapy, or for monitoring tumor progression or recurrence *(256–264)*. For example, EGF concentrations are significantly higher in cystic breast fluid from patients with associated proliferative benign or malignant breast pathology *(265,266)*. Reciprocally, expression of the EGFR in ductal ECs found in needle aspirates is significantly higher in women at high risk for BC development (e.g., first-degree relative with BC) than in low-risk women *(267)*.

The selective overexpression of GF receptors in tumors also offers the potential for therapeutic intervention, since humanized antireceptor mAbs, which can block the binding of a ligand to a receptor such as the EGFR or *erb*B-2, have been demonstrated to be efficacious in perturbing tumor cell growth in vitro and in vivo, particularly in breast and ovarian tumors that overexpress these receptors *(249–252,254,255,268–273)*. A prime example is Herceptin, which is a humanized anti-*erb*B-2 mAb that can block signaling through this receptor. Herceptin has significantly lengthened survival time in 16% of stage IV metastatic BC patients *(273)*. In addition to the use of antireceptor-blocking mAbs, anti-GF neutralizing mAbs, such as those directed against TGF-α, may also be equally as effective in directly or indirectly blocking tumor cell growth. In addition, combination or rotation therapy of these monoclonal antireceptor or anti-GF Abs or chimeric GF toxins with other more conventional chemotherapeutic drugs, such as *cis*-platinum, paclitaxel, or doxorubicin, may synergistically enhance the therapeutic efficacy of these drugs in breast and ovarian cancer. This may, therefore, reduce the systemic side effects of these drugs, because lower effective doses of these cytotoxic agents could be used *(274–277)*. For example, Herceptin in combination with paclitaxel produced an approx threefold increase in response rate (RR) in patients treated with Ab plus drug (45% RR), compared to the drug alone (16% RR) *(273)*. It may also be possible to construct synthetic peptide analogs of *erb*B receptor transmembrane region(s), which are involved in heterodimer formation, and which could sterically inhibit receptor dimerization in a manner similar to the mechanism by which dominant-negative receptor mutants abrogate normal receptor function. These peptides could be selectively introduced into tumor cells that are overexpressing a particular *erb*B receptor. Such an approach has already proven experimentally feasible, since expression vector constructs that produce short transmembrane *erb*B-2 proteins, which lack ligand binding or intracellular kinase domains, were able to significantly inhibit the in vitro growth and tumorigenicity of *erb*B-2 transformed cells *(278)*.

For radioimaging and for therapy, conjugation or genetic chimerization of radionuclides, bacterial or fungal toxins or drugs, to GFs or to different anti-*erb*B receptor or anti-GF mAbs may provide a mechanism for selectively delivering these cytotoxic agents to tumor cells that are overexpressing different *erb*B receptors or cell-associated EGF-like GFs. For example, chimeric toxins encoding GF genes, such as TGF-α, HB-EGF, or HRG, have been selectively chimerized to the II and III domains of *Pseudomonas* exotoxin A (PE). Some of these recombinant PE-peptides, such as HRGβ1-PE toxins, can selectively kill breast tumor cells in vitro and in vivo, which are expressing high numbers of *erb*B-3 or *erb*B-4 *(279–284)*.

Because members of the *erb*B family all possess an intracellular TK that is essential for signaling, specific inhibitors of this enzyme, such as the tryphostins and other quinazolone compounds, may also have potential for use as therapeutic drugs *(285–289)*. In fact, some of the newer pyrido–pyrimidine compounds are orally active against human breast tumor xenografts that overexpress EGFR *(289)*. A more provocative gene therapy approach might include the use of antisense RNA expression vectors, using ribozymes or chemically modified phosphorothioate or methylphosphonate antisense oligodeoxynucleotides *(290–297)*. This approach has already proven to be effective in blocking the expression of TGF-α, AR, CR-1, EGFR, and c-*erb*B-2 in breast carcinoma cell lines, and in significantly inhibiting the growth and tumorigenicity of these cells. Their potential use in vivo may be facilitated by their encapsulation into liposomes containing a mAb that is directed against a tumor-associated antigen, and that has been integrated into the liposome membrane bilayer *(298)*. Alternatively, it may be possible to immunize patients against tumor-associated antigens, using peptide vaccine immunotherapy. In this context, tumors expressing the type VIII mutant form of the EGFR could be effectively targeted by prior immunization of mice with a peptide derived from the fusion junction region of the type VIII EGFR *(299)*. Design of specific inhibitors that can disrupt the activity or function of specific signal transduction proteins may also yield novel drugs that can uncouple GF receptors from other downstream effectors in tumor cells, which possess a constitutively activated intracellular signal transduction pathway *(247,248, 253)*. For example, specific farnesyltransferase inhibitors (FPTIs) have been isolated, which can block the farnesylation of p21^{ras} and which can prevent association of p21^{ras} with plasma membrane, thereby perturbing its activity. These compounds are effective in blocking in vitro transformation induced by a point-mutated *ras* gene *(300–305)*. It is possible that cancer cells that possess an activated, point-mutated *ras* gene or that over-express p21^{ras} in an active guanosine triphosphate-bound state caused by chronic auto-crine GF-induced receptor TK activation, may be particularly sensitive to this new class of compounds. In this context, mammary tumor growth in vivo can be effectively blocked by FPTIs *(305)*. Finally, the availability of specific mitogen-activated protein kinase (MAPK) and phosphatidylinositol-3 kinase inhibitors now offers the possibility of target-ing these proteins, which are frequently engaged in *erb*B signaling pathways *(247,253,306)*.

CERVICAL CANCER

The incidence of invasive cervical cancer (CC) is relatively low in the United States, with 15,800 patients diagnosed and 4500 deaths occurring in 1995 *(307)*. It is clinically well established that the proliferation of normal squamous epithelium of the cervix is under the control of sex hormones during the menstrual cycle. Immunohistochemically, it has been shown that, during the proliferative phase, cervical cells are ER-negative *(308)*. As plasma E_2 levels increase, the basal and parabasal cell layers become ER-positive. Finally, in the secretory phase of the menstrual cycle, the nuclei of the super-ficial layers (stratum spinosum, granulosum et corneum) also express ER. Secondary estrogen responses on the cervical epithelium can be mediated by estrogen-dependent effects through the stroma *(309)*.

There are several studies that have assessed the presence of ER or PR in cervical carcinomas *(310–316)*. The reported presence of ER in cervical carcinomas ranges from 12 to 100%, depending on the method of assessment (for review, *see* ref. *317*). The pres-ence of functional ER seems to be higher in adenocarcinomas of the cervix than in squa-mous epithelial neoplasms *(315,318,319)*. In a study with 100 postmenopausal women with locally advanced cervical carcinomas, Battacharya et al. *(320)* demonstrated that estrogen treatment increased the S-phase fraction, but also increased ER and PR content, suggesting the need for use of estrogen in combination with other treatment modalities. There are no valid data demonstrating the prognostic value of ER or PR in CC *(311–315,321,322)*. However, the proportion of CC patients who might be expected to obtain objective benefit from endocrine therapy is only about 30% *(317)*. Since the regulation of EGF-related GFs, such as TGF-α and AR by estrogen could be demonstrated, the same mechanisms might be assumed for cervical tissues *(323–326)*.

Human Papilloma Virus and EGF-like GFs and Receptor Expression

The human papilloma virus (HPV-16, -18, -33) plays a dominant role in the etiology of cervical carcinogenesis *(327,328)*. The viral proteins, E6 and E7, which are expressed by the high-risk types of HPV, are able to bind to and inactivate the host tumor suppressor proteins p53 and Rb, which normally inhibit cell cycle progression *(329,330)*. Inactiva-tion of p53 and Rb by E6 and E7 leads to dysregulated entry of cells into the S-phase of the cell cycle *(307,331–333)*. However, only a minority of HPV-infected women actually develop invasive CC. Thus, additional environmental and/or genetic factors must be involved in cervical carcinogenesis.

Approximately 66% of cervical carcinomas and 100% of vulvar condylomas that are the result of HPV-infection express high levels of TGF-α mRNA *(325)*. Because HPV-16 and HPV-18 are associated with approx 60–90% of cervical intraepithelial neoplasias, and since these viruses have a major transforming potential, these data suggest that overexpression of TGF-α may be associated with the early stages of disease after HPV infection. In this context, the *E6* and *E7* genes are involved in the immortalization and transforming activities of HPV, and the effects of these genes are accentuated by the product of the *E5* gene *(334)*. The *E5* gene encodes for a small membrane-associated protein that can inhibit the downregulation and degradation of the EGFR in response to ligand binding. In addition, *E5* can induce hyperphosphorylation of the EGFR in a ligand-independent fashion, and can accelerate receptor recycling at the cell surface, thereby hypersensitizing infected cells to the effects of EGF-related ligands *(335)*. This observation is of clinical relevance, because EGFR expression can be detected in 85–100% of HPV-related cervical dysplasias or condylomas *(336–339)*. In a series of 97 HPV lesions of the uterine cervix, EGFR expression was found in 95/97 (98%) specimens, mostly in the basal or parabasal cells *(340)*. No associations were established between the EGFR or *erb*B-2 and the specific HPV types, grade of cervical intraepithelial neoplasia (CIN), or the clinical course of cervical HPV lesions. Therefore, assessment of these factors seems to be of limited value in explaining the development of HPV-associated CIN, and in predicting the prognosis of this disease.

The tumor growth rate in CC cells is related to the level of induction of HPV gene products, but increased proliferation is not associated with upregulation of EGFR levels *(341)*. This finding suggests that EGFR overexpression by itself may not be an important feature in the etiology of cervical carcinoma. However, Woodworth et al. *(342)* have found in HPV-immortalized and carcinoma-derived cervical ECs, that the proinflammatory cytokines, interleukin 1α (IL-1α) and tumor necrosis factor α (TNF-α), stimulate the autocrine expression of AR in vitro. In contrast, both cytokines only minimally stimulated TGF-α mRNA expression. Additionally, treatment with recombinant TGF-α or AR could stimulate the proliferation of CX16-2 cervical cells in the absence of EGF. Similar results were reported for five immortal or carcinoma cell lines. Those investigators also observed that IL-1- and TNF-α-induced mitogenesis is dependent on a functional EGFR, and is further dependent on autocrine stimulation by AR. Recently, Hu et al. *(343)* demonstrated that either the expression of antisense HPV E6/E7 or the Rb transcription unit results in decreased expression of EGFR protein. EGFR levels were not affected at the transcriptional level, but at the posttranscriptional level. Reduced cancer cell growth has now been shown to occur when the EGFR transduction pathway is turned off by a diverse set of therapeutic agents, including antisense E6/E7 constructs *(344,345)*, anti-EGFR neutralizing Abs *(346)*, and specific inhibitors of the EGFR kinase *(347)*. It has also been shown that EGF has a direct stimulatory effect on the expression of E6 and E7 genes by activating AP-1 transcription factor activation *(348)*.

Expression Patterns and Biological Effects of EGF-Related GFs

Recently, using semiquantitative reverse transcriptase-polymerase chain reactions, Pfeiffer et al. *(349)* investigated the mRNA expression pattern of several EGF-related peptides in the normal human cervical epithelium and in CC, and found that CR-1 mRNA was expressed only in the stroma of normal cervix and not in the epithelium. Expression of TGF-α mRNA was found in the stroma. EGF, AR, and BTC mRNA were equally expressed in epithelium and stroma. Furthermore, there were no significant differences in the mRNA expression of any EGF-related peptide between normal cervix and CC. In approx 10% of the carcinomas, overexpression of EGF, AR, and TGF-α mRNA was observed. In the majority of cervical carcinomas, the level of mRNA expression of EGF-related peptides seemed to decline with tumor progression. In undifferentiated stage II cervical carcinomas, the mRNA expression of TGF-α and HB-EGF was significantly reduced, in comparison with more differentiated stage I tumors *(349)*. Konishi et al. *(350)* demonstrated TGF-α expression in normal, benign, and malignant lesions of the cervix. Immunohistochemically, normal squamous cells of the exocervix were found to be TGF-α-negative; reserve cells and metaplastic squamous cells in the transformation zone were positive. Most cases of CIN, with or without koilocytotic atypias, were TGF-α-negative. In invasive carcinomas (SCC), TGF-α immunoreactivity was observed in 49% of squamous cell carcinomas, and in 100% of adenocarcinomas (ACs) and adenosquamous carcinomas. There was no significant correlation between TGF-α positivity and clinical stage of disease or degree of keratinization.

GFs have been implicated as agents that stimulate proliferation and enhance the possibility of malignant transformation in cervical cells *(351)*. In proliferation assays, EGF can enhance CC cell growth in a dose-dependent manner *(352,353)*. EGF may be stimulating proliferation by an EGF mitogenic pathway, and by indirectly reducing the levels of inhibitory insulin-like GF binding proteins. It has also been demonstrated that the autocrine production of IGF-II and the overexpression of IGF-IR, are important in controling the proliferation of CC cells, and that autocrine IGF-II production may also participate in the mitogenic signaling of EGF in these cells *(354)*. This might be an important mechanism, since Tonkin et al. *(355)* did not find evidence of amplification of the EGFR gene in four CC cell lines, using Southern blot analysis. Additionally, infection with multiple sexually transmitted pathogens has been associated with inflammation of the cervix and an increased risk of CC in women who are also infected with HPVs. Various studies have demonstrated that IL-1α and TNF-α stimulate the proliferation of immortal and malignant cervical cells by an EGFR-dependent pathway requiring autocrine stimulation by AR *(342)*. In addition, in the ME180 cervical carcinoma cell line, the expression and the TK activity of the EGFR may alter TNF-α cytotoxicity and signal transduction, and may therefore control TNF-α responsiveness *(356–358)*. In contrast, in the same cell line, retinoic acid reduces the synthesis of EGFR *(359)*. In SKG-III cervical carcinoma cells, EGF and TGF-α stimulate haptotactic migration, invasive activity, and type-IV collagenase activity *(360)*. In OMC-4 cervical AC cells, the production of laminin and collagen IV is inhibited by EGF; that of tissue plasminogen activator was significantly promoted at physiological concentrations of EGF *(361)*.

Clinical Use of erbB-Receptors as Prognostic Factors

There are a number of publications demonstrating the expression of EGFR or erbB-2 in normal and dysplastic crvical epithelim or CC. Generally, overexpression of EGFR is a hallmark of human SCC *(362)*. In 52 cervical carcinomas and 40 normal cervical epithelia, Pfeiffer et al. *(363)* found a higher expression of EGFR in homogenized malignant tissue than in the normal samples, using a ligand-binding technique. A high EGFR expression was associated with a poor prognosis. In contrast, Kimmig et al. *(364)* have shown that expression of EGFR in most cervical carcinomas is reduced, compared with the normal cervical epithelium, indicating that dedifferentiation of cells may be associated with a reduction of EGFR, instead of an increase. Using two-color flow cytometry in a prospective study on 73 primary cervical carcinomas and 11 normal controls, they found EGFR overexpression in only 10% of cervical carcinomas. They suggest that cervical carcinomas overexpressing EGFR represent a small, biologically distinct subgroup of this cancer, which exhibits an enhanced aggressiveness associated with poor prognosis. In this context, EGFR levels seem to be indicative of the biological aggressiveness of cervical carcinomas, and may provide additional information for the prediction of the prognosis of this disease *(363,365)*. Recently, Pfeiffer et al. *(366)* showed that EGFR levels per cell were high in the nondividing, upper cell layers of the normal human cervical epithelium, where a mitogenic function of EGF can be excluded. In the proliferative basal or parabasal strata, normal cells express intermediate or comparatively reduced levels of EGFR per cell. CC cells displayed a significant reduction of specific EGF binding and of EGFR levels per cell, compared with normal epithelium. A significant negative correlation of cell density and EGFR number per cell was obtained *(366)*. In a retrospective study, Hale et al. *(367,368)* found EGFR staining in approx 34% of human invasive CCs. EGFR expression in SCC, adenosquamous carcinomas, and ACs was 50, 33, and 19%, respectively. Overall, EGFR staining was correlated with poor prognosis, but, in the histological subgroups, the results were quite different. Thus, in SCCs, there was no correlation between EGFR staining intensity and patient outcome. In contrast, in adenosquamous carcinoma there was a significant correlation between EGFR expression and mortality, both overall and in those lacking lymph node metastases. When lymph node metastasis was present, no such correlation could be shown. No correlation between EGFR expression and outcome could be demonstrated in ACs. However, in ACs, there was a correlation of EGFR expression and the presence of lymph node metastasis. Hale et al. *(367,368)* concluded that IHC demonstration of EGFR expression may be useful in identifying those patients with a poor prognosis, particularly those with adenosquamous carcinomas that have not metastasized to the regional lymph nodes. These findings are supported by Hayashi et al. *(369)*, who found no correlation between EGFR expression and lymph node status in SCCs. On the other hand, patients with positive staining for $p21^{ras}$ had a significantly higher incidence of lymph node metastasis. This suggests that expression of the *ras* oncogene product may be associated with biological aggressiveness in cervical carcinoma.

An interesting diagnostic approach involved the use of lymphoscintigraphy, using EGF as a tumor-seeking agent, in CC *(370)*. However, labeled EGF did not localize to the regional lymph nodes, where metastases could be detected. In fresh-frozen tissue samples, Berchuck et al. *(337)* found EGFR expression in basal keratinocytes of normal epithelium; in carcinoma *in situ*, the EGFR expression was maintained throughout the entire thickness of the epithelium. They also found EGFR staining in many carcinomas, but the staining intensity did not appear to be significantly stronger than that seen in the basal layer of normal cervical epithelium. In another study, Berchuck et al. *(337)* analyzed EGFR levels in frozen tissues, using ^{125}I-labeled EGF with a computerized image analysis system. Among 54 cervical carcinomas, 23 (43%) had an increase in EGFR levels (<3-fold). High overexpression (>3-fold) was seen in 2/54 cases. Patients whose cancer had significant EGFR overexpression died of disease.

In 6/11 normal cervical tissue samples, Goeppinger et al. *(371)* found strong EGFR staining, using frozen tissues samples from punch biopsies. The staining reaction was confined to the basal and deep parabasal cell layers. Staining was independent of the day of the menstrual cycle, age, or the presence of inflammatory disease. In contrast to the normal epithelium, in all 27 CIN samples (with or without HPV association), homogenous EGFR staining could be observed. In CINs, all dysplastic cells exhibited stronger EGFR staining. No correlation between HPV infection and EGFR staining, localization, or intensity could be found. No EGFR staining could be detected in the more differentiated cell layers of the normal cervical epithelium. This finding suggests that there is an inhibition of EGFR expression in the terminal phase of squamous epithelium cell differentiation.

Using an enzyme-linked immunosorbent assay in fresh tissue samples, Kim et al. *(372)* found no EGFR overexpression (defined as EGFR level exceeding the 250 fmol/mg protein) in a control group of 10 chronic cervicitis, but EGFR overexpression was found in 25% of 20 CIN II/III samples. In 40 invasive cervical carcinomas, 72.5% showed EGFR overexpression. Lesions of 4 cm or more had significantly higher EGFR levels than those under 4 cm. There were no significant differences in EGFR levels when stratified according to clinical stage, histological cell type, age, or menopausal status. These data were confirmed by the IHC findings of Maruo et al. *(336)*, who found no EGFR expression in normal cervical epithelium, but 75% of dysplastic and 50% of malignant tissues were positive. Large-cell nonkeratinizing and keratinizing carcinomas contained high levels of EGFR; small-cell nonkeratinizing carcinomas lacked EGFR. Elevated expression of EGFR may be involved in the initial stage of tumorigenesis, and may be related to the differentiation or dedifferentiation of cervical squamous carcinoma cells.

Expression of erbB-2 has also been examined in cervical tissues *(373,374)*. Berchuck et al. *(337)* found erbB-2 expression primarily in the ectocervical basal squamous cells of the normal cervix. In contrast, in the endocervix, EGFR staining was seen primarily in stroma, and erbB-2 expression was observed only in the glandular epithelium. In the same study, 1/26 CCs was found to overexpress erbB-2: This was the only patient who presented with pulmonary metastasis at the time of diagnosis. Mitra et al. *(375)* found erbB-2 amplification in 22% of 50 cervical carcinomas. Overexpression of erbB-2 was observed in 25% of cervical ACs *(376)*. Using IHC in a retrospective clinical evaluation of 62 cases with CC (20 SCCs, 21 adenosquamous carcinomas, and 21 ACs), Hale et al. *(367)* detected erbB-2 membrane staining in 24/62 (38.7%) cases. Overall, a significant correlation between positive staining and poor outcome for patients, both with or without lymph node metastasis, was found. Additionally, a significant correlation between positive staining and poor prognosis was seen in all three tumor subtypes. No significant correlation was detected between lymph node status and erbB-2 staining, except in ACs, in which there was significantly more staining in the tumors of patients in whom lymph node metastasis had been identified. Where lymph node metastasis was absent, positive erbB-2 staining was significantly related to poor outcome in SCCs and in adenosquamous carcinomas; in ACs, all 14 tumors lacking lymph node metastasis were negative for erbB-2. Immunostaining for erbB-2 could be useful as a prognostic marker and may help identify those patients for whom early adjuvant treatment might be beneficial.

Using IHC, Brumm et al. *(377)* showed at least focal positivity for erbB-2 protein expression in 100% (17/17) of CINs and in 6/8 cervical SCCs. In a larger retrospective IHC study of 125 patients with SCCs, 21 ACs, and 4 adenosquamous carcinomas, Ndubisi et al. *(378)* noted erbB-2 expression in 22% of total cases. Semiquantitative scoring of erbB-2 expression did not show any correlation with stage, histology, grade, or patient age. There was no significant change in 5-yr survival rates in patients whose tumors expressed erbB-2. Lakshmi et al. *(379)*, using IHC in 150 normal cervical tissue samples, found erbB-2 and EGFR expression in 83.3 and 86.6% of this group, respectively. There was no difference between erbB-2 and EGFR expression in 100 low-grade squamous intraepithelial lesions (SILs) vs staining in 122 high-grade SILs. In 166 invasive carcinomas, erbB-2 and EGFR expression was observed in 96.8 and 93.7% of the cases, respectively. Also, there was a significant correlation between EGFR and erbB-2 expression in the different cell layers of the cervix. In normal tissue, immunoreactivity for EGFR expression was mostly confined to the basal and parabasal cell layers, suggesting that there is a reduction in EGFR expression during the terminal phase of squamous cell differentiation. In SIL, all dysplastic cells were found to exhibit a stronger EGFR expression. The expression intensity and the localization of EGFR are independent of the day of the menstrual cycle *(379)*.

Altavilla et al. *(380)* reported EGFR and erbB-2 expression in 43 cervical ACs, in which 41.5% were EGFR-positive and 53.5% were erbB-2 positive. There was no significant correlation between EGFR expression and stage of disease, lymph node status, vascular space invasion, isthmus infiltration, or overall survival. Additionally, there was no significant correlation between EGFR or erbB-2 expression and different histological subgroups (endometroide, mucinous, clear cell, serous, mesonephric, adenosquamous). For erbB-2 expression, a significant correlation was observed with lymph node status, vascular space involvement, and isthmus infiltration. In lymph-node-positive cases, erbB-2 was expressed in all the tumor samples. In a retrospective IHC analysis, Kristensen et al. *(381)* evaluated the expression of EGFR, erbB-2, and cathepsin D expression in 132 patients with International Federation of Gynecology and Obstetrics (FIGO) Institute of Biology (IB) cervical carcinomas that had been treated surgically, and in 10 control patients without cancer. Overexpression of the EGFR was observed in 25.8% *(34)* of the tumors, but no correlation with any histopathological variables was detected. Otherwise, the relapse-free survival was lower in patients whose tumor was overexpressing EGFR. erbB2 was positive in 12% of the cases. However, no correlation with relapse-free survival was found. In a multivariate analysis, expression of EGFR and cathepsin D obtained independent prognostic significance, and, when considered together, were the strongest prognostic factors, after tumor size. Of clinical interest is the finding of no relapse in a subgroup of patients with squamous cervical cancer smaller than 2 cm in dimension and not overexpressing the EGFR. In contrast to Hale et al. *(367)*, erbB-2 was not found to be useful in predicting prognosis in squamous cervical cancer. In 64 patients with SCC that had been treated with radiation therapy, Nakano et al. *(382)* found IHC positivity for erbB-2 in 42.4% of the cases. A significant increase in erbB-2 expression was observed with advanced stages, but no correlation between erbB-2 expression and histological subtypes was detectable. The mean growth fraction of erbB-2-positive tumors was significantly lower than of erbB-2-negative tumors (26.2 vs 38.3%). Otherwise, the mitotic index in erbB-2-positive tumors was significantly higher than in erbB-2-negative samples (3.7 vs 2.0%). The 5-yr survival rates for erbB-2-positive and erbB-2-negative patients were 44.4 and 74.8%, respectively, indicating a poorer prognosis in erbB-2-positive patients. A similar trend was observed in stage III patients, in which 5-yr survival rates for erbB-2-positive and erbB-2-negative tumors were 44.4 vs 69%, respectively. The 5-yr recurrence rate of erbB-2-positive patients after radiotherapy was 37.3%, significantly higher than the 8.3% rate for erbB-2-negative patients. The same trend was seen in stage III patients. Nakano et al. *(382)* concluded that erbB-2 expression was chiefly associated with radiation resistance.

ENDOMETRIAL CANCER

Cancer of the endometrium is the most common female genital tract malignancy *(383)*. It is estimated by the American Cancer Society that approx 35,000 women develop endometrial cancer per year in the United States, making it the fourth most common cancer in women. Multiple risk factors, such as late menopause, nulliparity, or obesity, have been identified, but the etiology of this disease is unknown. There have been several studies demonstrating the importance of EGF-related peptides and their receptors *(384–386)*, in normal, hyperplastic, and malignant endometrial tissues *(387–389)*.

Expression and Biological Effects of EGF-Like Peptides

GFs may play an important role in human endometrial cancer development, both alone or in combination with sex steroids. In endometrial carcinoma cell lines, EGF-related GFs play a major role in regulating proliferation *(390–392)*. EGF might exert its mitogenic effects by activating protein kinase C through increased breakdown of phosphatidylinositol *(393)*. In the poorly differentiated endometrial cancer cell line, KLE, EGF stimulation of cell growth is exerted through both protein kinase C-dependent and independent pathways *(394)*. In vitro, the phosphatidylinositol cascade appears to be an important signal transduction pathway that mediates the growth effects of EGF on HEC-1-A endometrial cancer cells *(393)*. This may be significant, since, in endometrial carcinoma, sex steroid hormones can regulate phospholipid turnover. TAM action can be mediated through an alteration of protein kinase C activation *(395)*. An inverse relationship was found between EGFR content and the percentage of EGF-induced stimulation of phospholipid turnover. A similar relationship was observed between EGFR content in EGFR-positive samples and the extent of P suppression of EGF-induced turnover *(396)*. In vitro, it has been demonstrated that EGF-like GFs and sex steroids have significant effects on migration and invasion of endometrial cells *(397)*, endometrial receptivity *(398)*, proliferation and regulation of protein tyrosine phosphatase 1D *(399)*, and malignant transformation *(400)*.

Bauknecht et al. *(401)* found that the EGFR and EGF or TGF-α can be detected in most epithelial tumors of the female genital tract, such as CC, endometrial cancer, Fallopian tube cancer *(402,403)*, and OC. Using an EGFR radioreceptor assay, 4/14 (28%) endometrial carcinomas exhibited enhanced levels of EGF-like activity.

Expression of mRNA for EGF, TGF-α, AR, HB-EGF, BTC, and CR-1 has been detected by Pfeiffer et al. *(349)* in normal human endometrium. In 19 endometrial cancers, the same authors found that mRNA levels of these EGF-related peptides were higher than in normal endometrium samples. The increase was significant for TGF-α and AR, but no correlation of EGF-related peptide mRNA expression and tumor stage or histological differentiation was observed. Using IHC, Niikura et al. *(404)* demonstrated positive immunoreactivity for EGFR, EGF, TGF-α, and CR-1 in 58.5, 66.7, 91.6, and 66.7% of normal endometrium samples, respectively. In hyperplasia of the endometrium, positive immunoreactivity for EGFR, EGF, TGF-α, and CR-1 was observed in 100, 15.4, 100, and 30.8% of the samples, respectively. In endometrial cancer, they detected positive immunoreactivity for EGFR, EGF, TGF-α, and CR-1 in 67.5, 32.5, 65, and 65% of tumor samples, respectively. AR was not detected in normal endometrium, hyperplasia, or endometrial carcinomas. In their study, Niikura et al. *(404)* demonstrated that TGF-α or EGFR expression correlated significantly with surgical stage, the depth of myometrial invasion, and peritoneal washings. CR-1 expression correlated more significantly with surgical stage than either EGFR or TGF-α, and there was no significant correlation between CR-1 immunoreactivity and EGFR, TGF-α, or EGF expression. Niikura et al. *(404)* also demonstrated that co-expression of EGFR and CR-1 or TGF-α, and CR-1 in endometrial carcinoma specimens significantly correlated with advanced surgical stage, deeper myometrial invasion, and positive peritoneal washing cytology. Jasonni et al. *(405)* investigated 44 primary endometrial carcinomas for TGF-α and EGFR expression. They found a differential staining pattern for TGF-α and EGFR. EGFR and TGF-α co-expression was a constant feature of benign squamous metaplasia. Reinartz et al. *(406)* found that positive TGF-α staining (41/128, or 32%) correlated with increased myometrial infiltration, reduced survival, and the presence of vascular invasion. In a multivariant analysis. TGF-α staining was not an independent predictor of survival.

Exogenous or unopposed estrogen is a known risk factor for the development of endometrial cancer. In several human endometrial carcinoma cell lines and primary tumors, EGFR is expressed and seems to be regulated by sex steroids *(392,405,407,408)*. Additionally, there is evidence demonstrating that human endometrial cancer cell lines may also have a regulatory system for their proliferation that is dependent on luteinizing hormone-releasing hormone (LH-RH) and EGF *(409)*. For example, LH-RH analogs can entirely block EGF-induced MAPK activity in endometrial carcinoma cells *(410)*. In benign endometrium, EGFR expression increases during the estrogen-dominant follicular phase, and decreases during the P-dominant luteal phase *(411)*. Haining et al. *(412)* suggested that EGF may play a role in estrogen-stimulated proliferation of normal and endometriotic endometrium. Estrogen can increase c-H-ras expression and total TK activity in endometrial fibroblasts and in Ishikawa endometrial carcinoma cells. In contrast, P diminishes c-H-ras expression and TK activity induced by estrogen in the fibroblasts, but not in the carcinoma cells, which persistently overexpress c-H-ras *(413)*. EGF increased c-H-ras expression, as did E_2. Thus, it may be that a TK activity can lead to an overexpression of c-H-ras in endometrial cancer cells after estrogen stimulation, which may therefore be associated with an increase in tumor cell growth potential *(413)*. On the other hand, mutated Ki-ras can cause a loss of responsiveness to EGF in endometrial Ishikawa cells, where EGFR function is dispensable for the growth of mutant Ki-ras-positive endometrial carcinoma cells *(414)*. In human RL95-2 endometrial carcinoma cells, there is also evidence for a differential effect of EGF on fos/jun and c-myc expression *(415)*.

In normal human endometrium and in different types of endometrial hyperplasia, Niikura et al. *(404)* found that only the distribution of TGF-α was concordant with that of ER expression. The correlation between ER or PR expression and AR, EGF, EGFR, or CR-1 expression was not significant. In the same study, a significant inverse correlation between IHC positivity for TGF-α and ER was detected in human endometrial carcinoma samples of different histology. Within the same histological subtype, no correlation was found. The correlation between ER or PR and EGF, AR, CR-1, or EGFR was not significant. Niikura et al. *(404)* suggested that an estrogen-independent, EGFR/TGF-α autocrine pathway may be operative in poorly differentiated endometrial neoplasms that express TGF-α, but not ER. However, some moderately or well-differentiated endometrial carcinomas apparently express TGF-α through an estrogen-dependent pathway *(416)*, similar to normal cycling endometrium or hyperplasia. In a total of 113 cases of endometrial carcinomas, Yokoyama et al. *(417)* found positive immunoreactivity for EGF, EGFR, and TGF-α in 25.6, 53.1, and 67% of the cases, respectively. EGF and EGFR expression was not correlated with histologic grade or clinical stage. Only TGF-α expression was found to correlate with poor grading and advanced FIGO stage. There was a significant negative association between E_2 and TGF-α status. Also, simultaneous expression of E_2, EGF, and EGFR, or E_2, TGF-α, and EGFR was detected in 6.8 and 15.9% of all tumor samples, respectively. Yokoyama et al. *(417)* suggested that a predominant number of endometrial carcinomas escape autocrine or paracrine growth regulation by EGF and E_2 or TGF-α and E_2. EGF and TGF-α are therefore expressed independent of E_2 status in endometrial cancer. The relative amount of TGF-α mRNA was significantly reduced by medroxyprogesterone acetate in estrogen-responsive Ishikawa cells, but not in estrogen-unresponsive HEC-50 endometrial carcinoma cells *(418,419)*. Exogenous TGF-α stimulated proliferation of both cell lines *(418)*. Neither E_2 nor TAM affected mRNA levels for TGF-α in HEC-50 cells. In Ishikawa cells, E_2 increased TGF-α mRNA and TAM lowered the TGF-α mRNA *(416)*.

The findings of Berchuck et al. *(338)* also showed that high-level erbB-2 expression is associated with the absence of ER expression, and with an increased mortality rate from endometrial cancer. No significant correlations were revealed between EGFR and ER/PR status in 26 patients *(396)*. Estrogens may enhance EGFR expression in the uterus; EGF may promote a number of phenotypic changes in uterine ECs, that are normally induced by estrogens, such as regulation of ER and PR expression *(420–422)*. EGFR expression has been detected in 91% of endometrial carcinomas; 30% of these carcinomas express erbB-2. In certain endometrial cell lines, the antiproliferative effects of P are associated with a reduction in TGF-α mRNA expression *(405,423)*. The growth inhibitory effects of P could be significantly reversed by exogenous TGF-α. Finally, an anti-EGFR blocking Ab could produce a 40–50% inhibition of anchorage-dependent growth of these cells, suggesting that TGF-α was functioning as an autocrine GF. Also, a majority of primary endometrial carcinomas (66%) were found to express TGF-α mRNA *(424)*. Treatment of endometrial carcinomas with a synthetic P, Danazol, results in a significant decrease in TGF-α and EGFR expression *(405)*. TGF-α expression was co-expressed with EGFR in endometroid ACs and ACs with benign squamous metaplasia. In the prognostically unfavorable mucinous and serous papillary ACs, EGFR and TGF-α immunostaining was not observed. EGFR and TGF-α coexpression appeared as a constant feature of benign squamous metaplasia *(405)*. Normal endometrial cells are growth-inhibited by EGF, TGF-α and IGF-I; endometrial carcinoma cells exhibit an increase in thymidine incorporation when treated with EGF, TGF-α or IGF-I *(411)*. These data are consistent with the autocrine stimulation hypothesis for malignant cells, and illustrate differences, compared to normal endometrial GF-mediated proliferation.

Expression of erbB Receptors and Clinical Outcome

Several studies have focused on the expression of EGFR and/or erbB-2 and their biological or clinical role in endometrial cancer *(338,406,425,426,428)*, or in mixed malignant Muellerian tumors *(427)*. Overexpression of erbB-2 occurs in approx 10–30% of endometrial tumors, and is associated with aggressive, poorly differentiated tumors *(377,428,429)*. Using a multiparameter flow-cytometric quantitation method, Van Dam et al. *(425)* found overexpression of EGFR or erbB-2 in 2/15 (13%) and 2/13 (15%) endometrial carcinomas, respectively. The expression of both receptors was significantly higher in the malignant tissue than in the corresponding normal endometrium, but was also higher in premenopausal than in postmenopausal patients. A direct correlation between the ploidy status and the expression of EGFR and erbB-2 has been found. Esteller et al. *(426)* examined the amplification of erbB-2 and EGFR in 50 normal endometrial tissues, 10 adenomatous hyperplasias, and 50 endometrial carcinomas, using genomic differential polymerase chain reaction. No EGFR gene amplification was found in normal, hyperplastic, or malignant tissues, suggesting that mechanisms other than gene amplification could be responsible for the reported EGFR overexpression. Amplification of erbB-2 was found in 14% of endometrial carcinomas. None of the 50 endometrial normal tissues or the 10 adenomatous hyperplasias showed *erb*B-2 gene amplification. Nyholm et al. *(407)* have shown that EGFR expression was not correlated with histologic grade, surgical stage, or ER/PR status evaluated immunohistochemically or biochemically in adjacent tissue sections of endometrial carcinomas. In 65 endometrial carcinomas, 71% expressed positive EGFR immunoreactivity. EGFR immunoreactivity was also observed in 77% of atrophic/inactive endometria and in 54% of adenomatous hyperplasias. EGFR immunoreactivity seems to be related to the endometrial cancer histotype, regardless of the tumor grade or extent of myometrial invasion *(405,408)*.

Strong or diffuse staining for EGFR was found in 41/128 (32%) of endometrial carcinomas, but EGFR did not correlate with any known prognostic variable *(406)*. Expression of erbB-2 was found to correlate with tumor type, but was not found to be a valuable prognostic indicator. In contrast, Berchuck et al. *(338)* and Hetzel et al. *(428)* found that erbB-2 overexpression may be a useful prognostic factor in endometrial cancer. In 95 patients with endometrial cancer and in 24 patients with normal endometrium, Berchuck et al. *(338)* found that 9% of endometrial ACs had more intense staining for erbB-2 than was observed in normal endometrium. High erbB-2 expression was detected in 27% of patients with metastatic disease, compared with 4% of patients with disease confined to the corpus uteri. In a very complete study representing 247 patients with endometrial cancer, Hetzel et al. *(428)* analyzed the expression of erbB-2. Strong overexpression of erbB-2 was associated with a poor overall survival. Multivariate analysis revealed that overexpression had independent significance in predicting progression-free and overall patient survival. In stage I patients, the 5-yr progression-free survival was significantly decreased in the erbB-2-overexpressing group, compared to the erbB-2-negative group (62 vs 97%). No correlation between *erb*B-2 gene amplification and FIGO stage, histologic grade, or lymph node metastasis were found by Seki et al. *(430)*, but there was a significant association between erbB-2 amplification and deep myometrial infiltration, suggesting that erbB-2 gene amplification may be involved in local progression, but is not closely related to the loss of differentiation and metastasis. In contrast, Rasty et al. *(389)* published a significant correlation between the level of *erb*B-2 oncogene expression and overall survival. They suggest that the association between *erb*B-2 oncogene expression, higher grade lesions, and poor survival in patients with endometrial cancer may also justify assessment of the *erb*B-2 oncogene as a reliable prognostic marker.

Recently, Ayhan et al. *(431)* have demonstrated that CR-1 was expressed in 71% of endometrial carcinomas, but there was no significant correlation between cripto immunoreactivity and major determinants of survival for endometrial cancer, such as grade, myometrial invasion, lymph node involvement, or lymphovascular space involvement.

CR-1 immunoreactivity was stronger in adenomatous hyperplasia with atypia than without hyperplasia, suggesting that CR-1 may play a role in the transition from atypical hyperplasia to carcinoma. Costa and Walls *(427)* examined 82 cases of malignant, mixed Muellerian tumors, including 61 endometrial tumors for EGFR and erbB-2 expression. Immunoreactivity for erbB-2 was present in 96.3, and 99% of carcinomatous and sarcomatous tumor components, respectively. No association between erbB-2 immunoreactivity and pathological features was observed. In contrast, EGFR immunoreactivity was present in the carcinomatous components only in 55% of the cases, in sarcomatous components in 18% of the cases, and in both components in 27% of the cases. EGFR immunoreactivity was associated with adenosquamous and heterologous rhabdomyosarcomatous differentiation. EGFR expression may be an indicator for aggressive biological behavior, but its prognostic utility was found to be limited.

OVARIAN CANCER

Because of the diagnostic difficulties and the high mortality rate, OC is the enigma of gynecological oncology. About 26,500 new cases are diagnosed each year in the United States, and about 14,500 deaths occur annually as a result of this disease. Approximately 12/1000 women in the United States, older than 40 yr, will develop OC *(383)*. The etiology of epithelial neoplasms of the ovary, but also of the other histological types, is unknown today. There is a urgent need for new diagnostic and therapeutic approaches in this malignancy and its possible premalignant lesions *(432)*.

Role of EGF-Like Peptides in Ovarian Carcinogenesis

EGF-related peptides and their receptors may be involved in the autonomous proliferation of ovarian carcinoma cells, and may play a role in ovarian carcinogenesis *(401, 432–440)*. EGF and TGF-α stimulate the growth of several human ovarian carcinoma cell lines *(441,442)*. The stimulatory effects of EGF and TGF-α are accompanied by changes in cell cycle distribution, as detected by flow cytometric analysis *(443)*. Like TGF-α, AR is also mitogenic, but has less pronounced effects on proliferation *(444)*. The growth of some ovarian carcinoma cells can be inhibited by EGF, which suggests that the EGF effect is not only dependent on concentration, but also on different postreceptor events in various cell lines *(445)*. Neutralizing Abs directed against EGF or TGF-α can inhibit ovarian cell proliferation in cells that possess functional EGFR, suggesting a major role of TGF-α/EGFR autocrine growth mechanisms in primary Ocs, but also in OC cell lines and in xenotransplants *(441,446–448)*. Individual primary OCs vary widely in their response to and production of known peptide GFs *(437,438)*. Expression patterns of different GFs is dependent on the culture conditions *(449)*. In a series of 174 ovarian carcinomas from 133 patients, EGF was detected in 27.6% samples and TGF-α was present in 88.5% of the specimens. The mean levels for TGF-α were at least 10-fold greater than those for EGF. No correlation between GF expression and tumor grading could be found *(450)*. In OC cell lines, EGF or TGF-α treatment leads to a significant reduction in erbB-2 expression *(451)*. A role for erbB-2 in the development of benign ovarian surface epithelium, and in the genesis of neoplastic epithelium in borderline and some malignant ACs, has been suggested *(452)*.

In normal cycling ovaries, TGF-α has been detected in 12/33 antral follicles in the follicular phase of the menstrual cycle, but not in follicles of the luteal phase. Immunoreactive EGF, AR, and CR-1 were not found in any follicles. EGFR has been demonstrated in 24/33 antral follicles of the follicular phase and in 2/18 follicles of the luteal phase. TGF-α is synthesized in theca cells of normal ovaries, and affects granulosa cells in a paracrine fashion *(453)*. TGF-α is found in ECs of nonmalignant tissues, as well as in different ovarian carcinomas *(435)*. No correlation between EGFR/TGF-α and *c-myc/c-jun* expression was found *(454,455)*.

EGF has been detected in 75% of normal ovarian surface epithelium; TGF-α, AR, and CR-1 can be detected in 86, 0, and 86% of these samples. EGFR was found in 86% and *erb*B-2 in 100% of the specimens. In benign human cystadenomas, EGF, TGF-α, AR, CR-1, EGFR, and erbB-2 were found in 65, 65, 10, 28.6, 53, and 90% of the lesions, respectively. In borderline tumors, an increase in the frequency of expression was demonstrated for EGF (100%), TGF-α (70%), AR (90%), CR-1 (100%), EGFR (100%), and erbB-2 (100%). In ovarian ACs, EGF is expressed in 71%, TGF-α in 64%, AR in 18%, CR-1 in 53%, EGFR in 100%, and erbB-2 in 94% of the cases. In other studies, EGF expression has been reported in 28–71% of the tumors, TGF-α in 50–100%, CR-1 in 52%, and AR in 18–24% of the specimens *(440,446,450,454,456)*. Co-expression of more than two EGF-related peptides or the EGFR significantly correlates with increased surgical stage in prognosticly unfavorable serous and clear cell carcinomas. AR expression seems to correlate with mucinous differentiation, rather than with advanced stage of disease *(440)*. Furthermore, EGF is present in 12.7% of normal ovaries and in 32% of benign tumors; TGF-α was found in 85% of normal ovaries and in 84% of benign ovarian lesions *(457)*. Thirty-one percent of ovarian carcinomas expressed EGF mRNA and 35% TGF-α mRNA; in borderline lesions, 17% expressed TGF-α mRNA and 0% EGF mRNA. In benign ovarian tumors, 40% expressed EGF mRNA and 7% expressed TGF-α mRNA *(458)*. The sequential increase in expression of EGF-related peptides and their receptors suggests a possible role in malignant progression in ovarian carcinoma *(440,442,459)*. The expression of EGFR in ovarian tumors is associated with TGF-α expression, but not with EGF expression. Neither EGF or TGF-α showed an association with histological subtypes or stage of disease, but EGFR mRNA expression was significantly associated with a serous histology, but not with stage or grade *(458)*.

TGF-α is a major GF present in normal ovaries and benign tumors *(456,457)*. In ovarian carcinoma cell lines, dexamethasone may increase the number of high- and low-affinity EGFR in a dose-dependent manner *(460)*. Recently, it has been demonstrated that HRG can stimulate proliferation in several ovarian carcinoma cell lines. Because interaction of HRG with erbB-3 and erbB-4 results in the transactivation of erbB-2, in this system, erbB-2 was a critical component in mediating HRG responsiveness *(461)*. In ER-positive ovarian carcinoma cells, E_2 may increase the production of TGF-α and decrease EGFR expression. In primary ovarian tumors, high concentrations of ER were also associated with an increased percentage of tumors expressing TGF-α mRNA and a decreased percentage of cells expressing EGFR *(462)*. P and E_2 significantly increase the release of EGF and TGF-α from human benign ovarian tumors, but not from normal ovaries and malignant tissues *(463)*. In several OC cell lines, human chorionic gonadotropin (hCG), human follicle-stimulating hormone and EGF increased cell growth in a dose- and time-dependent manner, but E_2 inhibited cell growth. EGF and hCG were able to block the E_2 inhibitory effect, suggesting that EGF, hCG, and E_2 may modulate growth of metastatic epithelial OC *(464,465)*. Emons et al. *(411)* suggested that LH-RH analogs can effectively block EGF-induced MAPK activity in OC and endometrial cancer cells. Cytotoxic analogs of LH-RH may therefore be useful for targeted Chemo in OC, endometrial cancer, and in choriocarcinomas *(410)*. Measurement of EGF and TGF-α content in the urine of patients with OC may serve as a tumor marker *(466–468)*.

TGF-α is able to increase the CA125 and tissue plasminogen activator secretion levels in EGFR-expressing OC cells *(469)*. By IHC, the stroma is TGF-α-negative in ovarian carcinomas *(436,456)*.

Certain OC cell lines may secrete and respond to EGF and TGF-α, suggesting that endogenous activation of EGFR through autocrine or paracrine mechanisms may contribute to the proliferative response. In vitro, the proliferation of both human primary cell lines or human OC cell lines can be inhibited by anti-EGFR or anti-TGF-α mAbs *(441, 442,446)*. Additionally, EGFR antisense mRNA expression reduces the expression of EGFR and suppresses the malignant phenotype *(470)*. Although the mitogenic response to EGF may be attenuated in several OC cell lines, loss of responsiveness to EGF does not appear to be caused by decreased EGFR expression *(471)*. In contrast, using neutralizing anti-EGFR Abs, Ottensmeier et al. *(472)* could show that EGFR activation through an autocrine pathway is not a major mechanism for the growth of several OC cell lines. Additionally, EGFR-independent pathways may limit the effectiveness of strategies designed to inhibit OC cell growth. Ovarian carcinomas with an activated EGFR/TGF-α system seem to be biologically different, compared to EGFR/TGF-α-negative tumors *(436)*. In vitro, EGFRs may be affected by cytostatic agents *(473)*. However, it has been demonstrated that EGF did not enhance the sensitivity of carcinoma cells to cisplatin, or alter morphology in cisplatin-resistant human carcinoma cells, despite the presence of functional EGFR, suggesting that cisplatin resistance may be associated with a defect in the EGFR signal transduction pathway *(474)*. These data are confirmed by the finding that human ovarian carcinomas with no or low expression of TGF-α, EGFR, myc, and jun do not respond to Chemo *(434,475)*.

EGF-Receptors as Prognostic Factors in Human OC

The prognostic value of the erbB receptor family in human OC is still controversial. Enhanced cytoplasmatic or membrane EGFR expression has been detected in approx 40–70% in OC cells *(476–482)*. No correlation between EGFR expression and histological type of the tumors has been observed *(477)*. Low EGFR immunoreactivity has been observed in stromal and endothelial cells in both normal and tumorous ovarian tissues. Two of 30 normal ovarian epithelium samples were positive for EGFR expression; 47/103 malignant tumors showed cytoplasmatic immunoreactivity for EGFR. No correlation between EGFR immunoreactivity and histological subtype could be detected *(479)*. Also, no correlation was found between EGFR expression and clinical stage or any of several other prognostic factors *(482,483)*. EGFR expression showed no significant impact on survival, and does not seem to have prognostic relevance *(484)*. In contrast, EGFR-positive, TGF-α-expressing ovarian carcinomas showed a high response rate to Chemo, and EGFR- or TGF-α-negative tumors exhibited no change, or actually had more progressive disease *(436)*. Survival was significantly reduced in patients with EGFR-positive tumors than in EGFR-negative tumors. However, unlike protein expression, the expression of TGF-α mRNA or EGF mRNA was unrelated to survival *(458)*. Irrespective of the method of determination, the level of EGFR showed a positive, but not significant, correlation with the risk for disease progression *(480)*. The assessment of EGFR status at the time of surgery may be helpful in identifying a subset of patients with

Table 4
Multiple Expression of Different
TK Type I Receptors in Ovarian Tumors

	%Tumors positive		
	Benign	Borderline	Malignant
EGFR	39	38	65
erbB-2	31	25	76
erbB–3	62	100	89
EGFR + erbB-2	23	13	50
EGFR + erbB–3	39	38	63
erbB-2 + erbB–3	23	25	74
EGFR + erbB-2 + erbB–3	23	13	50

Adapted with permission from ref. *481*.

a particularly poor prognosis in advanced ovarian carcinomas. Only the postoperative residual tumor and EGFR expression remained significantly associated with a high risk of progression *(478)*.

In ovarian carcinomas, an association between EGFR gene copy number and metastasis was associated in a multivariate analysis *(485)*. In 17 ovarian carcinomas, EGFR, erbB-2, erbB-3, but not erbB-4, was detected by Western blot analysis *(486)*. EGFR expression correlates with erbB-2 and erbB-3 levels, but the highest correlation was obtained between erbB-2 and erbB-3. An increase of erbB receptors in OC may mediate increased propensity for tumor development.

No significant correlations between either EGFR or erbB-3 and other prognostic factors was observed. However, erbB-2 was associated with favorable prognostic parameters *(481)*. Multiple expression of different TK type I receptors was significantly higher in malignant tumors than in borderline or benign ovarian lesions (Table 4).

Early-stage tumors are more likely to express multiple erbB-receptors than late stage tumors. Co-expression of EGFR with erbB-2, and erbB-2 with erbB-3, was significantly greater in carcinomas than in borderline or benign tumors. In the OC subgroup, a positive association between EGFR and erbB-3, and between erbB-2 and erbB-3, was observed. It was suggested that stimulation by the appropriate ligand may confer a selective advantage to cells expressing more than one receptor *(481)*. Additionally, an association between EGFR and the androgen receptor, which is expressed in over 80% of ovarian carcinomas, has been demonstrated *(487)*.

erbB-2 may be involved in the pathogenesis of OC, and overexpression of erbB-2 receptors seems to be correlated with aggressiveness of disease *(333,439,458,475,481, 488,489)*. erbB-2 gene amplification was found in normal ovaries and malignant tumors *(490)*. erbB-2 has been detected in 18% of ovarian carcinomas, where it was found to have a significant prognostic value *(484,489)*. Using IHC in a retrospective study, Rubin et al. *(491)* tested the hypothesis that there was prognostic significance to the level of erbB-2 in 105 patients with advanced OC. Overall, 24% of investigated tumors showed strong membrane staining. No correlation of erbB-2 expression with stage, grade, cell type, and residual tumor was found. Additionally, there was no significant survival differences between patients with staining intensity levels similar to those of normal ovarian epithelium and those with increased expression. The authors concluded that erbB-2 expression does not appear to be an important prognostic factor in patients with advanced OC. The same authors examined the prevalence and significance of erbB-2 expression in 40 early epithelial OCs (stage I or II), by immunoperoxidase technique in fresh-frozen tissue samples. Again, no statistically significant relationship was found between erbB-2 expression and survival, disease-free interval, stage, or grade, suggesting that it is unlikely that such overexpression is a general early event in ovarian carcinogenesis *(492)*. In 104 common ovarian epithelial carcinomas, only 22% showed cytoplasmatic staining and 9% cytoplasmatic and membrane immunoreactivity *(493)*. Using IHC, only 10/56 ovarian carcinomas showed overexpression of erbB-2 *(494)*, which did not correlate with histological type, grade, FIGO stage, or prognosis. In contrast, Felip et al. *(495)* showed, in a multivariant analysis, that, in residual tumors, size and erbB-2 overexpression are independent prognostic factors. However, no correlation was found between erbB-2 expression and age, grade, or histological subtype. The percentage of tumors with erbB-2 overexpression was higher in those with stage III/IV diseases, compared with those patients with stage I/II disease, and in patients who failed to respond to Chemo (carboplatin, cyclophosphamide), compared with those who responded. erbB-2 overexpression was correlated with worsening survival rates. These data were confirmed by Berchuck et al. *(437)*. Patients with tumors showing a high erbB-2 expression had a significantly shorter survival time than those with normal erbB-2 expression. Additionally, erbB-2-overexpressing tumors were significantly less likely to have a complete response to primary therapy, suggesting that *erb*B-2 expression may play a role as a prognostic marker in a subset of human OC. In serous ovarian carcinomas, expression of erbB-2 may be associated with high stage of disease, but it is not likely to identify the small fraction of patients with serous tumors of low malignant potential *(496)*. It is likely that more of the patients whose tumors showed strong membrane staining for erbB-2 suffer relapses of the disease by 3 and 4 yr than did patients whose tumor showed no or weak membrane staining *(452)*. Recently, it was suggested that the increase of EGFR expression appears to be associated with early stage of ovarian tumorigenesis. The enhancement of erbB-2 reactivity may interact with EGFR activation in the development and progression of ovarian carcinomas *(497)*.

REFERENCES

1. Knudson AG. Anti-oncogenes and human cancer. Proc Natl Acad Sci USA 1993;90:10,914–10,921.
2. Levine AJ. The tumor suppressor genes. Ann Rev Biochem 1993;62:623–651.
3. Carney D, Sikora K, eds. Genes and Cancer. John Wiley, New York, 1990.
4. Vogelstein B, Kinzler KW. The multi–step nature of cancer. Trends Genet 1993;9:138–141.
5. Eng C, Ponder B. Role of gene mutation in the genesis of familial cancers. Science 1992;256:668–670.
6. Weinberg RA. Oncogenes and the Molecular Origins of Cancer. Cold Spring Harbor Laboratory, Cold Spring Harbor, NY, 1989.
7. Kahn P, Graf T, eds. Oncogenes and Growth Control. Springer-Verlag, New York, 1986.
8. Hunter T. Oncogenes and cell proliferation. Curr Opin Genet Dev 1993;3:1–4.
9. Bishop JM. Molecular themes in carcinogenesis. Cell 1991;64:235–248.
10. Hunter T. Cooperation between oncogenes. Cell 1991;64:249–270.
11. Marshall CJ. Tumor suppressor genes. Cell 1991;64:313–326.
12. Harris CC. p53: at the crossroads of molecular carcinogenesis and risk assessment. Science 1993;262:1980,1981.
13. Goustin AS, Leof EB, Shipley GD, Moses HL. Growth factors and cancer. Cancer Res 1986;46:1015–1029.
14. Aaronson SA. Growth factors and cancer. Science 1991;254:1146–1153.

15. Sporn MB, Roberts AB. Autocrine secretion: 10 years later. Ann Intern Med 1992;117:408–414.
16. Pimentel E. Hormones, Growth Factors, and Oncogenes. CRC, Boca Raton, FL, 1987.
17. Salomon DS, Brandt R, Ciardiello F, Normanno N. Epidermal growth factor-related peptides and their receptors in human malignancies. Crit Rev Oncol/Hematol 1995;19:183–232.
18. Campbell ID, Bork P. Epidermal growth factor-like modules. Curr Opin Struct Biol 1993;3:385–392.
19. Perrimon N, Perkins LA. There must be 50 ways to rule the signal: the case of the Drosophila EGF receptor. Cell 1997;89:13–16.
20. Schweitzer R, Shilo B-Z. A thousand and one roles for the Drosophila EGF receptor. Trends Genet 1997;13:191–196.
21. Groenen LC, Nice EC, Burgess AW. Structure-function relationships for the EGF/TGF-α family of mitogens. Growth Factors 1994;11:235–257.
22. Alroy I, Yarden Y. The ErbB signaling network in embryogenesis and oncogenesis: signal diversification through combanitorial ligand-receptor interactions. FEBS Lett 1997;410:83–86.
23. Riese DJ III, Stern DF. Specificity within the EGF family/ErbB receptor family signaling network. BioEssays 1998;20:41–48.
24. Chang H, Riese DJ III, Gilbert W, Stern DF, McMahan UJ. Ligands for ErbB-family receptors encoded by a neuregulin-like gene. Nature 1997;387:509–516.
25. Zhang D, Sliwkowski MX, Mark M, Frantz G, Akita R, Sun Y, et al. Neuregulin-3 (NRG3): a novel neural tissue-enriched protein that binds and activates ErbB4. Proc Natl Acad Sci USA 1997;94:9562–9567.
26. Massagué J, Pandiella A. Membrane-anchored growth factors. Ann Rev Biochem 1993;62:515–541.
27. Carpenter G, Cohen S. Epidermal growth factor. J Biol Chem 1990;265:7709–7712.
28. Browne CA. Epidermal growth factor and transforming growth factor α. Baillière's Clin Endocrinol Metab 1991;5:553–569.
29. Carpenter G. EGF: new tricks for an old growth factor. Curr Opin Cell Biol 1993;5:261–264.
30. Shoyab M, Plowman GD, McDonald VL, Bradley JG, Todaro GJ. Structure and function of human amphiregulin: a member of the epidermal growth factor family. Science 1989;243:1074–1076.
31. Higashiyama S, Lau K, Besner GE, Abraham JA, Klagsbrun M Structure of heparin-binding EGF-like growth factor. J Biol Chem 1992;267:6205–6212.
32. Holmes WE, Sliwkowski MX, Akita RW, et al. Identification of heregulin, a specific activator of p185^{erbB2}. Science 1992;256:1205–1210.
33. Falls DL, Rosen KM, Corfas G, Lane WS, Fischbach GD. ARIA, a protein that stimulates acetylcholine receptor synthesis, is a member of the Neu ligand family. Cell 1993;72:801–815.
34. Marchionni MA, Goodearl ADJ, Chen MS, et al. Glial growth factors are alternatively spliced erbB2 ligands expressed in the nervous system. Nature 1993;362:312–318.
35. Peles E, Yarden Y. Neu and its ligands: from an oncogene to neural factors. Bioessays 1993;15:815–824.
36. Shing Y, Christofori G, Hanahan D, et al. Betacellulin: a mitogen from pancreatic beta cell tumors. Science 1993;259:1604–1607.
37. Ciccodicola A, Dono R, Obici S, Simeone A, Zollo M, Persico MG. Molecular characterization of a gene of the 'EGF family' expressed in undifferentiated human NTERA2 teratocarcinoma cells. EMBO J 1989;8:1987–1991.
38. Brandt R, Normanno N, Gullick WJ, Lin J-H, Harkins R, Schneider D, et al. Identification and biological characterization of an epidermal growth factor-related protein: cripto-1. J Biol Chem 1994;269:17,320–17,328.
39. Kinoshita N, Minshull J, Kirschner MW. The identification of two novel ligands of the FGF receptor by a yeast screening method and their activity in Xenopus development. Cell 1995;83:621–630.
40. Shen MM, Wang H, Leder P. A differential display strategy identifies Cryptic, a novel EGF-related gene expressed in the axial and lateral mesoderm during mouse gastrulation. Development 1997;124:429–442.
41. Zhang J, Talbot WS, Schier AF. Positional cloning identifies zebrafish one-eyed pinhead as a permissive EGF-related ligand required during gastrulation. Cell 1998;92:241–251.
42. Mason S, Gullick WJ. Type 1 growth factor receptors: an overview of recent developments. Breast 1995;4:11–18.
43. Hynes N, Stern DF. The biology of erbB–2/neu/HER–2 and its role in cancer. Biochim Biophys Acta 1994;1198:165–184.
44. Ullrich A, Coussens L, Hayflick JS, et al. Human epidermal growth factor receptor cDNA sequence and aberrant expression of the amplified gene in A431 epidermoid carcinoma cells. Nature 1984;309:418–425.

45. Coussens L, Yang–Feng TL, Liao YC, et al. Tyrosine kinase receptor with extensive homology to EGF receptor shares chromosomal location with Neu oncogene. Science 1985;230:1132–1139.

46. Plowman GD, Whitney GS, Neubauer MG, et al. Molecular cloning and expression of an additional epidermal growth factor receptor-related gene. Proc Natl Acad Sci USA 1990;87:4905–4909.

47. Kraus MH, Issing W, Miki T, Popescu NC, and Aaronson SA. Isolation and characterization of *ERBB3*: a third member of the *ERBB*/epidermal growth factor receptor family: evidence for over-expression in a subset of human mammary tumors. Proc Natl Acad Sci USA 1989;86:9193–9197.

48. Plowman GD, Culouscou J-M, and Whitney GS, et al. Ligand-specific activation of HER4/p180^{erbB4}, a fourth member of the epidermal growth factor receptor family. Proc Natl Acad Sci USA 1993;90: 1746–1750.

49. Baulida J, Kraus MH, Alimandi M, Di Fiore PP, Carpenter G. All ErbB receptors other than the epidermal growth factor receptor are endocytosis impaired. J Biol Chem 1996;271:5251–5257.

50. Beerli RR, Hynes NE. Epidermal growth factor-related peptides activate distinct subsets of ErbB receptors and differ in their biological activities. J Biol Chem 1996;271:6071–6076.

51. Elenius K, Paul S, Allison G, Sun J, Klagsbrun M. Activation of HER4 by heparin-binding EGF-like growth factor stimulates chemotaxis but not proliferation. EMBO J 1997;16:1268–1278.

52. Alimandi M, Wang L-M, Bottaro D, Lee C-C, Kuo A, Frankel M, et al. Epidermal growth factor and betacellulin mediate signal transduction through co-expressed ErbB2 and ErbB3 receptors. EMBO J 1997;16:5608–5617.

53. Kannan S, De Santis M, Lohmeyer M, Riese D, Hynes NE, Smith GH, et al. Cripto stimulates the tyrosine phosphorylation of Shc and activates MAP-kinase in mammary epithelial cells. J Biol Chem 1997; 272:3330–3335.

54. Tzahar E, Waterman H, Chen X, Levkowitz G, Karunagaran D, Lavi S, Ratzkin BJ, Yarden Y. Hierarchical network of interreceptor interaction determines signal transduction by neu differentiation factor/neuregulin and epidermal growth factor. Mol Cell Biol 1996;16:5276–5287.

55. Karunagaran D, Tzahar E, Beerli RR, Chen X, Graus-Porta D, Ratzkin BJ, et al. ErbB-2 is a common auxiliary subunit of NDF and EGF receptors: implications for breast cancer. EMBO J 1996;15:254–264.

56. Graus-Porta D, Beerli RR, Daly JM, Hynes NE. ErbB-2: the preferred heterodimerization partner of all ErbB receptors, is a mediator of lateral signaling. EMBO J 1997;16:1647–1655.

57. Ling-Mei W, Kuo Alimandi M, Veri MC, Lee C-C, Kapoor V, et al. ErbB2 expression increases the spectrum and potency of ligand-mediated signal transduction through ErbB4. Proc Natl Acad Sci USA 1998;95:6809–6814.

58. Tzahar E, Pinkas-Kramarski R, Moyer JD, Klapper LN, Alroy I, Levkowitz G, et al. Bivalence of EGF-like ligands drives the ErbB signaling network. EMBO J 1997;16,4938–4950.

59. Gamett DC, Pearson G, Cerione RA, and Friedberg I. Secondary dimerization between members of the epidermal growth factor receptor family. J Biol Chem 1997;272:12,052–12,056.

60. Barnard JA, Graves-Deal R, Pittelkow MR, DuBois R, Cook P, Ramsey GW, et al. Auto- and cross-induction within the mammalian epidermal growth factor-related peptide family. J Biol Chem 1994; 269:22,817–22,822.

61. Medina D, Daniel C, eds. Experimental models of development function and neoplasia. J Mammary Gland Biol Neoplasia 1996;1:1–135.

62. Dickson RB, Lippman ME. Growth factors in breast cancer. Endocr Rev 1995;16:559–589.

63. Borellini F, Oka T. Growth control and differentiation in mammary epithelial cells. Environ Health Perspect 1989;80:85–99.

64. Oka T, Yoshimura M, Lavandero S, et al. Control of growth and differentiation of the mammary gland by growth factors. J Dairy Sci 1991;74:2788–2800.

65. Clarke R, Dickson RB, Lippman ME. Hormonal aspects of breast cancer: growth factors, drugs and stromal interactions. Crit Rev Oncol/Hematol 1992;12:1–23.

66. Ethier SP. Growth factor synthesis and human breast cancer progression. J Natl Cancer Inst 1995;87: 964–973.

67. Normanno N, Ciardiello F, Brandt R, Salomon DS. Epidermal growth factor-related peptides in the pathogenesis of human breast cancer. Breast Cancer Res Treat 1994;29:11–27.

68. Medina D. Mammary gland: a unique organ for the study of development and tumorigenesis. J Mammary Gland Biol Neoplasia 1996;1:5–20.

69. Cunha GR, Hom YK. Role of mesenchymal-epithelial interactions in mammary gland development. J Mammary Gland Biol Neoplasia 1996;1:21–36.

70. Imagawa W, Bandyopadhyay GK, Nandi S. Regulation of mammary epithelial cell growth in mice and rats. Endocr Rev 1990;11:494–523.

71. DiAugustine RP. The epidermal growth factor family in the mammary gland and other target organs for ovarian steroids. In: Lippman ME, Dickson RB, eds. Mammary Tumorigenesis and Malignant Progression. Kluwer, Boston, 1994, pp. 131–160.
72. Normanno N, Ciardiello F. EGF-related peptides in the pathophysiology of the mammary gland. J Mammary Gland Biol Neoplasia 1997;2:143–151.
73. DiAugustine RP, Richards RG, Sebastian J. EGF-related peptides and their receptors in mammary gland development. J Mammary Gland Biol Neoplasia 1997;2:109–118.
74. Liscia DS, Merlo G, Ciardiello F, et al. Transforming growth factor-α messenger RNA localization in the developing adult rat and human mammary gland by in situ hybridization. Dev Biol 1990;140:123–131.
75. Snedecker SM, Brown CF, DiAugustine RP. Expression and functional properties of TGFa and EGF during mouse mammary gland ductal morphogenesis. Proc Natl Acad Sci USA 1991;88:276–280.
76. Ankrapp DP, Bennett JM, Haslam SZ. Role of epidermal growth factor in the acquisition of ovarian steroid hormone responsiveness in the normal mouse mammary gland. J Cell Physiol 1998;174:251–260.
77. Yang Y, Spitzer E, Meyer D, et al. Sequential requirement of hepatocyte growth factor and neuregulin in the morphogenesis and differentiation of the mammary gland. J Cell Biol 1995;131:215–226.
78. Schroeder JA, Lee DC. Dynamic expression and activation of ERBB receptors in the developing mouse mammary gland. Cell Growth Differ 1998;9:451–464.
79. Vonderhaar BK. Regulation of development of the normal mammary gland by hormones and growth factors. In: Lippman ME, Dickson RB, eds. Breast Cancer: Cellular and Molecular Biology. Kluwer, Boston, 1988, pp. 251–266.
80. Daniel CW, Silberstein GB. Local effects of growth factors. In: Lippman M, Dickson R, eds.Regulatory Mechanisms in Breast Cancer. Kluwer, Boston, 1991, pp. 79–93.
81. Kenney NJ, Smith GH, Rosenberg K, Cutler ML, Dickson RB. Induction of ductal morphogenesis and lobular hyperplasia by amphiregulin in the mouse mammary gland. Cell Growth Differ 1996;7:1769–1781.
82. Hilakivi-Clarke L, Cho E, Raygada M, et al. Alterations in mammary gland development following neonatal exposure to estradiol, transforming growth factor α, and estrogen receptor antagonist ICI 182,780. J Cell Physiol 1997;170:279–289.
83. Jones FE, Jerry DJ, Guarino BC, et al. Heregulin induces in vivo proliferation and differentiation of mammary epithelium into secretory lobuloalveoli. Cell Growth Differ 1996;7:1031–1038.
84. Kenney NJ, Huang R-P, Johnson GR, et al. Detection and location of amphiregulin and cripto-1 expression in the developing postnatal mouse mammary gland. Mol Reprod Dev 1995;41:277–286.
85. Kenney NJ, Smith GH, Johnson MD, et al. Cripto-1 activity in the intact and ovariectomized virgin mouse mammary gland. Pathogenesis 1997;1:57–71.
86. Xie W, Paterson AJ, Chin E, et al. Targeted expression of a dominant negative epidermal growth factor receptor in the mammary gland of transgenic mice inhibits pubertal mammary duct development. Mol Endocrinol 1997;11:1766–1781.
87. Spitzer E, Zschiesche W, Binas B, et al. EGF and TGFα modulate structural and functional differentiation of the mammary gland from pregnant mice in vitro: possible role of the arachidonic acid pathway. J Cell Biochem 1995;57:495–508.
88. Merlo GR, Graus-Porta D, Cella N, et al. Growth differentiation and survival of HC11 mammary epithelial cells: diverse effects of receptor tyrosine kinase-activating peptide growth factors. Eur J Cell Biol 1996;70:97–105.
89. De Santis ML, Kannan S, Smith GH, et al. Cripto-1 inhibits β-casein expression in mammary epithelial cells through a p21ras- and phosphatidylinositol-3 kinase-dependent pathway. Cell Growth Differ 1997;8:1257–1266.
90. Kenney NJ, Smith GH, Maroulakou IG, et al. Detection of amphiregulin and Cripto-1 in mammary tumors from transgenic mice. Mol Carcinog 1996;15:44–56.
91. Martin G, Cricco G, Davio C, et al. Epidermal growth factor in NMU-induced mammary tumors in rats. Breast Cancer Res Treat 1998;48:175–185.
92. Ethier SP, Langton BC, Dilts CA. Growth factor-independent proliferation of rat mammary carcinoma cells by autocrine secretion of neu-differentiation factor/heregulin and transforming growth factor-α. Mol Carcinog 1996;15:134–143.
93. Ciardiello F, Dono R, Kim N, Persico MG, and Salomon DS. Expression of *cripto*, a novel gene of the epidermal growth factor gene family, leads to *in vitro* transformation of a normal mouse mammary epithelial cell line. Cancer Res 1991;51:1051–1054.
94. Ciardiello F, McGeady ML, Kim N, et al. Transforming growth factor-α expression is enhanced in human mammary epithelial cells transformed by an activated c-Ha-ras proto-oncogene and overexpres-

sion of the transforming growth factor-α a complementary DNA leads to transformation. Cell Growth Differ 1990;1:407–420.

95. Davies BR, Warren JR, Schmidt G, et al. Induction of a variety of preneoplasias and tumours in the mammary glands of transgenic rats. Biochem Soc Symp 1998;63:167–184.

96. Krane IM, Leder P. NDF/heregulin induces persistence of terminal end buds and adenocarcinomas in the mammary glands of transgenic mice. Oncogene 1996;12:1781–1788.

97. Smith GH, Sharp R, Kordon EC, Jhappan C, Merlino G. Transforming growth factor-α promotes mammary tumorigenesis through selective survival and growth of secretory epithelial cells. Am J Pathol 1995; 147:1081–1096.

98. Halter SA, Dempsey P, Matsui Y, et al. Distinctive patterns of hyperplasia in transgenic mice with mouse mammary tumor virus transforming growth factor α: characterization of mammary gland and skin proliferations Am J Pathol 1992;140:1131–1146.

99. Guy CT, Webster MA, Schaller M, et al. Expression of the neu proto-oncogene in the mammary epithelium of transgenic mice induces metastatic disease. Proc Natl Acad Sci USA 1992;89:10,578–10,582.

100. Sandgren EP, Schroeder JA, Qui TH, et al. Inhibition of mammary gland involution is associated with transforming growth factor α but not c-myc-induced tumorigenesis in transgenic mice. Cancer Res 1995;55:3915–3927.

101. Schroeder JA, Lee DC. Transgenic mice reveal roles for TGFα and EGF receptor in mammary gland development and neoplasia. J Mammary Gland Biol Neoplasia 1997;2:119–130.

102. Cardiff RD. The biology of mammary transgenes: five rules. J Mammary Gland Biol Neoplasia 1996; 1:61–74.

103. Muller WJ, Arteaga CL, Muthuswamy SK, et al. Synergistic interation of the neu proto-oncogene product and transforming growth factor α in the mammary epithelium of transgenic mice. Mol Cell Biol 1996;16:5726–5736.

104. Amundadottir LT, Johnson MD, Merlino G, et al. Synergistic interaction of transforming growth factor α and c-myc in mouse mammary and salivary gland tumorigenesis. Cell Growth Differ 1995;6: 737–748.

105. Amundadottir LT, Nass SJ, Berchem GJ, et al. Cooperation of TGFα and c-Myc in mouse mammary tumorigenesis: coordinated stimulation of growth and suppression of apoptosis. Oncogene 1996;13: 757–765.

106. Mincione G, Bianco C, Kannan S, et al. Enhanced expression of heregulin in c-erbB-2 and c-Ha-ras transformed mouse and human mammary epithelial cells. J Cell Biochem 1996;60:437–446.

107. Salomon DS, Ciardiello F, Valverius EM, Kim N. The role of *ras* gene expression and transforming growth factor α production in the etiology and progression of rodent and human breast cancer. In: Lippman M, Dickson R, eds. Regulatory Mechanisms in Breast Cancer. Kluwer, Boston, 1991, pp. 107–157.

109. Ciardiello F, Kim N, Hynes NE, et al. Induction of transforming growth factor α expression in mouse mammary epithelial cells after transformation with a point mutated c-Ha-*ras* protooncogene. Mol Endocrinol 1988;2:1202–1216.

110. Martinez-Lacaci I, Saceda M, Plowman G, et al. Estrogen and phorbol esters regulate amphiregulin expression by two separate mechanisms in human breast cancer cells. Endocrinology 1995;136: 3983–3992.

111. Bates SE, Davidson N, Valverius EM, et al. Expression of transforming growth factor α and its messenger ribonucleic acid in human breast cancer: its regulation by estrogen and its possible functional significance. Mol Endocrinol 1988;2:543–555.

112. Murphy LC, Dotzlaw H. Regulation of transforming growth factor α transforming growth factor β messenger ribonucleic acid abundance in T-47D human breast cancer cells. Mol Endocrinol 1989;3: 611–616.

113. Saeki T, Cristiano A, Lynch MJ, et al. Regulation by estrogen through the 5'-flanking region of the transforming growth factor alpha gene. Mol Endocrinol 1991;5:1955–1963.

114. El-Ashry D, Chrysogelos S, Lippman ME, et al. Estrogen induction of TGF-α is mediated by an estrogen response element composed of two imperfect palindromes. J Steroid Biochem 1996;59:261–269.

115. Kenney N, Saeki T, Gottardis M, et al. Expression of transforming growth factor α (TGFα) antisense mRNA inhibits the estrogen-induced production of TGFα and estrogen-induced proliferation of estrogen-responsive human breast cancer cells. J Cell Physiol 1993;156:497–514.

116. Ignar-Trowbridge DM, Pimentel M, Teng CT, et al. Cross talk between peptide growth factor and estrogen receptor signaling systems. Environ Health Perspect 1995;103(Suppl):35–38.

117. Murphy LC, Dotzlaw H, Wong MSJ, et al. Epidermal growth factor: receptor and ligand expression in human breast cancer. Semin Cancer Biol 1994;1:305–315.

118. Murphy LC, Murphy LJ, Dubik D, Bell GI, Shiu RPC. Epidermal growth factor gene expression in human breast cancer cells: regulation of expression by progestins. Cancer Res 1988;48:4555–4560.

119. Normanno N, Selvam P, Qi C-F, et al. Amphiregulin as an autocrine growth factor for c-Ha-ras and c-erbB-2-transformed human mammary epithelial cells. Proc Natl Acad Sci USA 1994;91:2790–2794.

120. Normanno N, Qi C-F, Gullick WJ, et al. Expression of amphiregulin, cripto-1, and heregulin in human breast cancer cells. Int J Oncol 1993;2:903–911.

121. Salomon DS, Normanno N, Ciardiello F, et al. The role of amphiregulin in breast cancer. Breast Cancer Res Treat 1995;33:103–114.

122. Ram TG, Kokeny K, Dilts CA, et al. Mitogenic activity of neu differentiation factor/heregulin mimics that of epidermal growth factor and insulin-like growth factor I in human mammary epithelial cells. J Cell Physiol 1995;163:589–596.

123. Ram TG, Dilts CA, Dziubinski ML, et al. Insulin-like growth factor and epidermal growth factor independence in human mammary carcinoma cells with c-erbB-2 gene amplification and progressively elevated levels of tyrosine-phosphorylated p185erbB-2. Mol Carcinog 1996;15:227–238.

124. Normanno N, Ciardiello F. EGF-related peptides in the pathophysiology of the mammary gland. J Mammary Gland Biol Neoplasia 1997;2:143–152.

125. Dotzlaw H, Miller T, Karvelas J, Murphy LC. Epidermal growth factor gene expression in human breast cancer biopsy samples: relationship to estrogen and progesterone receptor gene expression. Cancer Res 1990;50:4204–4208.

126. Mizukami Y, Nonomura A, Noguchi M, et al. Immunohistochemical study of oncogene product *Ras* p21, c-*Myc* and growth factor EGF in breast carcinomas. Anticancer Res 1991;11:1485–1494.

127. Pirinen R, Lipponen P, Aaltomaa S, et al. Prognostic value of epidermal growth factor expression in breast cancer. J Cancer Res Clin Oncol 1997;123:63–68.

128. Murray PA, Barrett-Lee P, Travers M, Luqmani Y, Powles T, Coombes RC. The prognostic significance of transforming growth factors in human breast cancer. Br J Cancer 1993;67:1408–1412.

129. Ciardiello F, Kim N, Liscia DS, et al. Transforming growth factor α (TGFα) mRNA expression in human breast carcinomas and TGFα activity in the effusions of breast cancer patients. J Natl Cancer Inst 1989;81:1165–1171.

130. Murray PA, Barrett-Lee PJ, Travers MT, Lugmani Y, Powles T, Coombes RC The prognostic significance of transforming growth factors in breast cancer. Br J Cancer 1993;67:1408–1412.

131. Dublin EA, Barnes DM, Wang DY, King RJB, Levison DA. TGF alpha and TGF beta expression in mammary carcinoma. J Pathol 1993;170:15–22.

132. De Jong JS, Van Diest PJ, Van Der Valk P, et al. Expression of growth factors, growth inhibiting factors, and their receptors in invasive breast cancer. I: An inventory in search of autocrine and paracrine loops. J Pathol 1998;184:44–52.

133. Artagaveytia N, Le Penven S, Falette N, et al. Epidermal growth factor and transforming growth factor alpha mRNA expression in human breast cancer biopsies: analysis in relation to estradiol, progesterone and EGF receptor content. J Steroid Biochem Mol Biol 1997;60:221–228.

134. Auvinen PK, Lipponen PK, Kataja V, et al. Prognostic significance of TGF-α expression in breast cancer. Acta Oncol 1996;35:995–998.

135. Castellani R, Visscher DW, Wykes S, et al. Interaction of transforming growth factor-alpha and epidermal growth factor receptor in breast carcinoma. Cancer 1994;73:344–349.

136. Barrett-Lee P, Travers M, Luqmani Y, Coombes RC. Transcripts for transforming growth factors in human breast cancer: clinical correlates. Br J Cancer 1990;61:612–617.

137. Qi C, Liscia DS, Normanno N, Merlo G, et al. Expression of transforming growth factor alpha, amphiregulin, and cripto-1 in human breast carcinomas. Br J Cancer 1994;69:903–910.

138. Umekita Y, Enokizono N, Sagara Y, et al. Immunohistochemical studies on oncogene products (EGF-R, c-erbB-2) and growth factors (EGF, TGF-α) in human breast cancer: their relationship to oestrogen receptor status, histological grade, mitotic index and nodal status. Virchows Archiv A Pathol Anat Histopathol 1992;420:345–351.

139. Perroteau I, Salomon DS, Debortoli M, et al. Immunological detection and quantitation of alpha transforming growth factors in human breast carcinoma cells. Breast Cancer Res Treat 1986;7:201–210.

140. Parkam DH, Jankowski J. Transforming growth factor α in epithelial proliferative diseases of the breast. J Clin Pathol 1992;45:513–516.

141. Macias A, Perez R, Hagerstrom T, Skoog L. Transforming growth factor α in human mammary carcinomas and their metastases. Anticancer Res 1989;9:177–182.

142. Lundy J, Scuss A, Stanick D, McCormack ES, Kramer S, Sorvillo JM. Expression of *neu* protein, EGF and TGFα in breast cancer. Am J Pathol 1991;138:1527–1534.

143. Noguchi S, Motomura K, Inaji H, Imaoka S, Koyama H. Down-regulation of transforming growth factor-α by tamoxifen in human breast cancer. Cancer 1993;4096:18,428–18,432.

144. Gregory H, Thomas CE, Willshire TR, et al. Epidermal growth factor and transforming growth factor α in patients with breast tumors. Br J Cancer 1989;59:605–609.

145. Arteaga CL, Hanauske AR, Clark GM, et al. Immunoreactive α transforming growth factor activity in effusions from cancer patients as a marker of tumor burden and patients prognosis. Cancer Res 1988; 48:5023–5028.

146. Kenney N, Johnson GR, Selvan MP, et al. Transforming growth factor alpha (TGFα) and amphiregulin (AR) as autocrine growth factors in nontransformed, immortalized 184A1N4 human mammary epithelial cells. Mol Cell Differ 1993;1:163–184.

147. Normanno N, Selvan MP, Qi C, et al. Amphiregulin as an autocrine growth factor for c-Ha-*ras* and c-*erb* B-2 transformed human mammary epithelial cells. Proc Natl Acad Sci USA 1994;91:2790–2794.

148. Li S, Plowman GD, Buckley SD, Shipley GD. Heparin inhibition of autonomous growth implicates amphiregulin as an autocrine growth factor for normal human mammary epithelial cells. J Cell Physiol 1992;153:103–111.

149. Li W, Park JW, Nuijens A, et al. Heregulin is rapidly translocated to the nucelus and its transport is correlated with c-myc induction in breast cancer cells. Oncogene 1996;12:2473–2477.

150. LeJeune S, Leek R, Horak E, Plowman GD, Greenall M, Harris AL. Amphiregulin, epidermal growth factor receptor, and estrogen receptor expression in human primary breast cancer. Cancer Res 1993;53: 3597–3602.

151. Visscher D, Sarkar FH, Kasunic TC, et al. Clinicopathologic analysis of amphiregulin and heregulin immunostaining in breast neoplasia. Breast Cancer Res Treat 1997;45:75–80.

152. Peles E, Bacus SS, Koski RA, et al. Isolation of the *neu*/HER-2 stimulatory ligand: a 44 kd glycoprotein that induces differentiation of mammary tumor cells. Cell 1992;69:205–216.

153. Holmes WE, Sliwkowski MX, Akita RW, et al. Identification of heregulin, a specific activator of p185 *erb* B-2. Science 1992;256:1205–1210.

154. Bacus SS, Gudkov AV, Zelnick CR, et al. Neu differentiation factor (heregulin) induces expression of intercellular adhesion molecule 1: implications for mammary tumors. Cancer Res 1993;53:5251–5261.

155. Bacus SS, Zelnick CR, Plowman G, et al. Expression of the erbB-2 family of growth factor receptors and their ligands in breast cancers. Am J Clin Pathol 1994;102(Suppl 1):S13–S24.

156. Normanno N, Kim N, Wen D, et al. Expression of messenger RNA for amphiregulin, heregulin and cripto-1, three new members of the epidermal growth factor family, in human breast carcinomas. Breast Cancer Res Treat 1995;35:293–297.

157. Tang CK, Perez C, Grunt T, et al. Involvement of heregulin-B2 in the acquisition of the hormone-independent phenotype of breast cancer cells. Cancer Res 1996;56:3350–3358.

158. Mueller H, Kueng W, Schoumacher F, et al. Selective regulation of steroid receptor expression in MCF-7 breast cancer cells by a novel member of the heregulin family. Biochem Biophys Res Commun 1995;26:1271–1278.

159. Pietras RJ, Arboleda J, Reese DM, et al. HER-2 tyrosine kinase pathway targets estrogen receptor and promotes hormone-independent growth in human breast cancer cells. Oncogene 1995;10: 2435–2447.

160. Grunt TW, Saceda M, Martin MB, et al. Bidirectional interactions between the estrogen receptor and the cerbB-2 signaling pathways: heregulin inhibits estrogenic effects in breast cancer cells. Int J Cancer 1995;63:560–567.

161. Daly JM, Jannot CB, Beerli RR, et al. Neu differentiation factor induces ErbB2 down-regulation and apoptosis of ErbB2-overexpressing breast tumor cells. Cancer Res 1997;57:3804–3811.

162. Dublin EA, Bobrow LG, Barnes DM, et al. Amphiregulin and cripto overexpression in breast cancer: relationship with prognosis and clinical and molecular variables. Int J Oncol 1995;7:617–622.

163. Panico L, D'Antonio A, Salvatore G, et al. Differential immunohistochemical detection of transforming growth factor α, amphiregulin and cripto in normal and malignant breast tissues. Int J Cancer 1996; 65:51–56.

164. Fox SB, Harris Adrian L. The epidermal growth factor receptor in breast cancer. J Mammary Gland Biol Neoplasia 1997;2:131–142.

165. Davidson NE, Gelmann EP, Lippman ME, Dickson RB. Epidermal growth factor receptor gene expression in estrogen receptor-positive and negative human breast cancer cell lines. Mol Endocrinol 1987;1:216–223.

166. Valverius EM, Velu T, Shankar V, Ciardiello F, Kim N, Salomon DS. Over-expression of the epidermal growth factor receptor in human breast cancer cells fails to induce an estrogen-independent phenotype. Int J Cancer 1990;46:712–718.

167. Klijn JGM, Berns PMJJ, Schmitz PIM, Foekens JA. The clinical significance of epidermal growth factor receptor (EGF-R) in human breast cancer: a review on 5,232 patients. Endocr Rev 1992;13:3–17.

168. Harris AL, Nicholson S. Epidermal growth factor receptors in human breast cancer. In: Lippman ME, Dickson RB, eds. Breast Cancer: Cellular and Molecular Biology. Kluwer, Boston, 1987, pp. 93–118.

169. Moscatello DK, Holdago-Madruga M, Godwin A, et al. Frequent expression of a mutant epidermal growth factor receptor in multiple human tumors. Cancer Res 1995;55:5536–5539.

170. Sainsbury JRC, Farndon JR, Needham GK, Malcolm AJ, Harris AL. Epidermal-growth-factor receptor status as predictor of early recurrence of and death from breast cancer. Lancet 1987;1:1398–1402.

171. Nicholson S, Richard J, Sainsbury C, et al. Epidermal growth factor receptor (EGFr); results of a 6 year follow-up study in operable breast cancer with emphasis on the node negative subgroup. Br J Cancer 1991;63:146–150.

172. Koenders PG, Beex LVAM, Kienhuis CBM, Kloppenborg PWC, Benraad TJ. Epidermal growth factor receptor and prognosis in human breast cancer: a prospective study. Breast Cancer Res Treat 1993;25: 21–27.

173. Harlozinska A, Bar JK, Wenderski R, et al. Relationship between c-erbB-2 oncoprotein, epidermal growth factor receptor, and estrogen receptor expression in patients with ductal breast carcinoma: association with tumor phenotypes. In Vivo 1996;10:217–222.

174. Nicholson S, Halcrow P, Sainsbury JRC, et al. Epidermal growth factor receptor (EGFr) status associated with failure of primary endocrine therapy in elderly postmenopausal patients with breast cancer. Br J Cancer 1988;58:810–814.

175. Nicholson RI, Gee JMW, Jones H, et al. erbB signalling and endocrine sensitivity of human breast cancer. In: Hurbin RN, et al., eds. EGF Receptor in Tumor Growth and Progression. Einstein-Schering Foundation Workshop, Springer-Verlag, Boston, 1997.

176. Nicholson S, Sainsbury JRC, Halcrow P, Chambers P, Farndon JR, Harris AL. Expression of epidermal growth factor receptors associated with lack of response to endocrine therapy in recurrent breast cancer. Lancet 1989;1:182–186.

177. Gullick WJ. The role of the epidermal growth factor receptor and the c-erbB-2 protein in breast cancer. Int J Cancer 1990;5(Suppl):55–61.

178. Bargmann CI, Weinberg RA. Oncogenic activation of the *neu*-encoded receptor protein by point mutation and deletion. EMBO J 1988;7:2043–2052.

179. DiFiore PP, Pierce JH, Kraus MH, Segatto O, King CR, Aaronson SA. erbB-2 is a potent oncogene when overexpressed in NIH/3T3 cells. Science 1987;237:178–182.

180. Hudziak RM, Schlessinger J, Ullrich A. Increased expression of the putative growth factor receptor p185^{HER2} causes transformation and tumourigenesis of NIH 3T3 cells. Proc Natl Acad Sci USA 1987; 84:7159–7163.

181. Lemoine NR, Staddon S, Dickson C, Barnes DM, Gullick WJ. Absence of activating transmembrane mutations in the c-erbB-2 proto-oncogene in human breast cancer. Oncogene 1989;5:237–239.

182. Rilke F, Colnaghi MI, Cascinelli N, et al. Prognostic significance of HER-2/*neu* expression in breast cancer and its relationship to other prognostic factors. Int J Cancer 1991;49:44–49.

183. Revillion F, Bonneterre J, Peyrat JP. ERBB2 oncogene in human breast cancer and its clinical significance. Eur J Cancer 1998;34:791–808.

184. Bacus SS, Chin D, Yarden Y, et al. Type 1 receptor tyrosine kinases are differentially phosphorylated in mammary carcinoma and differentially associated with steroid receptors. Am J Pathol 1996;148: 549–558.

185. DiGiovanna MP, Carter D, Flynn SD, et al. Functional assay for HER-2/neu demonstrates active signalling in a minority of HER-2/neu-overexpressing invasive human breast tumours. Br J Cancer 1996; 74:802–806.

186. Slamon DJ, Clark GM, Wong SG, et al. Human breast cancer: correlation of relapse and survival with amplification of the HER-2/neu oncogene. Science 1987;235:177–182.

187. Antoniotti S, Maggioar P, Dati C, et al. Tamoxifen up-regulates c-erbB-2 expression in oestrogen-responsive breast cancer cells in vitro. Eur J Cancer 1992;28:318–321.

188. Yu D, Liu B, Jing T, et al. Overexpression of both p185$^{c-erbB2}$ and p170^{mdr-1} renders breast cancer cells highly resistant to taxol. Oncogene 1998;16:2087–2094.

189. Gusterson BA, Machin LG, Gullick WJ, et al. c-erbB-2 expression in benign and malignant breast disease. Br J Cancer 1988;58:453–457.

190. Tsutsumi Y, Naber SP, DeLellis RA, et al. *neu* oncogene protein and epidermal growth factor receptor are independently expressed in benign and malignant breast tissues. Hum Pathol 1990;21: 750–758.

191. Van De Vijer MJ, Peterse JL, Mooi WJ, et al. Neu-protein overexpression in breast cancer. Association with comedo-type ductal carcinoma in situ and limited prognostic value in stage II breast cancer. N Engl J Med 1988;319:1239–1242.

192. Barnes DM, Bartkova J, Camplejohn RS, Gullick WJ, Smith PJ, Millis RR. Overexpression of the c-*erb*B-2 oncoprotein: why does this occur more frequently in ductal carcinoma *in situ* than in invasive mammary carcinoma and is this of prognostic significance? Eur J Cancer 1992;28:644–648.

193. Guerin M, Gabillot M, Mathieu M-C, et al. Structure and expression of c-erbB-2 and EGF receptor genes in inflammatory and non-inflammatory breast cancer: prognostic significance. Int J Cancer 1989;43:201–208.

194. Garcia I, Dietrich P-Y, Aapro M, Vauthier G, Vadas L, Engel E. Genetic alterations of c-*myc* c-erbB-2 and c-Ha-*ras* proto-oncogenes and clinical associations in human breast carcinomas. Cancer Res 1989;49:6675–6679.

195. Dati C, Antoniotti S, Taverna D, Perroteau I, De Bortoli M. Inhibition of c-*erb*B-2 oncogene expression by estrogens in human breast cancer cells. Oncogene 1990;5:1001–1006.

196. Gullick WJ, Love SB, Wright C, et al. c-erbB-2 protein overexpression in breast cancer is a risk factor in patients with involved and uninvolved lymph nodes. Br J Cancer 1992;63:434–438.

197. Richter King C, Kraus MH, DiFiore PP, Paik S, Kasprzyk PG. Implications of *erbB-2* overexpression for basic science and clinical medicine. Semin Cancer Biol 1990;1:329–337.

198. Harris AL, Nicholson S, Sainsbury JRC, Farndon J, Wright C. Epidermal growth factor receptors in breast cancer: association with early relapse and death, poor response to hormones and interactions with *neu*. J Steroid Biochem 1989;34:123–131.

199. Osaki A, Toi M, Yamada H, Kawami H, Kuroi K, Toge T. Prognostic significance of co-expression of c-*erb*B-2 oncoprotein and epidermal growth factor receptor in breast cancer patients. Am J Surg 1992;164:323–326.

200. Prigent SA, Lemoine NR, Hughes CM, Plowman GD, Selden C, Gullick WJ. Expression of the c-*erb*B-3 protein in normal human adult and fetal tissues. Oncogene 1992;7:1273–1278.

201. Kraus MH, Issing W, Miki T, Popescu NC, Aaronson SA. Isolation and characterization of *ERBB3*, a third member of the *ERBB*/epidermal growth factor receptor family: evidence for overexpression in a subset of human mammary tumors. Proc Natl Acad Sci USA 1989;86:9193–9197.

202. Lemoine NR, Barnes DM, Hollywood DP, et al. Expression of the *ERBB3* gene product in breast cancer. Br J Cancer 1992;66:1116–1121.

203. Gasparini G, Gullick WJ, Maluta S, et al. c-erbB-3 and c-erbB-2 protein expression in node-negative breast carcinoma: an immunocytochemical study. Eur. J Cancer 1994;30A:16–22.

204. Quinn CM, Ostrowski JL, Lane SA, et al. c-erbB-3 protein expression in human breast cancer: comparison with other tumour variables and survival. Histopathology 1994;25:247–252.

205. Travis A, Pinder SE, Robertson JFR, Bell JA, Wencyk P, Gullick WJ, et al. C-erbB-3 in human breast carcinoma: expression and relation to prognosis and established prognostic indicators. Br J Cancer 1996;74:229–233.

206. Carter HB, Coffey D. Magnitude of the problem in the United States. In: Coffey D, Resnick M, Dorr F, eds. A Multidisciplinary Analysis of Controversies in the Management of Prostate Cancer. Plenum, New York, 1988, pp. 1–9.

207. Carter HB, Piantadosi S, Isaacs JT. Clinical evidence for and implications of the multistep development of prostate cancer. J Urol 1990;143:742–746.

208. Russell PJ, Bennett S, Stricker P. Growth factor involvement in progression of prostate cancer. Clin Chem 1998;44:705–723.

209. Sherwood ER, Lee C. Epidermal growth factor-related peptides and the epidermal growth factor receptor in normal and malignant prostate. World J Urol 1995;13:290–296.

210. Culig Z, Hobisch A, Cronauer MV. Regulation of prostatic growth and function by peptide growth factors. Prostate 1996;28:392–405.

211. Ching KZ, Ramsey E, Pettigrew N, et al. Expression of mRNA for epidermal growth factor, transforming growth factor–alpha and their receptor in human prostate tissue and cell lines. Mol Cell Biochem 1993;126:151–158.

212. Myers RB, Kudlow JE, Grizzle WE. Expression of transforming growth factor-α, epidermal growth factor and epidermal growth factor receptor in adenocarcinoma of the prostate and benign prostatic hyperplasia. Modern Pathol 1993;6:733–737.

213. Leav I, McNeal JE, Ziar J, et al. The localization of transforming growth factor alpha and epidermal growth factor receptor in stromal and epithelial compartments of developing human prostate and hyperplastic, dysplastic, and carcinomatous lesions. Hum Pathol 1998;29:668–675.

214. Hiramatsu M, Kashimata M, Minami N, et al. Androgenic regulation of epidermal growth factor in the mouse ventral prostate. Biochem Int 1988;17:311–317.

215. Connolly JM, Rose DP. Production of epidermal growth factor and transforming growth factor α by the adrenogen-responsive LNCaP human prostate cancer cell line. Prostate 1990;16:209–218.

216. McKeehan WL, Adams PS, Rosser MP. Direct mitogenic effects of insulin, epidermal growth factor, glucocorticoid, cjoleratoxin, unknown pituitary factors and possibly prolactin, but not androgen, on normal rat prostate epithelial cells in serum-free, primary cell culture. Cancer Res 1984;44:4998–5010.

217. Peehl DM, Stamey TA. Serum-free growth of adult human prostatic carcinoma. In Vitro Cell Dev Biol 1986;22:82–90.

218. Schuurmans ALG, Bolt J, Mulder E. Androgens and transforming growth factor modulate the growth response to epidermal growth factor in human prostatic tumor cells. Mol Cell Endocrinol 1988;60:101–104.

219. Nishi N, Oya H, Matsumoto K, et al. Changes in gene expression of growth factors and their receptors during castration-induced involution and androgen-induced regrowth of rat prostates. The Prostate 1996;28:139–152.

220. Sehgal I, Bailey J, Hitzemann K, et al. Epidermal growth factor receptor-dependent stimulation of amphiregulin expression in androgen-stimulated human prostate cancer cells. Mol Biol Cell 1994;5:339–347.

221. Liu X–H, Wiley HS, Meikle AW. Androgens regulate proliferation of human prostate cancer cells in culture by increasing transforming growth factor-α (TGF-α) and epidermal growth factor (EGF)/TGF-α receptor. J Clin Endocrinol Metab 1993;77:1472–1478.

222. Morris GL, Dodd JG. Epidermal growth factor receptor mRNA levels in human prostatic tumors and cell lines. J Urol 1990;143:1272–1274.

223. Wilding GE, Valverius C, Knabbe C, et al. Role of transforming growth factor-alpha in human prostate cancer cell growth. Prostate 1989;15:1–12.

224. Hofer DR, Sherwood ER, Bromberg WD, et al. Autonomous growth of androgen-independent human prostatic carcinoma cells: role of transforming growth factor α. Cancer Res 1991;51:2780–2785.

225. Rubenstein M, Mirochnik Y, Chou P, et al. Antisense oligonucleotide intralesional therapy for human PC-3 prostate tumors carried in athymic nude mice. J Surg Oncol 1996;62:194–200.

226. Schuurmans AL, Bolt J, Veldscholte J, et al. Regulation of growth of LNCaP human prostate tumor cells by growth factors and steroid hormones. J Steroid Biochem Mol Biol 1991;40:193–197.

227. Grasso AW, Wen D, Miller CM, et al. ErbB kinases and NDF signaling in human prostate cancer cells. Oncogene 1997;15:2705–2716.

228. Knabbe C, Kellner U, Schmahl M, et al. Growth factors in human prostate cancer cells: implications for an improved treatment of prostate cancer. J Steroid Biochem Mol Biol 1991;40:185–192.

229. Kim JH, Sherwood ER, Sutkowski DM, et al. Inhibition of prostatic tumor cell proliferation by suramin: alterations in TGF alpha-mediated autocrine growth regulation and cell cycle distribution. J Urol 1991;146:171–176.

230. Yang Y, Chisholm GD, Habib FK. Epidermal growth factor and transforming growth factor α concentrations in BPH and cancer of the prostate: their relationships with tissue androgene levels. Br J Cancer 1993;67:152–155.

231. Leav I, McNeal JE, Ziar J, et al. The localization of transforming growth factor alpha and epidermal growth factor receptor in stromal and epithelial compartments of developing human prostate and hyperplastic, dysplastic, and carcinomatous lesions. Human Pathol 1998;29:668–675.

232. Leung HY, Weston J, Gullick WJ, et al. A potential autocrine loop between heregulin-alpha and erbB-3 receptor in human prostatic adenocarcinoma. Br J Urol 1997;79:212–216.

233. Myers RB, Srivastava S, Oelschlager DK, et al. Expression of p160erbB-3 and p185erbB-2 in prostatic intraepithelial neoplasia and prostatic adenocarcinoma. J Natl Cancer Inst 1994;86:1140–1145.

234. Lyne JC, Melhern MF, Finley GG, et al. Tissue expression of neu differentiation factor/heregulin and its receptor complex in prostate cancer and its biologic effects on prostate cancer cells in vitro. Cancer J Sci Am 1997;3:21–30.

235. Harper ME, Goddard L, Glynne-Jones E, et al. Epidermal growth factor receptor expression by northern analysis and immunohistochemistry in benign and malignant prostatic tumours. Eur J Cancer 1995;31A:1492–1497.

236. Davies P, Eaton C, France C, et al. Growth factor receptors and oncogene expression in prostate cells. Am J Clin Oncol 1988;11:1–6.

237. Davies P, Eaton CL. Binding of epidermal growth factor by human normal, hypertrophic and carcinomatous prostate. Prostate 1989;14:123–132.

238. Ibrahim GK, Kerns BM, MacDonald JA, et al. Differential immunoreactivity of epidermal growth factor receptor in benign, dysplastic and malignant prostatic tissues. J Urol 1993;149:170–173.

239. McCann A, Dervan PA, Gullick WJ, et al. c-erbB-2 oncoprotein expression in malignant and nonmalignant tissues. Proc Am Assoc Cancer Res 1989;30:914(Abstract).

240. Ware JL, Maygarden SJ, Koontz WW, et al. Differential reactivity with anti-erb-B2 antiserum among human malignant and benign prostatic tissue. Proc Am Assoc Cancer Res 1989;30:1737(Abstract).

241. Zhau HE, Wan DS, Zhou J, et al. Expression of e-erb B-2/neu proto-oncogene in human prostatic cancer tissues and cell lines. Mol Carcinog 1992;5:320–327.

242. Kuhn EJ, Kurnot RA, Sesterhenn IA, Chang EH, Moul JW. Expression of the c-erbB-2 (HER-2/neu) oncoprotein in human prostatic carcinoma. J Urol 1993;150:1427–1433.

243. Schwartz S, Caceres C, Morote J, et al. Over-expression of epidermal growth factor receptor and c-erbB2/neu but not of int-2 genes in benign prostatic hyperplasia by means of semi-quantitative PCR. Int J Cancer 1998;76:464–467.

244. Ross JS, Sheehan C, Hayner-Buchan AM, et al. HER-2/neu gene amplification status in prostate cancer by fluorescence in situ hybridization. Hum Pathol 1997;28:827–833.

245. Ross JS, Sheehan CE, Hayner-Buchan AM, et al. Prognostic significance of HER-2/neu gene amplification status by fluorescence in situ hybridization of prostate carcinoma. Cancer 1997;79:2162–2170.

246. Gullick WJ. Inhibitors of growth factor receptors. In: Carney D, Sikora K, eds. Genes and Cancer. Wiley, New York, 1990, pp. 263–273.

247. Powis G, Kozikowski A. Growth factor and oncogene signalling pathways as targets for rational anti-cancer drug development. Clin Biochem 1991;24:385–397.

248. Garner A. Therapeutic potential of growth factors and their antagonists. Yale J Biol Med 1992;65:715–723.

249. Shepard HM, Lewis GD, Sarup JC, et al. Monoclonal antibody therapy of human cancer: taking the HER2 protooncogene to the clinic. J Clin Immunol 1991;11:117–127.

250. Stancovski I, Peles E, Ben Levy R, et al. Signal transduction by the neu/erbB-2 receptor: a potential target for anti-tumor therapy. J Steroid Biochem Mol Biol 1992;43:95–103.

251. Hynes NE. Amplification and overexpression of the erbB-2 gene in human tumors: its involvement in tumor development, significance as a prognostic factor, and potential as a target for cancer therapy. Semin Cancer Biol 1993;4:19–26.

252. Baselga J, Mendelsohn J. Type I receptor tyrosine kinase as target for therapy in breast cancer. J Mammary Gland Biol Neoplasia 1997;2:165–174.

253. Yang D, Wang S. Small molecule antagonsists targeting growth factors/receptors. Curr Pharm Design 1997;3:335–354.

254. Rusch V, Mendelsohn J, Dmitrovsky E. The epidermal growth factor receptor and its ligands as therapeutic targets in human tumors. Cytokine Growth Factor Revs 1996;7:133–141.

255. O'Rourke DM, Greene MI. Immunologic approaches to inhibiting cell-surface-residing oncoproteins in human tumors. Immunol Res 1998;17:179–189.

256. Mori S, Mori Y, Mukaiyama T, et al. In vitro and in vivo release of soluble erbB-2 protein from human carcinoma cells. Jpn J Cancer Res 1990;81:489–494.

257. Carney WP, Hamer PJ, Petit D, et al. Detection and quantitation of the human neu oncoprotein. J Tumor Marker Oncol 1991;6:53–72.

258. Breuer B, Luo J-C, DeVivo I, et al. Detection of elevated c-erbB-2 oncoprotein in the serum and tissue in breast cancer. Med Sci Res 1993;21:383,384.

259. Fleisher M. Prognostic markers other than hormone receptors in breast cancer. J Clin Ligand Assay 1998;21:41–46.

260. Brandt-Rauf PW. The c-erbB transmembrane growth factor receptors as serum biomarkers in human cancer studies. Mutation Res 1995;333:203–208.

261. Müller-Newen G, Köhne C, Heinrich PC. Soluble receptors for cytokines and growth factors. Int Arch Allergy Immunol 1996;111:99–106.

262. Arai Y, Yoshiki T, Yoshida O. c-erbB-2 oncoprotein: a potential biomarker of advanced prostate cancer. Prostate 1997;1530:195–201.
263. Myers RB, Brown D, Oelschlager DK, et al. Elevated serum levels of p105 (erbB-2) in patients with advanced-stage prostatic adenocarcinoma. Int J Cancer 1996;69:398–402.
264. Mehta RR, McDermott JH, Hieken TJ, et al. Plasma c-erbB-2 levels in breast cancer patients: prognostic significance in predicting response to chemotherapy. J Clin Oncol 1998;16:2409–2416.
265. Torrisi R, Zanardi S, Pensa F, et al. Epidermal growth factor content of breast cyst fluids from women with breast cancer or proliferative disease of the breast. Breast Cancer Res Treat 1995;33:219–224.
266. Gann P, Chatterton R, Vogelsong K, et al. Mitogenic growth factors in breast fluid obtained from healthy women: evaluation of biological and extraneous sources of variability. Cancer Epidemiol Biomarkers Prev 1997;6:421–428.
267. Fabian CJ, Zalles C, Kamel S, et al. Breast cytology and biomarkers obtained by random fine needle aspiration: use in risk assessment and early chemoprevention trials. J Cell Biochem 1997;28/29(Suppl): 101–110.
268. Baselga J, Tripathy J, Mendelsohn J, et al. Phase II study of weekly intravenous recombinant humanized anti-p185HER2 monoclonal antibody in patients with HER2/neu overexpressing metastatic breast cancer. J Clin Oncol 1996;14:737–744.
269. Schroeder W, Biesterfeld S, Zillessenm S, et al. Epidermal growth factor receptor-immunohistochemical detection and clinical significance for treatment of primary breast cancer. Anticancer Res 1997;17: 2799–2802.
270. Wikstrand CJ, Hale LP, Batra SK, et al. Monoclonal antibodies against EGFRvIII are tumor specific and react with breast and lung carcinomas and malignant gliomas. Cancer Res 1995;55:3140–3148.
271. Viloria Petit AM, Rak J, Hung M-C, et al. Neutralizing antibodies against epidermal growth factor and ErbB-2/neu receptor tyrosine kinases down-regulate vascular endothelial growth factor production by tumor cells in vitro and in vivo. Am J Pathol 1997;151:1523–1530.
272. Di Massimo AM, Di Loreto M, Pacilli A, et al. Immunoconjugates made of an anti-EGF receptor monoclonal antibody and type 1 ribosome-inactivating proteins from *Saponaria ocymoides* or *Vaccaria pyramidata*. Br. J Cancer 1997;75:822–828.
273. McNeil C. Herceptin raises its sights beyond advanced breast cancer. J Natl Cancer Inst 1998;90: 882,883.
274. Hancock MC, Langton BC, Chan T. A monoclonal antibody against the c-*erbB*-2 protein enhances the cytotoxicity of *cis*-diamminedichloroplatinum against human breast and ovarian tumor cell lines. Cancer Res 1991;51:4575–4580.
275. Lan I, Baselga J, Masui H, and Mendelsohn J. Antitumor effect of anti-epidermal growth factor receptor monoclonal antibodies plus *cis*-diamminedichloroplatinum on well established A431 cell xenografts. Cancer Res 1993;53:4637–4642.
276. Baselga J, Norton L, Masui H, et al. Antitumor effects of doxorubicin in combination with anti-epidermal growth factor receptor monoclonal antibodies. J Natl Cancer Inst 1998;85:1327–1333.
277. Baselga J, Norton L, Albanell J, et al. Recombinant humanized anti-HER2 antibody (Herceptin™) enhances the antitumor activity of paclitaxel and doxorubicin against HER2/neu overexpressing human breast cancer xenografts. Cancer Res 1998;58:2825–2831.
278. Lofts FJ, Hurst HC, Sternberg MJE, Gullick WJ. Specific short transmembrane sequences can inhibit transformation by the mutant *neu* growth factor receptor *in vitro* and *in vivo*. Oncogene 1993;8: 2813–2820.
279. Theuer CP, Pastan I. Immunotoxin and recombinant toxins in the treatment of solid carcinomas. Am J Surg 1993;166:284–288.
280. Jeschke M, Wels W, Dengler W, et al. Targeted inhibition of tumor-cell growth by recombinant heregulin-toxin fusion proteins. Int. J Cancer 1995;60:730–739.
281. Fiddes RJ, Janes PW, Sanderson GM, et al. Heregulin (HRG)-induced mitogenic signaling and cytotoxic activity of a HRG/PE40 ligand toxin in human breast cancer cells. Cell Growth Differ 1995;6: 1567–1577.
282. Groner B, Wick B, Jeschke M, et al. Intra-tumoral application of a heregulin-exotoxin-a fusion protein causes rapid tumor regression without adverse systemic or local effects. Int J Cancer 1997;70:682–687.
283. Fominaya J, Uherek C, Wels W. A chimeric fusion protein containing transforming growth factor-alpha mediates gene transfer via binding to the EGF receptor. Gene Ther 1998;5:521–530.
284. Yang D, Kuan C-T, Payne J. Recombinant heregulin-pseudomonas exotoxin fusion proteins: interactions with the heregulin receptors and antitumor activity in vivo. Clin Cancer Res 1998;4:993–1004.

285. Osherov N, Gazit A, Gilon C, Levitzki A. Selective inhibition of the epidermal growth factor and HER2/neu receptors by tyrphostins. J Biol Chem 1993;268:11,134–11,142.

286. Fry DW, Nelson JM, Slintak V, et al. Biochemical and antiproliferative properties of 4-[ar(alk)ylamino] pyridopyrimidines, a new chemical class of potent and specific epidermal growth factor receptor tyrosine kinase inhibitor. Biochem Pharmacol 1997;54:877–887.

287. Kelloff GJ, Fay JR, Steele VE, et al. Epidermal growth factor receptor tyrosine kinase inhibitors as potential cancer chemopreventives. Cancer Epidemiol Biomarkers Prev 1996;5:657–666.

288. Bos M, Mendelsohn J, Kim Y-M, et al. PD153035, a tyrosine kinase inhibitor, prevents epidermal growth factor receptor activation and inhibits growth of cancer cells in a receptor number-dependent manner. Clin Cancer Res 1997;3:2099–2106.

289. Lydon NB, Mett H, Mueller M, et al. A potent protein-tyrosine kinase inhibitor which selectively blocks proliferation of epidermal growth factor receptor-expressing tumor cells in vitro and in vivo. Int J Cancer 1998;76:154–163.

290. Sizeland AM, Burgess AW. Anti-sense transforming growth factor α oligonucleotides inhibit autocrine stimulated proliferation of a colon carcinoma cell line. Mol Biol Cell 1992;3:1235–1243.

291. Moroni MC, Willingham MC, Beguinot L. EGF-R antisense RNA blocks expression of the epidermal growth factor receptor and suppresses the transforming phenotype of a human carcinoma cell line. J Biol Chem 1992;267:2714–2722.

292. Trojan J, Blossey BK, Johnson TR, et al. Loss of tumorigenicity of rat glioblastoma directed by episome-based antisense cDNA transcription of insulin-like growth factor I. Proc Natl Acad Sci USA 1992;89:4874–4878.

293. Shaw Y-T, Chang S-H, Chiou S-T, Chang W-C, Lai M-D. Partial reversion of transformed phenotype of B104 cancer cells by antisense nucleic acids. Cancer Lett 1993;69:27–32.

294. Rubenstein M, Mirochnik Y, Ray V, et al. Lack of toxicity associated with the systemic administration of antisense oligonucleotides for treatment of rats bearing LNCaP prostate tumors. Med Oncol 1997; 14:131–136.

295. Dixit M, Yang J-L, Poirier MC, et al. Abrogation of cisplatin-induced programmed cell death in human breast cancer cells by epidermal growth factor antisense RNA. J Natl Cancer Inst 1997;89:365–373.

296. Sacco MG, Barbieri O, Piccini D, et al. In vitro and in vivo antisense-mediated growth inhibition of a mammary adenocarcinoma from MMTV-neu transgenic mice. Gene Ther 1998;5:388–393.

297. Yamazaki H, Kijima H, Ohnishi Y, et al. Inhibition of tumor growth by ribozyme-mediated suppression of aberrant epidermal growth factor receptor gene expression. J Natl Cancer Inst 1998;90:581–587.

298. Asano T, Kleinerman ES. Liposome-encapsulated MTP-PE: a novel biologic agent for cancer therapy. J Immunother 1993;14:286–292.

299. Moscatello DK, Ramirez G, Wong AJ. A naturally occurring mutant human epidermal growth factor receptor as a target for peptide vaccine immunotherapy of tumors. Cancer Res 1997;57:1419–1424.

300. Travis J. Novel anticancer agents move closer to reality. Science 1993;260:1877,1878.

301. Kohl NE, Mosser SD, deSolms SJ, et al. Selective inhibition of *ras*-dependent transformation by a farnesyltransferase inhibitor. Science 1993;260:1934–1936.

302. James GL, Goldstein JL, Brown MS, et al. Benzodiazepine peptidomimetics: potent inhibitors of Ras farnesylation in animal cells. Science 1993;260:1937–1942.

303. Kelloff GJ, Lubet RA, Fay JR, et al. Farnesyl protein transferase inhibitors as potential cancer chemopreventives. Cancer Epidermiol Biomarkers Prev 1997;6:267–282.

304. Gibbs JB, Oliff A. The potential of farnesyltransferase inhibitors as cancer chemotherapeutics. Ann Rev Pharmacol Toxicol 1997;37:143–166.

305. Mangues R, Corral T, Kohl NE, et al. Antitumor effect of a farnesyl protein transferase inhibitor in mammary and lymphoid tumors overexpressing N-ras in transgenic mice. Cancer Res 1998;58:1253–1259.

306. Li N, Batzer A, Daly R, et al. Guanine-nucleotide-releasing factor hSos1 binds to Grb2 and links receptor tyrosine kinases to Ras signalling. Nature 1993;363:15–16.

307. Cannistra SA, Niloff JM. Cancer of the uterine cervix. N Engl J Med 1996;334:1030–1038.

308. Mosny DS, Herholtz J, Degan W, Bender HG. Immunhistochemical investigations of steroid receptors in normal and neoplastic squamous epithelium of the uterine cervix. Gynecol Oncol 1989;35:373–377.

309. Ciocca DR, Roig LM. Estrogen receptors in human nontarget tissues: biological and clinical implications. Endocr Rev 1995;16:35–62.

310. Soutter WP, Pegoraro RJ, Green-Thompson RW, Naidoo DV, Joubert SM, Philpott RM. Nuclear and cytoplasmatic oestrogen receptors in squamous carcinoma of the cervix. Br J Cancer 1981;44:154–159.

311. Martin JD, Hahnel R, McCartney AJ, Woodings T. Prognostic value of estrogen receptors in cancer of the uterine cervix. New Engl J Med 1982;306:485.

312. Martin JD, Hahnel R, McCartney AJ, DeKlerk N. The influence of estrogen and progesterone receptors on survival in patients with carcinoma of the uterine cervix. Gynecol Oncol 1986;23:329–335.

313. Darne J, Soutter WP, Ginsberg R, Sharp F. Nuclear and "cytoplasmatic" estrogen and progsterone receptors in squamous cell carcinoma of the cervix. Gynecol Oncol 1990;38:216–219.

314. Hunter RE, Longcope C, Keough P. Steroid hormone receptors in carcinoma of the cervix. Cancer 1987;60:392–396.

315. Harding M, McIntosh J, Paul J, Symonds RP, Reed N, Habeshaw T, Stewart M, Leake RE. Oestrogen and progesterone receptors in carcinoma of the cervix. Clin Oncol 1990;2:313–317.

316. Syrjala P, Kontula K, Janne O, Kuppila A, Vihko R. Steroid receptors in normal and neoplastic human uterine tissue. In: Brush MG, King RJB, Taylor R, eds. Endometrial Cancer. Bailliere Tindall, London, 1978, pp. 242–260.

317. Leake R. Cervical cancer: hormones growth factors and cytokines. In: Langdon SP, Miller WR, Berchuck A, eds. Biology of Female Cancer. CRC, Boca Raton, FL, 1997, pp. 245–250.

318. Gao YL, Twiggs LB, Leung BS, Yu WCY, Potish RA, Okagaki T, Adcock LL, Prem KA. Cytoplasmatic estrogen and progesterone receptors in primary cercival carcinoma: clinical and histopathologic correlates. Am J Obstet Gynecol 1983;146:299–306.

319. Ghandour FA, Attanoos R, Nahar K, Gee JW, Brigrigg A, Ismail SM. Immunocytochemical localization of oestrogen and progesterone receptors in primary adenocarcinoma of the cervix. Histopathology 1994;24:49–55.

320. Bhattacharya D, Redkar A, Mittra I, Sutaria U, MacRae KD. Oestrogen increases S-phase fraction and oestrogen and progesterone receptors in human cervical cancer in vitro. Br J Cancer 1997;75:554–558.

321. Twiggs LB, Potish RA, Leung BS, Carson LF, Adcock LL, Savage JE, Prem JE. Cytosolic estrogen and progesterone receptors as prognostic parameters in stage IB cervical carcinoma. Gynecol Oncol 1987;28:156–160.

322. Fujimoto J, Fujita H, Hosoda S, Okada H, Tamaya T. Prognosis of cervical cancers with reference to steroid receptors. Nippon Gan Chiryo Gakkai Shi 1989;24:21–31.

323. Bates SE, Davidson NE, Valverius EM, Freter CE, Dickson RB, Tam JP, et al. Expression of transforming growth factor alpha and its messenger ribonucleic acid in human breast cancer: its regulation by estrogen and its possible functional significance. Mol Endocrinol 1988;2:543–555.

324. Salomon DS, Kidwell WR, Kim N, Ciardiello F, Bates SE, Valverius E, et al. Modulation by estrogen and growth factors of transforming growth factor-alpha and epidermal growth factor receptor expression in normal and malignant human mammary epithelial cells. Recent Res Cancer Res 1989;113:57–69.

325. Salomon DS, Brandt R, Ciardiello F, Normanno N. Epidermal growth factor-related peptides and their receptors in human malignancies. Crit Rev Oncol Hematol 1995;19:83–232.

326. Martinez-Lacaci I, Saceda M, Plowman GD, Johnson GR, Normanno N, Salomon DS, Dickson RB. Estrogen and phorbol esters regulate amphiregulin expression by two separate mechanisms in human breast cancer cell lines. Endocrinology 1995;136:3983–3992.

327. Rorke EA. Antisense human papillomavirus (HPV) E6/E7 expression, reduced stability of epidermal growth factor, and diminished growth of HPV-positive tumor cells. J Natl Cancer Inst 1997;89:1243–1246.

328. Arends MJ, Buckley CH, Wells M. Aetiology, pathogenesis, and pathology of cervical neoplasia. J Clin Pathol 1998;51:96–103.

329. Stöppler H, Conrad Stöppler M, Schlegel R. Transforming proteins of the papilloma viruses. Intervirology 1994;37:168–179.

330. Kubbutat MHG, Vousden KH. Role of E6 and E7 oncoproteins in HPV-induced anogenital malignancies. Semin Virol 1996;7:295–304.

331. Galloway DA, McDougall JK. The disruption of cell cycle checkpoints by papillomavirus oncoproteins contributes to anogenital neoplasia. Semin Cancer Biol 1996;7:309–315.

332. Jones DL, Münger K. Interactions of the human papillomavirus E7 protein with cell cycle regulators. Semin Cancer Biol 1996;7:327–337.

333. Huibregtse JM, Beaudenon SL. Mechanism of HPV E6 proteins in cellular transformation. Semin Cancer Biol 1996;7:317–326.

334. Leechanachai P, Banks L, Moreau F, Matlashewski G. The E5 gene from human papillomavirus type 16 is an oncogene which enhances growth factor-mediated signal transduction to the nucleus. Oncogene 1992;7:19–25.

335. Straight SW, Hinkle PM, Jewers RJ, McCance DJ. The E5 oncoprotein of human papillomavirus type 16 transforms fibroblasts and effects the downregulation of the epidermal growth factor receptor in keratinocytes. J Virol 1993;67:4521–4532.

336. Maruo T, Yamasaki M, Ladines-Llave CA, Mochizuki M. Immunohistochemical demonstration of elevated expression of epidermal growth factor receptor in the neoplastic changes of cervical squamous epithelium. Cancer 1992;69:1182–1187.

337. Berchuck A, Rodriguez G, Kamel A, Soper JT, Clark-Pearson DL, Bast RC. Expression of epidermal growth factor receptor and ErbB-2 in normal and neoplastic cervix, vulva and vagina. Obstet Gynecol 1990;76:381–387.

338. Berchuck A, Rodriguez G, Kinney RB, Soper JT, Dodge RK, Clarke-Pearson DL, Bast RC Jr. Overexpression of HER-2/neu in endometrial cancer is associated with advanced stage disease. Am J Obstet Gynecol 1991;164:15–21.

339. Gullick WJ, Marsden JJ, Whittle N, Ward B, Bobrow L, Waterfield M. Expression of epidermal growth factor receptors on human cervical, ovarian and vulvar carcinomas. Cancer Res 1986;46:285–292.

340. Tervahauta A, Syrjanen S, Syrjanen K. Epidermal growth factor receptor, c-berbB-2 proto-oncogene and estrogen receptor expression in human pillomavirus lesions of the uterine cervix. Int J Gynecol Pathol 1994;13:234–240.

341. Doeberitz M, Gissmann L, Zur Hausen H. Growth-regulating functions of human papillomavirus early gene products in cervical cancer cells acting dominant over enhanced epidermal growth factor receptor expression. Cancer Res 1990;50:3730–3736.

342. Woodworth CD, McMullin E, Iglesias M, Plowman GD. Interleukin 1a and tumor necrosis factor a stimulate autocrine amphiregulin expression and proliferation of human papillomavirus-immortalized and carcinoma-derived cervical epithelial cells. Proc Natl Acad Sci USA 1995;92:2840–2844.

343. Hu G, Liu W, Mendelsohn J, Ellis LM, Radinsky R, Andreeff M, Deisseroth AB. Expression of epidermal growth factor receptor and human papillomavirus E6/E7 proteins in cervical carcinoma cells. J Natl Cancer Inst 1997;89:1271–1276.

344. Von Knebel–Doeberitz M, Rittmuller C, zur Hausen H, Durst M. Inhibition of tumorigenicity of cervical cancer cells in nude mice by HPV E6/E7 antisense RNA. Int J Cancer 1992;51:51,831–51,834.

345. Hamada K, Sakaue M, Alemany R, Zhang WW, Horio Y, Roth JA, et al. Adenovirus-mediated transfer of HPV 16 E6/E7 antisense RNA to human cervical cancer cells. Gynecol Oncol 1996;63:219–227.

346. Rusch V, Mendelsohn J, Dmitrovsky E. The epidermal growth factor receptor and its ligands as therapeutic targets in human tumors. Cytokine Growth Factor Rev 1996;7:133–141.

347. Brunton VG, Carlin S, Workman P. Alterations in EGF–dependent proliferative and phosphorylation events in squamous cell carcinoma cell lines by a tyrosine kinase inhibitor. Anticancer Drug Des 1994; 9:311–329.

348. Peto M, Tolle-Ersu I, Krysch HG, Klock G. Epidermal growth factor induction of human papillomavirus type 16 E6/E7 mRNA in tumor cells involves two AP-1 binding sites in the viral enhancer. J Gen Virol 1995;76:1945–1958.

349. Pfeiffer D, Spranger J, Al-Deiri M, Kimmig R, Fisseler–Eckhoff A, Scheidel P, Schatz H, Jensen A, Pfeiffer A. mRNA expression of ligands of the epidermal-growth-factor-receptor in the uterus. Int J Cancer 1997;72:581–586.

350. Konishi I, Ishikawa Y, Wang S-Y, Wang D-P, Koshiyama M, Mandai M, Komatsu T, Yamamoto S, Mori T. Expression of transforming growth factor-α in the normal cervix and in benign and malignant lesions of the uterine cervix. Br. J Obstet Gynaecol 1994;101:325–329.

351. Hembree JR, Agarwal C, Eckert RL. Epidermal growth factor suppresses insulin–like growth factor binding protein 3 level in human papillomavirus type 16-immortalized cervical epithelial cells and thereby potentiates the effects of insulin-like growth factor-1. Cancer Res 1994;54:3160–3166.

352. Ueda M, Ueki M, Yamada T, Okamoto Y, Maeda T, Sugimoto O, Otsuki Y. Scatchard analysis of EGF receptor and effects of EGF on growth and TA-4 production of newly established uterine cervical cancer cell line (OMC-1). Hum Cell 1989;2:401–410.

353. Steller MA, Delgado CH, Zou Z. Insulin-like growth factor II mediates epidermal growth factor-induced mitogenesis in cervical cancer cells. Proc Natl Acad Sci USA 1995;92:11,970–11,974.

354. Steller MA, Delgado CH, Bartels CJ, Woodworth CD, Zou Z. Overexpression of the insuline-like growth factor-1 receptor and autocrine stimulation in human cervical cancer cells. Cancer Res 1996; 56:1761–1765.

355. Tonkin KS, Berger M, Ormerod M. Epidermal growth factor status in four carcinoma of the cervix cell lines. Int J Gynecol Cancer 1991;1:185–192.
356. Donato NJ, Gallick GE, Steck PA, Rosenblum MG. Tumor necrosis factor modulates epidermal growth factor receptor phosphorylation and kinase activity in human tumor cells. Correlation with cytotoxicity. J Biol Chem 1989;264:20,474–20,481.
357. Nishikawa K, Rosenblum MG, Newman RA, Pandita TK, Hittelman WN, Donato NJ. Resistance of human cervical carcinoma cells to tumor necrosis factor correlates with their increased sensitivity to cisplatin: evidence of a role for DNA repair and epidermal growth factor receptor. Cancer Res 1992;52: 4758–4765.
358. Donato NJ, Yan DH, Hung MC, Rosenblum MG. Epidermal growth factor receptor expression and function control cytotoxic responsiveness to tumor necrosis factor in ME-180 squamous carcinoma cells. Cell Growth Differ 1993;4:411–419.
359. Zheng ZS, Goldsmith LA. Modulation of epidermal growth factor receptors by retinoic acid in ME 180. Cancer Res 1990;50:1201–1205.
360. Ueda M, Ueki M, Terai Y, Morimoto A, Fujii H, Yoshizawa K, Yanagihara T. Stimulatory effects of EGF and TGF-α on invasive activity and 5-deoxy-5-fluorouridine sensitivity in uterine cervical-carcinoma SKG-IIIB cells. Int J Cancer 1997;72:1027–1033.
361. Ueda M, Ueki M, Sugimoto O. Characterization of epidermal growth factor (EGF) receptor and biological effect of EGF on human uterine cervical adenocarcinoma cell line OMC-4. Hum Cell 1993; 6:218–225.
362. Ozanne B, Richards CS, Hendler F, Burns D, Gusterson B. Overexpression of the EGF receptor is a hall mark of squamous cell carcinomas. J Pathol 1986;149:9–14.
363. Pfeiffer D, Stellwag B, Pfeiffer A, Borlinghaus P, Meier W, Scheidel P. Clinical implications of the epidermal growth factor receptor in the squamous cell carcinoma of the uterine cervix. Gynecol Oncol 1989;33:146–150.
364. Kimmig R, Pfeiffer D, Landsmann H, Hepp H. Quantitative determination of the epidermal growth factor receptor in cervical cancer and normal cervical epithelium by 2-color flow cytometry: evidence for downregulation in cervical cancer. Int J Cancer 1997;74:365–373.
365. Stellwag B, Scheidel P, Pfeiffer D, Hepp H. EGF receptor and EGF-like activity as prognostic factors in cervix cancer. Geburtsh Frauenheilkd 1993;53:177–181.
366. Pfeiffer D, Kimmig R, Herrmann J, Ruge M, Fisseler-Eckhoff A, Scheidel P, et al. Epidermal growth factor receptor correlates negatively with cell density in cervical squamous epithelium and is down-regulated in cancers of the uterus. Int J Cancer 1998;79:49–55.
367. Hale RJ, Buckley CH, Fox H, Williams J. Prognostic value of c-erbB-2 expression in uterine cervical carcinoma. J Clin Pathol 1992;45:594–596.
368. Hale RJ, Buckley CH, Gullick WJ, Fox H, Williams J, Wilcox FL. Prognostic value of epidermal growth factor expression in cervical carcinoma. J Clin Pathol 1993;46:149–153.
369. Hayashi Y, Hachisuga T, Iwasaka T, Fukada K, Okuma Y, Yokoyama M, Sugimori H. Expression of ras oncogene product and EGF receptor in cervical lymph node involvement. Gynecol Oncol 1991; 40:147–151.
370. Pateisky N, Schatten C, Vavra N, Ehrebock P, Angelberger P, Barrada M, Epenetos A. Lymphoscintigraphy using epidermal growth factor as tumour-seeking agent in uterine cervical cancer. Wien Klin Wochenschr 1991;103:654–656.
371. Goeppinger A, Wittmaack FM, Wintzer HO, Ikenberg H, Bauknecht T. Localization of human epidermal growth factor receptor in cervical intraepithelial neoplasias. J Cancer Res Clin Oncol 1989;115: 259–263.
372. Kim JW, Kim YT, Kim DK, Song CH, Lee JW. Expression of epidermal growth factor receptor in carcinoma of the cervix. Gynecol Oncol 1996;60:283–287.
373. Costa MJ, Walls J, Trelford JD. c-erbB-2 oncoprotein overexpression in uterine cervix carcinoma with glandular differentiation. A frequent event but not an independent prognostic marker because it occurs late in the disease. Am J Clin Pathol 1995;104:634–642.
374. Langlois NE, Skinner L, Miller ID. C-erbB-2 in cervical carcinoma. Am J Clin Pathol 1996;106: 556,557.
375. Mitra AB, Murty VV, Pratap M, Sodhani P, Chaganti RS. ErbB2 (HER2/neu) oncogene is frequently amplified in squamous cell carcinoma of the uterine cervix. Cancer Res 1994;54:637–639.
376. Kihana T, Tsuda H, Teshima S, Nomoto K, Tsugane S, Sonoda T, Matsuura S, Hirohashi S. Prognostic significance of the overexpression of c-erbB-2 protein in adenocarcinoma of uterine cervix. Cancer 1994;73:148–153.

377. Brumm C, Riviere A, Wilckens C, Loning T. Immunohistochemical investigation and northern blot analysis of c-erbB-2 expression in normal, premalignant and malignant tissues of the corpus and cervix uteri. Virchows Arch A Pathol Anat Histopathol 1990;417:477–484.

378. Ndubisi B, Sanz S, Lu L, Podczaski E, Benrubi G, Masood S. The prognostic value of HER-2/neu oncogene in cervical cancer. Ann Clin Lab Sci 1997;27:396–401.

379. Lakshmi S, Balaraman Nair M, Jayaprakash PG, Rajalekshmy TN, Krishnan Nair M, Radhakrishna Pillai M. c-erbB-2 oncoprotein and epidermal growth factor receptor in cervical lesions. Pathobiology 1997;65:163–168.

380. Altavilla G, Castellan L, Wabersich J, Marchetti M, Onnis A. Prognostic significance of epidermal growth factor receptor (EGFR) and c-erbB-2 protein, overexpression in adenocarcinoma of the uterine cervix. Eur J Gynaecol Oncol 1996;XVII:267–270.

381. Kristensen GB, Holm R, Abeler VM, Trope CG. Evaluation of the prognostic significance of cathepsin D epidermal growth factor receptor, and c-erbB-2 in early cervical squamous cell carcinoma. Cancer 1996;78:433–440.

382. Nakano T, Oka K, Ishikawa A, Morita S. Correlation of cervical carcinoma c-erbB-2 oncogene with cell proliferation parameters in patients treated with radiation therapy for cervical carcinoma. Cancer 1997;79:513–520.

383. DiSaia PJ, Creasman WT. Clinical Gynecologic Oncology. Mosby, St. Louis, 1997.

384. Nelson KG, Takahashi T, Bossert NL, Walmer DK, McLachlan JA. Epidermal growth factor replaces estrogen in the stimulation of female genital tract growth and differentiation. Proc Natl Acad Sci USA 1991;88:21–25.

385. Horowitz GM, Scott RT, Drews MR, Mavot D, Hofmann GE. Immunohistochemical localization of transforming growth factor a in human endometrium, decidua, and trophoblast. J Clin Endocrinol Metab 1993;76:786–792.

386. Konopka B, Sasko E, Kluska A, Goluda M, Janiec-Jankowska A, Paszko Z, Ujec M. Changes in the concentrations of receptors of insuline-like growth factor-1, epithelial growth factor, oestrogens and progestagens in adenomyosis foci, endometrium and myometrium of women during menstrual cycle. Eur J Gynaecol Oncol 1998;19:93–97.

387. Hom YK, Young P, Wiesen JF, Miettinen PJ, Derynck R, Werb Z, Cunha GR. Uterine and vaginal organ growth requires epidermal growth factor receptor signaling from stroma. Endocrinology 1998; 139:913–921.

388. Miturski R, Semczuk A, Jakowicki JA. C-erbB-2 expression in human proliferative and hyperplastic endometrium. Int J Gynecol Obstet 1998;61:73,74.

389. Rasty G, Murray R, Lu L, Kubilis P, Benrubi G, Masood S. Expression of HER-2/neu oncogene in normal, hyperplastic and malignant endometrium. Ann Clin Lab Science 1998;28:138–143.

390. Pearl ML, Talavera F, Gretz HF, Roberts JA, Menon KM. Mitogenic activity of growth factors in the human endometrial adenocarcinoma cell lines HEC-1-A and KLE. Gynecol Oncol 1993;49:325–332.

391. Lelle RJ, Talavera F, Gretz H, Roberts JA, Menon KM. Epidermal growth factor receptor expression in three different human endometrial cancer cell lines. Cancer 1993;72:519–525.

392. Watson H, Franks S, Bonney RC. The epidermal growth factor receptor in the human endometrial adenocarcinoma cell line HEC-1-B. J Steroid Biochem Mol Biol 1994;51:41–45.

393. Connor P, Talavera F, Kang JS, Burke J, Roberts J, Menon KM. Epidermal growth factor activates protein kinase C in the human endometrial cancer cell line HEC-1A. Gynecol Oncol 1997;67:46–50.

394. Gretz HF, Talavera F, Connor P, Pearl M, Lelle RJ, Roberts JA, Menon KM. Protein kinase C-dependent and -independent pathways mediate epidermal growth factor (EGF) effects in human endometrial adenocarcinoma cell line KLE. Gynecol Oncol 1994;53:228–233.

395. Krasilnikov MA, Shatskaya VA, Kuzmina ZV, Barinov VV, Letyagin VP, Bassalyk LS. Regulation of phospholipid turnover by steroid hormones in endometrial carcinoma and breast cancer cells. Acta Endocrinol 1993;128:543–548.

396. Gershtein ES, Shatskaya VA, Kostyleva OI, Ermilova VD, Kushlinsky NE, Krasilnikov MA. Comparative analysis of the sensitivity of endometrial cancer cells to epidermal growth factor and steroid hormones. Cancer 1995;76:2524–2529.

397. Ueda M, Fujii H, Yoshizawa K, Abe F, Ueki M. Effects of sex steroids and growth factors on migration and invasion of endometrial adenocarcinoma SNG-M cells in vitro. Jpn J Cancer Res 1996;87:524–533.

398. Somkuti SG, Yuan L, Fritz MA, Lessey BA. Epidermal growth factor and sex steroids dynamically regulate a marker of endometrial receptivity in Ishikawa cells. J Clin Endocrinol Metab 1997;82:2192–2197.

399. Burke JJ, Talavera F, Menon KM. Regulation of PTP1D mRNA by peptide growth factors in the human endometrial cell line HEC-1-A. J Soc Gynecol Investig 1997;4:310–315.

400. Bolufer P, Lluch A, Molina R, Alberola V, Vazquez C, Padilla J, et al. Epidermal growth factor in human breast cancer, endometrial carcinoma and lung cancer. Its rela-tionship to epidermal growth factor receptor estradiol receptor, and tumor TNM. Clin Chim Acta 1993;215:51–61.

401. Bauknecht T, Kohler M, Janz I, Pfleiderer A. The occurrence of epidermal growth factor receptors and the characterization of EGF-like factors in human ovarian endometrial, cervical and breast cancer. EGF receptors and factors in gynecological carcinomas. J Cancer Res Clin Oncol 1989;115:193–199.

402. Adachi K, Kurachi H, Homma H, Adachi H, Imai T, Sakata M, et al. Estrogen induces epidermal growth factor (EGF) receptor and its ligands in human Fallopian tube: involvement of EGF but not transforming growth factor-a in estrogen-induced tubal cell growth in vitro. Endocrinology 1995; 136: 2110–2119.

403. Adachi K, Kurachi H, Adachi H, Imai T, Sakata M, Homma H, et al. Menstrual cycle specific expression of epidermal growth factor receptors in human fallopian tube epithelium. J Endocrinol 1995;147: 553–563.

404. Niikura H, Sasano N, Kaga K, Sato S, Yajima A. Expression of epidermal growth factor family proteins and epidermal growth factor receptor in human endometrium. Hum Pathol 1996;27:282–289.

405. Jasonni VM, Amadori A, Santini D, Ceccarelli C, Naldi S, Flamigni C. Epidermal growth factor receptor (EGF-R) and transforming growth factor alpha (TGFA) expression in different endometrial cancers. Anticancer Res 1995;15:1327–1332.

406. Reinartz JJ, George E, Lindgren BR, Niehans GA. Expression of p53, transforming growth factor alpha, epidermal growth factor receptor, and c-erbB-2 in endometrial carcinoma and correlation with survival and known predictors of survival. Hum Pathol 1994;25:1075–1083.

407. Nyholm HC, Nielsen AL, Ottesen B. Expression of epidermal growth factor receptors in human endo-metrial carcinomas. Int J Gynecol Pathol 1993;12:241–245.

408. Jasonni VM, Santini D, Amadori A, Ceccarelli C, Naldi S. Epidermal growth factor receptor expres-sion and endometrial cancer histotypes. Ann NY Acad Sci 1994;734:298–305.

409. Lamharzi N, Halmos G, Armatis P, Schally AV. Expression of mRNA for luteinizing hormone-releas-ing hormone receptors and epidermal growth factor receptors in human cancer cell lines. Int J Oncol 1998;12:671–675.

410. Emons G, Muller V, Ortmann O, Schultz KD. Effects of LHRH-analogues on mitogenic signal trans-duction in cancer cells. J Steroid Biochem Mol Biol 1998;65:199–206.

411. Reynolds RK, Owens CA, Roberts JA. Cultured endometrial cancer cells exhibit autocrine growth factor stimulation that is not observed in cultured normal endometrial cells. Gynecol Oncol 1996;60: 380–386.

412. Haining RE, Cameron IT, van Papendorp C, Davenport AP, Prentice A, Thomas EJ, Smith SK. Epi-dermal growth factor in human endometrium: proliferative effects in culture and immunocytochemical localization in normal and endometriotic tissues. Hum Reprod 1991;6:1200–1205.

413. Fujimoto J, Ichigo S, Hori M, Morishita S, Tamaya T. Estrogen induces c-Ha-ras expression via activation of tyrosine kinase in uterine endometrial fibroblasts and cancer cells. J Steroid Biochem Mol Biol 1995;55:25–33.

414. Kato K, Ueoka Y, Kato K, Tamura T, Nishida J, Wake N. Oncogenic Ras modulates epidermal growth factor responsiveness in endometrial carcinomas. Eur J Cancer 1998;34:737–744.

415. Sallot M, Ordener C, Lascombe I, Propper A, Adessi GL, Jouvenot M. Differential EGF action on nuclear proto-oncogenes in human endometrial carcinoma RL95-2 cells. Anticancer Res 1996;16: 401–406.

416. Anzai Y, Gong Y, Holinka CF, Murphy LJ, Murphy LC, Kuramoto H, Gurpide E. Effects of transform-ing growth factors and regulation of their mRNA levels in two human endometrial adenocarcinoma cell lines. J Steroid Biochem Mol Biol 1992;42:449–455.

417. Yokoyama Y, Takahashi Y, Hashimoto M, Morishita S, Tamaya T. Immunhistochemical study of estradiol, epidermal growth factor, transforming growth factor alpha and epidermal growth factor receptor in endometrial neoplasia. Jpn J Clin Oncol 1996;26:411–416.

418. Murphy LC, Dotzlaw H, Alkhalaf M, Coutts A, Miller T, Wong MS, Gong Y, Murphy LJ. Mechanisms of growth inhibition by antiestrogens and progestins in human breast and endometrial cancer cells. J Steroid Biochem Mol Biol 1992;43:117–121.

419. Murphy LJ, Gong Y, Murphy LC. Regulation of transforming growth factor gene expression in human endometrial adenocarcinoma cells. J Steroid Biochem Mol Biol 1992;41:309–314.

420. Ignar-Trowbridge DM, Nelson KG, Bidwell MC, Curtis SW, Washburn TF, McLachlan JA, Korach KS. Coupling of dual signalingpathways: epidermal growth factor action involves the estrogen recep-tor. Proc Natl Acad Sci USA 1992;89:4658–4662.

421. Ignar-Trowbridge DM, Pimentel M, Teng CT, Korach KS, McLachlan JA. Cross talk between peptide growth factor and estrogen receptor signaling systems. Environ Health Perspect 1995;103(Suppl 7): 35–38.

422. Ignar-Trowbridge DM, Pimentel M, Parker MG, McLachlan JA, Korach KS. Peptide growth factor cross-talk with the estrogen receptor requires the A/B domain and occurs independently of protein kinase C or estradiol. Endocrinology 1996;137:1735–1744.

423. Gong Y, Anzai Y, Murphy LC, Ballejo G, Holinka CF, Gurpide E, Murphy LJ. Transforming growth factor gene expression in human endometrial adenocarcinoma cells: regulation by progestins. Cancer Res 1991;51:5476–5481.

424. Xynos FP, Klos DJ, Hamilton PD, Schuette V, Fernandez-Pol JA. Expression of transforming growth factor alpha mRNA in benign and malignant tissues derived from gynecologic patients with various proliferative conditions. Anticancer Res 1992;12:1115–1120.

425. Van Dam PA, Lowe G, Watson JV, James M, Chard T, Hudson CN, Shepherd JH. Multiparameter flow-cytometric quantitation of epidermal growth factor receptor and c-erbB-2 oncoprotein in normal and neoplastic tissues of the female genital tract. Gynecol Oncol 1991;42:256–264.

426. Esteller M, Garcia A, Martinez I, Palones JM, Cabero A, Reventos J. Detection of c-erbB-2/neu and fibroblast growth factor-3/INT-2 but not epidermal growth factor gene amplification in endometrial cancer by differential polymerase chain reaction. Cancer 1995;75: 2139–2146.

427. Costa MJ, Walls J. Epidermal growth factor receptor and c-erbB-2 oncoprotein expression in female genital tract carcinosarcomas (malignant mixed mullerian tumors). Clinicopathologic study of 82 cases. Cancer 1995;77:533–542.

428. Hetzel DJ, Wilson TO, Keeney GL, Roche PC, Cha SS, Podratz KC. HER-2/neu expression: a major prognostic factor in endometrial cancer. Gynecol Oncol 1992;47:179–185.

429. Kohlberger P, Loesch A, Koelbl H, Breitenecker G, Kainz C, Gitsch G. Prognostic value of immunohistochemically detected HER-2/neu oncoprotein in endometrial cancer. Cancer Lett 1996;98:151–155.

430. Seki A, Nakamura K, Kodama J, Miyagi Y, Yoshinouchi M, Kudo T. A close correlation between c-erbB-2 gene amplification and local progression in endometrial adenocarcinoma. Eur J Gynaecol Oncol 1998;19:90–92.

431. Ayhan A, Tuncer ZS, Ruacan S, Ayhan A, Yasui W, Tahara E. Abnormal expression of cripto and p53 protein in endometrial carcinoma and its precursor lesions. Eur J Gynaecol Oncol 1998;19:316–318.

432. Berchuck A, Kohler MF, Bast RC. Oncogenes in ovarian cancer. Hematol Oncol Clin North Am 1992; 6:813–827.

433. Bauknecht T, Janz I, Kohler M, Pfleiderer A. Human ovarian carcinomas: correlation of malignancy and survival with the expression of epidermal growth factor receptors (EGF-R) and EGF-like faktors (EGF-F). Med Oncol Tumor Pharmacother 1989;6:121–127.

434. Bauknecht T, Angel P, Kohler M, Kommoss F, Birmelin G, Pfleiderer A, Wagner E. Gene structure and expression analysis of the epidermal growth factor receptor, transforming growth factor-alpha, myc, jun, and metallothionein in human ovarian carcinomas. Classification of malignant phenotypes. Cancer 1993;71:419–429.

435. Bauknecht T, Birmelin G, Kommoss F. Clinical significance of oncogenes and growth factors in ovarian carcinomas. J Steroid Biochem Mol Biol 1990;37:855–862.

436. Bauknecht T, Kommoss F, Birmelin G, von Kleist S, Kohler M, Pfleiderer A. Expression analysis of EGF-R and TGF-α in human ovarian carcinomas. Anticancer Res 1991;11:1523–1528.

437. Berchuck A, Kamel A, Whitaker R, Kerns B, Olt G, Kinney R, et al. Overexpression of HER-2/neu is associated with poor survival in advanced epithelial ovarian cancer. Cancer Res 1990;50:4087–4091.

438. Berchuck A, Olt GJ, Everitt L, Soisson AP, Bast RC, Boyer CM. Role of peptide growth factors in epithelial ovarian cancer. Obstet Gynecol 1990;75:255–262.

439. Westermann AM, Beijnen JH, Moolenaar WH, Rodenhuis S. Growth factors in human ovarian cancer. Cancer Treat Rev 1997;23:113–131.

440. Niikura H, Sasano H, Sato S, Yajima A. Expression of epidermal growth factor-related proteins and epidermal growth factor receptor in common epithelial ovarian tumors. Int J Gynecol Pathol 1997; 16:60–68.

441. Morishige K, Kurachi H, Amemiya K, Adachi H, Inoue M, Miyake A, Tanizawa O, Sakoyama Y. Involvement of transforming growth factor alpha/epidermal growth factor receptor autocrine growth mechanism in an ovarian cancer cell line in vitro. Cancer Res 1991;51:5951–5955.

442. Stromberg K, Johnson GR, O'Connor DM, Sorensen CM, Gullick WJ, Kannan B. Frequent immuno-histochemical detection of EGF supergene family members in ovarians carcinogenesis. Int J Gynecol Pathol 1994;13:342–347.

443. Crew AJ, Langdon SP, Miller EP, Miller WR. Mitogenic effects of epidermal growth factor and transforming growth factor-alpha on EGF-receptor positive human ovarian carcinoma cell lines. Eur J Cancer 1992;28:337–341.

444. Shoyab M, McDonald VL, Bradley JG, Todaro GJ. Amphiregulin: a bifunctional growth-modulating glycoprotein produced by the phorbol 12-myristate 13-acetate-treated human breast adenocarcinoma cell line MCF-7. Proc Natl Acad Sci USA 1988;85:6528–6532.

445. Zhou L, Leung BS. Growth regulation of ovarian cancer cells by epidermal growth factor and transforming growth factors alpha and beta 1. Biochim Biophys Acta 1992;1180:130–136.

446. Morishige K, Kurachi H, Amemiya K, Fujita Y, Yamamoto T, Miyake A, Tanizawa O. Evidence for the involvement of transforming growth factor alpha and epidermal growth factor receptor autocrine growth mechanism in primary human ovarian cancers in vitro. Cancer Res 1991;51:5322–5328.

447. Kurachi H, Morishige K, Amemiya K, Adachi H, Hirota K, Miyake A, Tanizawa O. Importance of transforming growth factor alpha/epidermal growth factor receptor autocrine growth mechanism in an ovarian cancer cell line in vivo. Cancer Res 1991;51:5956–5959.

448. Kurachi H, Morishige K, Adachi H, Adachi K, Tasaka K, Sawada M, Miyake A. Implantation and growth of epidermal growth factor (EGF) receptor expressing human ovarian xenografts in nude mice is dependent on EGF. Cancer 1994;74:2984–2990.

449. Gordon AW, Pegues JC, Johnson GR, Kannan B, Auersperg N, Stromberg K. mRNA phenotyping of the major ligands and receptors of the EGF supergene family in human ovarian epithelial cells. Cancer Lett 1995;89:63–71.

450. Owens OJ, Stewart C, Leake RE. Growth factors in ovarian cancer. Br J Cancer 1991;64:1177–1181.

451. Marth C, Lang T, Cronauer MV, Doppler W, Zeimet AG, Bachmair F, Ullrich A, Daxenbichler G. Epidermal growth factor reduces HER-2 protein level in human ovarian carcinoma cells. Int J Cancer 1992;52:311–316.

452. Kacinski BM, Mayer AG, King BL, Carter D, Chambers SK. NEU protein overexpression in benign, borderline, and malignant ovarian neoplasms. Gynecol Oncol 1992;44:245–253.

453. Tamura M, Sasano H, Suzuki T, Fukaya T, Funayama Y, Takayama K, Takaya R, Yajima A. Expression of epidermal growth factors and epidermal growth factor receptor in normal cycling human ovaries. Hum Reprod 1995;10:1891–1896.

454. Kommoss F, Bauknecht T, Birmelin G, Kohler M, Tesch H, Pfleiderer A. Oncogene and growth factor expression in ovarian cancer. Acta Obstet Gynecol Scand 1992;155:19–24.

455. Kommoss F, Wintzer HO, von Kleist S, Kohler M, Walker R, Langdon B, van Tran K, Pfleiderer A. In situ distribution of transforming growth factor alpha in normal tissues and malignant tumours of the ovary. J Pathol 1992;162:223–228.

456. Kohler M, Bauknecht T, Grimm M, Birmelin G, Kommoss F, Wagner E. Epidermal growth factor receptor and transforming growth factor alpha expression in human ovarian carcinomas. Eur J Cancer 1992;28A:1432–1437.

457. Owens OJ, Leake RE. Growth factor content in normal and benign ovarian tumours. Eur J Obstet Gynecol Reprod Biol 1992;47:223–228.

458. Bartlett JM, Langdon SP, Simpson BJ, Stewart M, Katsaros D, Sismondi P, et al. Prognostic value of epidermal growth factor receptor mRNA expression in primary ovarian cancer. Br J Cancer 1996;73:301–306.

459. Yeh J, Yeh YC. Transforming growth factor-alpha and human cancer. Biomed Pharmacother 1989;43:651–659.

460. Ferrandina G, Scambia G, Benedetti-Pancini P, Bonanno G, De Vincenzo R, Rumi C, et al. Effects of dexamethasone on the growth and epidermal growth factor expression of the OVCA 433 ovarian cancer cells. Mol Cell Endocrinol 1992;83:183–193.

461. Lewis GD, Lofgren JA, McMurtrey AE, Nuijens A, Fendly BM, Bauer KD, Sliwkowski MX. Growth regulation of human breast and ovarian tumor cells by heregulin: evidence for the requirement of ErbB2 as a critical component in mediating heregulin responsiveness. Cancer Res 1996;56:1457–1465.

462. Simpson BJ, Langdon SP, Rabiasz GJ, Macleod KG, Hirst GL, Bartlett JM, et al. Estrogen regulation of transforming growth factor-alpha in ovarian cancer. J Steroid Biochem Mol Biol 1998;64:137–145.

463. Ridderheim M, Stendahl U, Backstrom T. Progesterone and estradiol stimulate release of epidermal growth factor/transforming growth factor alpha by ovarian tumours in vitro. Anticancer Res 1994;14:2763–2768.

464. Wimalasena J, Dostal R, Meehan D. Gonadotropins, estradiol, and growth factors regulate epithelial ovarian cancer cell growth. Gynecol Oncol 1992;46:345–350.

465. Wimalasena J, Meehan D, Dostal R, Foster JS, Cameron M, Smith M. Growth factors interact with estradiol and gonadotropins in the regulation of ovarian cancer cell growth and growth factor receptors. Oncol Res 1993;5:325–337.
466. Ridderheim M, Cajander S, Tavelin B, Stendahl U, Bachstrom T. EGF/TGF-alpha and progesterone in urine of ovarian cancer patients. Anticancer Res 1994;14:2119–2123.
467. Feldkamper M, Enderle–Schmitt U, Hackenberg R, Schulz KD. Urinary excretion of growth factors in patients with ovarian cancer. Eur J Cancer 1994;30A:1851–1858.
468. Shah NG, Bhatavdekar JM, Doctor SS, Suthar TP, Balar DB, Dave RS. Circulating epidermal growth factor (EGF) and insulin-like growth factor-I (IGF-I) in patients with epithelial ovarian carcinoma. Neoplasma 1994;41:241–243.
469. Kurachi H, Adachi H, Morishige K, Adachi K, Takeda T, Homma H, Yamamoto T, Miyake A. Transforming growth factor-alpha promotes tumor markers secretion from human ovarian cancers in vitro. Cancer 1996;78:1049–1054.
470. Brader KR, Wolf JK, Chakrabarty S, Price JE. Epidermal growth factor receptor (EGFR) antisense transfection reduces the expression of EGFR and suppresses the malignant phenotype of a human ovarian cancer cell line. Oncol Rep 1998;5:1269–1274.
471. Rodriguez GC, Berchuck A, Whitaker RS, Schlossman D, Clarke-Pearson DL, Bast RC. Epidermal growth factor receptor expression in normal ovarian epithelium and ovarian cancer. II. Relationship between receptor expression and response to epidermal growth factor. Am J Obstet Gynecol 1991;164:745–750.
472. Ottensmeier C, Swanson L, Strobel T, Druker B, Niloff J, Cannistra SA. Absence of constitutive EGF receptor activation in ovarian cancer cell lines. Br J Cancer 1996;74:446–452.
473. Lang T, Daxenbichler G, Merth C. Effects of cytostatic agents on the expression of epidermal growth factor receptor in ovarian cancer cells. Anticancer Res 1994;14:1871–1874.
474. Christen RD, Hom DK, Porter DC, Andrews PA, MacLeod CL, Hafstrom L, Howell SB. Epidermal growth factor regulates the in vitro sensitivity of human ovarian carcinoma cells to cisplatin. J Clin Invest 1990;86:1632–1640.
475. Kohler M, Janz I, Wintzer HO, Wagner E, Bauknecht T. The expression of EGF receptors, EGF-like factors and c-myc in ovarian and cervical carcinomas and their potential clinical significance. Anticancer Res 1989;9:1537–1547.
476. Berns EM, Klijn JG, Henzen-Logmans SC, Rodenburg CJ, van der Burg ME, Foekens JA. Receptors for hormones and growth factors and (onco)-gene amplification in human ovarian cancer. Int J Cancer 1992;52:218–224.
477. Henzen-Logmans SC, van der Burg ME, Foekens JA, Berns PM, Brussee R, Fieret JH, et al. Occurrence of epidermal growth factor receptors in benign and malignant ovarian tumors and normal ovarian tissues: an immunohistochemical study. J Cancer Res Clin Oncol 1992;118:303–307.
478. Scambia G, Benedetti-Panici P, Battaglia F, Ferrandin G, Baiocchi G, Greggi S, De Vincenzo R, Mancuso S. Significance of epidermal growth factor receptor in advanced ovarian cancer. J Clin Oncol 1992;10:529–535.
479. Stewart CJ, Owens OJ, Richmond JA, McNicol AM. Expression of epidermal growth factor receptor in normal ovary and in ovarian tumors. Int J Gynecol Pathol 1992;11:266–272.
480. Van der Burg ME, Henzen-Logmans SC, Foekens JA, Berns EM, Rodenburg CJ, van Putten WL, Klijn JG. The prognostic value of epidermal growth factor receptors, determined by both immunohistochemistry and ligand binding assays, in primary epi thelial ovarian cancer: a pilot study. Eur J Cancer 1993;29A:1951–1957.
481. Simpson BJ, Phillips HA, Lessells AM, Lamgdon SP, Miller WR. C-erbB growth-factor-receptor proteins in ovarian tumours. Int J Cancer 1995;64:202–206.
482. Minguillon C, Schönborn I, Reles A, Bartel U, Lichtenegger W. EGF-R and PCNA expression in ovarian carcinomas: correlation with classic prognostic factors. Gen Diagn Pathol 1996;141:197–201.
483. Janinis J, Nakopoulou L, Panagos G, Davaris P. Immunohistochemical expression of EGF-R in malignant surface epithelial ovarian neoplasms (SEON). Eur J Gynaecol Oncol 1994;15:19–23.
484. Meden H, Marx D, Raab T, Kron M, Schauer A, Kuhn W. EGF-R and overexpression of the oncogene c-erbB-2 in ovarian cancer: immunohistochemical findings and prognostic value. J Obstet Gynecol 1995;21:167–178.
485. Brandt B, Vogt U, Schlotter CM, Jakisch C, Werkmeister R, Thomas M, et al. Prognostic relevance of abberations in the c-erbB oncogenes from breast, ovarian, oral and lung cancers: double-differential polymerase chain reaction (ddPCR) for clinical diagnosis. Gene 1995;159:35–42.

486. Scoccia B, Lee YM, Niederberger C, Ilekis JV. Expression of the ErbB family of receptors in ovarian cancer. J Soc Gynecol Invest 1998;5:161–165.
487. Ilekis JV, Connor JP, Prins GS, Ferrer K, Niederberger C, Scoccia B. Expression of epidermal growth factor and androgen receptors in ovarian cancer. Gynecol Oncol 1997;66:250–254.
488. Slamon DJ, Godolphin W, Jones LA, Holt JA, Wong SG, Keith DE, et al. Studies of the HER-2/neu proto-oncogene in human breast and ovarian cancer. Science 1989;244:707–712.
489. Meden H, Kuhn W. Overexpression of the oncogene c-erbB-2 (HER2/neu) in ovarian cancer: a new prognostic factor. Eur J Obstet Gynecol Reprod Biol 1997;71:173–179.
490. Mileo AM, Fanuele M, Battaglia F, Scambia G, Benedetti-Panici C, Mattei E, Mancuso S, Delpino A. Preliminary evaluation of HER-2/neu oncogene and epidermal growth factor receptor expression in normal and neoplastic human ovaries. Int J Biol Markers 1992;7:114–118.
491. Rubin SC, Finstad CL, Wong GY, Almadrones L, Plante M, Lloyd KO. Prognostic significance of HER-2/neu expression in advanced epithelial ovarian cancer: a multivariate analysis. Am J Obstet Gynecol 1993;168:162–169.
492. Rubin SC, Finstad CL, Federici MG, Scheiner L, Lloyd KO, Hoskins WJ. Prevalence and significance of HER-2/neu expression in early epithelial ovarian cancer. Cancer 1994;73:1456–1459.
493. Haldane JS, Hird V, Hughes CM, Gullick WJ. C-erbB-2 oncogene expression in ovarian cancer. J Pathol 1990;162:231–237.
494. Singleton TP, Perrone T, Oakley G, Niehans GA, Carson L, Cha SS, Strickler JG. Activation of c-erbB-2 and prognosis in ovarian carcinoma. Cancer 1994;73:1460–1466.
495. Felip E, Del Campo JM, Rubio D, Vidal MT, Colomer R, Bermejo B. Overexpression of c-erbB-2 in epithelial ovarian cancer. Cancer 1995;75:2147–2152.
496. Seidman JD, Frisman DM, Norris HJ. Expression of the HER-2/neu proto-oncogene in serous ovarian neoplasms. Cancer 1992;70:2857–2860.
497. Harlozinska A, Bar JK, Sobanska E, Goluda M. Epidermal growth factor receptor and c-erbB-2 onco-proteins in tissue and tumor effusion cells of histopathologically different ovarian neoplasms. Tumor Biol 1998;19:364–373.

10

Insulin-Like Growth Factors and Endocrine Neoplasia

Douglas Yee, PHD and Adrian V. Lee, PHD

Contents

INTRODUCTION

The observation that breast (BC) and prostate cancer (PC) are regulated by sex hormones provided a paradigm for treatment of these diseases *(1,2)*. Despite the accumulation of multiple genetic abnormalities, the cancer cell is still responsive to extracellular signals that were previously required for normal growth and development of the organ. Blockade of steroid hormone receptors, or inhibition of the synthesis of the ligands for the receptors, are successful and relatively nontoxic therapeutic modalities for treatment of virtually all stages of BC and PC *(3,4)*. Thus, it is a worthwhile effort to define other growth regulatory pathways important for cancer cells, with the long-term goal of developing additional specific therapies. This chapter discusses the evidence that the insulin-like growth factors (IGFs) regulate cancer cell growth, and that strategies directed at inhibition of IGF action could be useful therapeutic strategies for cancer treatment.

THE IGF SYSTEM

Like other growth factors (GFs), the IGF system is composed of an interacting network of ligand and receptors. In addition, there are high-affinity binding proteins (IGFBPs) that bind the ligands with equal or higher affinity than the receptors, and have the potential to influence ligand–receptor interactions.

From: *Contemporary Endocrinology: Endocrine Oncology*
Edited by: S. P. Ethier © Humana Press Inc., Totowa, NJ

IGF Ligands

Two well-characterized ligands, IGF-I and IGF-II, exist. Both ligands have a high degree of homology to insulin, with a disulfide linkage between the amino and carboxy terminii (A and B domains), but, unlike insulin, both IGF-I and IGF-II retain the middle portion of the molecule (C domain). It is well-known that IGF-I is an important determinant of linear skeletal growth that accompanies puberty *(5,6)*. Pituitary release of growth hormone (GH) results in increased gene expression of IGF-I by the liver, and people who have mutations in GH receptor are dwarfs with no detectable circulating IGF-I *(7)*. In addition to the endocrine function of IGF-I, mouse models have suggested that IGF-I also has an important role in prenatal growth. Mice with a homozygous deletion of the IGF-I gene have a birthweight of less than 60% of their wild-type littermates, and do not survive, because of hypodevelopment of the lungs and diaphragm *(8–10)*. Recent data suggest that this perinatal lethality can be controlled by reducing the level of gene deletion, using the *cre* recombinase system *(11)*. A human with partial homozygous deletion of the IGF-I gene has also been described *(12)*. Although this person's gene deletion could encode for a truncated protein, he still has significant growth retardation and abnormalities of the nervous system, compatible with observations made in the mouse *(13)*. These data support an important role for the local (paracrine or autocrine) expression of IGF-I, in addition to its endocrine function during normal growth and development of the entire organism. Moreover, the data suggest that the function of IGF-I during fetal development cannot easily be substituted by other related GFs.

Mouse models have also suggested a role for IGF-II during prenatal development *(14)*. When the paternal allele is deleted, animals are also growth-retarded at birth. However, they may survive postnatally and remain consistently smaller than their wild-type littermates, suggesting that the growth effects of IGF-II occur during embryonic life. These gene-knockout studies led to the observation that the IGF-II gene is imprinted, i.e., only the paternal allele is expressed *(15)*. In humans, the function of IGF-II is less well understood. Unlike mice, whose IGF-II levels decline shortly after birth, humans retain high levels of IGF-II throughout life *(16)*. Humans lacking IGF-II expression have not been described.

IGF Receptors

There are two well-defined receptors that have high affinity for the IGFs: the type I and type II IGF receptor. However, these high-affinity receptors are completely different in their structure and function. The type II IGF receptor (IGF-IIR) is a multifunctional receptor that binds IGF-II, transforming growth factor β, leukemia inhibitory factor, retinoic acid, and lysosomal enzymes bearing mannose-6-phosphate moieties *(17–19)*. The receptor is 300 kDa, with a small intracellular domain and a large extracellular domain containing 15 repeated motifs. Initial reports suggested that this receptor may signal through a G-protein-coupled signal transduction pathway *(20–22)*, but subsequent reports have not shown this to be the case *(23)*. It appears that ligands that bind IGF-IIR are sorted to lysosomal compartments. However, there are distinct domains within the receptor responsible for binding lysosomal enzymes, or IGF-II, with binding of IGF-II localized to the eleventh repeat *(24,25)*. In mice, the IGF-IIR gene is also imprinted with expression of the maternal allele only *(26,27)*. Mice that fail to express IGF-IIR, because of deletion of the maternal allele, are actually 30% larger at birth than their littermates;

however, this results from accumulation of extracellular fluid, and is generally lethal. In humans, imprinting of IGF-IIR seems to be less frequent, and its imprinting may be a polymorphic trait *(28–32)*. It is possible that IGF-IIR functions as a sink for IGF-II, thereby regulating its interaction with the type I IGF receptor (IGF-IR).

Most evidence suggests that the IGF-IR, or insulin receptor–IGF-IR hybrids, mediate IGF action. The IGF-IR is transcribed from a single gene, and is processed into α- and β-subunits *(33)*. The α-subunits are extracellular and contain ligand binding domains. The β-subunit spans the membrane and has tyrosine kinase (TK) activity, and αβ dimers are assembled into a tetrameric structure, which is required for receptor function, because transphosphorylation of one β-chain by the other chain is necessary for activation of downstream signaling pathways *(34)*. Specific tyrosine residues have been identified in the β-subunit, which are associated with phenotypes important for cancer, such as transformation, proliferation, and protection from apoptosis *(35–40)*. This observation suggests that IGF-IR can signal through a variety of different pathways, and this has indeed been shown, with multiple adaptor proteins binding directly to phosphorylated IGF-IR *(41–45)*. Moreover, the insulin receptor substrate (IRS) family of adapter proteins are substrates for both IR and IGF-IR, and can also couple signals generated from either receptor to many downstream activators *(46)*. Thus, activation of IGF-IR can initiate a myriad of signaling pathways that could contribute to the maintenance of the malignant phenotype.

In addition to IGF-IR, it is clear that hybrids between the IR and IGF-IR also exist *(47–54)*. These hybrids contain an αβ dimer from each subtype. Studies suggest that these hybrids behave like IGF-IR in their ligand affinity *(55)*. In addition, the IR can also bind IGF-II with fairly high affinity, providing yet another way in which IGFs may stimulate signal transduction *(38,56)*.

IGF Binding Proteins

Both IGF-I and IGF-II are found complexed to high affinity binding proteins, when examined in all extracellular fluids. Six distinct species have been cloned, and an additional four have homologous structures and are termed IGFBP-related proteins (IGFBP-rP) *(57)*. Obviously, the presence of IGFBPs lend another level of complexity to the regulation of IGF action. It is felt that most IGFBP species function to regulate access of the IGF ligands to the IGF receptors. For example, in the circulation, most IGF-I and IGF-II are complexed in a high-mol wt complex composed of the IGF, IGFBP-3, and an additional protein called the "acid labile subunit" *(58)*. In this ternary complex, IGF-I is unable to initiate receptor signaling. However, during certain physiologic states (stress, pregnancy), IGFBP-3 is cleaved by a protease, freeing IGF-I to interact with its receptor *(59,60)*. These data suggest that the IGFBPs play a critical role in IGF storage, transport, and tissue distribution. At the tissue level, IGFBPs could be a major determinant of IGF action. It is likely that IGFBP interactions with specific proteases are also critical in regulating ligand–receptor interactions *(61)*.

However, it is clear that the IGFBPs have physiologic functions that do not require their interaction with the IGFs or the IGF-IR. For example, IGFBP-3 can induce apoptosis in cells that do not express IGF-IR *(62)*. Furthermore, specific cell surface binding of IGFBP-3 has been suggested *(63,64)*. Although the exact nature of the IGFBP-3 receptor has not been unambiguously identified, it is clear that IGFBP-3 can interact with the cell

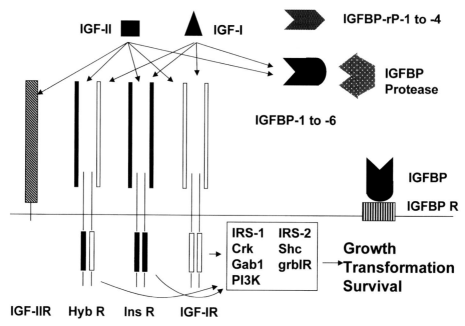

Fig. 1. Schematic representation of the IGF system. Four receptors: type I IGF receptor (IGF-IR), insulin receptor (Ins R), hybrid insulin/type I IGF receptors (Hyb R), and type II IGF receptor (IGF-IIR), all have the potential to interact with the two IGF ligands (IGF-I and IGF-II). In addition, the six IGFBPs and four IGFBP-rPs can interact with the ligands. Once the TK receptors are activated, numerous downstream signaling molecules are phosphorylated, which convey the growth, transformation, and survival signals mediated by both IGF-I and IGF-II.

membrane. Likewise, IGFBP-1 has been shown to interact with the α5β1 integrin, to mediate cell motility *(65)*. Certain IGFBPs appear to be transported to the nucleus *(66)* in human BC cells. Their role as intranuclear proteins has not yet been defined; however, this location would suggest an extra-IGF function. Thus, it appears that the IGFBPs are multifunctional proteins: In addition to binding IGFs with high affinity, they appear to have additional functions that have nothing to do with IGF signaling

The IGFBP-rPs have only recently been described. These proteins were identified based on their structural similarity to known IGFBPs; like the IGFBPs, they share a series of conserved cysteine residues in their amino terminii *(67)*. It has not yet been determined if these IGFBP-rPs have high affinity for the IGFs, thus they are called "related proteins." Some of these proteins have interesting functions. For example, one of these species (initially called IGFBP-7/mac25, now referred to as IGFBP-rP1), appears to have high affinity for insulin *(68)*. Moreover, fragments of IGFBP-rP1 also bind insulin with high affinity, as do fragments of other IGFBPs. Thus, both the IGFBPs and IGFBP-rPs appear to be multifunctional proteins.

The IGF System in Perspective

It is obvious that the potential for cellular regulation by the IGF system components is complex and incompletely understood. Figure 1 demonstrates the potential for interactions. For example, IGF-II can potentially bind to four different receptors (IGF-IR, IGF-IIR, insulin/IGF-IR, and IRs) and this ligand–receptor interaction can be regulated by six specific IGFBPs, which is influenced further by specific IGFBP proteases. In addition to the IGFBPs' ability to influence IGF action, both the intact IGFBP and IGFBP proteolytic fragments may also influence cell behavior through IGF-independent pathways. There are also IGFBP-rPs that may also influence IGF action. Thus, research during the past several years has added significant detail concerning the identity of the components involved in the IGF system. However, this detail has also enhanced the potential complexity of this system. In order to understand IGF action in tumor cells, an understanding of the key elements responsible for IGF action also needs to be elucidated.

IGF SYSTEM COMPONENTS AND RISK OF CANCER

Many proteins that regulate proliferation of the normal cell (Ras, Myc, cyclin D1, and so on) are also intimately associated with malignant transformation. Because the IGFs are key extracellular triggers involved in progression through the cell cycle, it is also possible that the IGFs also function in malignant transformation. Recent evidence suggests that this may be the case, because in vitro, animal, and human studies have all linked IGF action to cancer.

Malignant Transformation and IGF-IR

Although homozygous deletion of IGF-IIR is lethal to the animal, fibroblasts obtained from the embryos have been created *(8)*. Work from the laboratory of Baserga has shown that these cells are refractory to transformation by a variety of known oncogenes *(69–72)*. Specific tyrosine residues of the receptor have also been shown to be required for the ability of the IGF-IR to cooperate with oncogenes *(36,73)*, suggesting that specific signal transduction pathways engaged by the receptor are associated with transformation. Although IGF-IR overexpression has been shown to transform cells in a NIH 3T3 focus-forming assay, in a ligand-dependent manner *(74)*, gene amplification of IGF-IR is uncommon, at least in BC *(75)*. Moreover, not all oncogenes require IGF-IR action to transform cells in these model systems *(76)*.

It is obvious that the in vivo transformation of human epithelial cells (ECs) is much more complex than these simple model systems performed in fibroblast cells. However, these experiments suggest that the genetically transformed cell may still require normal signals required for controlled proliferation to fully display the transformed phenotype of unregulated cellular proliferation. As noted in all of the studies examining the role of IGF-IR in malignant transformation, stimulation of the receptor by ligand is required. Unlike other TK growth factor receptors (such as the epidermal growth factor [EGF] receptor family), overexpression of IGF-IR alone is insufficient to activate signal transduction. Thus, it appears that both receptor function and ligand action could have a role in transformation. Studies examining the control of systemic IGF-I levels have supported this concept.

IGF Serum Levels and Malignant Transformation

Serum IGF-I levels are controlled by a number of factors, one of which is diet *(77,78)*, which may account for up to 30% of all cancer-related deaths, and diet restriction can reduce cancer progression and incidence in animal systems *(79)*. Hursting et al. *(80)* reported that serum IGF-I levels are decreased in rats that are diet-restricted (DR), and that this is associated with a decrease in mononuclear cell leukemia. Further studies have recently shown that DR can inhibit progression of chemically induced bladder carcinoma in p53 heterozygous mice, and that restoration of serum IGF-I levels, by administration of recombinant IGF-I, relieved the DR inhibition, resulting in an increase in stage and incidence of bladder carcinoma *(81)*. An insight into the mechanism of these effects comes from measurements of proliferative and apoptotic indices in hyperplastic foci within the bladder. DR resulted in a 10-fold decrease in proliferative index and a 10-fold increase in apoptotic index. Administration of IGF-I increased proliferation and decreased apoptosis, reverting to levels seen in rats fed ad libidum. These results directly implicate circulating IGFs in bladder cancer growth, and suggest that approaches to lowering serum IGF-I levels may be beneficial for cancer prevention and treatment.

IGF-IIR and Malignant Transformation

As noted above, most evidence suggests that interaction of IGF-IR with its ligand, either IGF-I or IGF-II, is required for transformation. The ability of IGF-IIR to function in a signaling pathway has been brought into question *(23)*. It is possible that the high-affinity binding of IGF-II to this class of receptors represents a sink for inhibition of IGF-II action.

Recent data have shown that the IGF-IIR demonstrates frequent loss of heterozygosity (LOH) in hepatocellular and BC, a finding compatible with its function as a tumor suppressor gene *(82–84)*. Since IGF-IIR is a multifunctional protein that binds several secreted proteins, and also plays a key role in intracellular protein trafficking, there are many potential explanations for this finding. However, one possible explanation for its role as a tumor suppressor gene is that it normally functions to suppress a proliferative signal mediated by an IGF-II–IGF-IR interaction. When LOH occurs, and the remaining allele is subsequently mutated to disrupt its function as an IGF-II receptor, unopposed action of IGF-II at IGF-IR results. IGF-II gene expression is often found adjacent to transformed ECs (*see* below), making it theoretically possible that the dysfunction of IGF-IIR could influence IGF-II action in a paracrine manner at the tumor microenvironment. Additional experimentation using intact animals will be required to prove whether or not this model is correct.

IGF-II and Risk of Cancer

As mentioned, IGF-II is an imprinted gene with the paternal allele normally expressed in adult tissues *(27,85,86)*. Loss of imprinting was initially shown in several childhood cancers *(87–90)*, with the idea that loss of imprinting would allow increased expression of IGF-II from two alleles, rather than only one allele. Similar findings have also been made in adult cancers, including BC *(91–96)*, although the frequency and relevance of these observations are somewhat controversial. Nonetheless, these findings add further credence to the idea that dysregulation of IGF action at the tissue level could function to promote malignant transformation.

Serum IGF-I Levels and Risk of PC and BC

Recent evidence taken from two prospective studies have shown that high IGF levels are associated with an increased risk of BC and PC *(97,98)*. In PC, data from the Physician's Health Study demonstrated that men with the highest quartile of serum IGF-I levels had 4.3-fold increased relative risk, compared to men in the lowest quartile. In addition, there was a strong positive association between serum IGF-I levels and PC risk. These data are compatible with several other studies linking IGF-I levels and PC risk (reviewed in ref. *99*). Some of the earlier studies could be criticized for using an older method of IGF-I analysis, which did not completely exclude interference of IGFBPs, but the two newest studies *(97,100)* have used assays that eliminated this confounding variable.

In the Nurses Health Study, a similar prospective analysis of IGF-I levels and BC risk was performed. In contrast to the PC study, no association between IGF-I levels and the risk of BC for the entire group was observed. However, when only premenopausal women were studied, it was found that the top tertile had a relative risk of 2.33, compared to the lowest tertile. When women under age 50 yr were analyzed further, there was a further increase in relative risk (4.58) in the highest quintile, compared to the lowest. If IGF-I levels were normalized for alterations in IGFBP-3 levels, then the relative risk was further enhanced to more than sevenfold in the youngest cohort of women studied. No such relationship between IGF-I and BC risk was found in postmenopausal women. Although these studies have been criticized on statistical grounds *(101–105)*, they do provide evidence that serum levels are at least associated with BC and PC. However, because the interactions between the IGF system components are complex, it remains to be shown that these changes are indeed causative and not a marker for another risk factor, such as nutritional status. Moreover, further study, accounting for the other key regulators of endocrine IGF action (IGFBPs, serum IGF-I and IGF-II levels, and IGFBP proteases), will need to be performed to fully explain the increased risk for cancer.

IGFS AND PC

IGFs and Normal Prostate Epithelium

We have suggested that the normal EC at risk for transformation is likely to be responsive to IGF-mediated mitogenesis. IGF-I has been shown to be a potent mitogen for prostate ECs in culture *(106,107)*, but it is always of concern that these types of cells removed from the host are not actually representative of the behavior of the cell in the organ. However, recently it has been shown that a 7-d administration of IGF-I, but not EGF, to Wistar rats, causes increased mean wet weight of the ventral prostate *(108)*. Although it is likely that the doses used in this study are superphysiologic (400 µg/d), it does show that the same responsiveness to IGF-I observed in vitro is also evident in vivo. It has also been shown that inhibition of prostate growth by the 5α-reductase inhibitor, finasteride, reduces IGF-I and IGF-IR expression in the ventral prostate of the rat *(109)*. Thus, both increased and decreased IGF action is associated with normal prostate growth in the rat. Moreover, it is possible that autocrine or paracrine expression of IGF-I in the prostate can regulate normal growth.

IGF as an Autocrine GF for PC

It has long been suggested that production of peptide GFs by cancer cells could lead to autocrine growth characteristic of cancer cells *(110)*. Several groups have studied human PC cells in vitro, and have found that they indeed do express IGFs, and are implicated in autocrine growth *(111–116)*. Furthermore, inhibition of IGF action inhibits growth in vitro *(113,117–119)*. Most of these in vitro studies have documented IGF-II, but not IGF-I, gene expression. Thus, autocrine production of IGF-II is well documented in transformed prostate ECs.

In vivo, tumor growth of DU-145 human PC cell xenograft tumors are suppressed by a growth-hormone-releasing hormone (GH-RH) antagonist *(120)*. In these animals, the GH-RH antagonist suppressed serum IGF-I levels as expected; however, significant downregulation of tumor-expressed IGF-II was also seen. Thus, both endocrine and autocrine sources of IGFs may be important for PC growth.

Strategies designed to interrupt IGF-IR function have also been successful in inhibiting PC growth. Burfeind et al. *(121)* demonstrated that rat PC cells, transfected with an antisense IGF-IR, grow poorly in rats. However, there is also evidence that IGF-IR may oppose the expression of the malignant phenotype. Plymate et al. *(122)* found that prostate ECs, transformed with SV40T antigen, lost IGF-IR expression. When IGF-IR was re-expressed in these cells, decreased cell growth was seen, suggesting that, in this context, loss of IGF-IR was associated with progression of PC. Similarly, this group observed that IGF-IR gene expression is decreased in human PC, compared to benign prostatic hypertrophy *(123)*. These results may seem contradictory, but it is possible that the different model systems account for the conflicting results. Moreover, it is possible that appropriate regulation of IGF-IR gene expression, rather than unregulated expression, ultimately determines IGF action. For example, it is possible that high levels of constitutive expression, obtained by transfection, are toxic to cells, because appropriately regulated receptor function, as seen with the endogenous receptor, is required for coupling to signal transduction pathways required for growth.

It has also been shown that the IGFs can stimulate transactivation of the androgen receptor *(124,125)* in culture model systems. In these studies, transfection of androgen-receptor-negative cells with the androgen receptor and a reporter construct showed that IGF-I could activate the androgen receptor in an androgen-independent manner. Although similar studies have not been done for PC cells that express endogenous androgen receptor, as have been done for BC (*see* below), these studies suggest that dual blockade of both androgen and IGF pathways could combine to inhibit PC cell growth.

Direct Effects of IGFBPs in PC

The original view of the IGFBPs is that they influenced the cell by influencing IGF ligand–receptor interactions. It is now clear that the term "binding protein" only partially describes the functions of the IGFBPs *(126)*. In particular, IGF-independent effects of the binding proteins are well-characterized in several model systems.

It has been suggested that a high-affinity cell surface receptor for IGFBP-3 exists *(63,64)*. Moreover, cells lacking IGF-IR can be affected by IGFBP-3, highlighting the IGF-independent effects of this protein *(62)*.

In PC cells, it has been shown that IGFBP-3 can directly induced apoptosis *(127)*. Moreover, induction of apoptosis by TGF-β in PC-3 PC cells is mediated by induction of IGFBP-3. Fragments of IGFBP-3 generated by proteases also have activity in this assay *(128,129)*. Since prostate-specific antigen is an IGFBP-3 protease *(130,131)*, the interplay between cell growth, IGFBP-3 expression, and protease production is likely to be quite complex. This situation may be even more complicated when also considering the IGF-dependent functions of IGFBP-3.

Expression of IGF System Components in Human Prostate Tissues

Expression of IGF system components in vitro supports the idea that this GF system can regulate prostate EC growth, but expression in human tissue specimens must also be shown to prove that this pathway is relevant. In both benign and malignant prostate tissues, a number of studies have shown that the ligands, receptors, and binding proteins are present *(106,123,132–137)*.

In benign disease of the prostate, stromal cells produce IGF-II, and have upregulated IGF-IR, thus leading to a potential hyperproliferative state *(137,138)*. In PC cells, IGF-II expression has been found to be enhanced *(123,136)*. Although IGF-IR is present, levels appear to be reduced *(123)*. However, this apparent decrease of receptor levels in malignant cells, compared to normal cells, may reflect IGF-II-induced downregulation of the receptor, when the cells are undergoing autocrine growth stimulation. Thus, the key components required for autocrine growth regulation of PC by IGF-II are expressed. Taken together with the data obtained from in vitro systems, inhibition of the IGF axis may result in inhibition of PC growth.

IGFs AND BC

IGFs Effects on BC Cells

Estrogen receptor (ER)-positive BC cells (e.g., MCF-7, ZR-75, and T47D) are stimulated to proliferate by pico- to nanomolar concentrations of IGF-I and IGF-II *(139)*. In contrast, ER-negative cells (e.g., MDA-435, MDA-231, or MDA-468) tend not to proliferate, or are minimally responsive to IGF stimulation. Expression of practically all members of the IGF family are under the control of the ER, including IGF-I *(140)*, IGF-II *(141,142)*, IGF-IR *(143)*, and IGFBPs *(144)*, possibly accounting for IGF action within cells that contain an active ER. Additionally, the ability of the ER to regulate IGF signaling molecule expression may account for the apparent growth synergism between estradiol (E_2) and IGF *(145)*. However, it is not known at present whether ER is a requisite for IGF-stimulated growth, or whether ER is simply an indicator of a cell line that has a relatively intact growth signaling pathway (ER-positive cells are less aggressive and more differentiated than ER-negative tumors). For example, ER-negative cells have been shown to have defects in either IGF-IR action *(146)* or downstream signaling through IRS-1 *(147)*, and often have other constitutively active GF pathways.

The majority of studies have concentrated on the mitogenic ability of the IGFs, but, as discussed above, the IGF system can mediate a number of different responses. Many reports have documented the ability of IGF to protect cells from apoptosis *(148)*, and it has recently been shown that IGF-I can protect BC cells from chemotherapy-induced cell death *(149,150)*. IGFs are chemoattractants for BC cells *(151)*, possibly through interaction with integrins *(152)*. Finally, IGFs may be involved in cell migration and invasion, because dominant-negative IGF-IR constructs inhibit invasion and metastasis of MDA-435 BC cells in vitro and in vivo *(153)*.

IGF Signaling Pathways in BC

Because expression of most of the IGF family members is regulated by estrogen, it is not surprising that overexpression of IGFs in ER-positive BC cells results in reduced estrogen requirements or estrogen-independent growth. Overexpression of IGF-II in MCF-7 cells results in estrogen-independent growth *(154,155)*. It is surprising, however, that overexpression of IGF-IR does not result in dramatic phenotypic changes, with only slight changes in IGF, estrogen responsiveness *(156)*, and E-cadherin association *(157)*. In contrast, overexpression of IRS-1 in the same cell line results in a large increase in autocrine-mediated growth and reduced estrogen responsiveness *(158)*, suggesting that IRS-1 may be the rate-limiting step in IGF action in BC cells.

In many other cell systems, the contribution of the various IGF signaling pathways to cell proliferation has been analyzed by transfecting signaling components into cells that do not normally express them. This has undoubtedly furthered knowledge of IGF signaling pathways, but the relevance of these results to cells that normally express and respond to IGFs is only now being discovered. In BC cells that respond to IGF (ER-positive cells), IRS-1 is the predominant activated downstream signaling molecule *(159)*. IRS-1 activation results in downstream activation of mitogen activated protein kinase (MAPK) and phosphatidylinositol-3-kinase (PI-3-K). Inhibition of both of these pathways, using the specific inhibitors, PD90859 (MAPK) and wortmannin (PI-3-K), can reduce IGF-mediated growth *(159,160)*. However, the inability of either inhibitor to completely abolish IGF-mediated growth suggests the involvement of other signaling pathways.

One consequence of IGF signaling that has particular importance in BC is the ability of IGF to activate the ER. Expression of progesterone receptor (PR), an estrogen-responsive gene, is regulated by many factors including E_2 and IGF-I in BC cells *(161)*, and this occurs at the level of gene expression *(162)*. Further studies have shown transcriptional activation and phosphorylation of the ER by IGF-I *(163–165)*. The authors have shown that IGF-I can activate the ER in ER-positive BC cells *(166)*, and further, like others, that IGF-I can increase expression of estrogen-inducible genes, such as pS2 and PR in vitro, indicating that crosstalk between GF pathways and nuclear steroid hormone receptors can occur within cells that normally express ER. Indeed, there is evidence that GF crosstalk with hormone receptors may occur in vivo. It is well established that EGF can elicit an estrogen-like uterotropic response in vivo. However, in ER knockout mice, EGF fails to cause this response, indicating in vivo GF crosstalk *(167)*. The mechanism for IGF activation of the ER remains unclear, which is, in part, because of the cell type and promoter specificity of the ER and the recent identification of a family of ER co-activators and co-repressors that can affect ER action *(168)*.

IGF Expression in Human Tissue

Analysis of IGF ligand expression has historically been hampered by the presence of IGFBPs, which interfere with radioimmunoassays *(169)*. Although IGF can be separated from IGFBP by acid extraction and chromatography, a large portion of the IGF can be lost. Furthermore, analysis of tumor extracts does not indicate where the IGF originated. For these two reasons, immunohstochemistry (IHC) and *in situ* hybridization studies have given an insight into IGF expression in BC. IGF-I is rarely expressed in breast ECs, but is expressed in the stroma *(170)*. IGF-II is also expressed mostly in the stroma *(171)*, but may ocasionally be found in ECs *(172)*. IHC studies have confirmed these observations, which suggest a paracrine role for IGF action in BC *(173)*. Strengthening this hypothesis is the fact that IGF-II expression is increased in breast stroma associated with a malignancy, compared to benign and normal breast *(174)*. Furthermore, malignant breast ECs can induce IGF-II expression in breast stroma in vitro *(175)*.

In contrast to other GF families, which can only act by autocrine and paracrine mechanisms, the IGFs can also act in an endocrine manner. Recent evidence has shown that circulating IGFs can effect xenograft breast tumor growth *(176)* and tumor growth in p53 heterozygous mice *(81)*. Several retrospective studies have shown that circulating IGF levels are higher in BC patients than in normal controls *(177)*, which is strengthened by the recent finding that circulating IGF levels are a strong predictive risk factor for BC *(98)*. Of further importance is the large body of evidence showing that the major therapy in BC, antiestrogens, consistently reduces serum IGF-I levels in patients *(177)*. Furthermore, in vitro evidence suggests that part of the action of antiestrogens may be through anti-IGF mechanisms *(178,179)*.

IGF-IR mRNA expression is detected in the majority of breast tumors *(174)*. Protein analysis has revealed similar results (50–93% BCs express IGF-IR), and that IGF-IR expression correlates with ER status *(180,181)*. BCs express higher levels of IGF-IR than benign or normal tissue. Recent evidence suggests that radioresistant BCs express high IGF-IR levels *(182)*, supporting the role for IGF-IR in antiapoptotic signaling pathways. Furthermore, IGF-IR from BCs has higher intrinsic TK activity than that from normal breast *(183)*, suggesting that the IGF-IR is in an active signaling cascade.

Very few studies have examined IGF-IIR expression in BC. However, it has been shown that there is significant LOH at the IGF-IIR locus in BC, and that this is associated with a mutation in the other allele of IGF-IIR *(82)*. Although it has yet to be shown that these mutations disrupt IGF-IIR action, they do appear in the ligand binding domain, and so possibly could disrupt IGF-II binding to IGF-IIR. Hypothetically, this could release IGF-II, that would then be able to act through IGF-IR. Thus, IGF-IIR may represent a tumor suppressor gene in BC. Further studies are underway to confirm these observations.

The role of IGFBPs in IGF signaling remains unclear, but the authors have examined their expression in BC cell lines and tissue. ER-positive BC cells generally express IGFBP-2, -4, and -5; while ER-negative cell lines express IGFBP-1 and -3 *(144)*. A similar pattern of expression was seen in BCs, with all BCs expressing at least some of the IGFBPs, and IGFBP expression correlating with ER status *(184)*. Because the cloning and characterization of the six high-affinity binding proteins (IGFBP1–6), four more proteins that share some homology, and can bind IGF with lower affinity, have been identified *(67)* and termed IGFBP-related proteins (IGFBP-rP). The first discovered was MAC25/IGFBP-7/TIA (IGFBP-rP1), which has been found to be expressed in normal breast tissue, but not BC specimens, suggesting a tumor-suppressor-like function *(185)*. Additionally, there is frequent LOH (50%) at the chromosomal locus of IGFBP-rP1 *(186)* in human BC. Studies have yet to be performed that examine expression of the other IGFBP-rPs in human BC.

If IGFs are important in BC growth and progression, then their expression should be an indicator of the prognosis of the disease. The authors and others have therefore examined IGF expression in breast tumors. High IGF-II expression, measured by enzyme-linked immunosorbent assay, is associated with poor prognostic features *(187)*. However, IGF-II expression measured by IHC is weakly, inversely related to poor prognostic features *(173)*, perhaps reflecting the difficulty in measuring IGF ligand expression and the weakness of the correlations. IGF-IR is expressed in a high number of BCs, and expression is an indication of good prognosis *(188,189)*. IGFBP-3 expression is associated with poor prognostic features (ER-negative, high S-phase, and so on) as is IGFBP-4 in a small subset of tumors *(184,190)*. Finally the authors examined the prognostic potential of the IGF downstream signaling molecule, IRS-1, in BC patients. Examination of IRS-1 expression in 200 node-negative patients revealed that IRS-1 expression was significantly correlated with ER status, and that, in a subset of patients with small tumors, IRS-1 expression predicted a shorter disease-free survival *(190)*. Thus, expression of nearly all of the IGF family members is associated or correlated with prognostic features, suggesting a role for the IGFs in BC pathogenesis.

Inhibition of IGF Signaling as a Therapy for BC

Substantial circumstantial evidence implicates IGFs in breast tumor growth, but inhibition of IGF signaling in vitro, and translation of these finding to in vivo and clinical studies, has been problematic. Clearly, the IGF system is an ideal target *(191,192)*, because the IGF-IR can provide signals for proliferation, survival, and transformation, which are critical for tumor growth. Thus, it can be envisioned that inhibition of IGF-IR signaling, or removal of IGF ligand, would have profound effects on tumors cells, and this is indeed the case in most model systems.

Several different strategies have been employed to inhibit IGF signaling in BC, including dominant-negative IGF-IR *(153)*, soluble IGF-IR *(193)*, antisense IGF-IR *(194)*, overexpression of IGFBP-1 *(195)*, antisense IRS-1 *(158)*, and blocking antibody against IGF-IR *(196–198)*. All of these mechanisms can inhibit BC cell growth in vitro, and some have also been shown to inhibit xenograft tumor growth.

Despite the wealth of evidence implicating the IGFs in breast tumor growth, very few clinical trials have attempted to target IGFs. This is probably because of the difficulty in inhibiting autocrine, paracrine, and endocrine IGF action. Furthermore, the IGFs are important in several other physiological responses within the body, making targeting of IGF action within tumor tissue imperative. Estrogen was discovered as a mediator of breast tumor growth over 100 yr ago by simple ovariectomy of BC patients *(2)*. Because production of circulating IGF is controlled by the hypothalamus, ablation of circulating IGF-I by hypophysectomy is not practical. Despite this, there is evidence that hypophysectomy is an effective treatment of metastatic BC *(199)*.

Clinical trials have already been performed, or are currently underway, examining the efficacy of somatostatin analogies on lowering IGF-I level as a therapy for BC. A trial of lanreotide failed to decrease GH levels in BC patients *(200)*; a trial of somatuline lowered IGF-I levels, but had no effect on GH levels *(201)*. Perhaps the most exciting drug studied thus far is octreotide, which, in combination with tamoxifen (TAM), has been shown to be effective in lowering circulating IGF-I levels, both experimentally and clinically. In the 1,2-dimethylbenz[a]anthracene model of breast carcinogenesis, the combination of octreotide and TAM was more potent than TAM alone at inhibiting tumor growth *(202)*. In a small feasibility study involving 22 women, the combination of TAM, octreotide, and an antiprolactin gave a higher objective response rate (55%) than TAM alone (36%), and gave a longer time to disease progression (84 vs 33 wk) *(203)*. The combination of octreotide and TAM is being tested in two randomized clinical trials (National Surgical Adjuvant Breast and Bowel Project B29 and National Cancer Institute of Canada MA14).

SUMMARY AND FUTURE DIRECTIONS

It is clear that the IGF system is complex and the biological effects of the IGFs are determined by diverse interactions between many different molecules. However, most of the data suggest that both BC and PC are responsive to the IGFs in many model systems. Moreover, the IGFs may have a role in malignant transformation of normal breast and prostate epithelium.

In these endocrine-sensitive cancers, a major advance was the demonstration that agents that interfered with steroid hormone receptor function had significant clinical activity. In clinical oncology, the selective ER modulators (antiestrogens) for BC and strategies to deprive the PC of androgens are clearly the most successful therapies available. Neither antihormonal strategy is curative for patients with advanced cancer, but they are effective and well-tolerated.

It is hoped that other hormonal pathways are also active in human cancer and can be targeted for therapy. This argument is validated by the recent demonstration that a humanized antibody directed against the epidermal growth factor receptor, HER2/neu, has modest activity in BC (204,205). In fact, this antibody strategy has been approved for treatment in a relatively short period of time, because its relevance was demonstrated in BC as a prognostic factor (206).

What is needed to prove that the IGF system is also a relevant growth regulatory system in BC and PC? IGF system components have been shown to be expressed in these cancers, growth regulation in vitro and in vivo is well documented, prognostic significance of some of the IGF system components has been demonstrated, and strategies designed to inhibit IGF action clearly reduced tumor growth in animals. Thus, the remaining proof required is the development of a therapeutic strategy demonstrating activity in BC and PC patients. The knowledge gained about the IGF system may soon translate into clinical strategies.

REFERENCES

1. Huggins C, Hodges CV. Studies on prostatic cancer: effect of castration, of estrogen and of androgen injection on serum phosphtases in metastatic carcinoma of the prostate. Cancer Res 1941;1:293–297.
2. Beatson GT. On the treatment of inoperable cases of carcinoma of the mamma. Suggestions for a new method of treatment with illustrative cases. Lancet 1896;2:104–107.
3. Small EJ. Update on the diagnosis and treatment of prostate cancer. Curr Opin Oncol 1998;10: 244–252.
4. Hortobagyi GN. Treatment of breast cancer. N Engl J Med 1998;339:974–984.
5. Salmon WD, Daughaday WH. A hormonally controlled serum factor which stimulates sulfate incorporation by cartilage in vitro. J Lab Clin Med 1957;49:825–836.
6. Daughaday WH, Rotwein P. Insulin-like growth factors I and II. Peptide, messenger ribonucleic acid and gene structures, serum, and tissue concentrations. Endocr Rev 1989;10:68–91.
7. Laron Z. Laron-type dwarfism (hereditary somatomedin deficiency): a review. Adv Intern Med Pediatr 1984;51:117.
8. Liu JP, Baker J, Perkins AS, Robertson EJ, Efstratiadis A. Mice carrying null mutations of the genes encoding insulin-like growth factor-I (IGF-1) and type-1 IGF receptor (IGF1r). Cell 1993;75:59–72.
9. Baker J, Liu JP, Robertson EJ, Efstratiadis A. Role of insulin-like growth factors in embryonic and postnatal growth. Cell 1993;75:73–82.
10. Powell-Braxton L, Hollingshead P, Warburton C, Dowd M, Pittsmeek S, Dalton D, Gillett N, Stewart TA. IGF-I is required for normal embryonic growth in mice. Gene Dev 1993;7:2609–2617.
11. Liu JL, Grinberg A, Westphal H, Sauer B, Accili D, Karas M, LeRoith D. Insulin-like growth factor-I affects perinatal lethality and postnatal development in a gene dosage-dependent manner: manipulation using the Cre/loxP system in transgenic mice. Mol Endocrinol 1998;12:1452–1462.
12. Woods KA, Camacho-Hubner C, Barter D, Clark AJ, Savage MO. Insulin-like growth factor I gene deletion causing intrauterine growth retardation and severe short stature. Acta Paediatr 1997;423(Suppl): 39–45.
13. Beck KD, Powellbraxton L, Widmer HR, Valverde J, Hefti F. Igf1 gene disruption results in reduced brain size, CNS hypomyelination, and loss of hippocampal granule and striatal parvalbumin-containing neurons. Neuron 1995;14:717–730.
14. DeChiara TM, Efstratiadis A, Robertson EJ. A growth deficiency phenotype in heterozygous mice carrying an insulin-like growth factor II gene distributed by targeting. Nature 1990;345:78–80.

15. DeChiara TM, Robertson EJ, Efstratiadis A. Parental imprinting of the mouse insulin-like growth factor II gene. Cell 1991;64:849–859.

16. LeRoith D. Seminars in medicine of the Beth Israel Deaconess Medical Center: insulin-like growth factors. N Engl J Med 1997;336:633–640.

17. Morgan DO, Edman JC, Standring DN, Fried VA, Smith MC, Roth RA, Rutter WJ. Insulin-like growth factor II receptor as a multifunctional binding protein. Nature 1987;329:301–307.

18. Blanchard F, Raher S, Duplomb L, Vusio P, Pitard V, Taupin JL, et al. The mannose 6-phosphate/insulin-like growth factor II receptor is a nanomolar affinity receptor for glycosylated human leukemia inhibitory factor. J Biol Chem 1998;273:20,886–20,893.

19. Kang JX, Li YY, Leaf A. Mannose-6-phosphate/insulin-like growth factor-II receptor is a receptor for retinoic acid. Proc Natl Acad Sci USA 1997;94:13,671–13,676.

20. Nishimoto I, Murayama Y, Katada T, Ui M, Ogata E. Possible direct linkage of insulin-like growth factor II receptor with guanine nucleotide-binding protein. J Biol Chem 1989;264:14,029–14,038.

21. Kojima I, Nishimoto I, Iiri T, Ogata E, Rosenfeld R. Evidence that type II insulin-like growth factor receptor is coupled to calcium gating system. Biochem Biophys Res Commun 1988;154:9–19.

22. Okamoto T, Katada T, Murayama Y, Ui M, Ogata E, Nishimoto I. A simple structure encodes G protein-activating function of the IGF-II/mannose 6-phosphate receptor. Cell 1990;62:709–717.

23. Korner C, Nurnberg B, Uhde M, Braulke T. Mannose 6-phosphate insulin-like growth factor II receptor fails to interact with G-proteins: analysis of mutant cytoplasmic receptor domains. J Biol Chem 1995;270:287–295.

24. Schmidt B, Kieckesiemsen C, Waheed A, Braulke T, von Figura K. Localization of the insulin-like growth factor II binding site to amino acids 1508-1566 in repeat 11 of the mannose 6-phosphate/insulin-like growth factor II receptor. J Biol Chem 1995;270:14,975–14,982.

25. Braulke T, Causin C, Waheed A, Junghans U, Hasilik A, Maly P, Humbel RE, vonFigura K. Mannose 6-phosphate/insulin-like growth factor II receptor: distinct binding sites for mannose 6-phosphate and insulin-like growth factor II. Biochem Biophys Res Commun 1988;150:1287–1293.

26. Barlow DP, Stoger R, Herrmann BG, Saito K, Schweifer N. The mouse insulin-like growth factor type-2 receptor is imprinted and closely linked to the Tme locus. Nature 1991;349:84–87.

27. Stoger R, Kubicka P, Liu CG, Kafri T, Razin A, Cedar H, Barlow DP. Maternal-Specific methylation of the imprinted mouse igf2r locus identifies the expressed locus as carrying the imprinting signal. Cell 1993;73:61–71.

28. Xu Y, Goodyer CG, Deal C, Polychronakos C. Functional polymorphism in the parental imprinting of the human IGF2R gene. Biochem Biophys Res Commun 1993;197:747–754.

29. Smrzka OW, Fae I, Stoger R, Kurzbauer R, Fischer GF, Henn T, Weith A, Barlow DP. Conservation of a maternal-specific methylation signal at the human IGF2R locus. Hum Mol Genet 1995;4:1945–1952.

30. Giannoukakis N, Deal C, Paquette J, Kukuvitis A, Polychronakos C. Polymorphic functional imprinting of the human IGF2 gene among individuals, in blood cells, is associated with H19 expression. Biochem Biophys Res Commun 1996;220:1014–1019.

31. Kalscheuer VM, Mariman EC, Schepens MT, Rehder H, Ropers HH. Insulin-like growth factor type-2 receptor gene is imprinted in the mouse but not in humans. Nature Genet 1993;5:74–78.

32. Ogawa O, McNoe LA, Eccles MR, Morison IM, Reeve AE. Human insulin-like growth factor type I and type II receptors are not imprinted. Hum Mol Genet 1993;2:2163–2165.

33. Ullrich A, Gray A, Tam AW, Yang FT, Tsubokawa M, Collins C, et al. Insulin-like growth factor I receptor primary structure: comparison with insulin receptor suggests structural determinants that define hormonal specificity. EMBO J 1986;5:2503–2512.

34. Tollefsen SE, Stoszek RM, Thompson K. Interaction of the alpha-beta dimers of the insulin-like growth factor I receptor is required for receptor autophosphorylation. Biochemistry 1991;30:48–54.

35. Blakesley VA, Stannard BS, Kalebic T, Helman LJ, LeRoith D. Role of the IGF-I receptor in mutagenesis and tumor promotion. J Endocrinol 1997;152:339–344.

36. Esposito DL, Blakesley VA, Koval AP, Scrimgeour AG, LeRoith D. Tyrosine residues in the C-terminal domain of the insulin-like growth factor-I receptor mediate mitogenic and tumorigenic signals. Endocrinology 1997;138:2979–2988.

37. Xu SQ, Tang DH, Chamberlain S, Pronk G, Masiarz FR, Kaur S, et al. The granulin/epithelin precursor abrogates the requirement for the insulin-like growth factor 1 receptor for growth in vitro. J Biol Chem 1998;273:20,078–20,083.

38. Morrione A, Valentinis B, Xu SQ, Yumet G, Louvi A, Efstratiadis A, Baserga R. Insulin-like growth factor II stimulates cell proliferation through the insulin receptor. Proc Natl Acad Sci USA 1997;94:3777–3782.

39. Morrione A, Valentinis B, Li SW, Ooi JYT, Margolis B, Baserga R. Grb10: a new substrate of the insulin-like growth factor i receptor. Cancer Res 1996;56:3165–3167.

40. Resnicoff M, Abraham D, Yutanawiboonchai W, Rotman HL, Kajstura J, Rubin R, Zoltick P, Baserga R. The insulin-like growth factor I receptor protects tumor cells from apoptosis in vivo. Cancer Res 1995;55:2463–2469.

41. Dey BR, Frick K, Lopaczynski W, Nissley SP, Furlanetto RW. Evidence for the direct interaction of the insulin-like growth factor I receptor with IRS-1, shc, and grb10. Mol Endocrinol 1996;10:631–641.

42. Sun XJ, Wang L-M, Zhang Y, Yenush L, Myers MG Jr, Glasheen E, et al. Role of IRS-2 in insulin and cytokine signalling. Nature 1995;377:173–177.

43. Beitner-Johnson D, Leroith D. Insulin-like growth factor-I stimulates tyrosine phosphorylation of endogenous c-Crk. J Biol Chem 1995;270:5187–5190.

44. Koval AP, Karas M, Zick Y, LeRoith D. Interplay of the proto-oncogene proteins CrkL and CrkII in insulin-like growth factor-I receptor-mediated signal transduction. J Biol Chem 1998;273:14,780–14,787.

45. O'Neill TJ, Rose DW, Pillay TS, Hotta K, Olefsky JM, Gustafson TA. Interaction of a GRB-IR splice variant (a human GRB10 homolog) with the insulin and insulin-like growth factor I receptors: evidence for a role in mitogenic signaling. J Biol Chem 1996;271:22,506–22,513.

46. White MF. IRS-signaling system: a network of docking proteins that mediate insulin action. Mol Cell Biochem 1998;182:3–11.

47. Federici M, Zucaro L, Porzio O, Massoud R, Borboni P, Lauro D, Sesti G. Increased expression of insulin/insulin-like growth factor-I hybrid receptors in skeletal muscle of noninsulin-dependent diabetes mellitus subjects. J Clin Invest 1996;98:2887–2893.

48. Federici M, Porzio O, Zucaro L, Fusco A, Borboni P, Lauro D, Sesti G. Distribution of insulin/insulin-like growth factor-I hybrid receptors in human tissues. Mol Cell Endocrinol 1997;129:121–126.

49. Garrouste FL, RemacleBonnet MM, Lehmann MMA, Marvaldi JL, Pommier GJ. Up-regulation of insulin/insulin-like growth factor-I hybrid receptors during differentiation of HT29-D4 human colonic carcinoma cells. Endocrinology 1997;138:2021- 2032.

50. Kasuya J, Paz IB, Maddux BA, Goldfine ID, Hefta SA, Fujita-yamaguchi Y. Characterization of human placental insulin-like growth factor-I/insulin hybrid receptors by protein microsequencing and purification. Biochemistry 1993;32:13,531–13,536.

51. Langlois WJ, Sasaoka T, Yip CC, Olefsky JM. Functional characterization of hybrid receptors composed of a truncated insulin receptor and wild type insulin-like growth factor 1 or insulin receptors. Endocrinology 1995;136:1978–1986.

52. Moxham CP, Duronio V, Jacobs S. Insulin-like growth factor I receptor a-subunit heterogeneity, evidence for hybrid tetramers composed of insulin-like growth factor I and insulin receptor heterodimers. J Biol Chem 1989;264:13,238–13,244.

53. Seely BL, Reichart DR, Takata Y, Yip C, Olefsky JM. A functional assessment of insulin/insulin-like growth factor-I hybrid receptors. Endocrinology 1995;136:1635–1641.

54. Soos MA, Whittaker J, Lammers R, Ullrich A, Siddle K. Receptors for insulin and insulin-like growth factor-I can form hybrid dimers, characterisation of hybrid receptors in transfected cells. Biochem J 1990;270:383–390.

55. Soos MA, Field CE, Siddle K. Purified hybrid insulin/insulin-like growth factor-I receptors bind insulin-like growth factor-I, but not insulin, with high affinity. Biochem J 1993;290:419–426.

56. Sakano K, Enjoh T, Numata F, Fujiwara H, Marumoto Y, Higashihashi N, et al. The design, expression, and characterization of human insulin-like growth factor II (IGF-II) mutants specific for either the IGF-II/cation-independent mannose 6-phosphate receptor or IGF-I receptor. J Biol Chem 1991;266: 20,626–20,635.

57. Baxter RC, Binoux MA, Clemmons DR, Conover CA, Drop SLS, Holly JMP, et al. Recommendations for nomenclature of the insulin-like growth factor binding protein superfamily. J Clin Endocrinol Metab 1998;83:3213–3213.

58. Leong SR, Baxter RC, Camerato T, Dai J, Wood WI. Structure and functional expression of the acid-labile subunit of the insulin-like growth factor-binding protein complex. Mol Endocrinol 1992;6:870–876.

59. Kubler B, Cowell S, Zapf J, Braulke T. Proteolysis of insulin-like growth factor binding proteins by a novel 50-kilodalton metalloproteinase in human pregnancy serum. Endocrinology 1998;139:1556–1563.

60. Hossenlopp P, Segovia B, Lassarre C, Roghani M, Bredon M, Binoux M. Evidence of enzymatic degradation of insulin-like growth factor-binding proteins in the 150K complex during pregnancy. J Clin Endocrinol Metab 1990;71:797–805.

61. Clemmons DR, Busby W, Clarke JB, Parker A, Duan C, Nam TJ. Modifications of insulin-like growth factor binding proteins and their role in controlling IGF actions. Endocr J 1998;45:S1–S8.

62. Valentinis B, Bhala A, Deangelis T, Baserga R, Cohen P. The human insulin-like growth factor (IGF) binding protein-3 inhibits the growth of fibroblasts with a targeted disruption of the IGF-I receptor gene. Mol Endocrinol 1995;9:361–367.

63. Oh Y, Mueller HL, Pham Y, Rosenfeld RG. Demonstration of receptors for insulin-like growth factor binding protein-3 on Hs578T human breast cancer cells. J Biol Chem 1993;268:26,045–26,048.

64. Leal SM, Liu Q, Huang SS, Huang JS. The type V transforming growth factor beta receptor is the putative insulin-like growth factor-binding protein 3 receptor. J Biol Chem 1997;272:20,572–20,576.

65. Jones JI, Gockerman A, Busby WH Jr, Wright G, Clemmons DR. Insulin-like growth factor binding protein-1 stimulates cell migration and binds alpha5beta1 integrin by means of its arg-gly-asp sequence. Proc Natl Acad Sci USA 1993;90:10,553–10,557.

66. Schedlich LJ, Young TF, Firth SM, Baxter RC. Insulin-like growth factor-binding protein (IGFBP)-3 and IGFBP-5 share a common nuclear transport pathway in T47D human breast carcinoma cells. J Biol Chem 1998;273:18,347–18,352.

67. Kim HS, Nagalla SR, Oh Y, Wilson E, Roberts CT Jr, Rosenfeld RG. Identification of a family of low-affinity insulin-like growth factor binding proteins (IGFBPs): characterization of connective tissue growth factor as a member of the IGFBP superfamily. Proc Natl Acad Sci USA 1997;94:12,981–12,986.

68. Yamanaka Y, Wilson EM, Rosenfeld RG, Oh Y. Inhibition of insulin receptor activation by insulin-like growth factor binding proteins. J Biol Chem 1997;272:30,729–30,734.

69. Sell C, Dumneil G, Deveaud C, Miura M, Coppola D, DeAngeli T, et al. Effect of a null mutation of the type 1 IGF receptor gene on growth and transformation of mouse embryo fibroblasts. Mol Cell Biol 1994;14:3604–3612.

70. Sell C, Rubini M, Rubin R, Liu JP, Efstratiadis A, Baserga R. Simian virus-40 large tumor antigen is unable to transform mouse embryonic fibroblasts lacking type-1 insulin-like growth factor receptor. Proc Natl Acad Sci USA 1993;90:11,217–11,221.

71. Valentinis B, Porcu P, Quinn K, Baserga R. The role of the insulin-like growth factor I receptor in the transformation by simian virus 40 T antigen. Oncogene 1994;9:825- 831.

72. Coppola D, Ferber A, Miura M, Sell C, Dambrosio C, Rubin R, Baserga R. A functional insulin-like growth factor I receptor is required for the mitogenic and transforming activities of the epidermal growth factor receptor. Mol Cell Biol 1994;14:4588–4595.

73. Li SW, Resnicoff M, Baserga R. Effect of mutations at serines 1280-1283 on the mitogenic and transforming activities of the insulin-like growth factor I receptor. J Biol Chem 1996;271:12,254–12,260.

74. Kaleko M, Rutter WJ, Miller AD. Overexpression of the human insulin-like growth factor I receptor promotes ligand-dependent neoplastic transformation. Mol Cell Biol 1990;10:464–473.

75. Berns EMJJ, Klign JGM, van Staveren IL, Portengen H, Foekens JA. Sporadic amplification of the insulin-like growth factor I receptor gene in human breast tumors. Cancer Res 1992;52:1036–1039.

76. Valentinis B, Morrione A, Taylor SJ, Baserga R. Insulin-like growth factor I receptor signaling in transformation by src oncogenes. Mol Cell Biol 1997;17:3744–3754.

77. Parr T. Insulin exposure controls the rate of mammalian aging. Mech Ageing Dev 1996;88:75–82.

78. Clemmons DR, Underwood LE. Nutritional regulation of IGF-I and IGF binding proteins. Annu Rev Nutr 1991;11:393–412.

79. Doll R, Peto R. The causes of cancer: quantitative estimates of avoidable risks of cancer in the United States today. J Natl Cancer Inst 1981;66:1191–1308.

80. Hursting SD, Perkins SN, Brown CC, Haines DC, Phang JM. Calorie restriction induces a p53-independent delay of spontaneous carcinogenesis in p53-deficient and wild-type mice. Cancer Res 1997;57: 2843–2846.

81. Dunn SE, Kari FW, French J, Leininger JR, Travlos G, Wilson R, Barrett JC. Dietary restriction reduces insulin-like growth factor I levels, which modulates apoptosis, cell proliferation, and tumor progression in p53-deficient mice. Cancer Res 1997;57:4667–4672.

82. Hankins GR, Desouza AT, Bentley RC, Patel MR, Marks JR, Iglehart JD, Jirtle RL. M6P/IGF2 receptor: a candidate breast tumor suppressor gene. Oncogene 1996;12:2003–2009.

83. Desouza AT, Hankins GR, Washington MK, Orton TC, Jirtle RL. M6P/IGF2R gene is mutated in human hepatocellular carcinomas with loss of heterozygosity. Nature Genet 1995;11:447–449.

84. Desouza AT, Hankins GR, Washington MK, Fine RL, Orton TC, Jirtle RL. Frequent loss of heterozygosity on 6q at the mannose 6-phosphate/insulin-like growth factor II receptor locus in human hepatocellular tumors. Oncogene 1995;10:1725–1729.

85. Rappolee DA, Sturm KS, Behrendtsen O, Schultz GA, Pedersen RA, Werb Z. Insulin-like growth factor-II acts through an endogenous growth pathway regulated by imprinting in early mouse embryos. Gene Dev 1992;6:939–952.

86. Haig D, Graham C. Genomic imprinting and the strange case of the insulin-like growth factor II receptor. Cell 1991;64:1045,1046.

87. Ogawa O, Eccles MR, Szeto J, McNoe LA, Yun K, Maw MA, Smith PJ, Reeve AE. Relaxation of insulin-like growth factor-II gene imprinting implicated in Wilms' tumour. Nature 1993;362:749–751.

88. Zhan SL, Shapiro DN, Helman LJ. Activation of an imprinted allele of the insulin-like growth factor II gene implicated in rhabdomyosarcoma. J Clin Invest 1994;94:445–448.

89. Rainier S, Dobry CJ, Feinberg AP. Loss of imprinting in hepatoblastoma. Cancer Res 1995;55:1836–1838.

90. Zhan SL, Shapiro DN, Helman LJ. Loss of imprinting of IGF2 in ewing's sarcoma. Oncogene 1995;11:2503–2507.

91. Zhan SL, Shapiro D, Zhan SX, Zhang LJ, Hirschfeld S, Elassal J, Helman LJ. Concordant loss of imprinting of the human insulin-like growth factor II gene promoters in cancer. J Biol Chem 1995;270:27,983–27,986.

92. Vu TH, Yballe C, Boonyanit S, Hoffman AR. Insulin-like growth factor II in uterine smooth-muscle tumors: maintenance of genomic imprinting in leiomyomata and loss of imprinting in leiomyosarcomata. J Clin Endocrinol Metab 1995;80:1670–1676.

93. Doucrasy S, Barrois M, Fogel S, Ahomadegbe JC, Stehelin D, Coll J, Riou G. High incidence of loss of heterozygosity and abnormal imprinting of h19 and IGF2 genes in invasive cervical carcinomas. Uncoupling of h19 and IGF2 expression and biallelic hypomethylation of h19. Oncogene 1996;12:423–430.

94. Yballe CM, Vu TH, Hoffman AR. Imprinting and expression of insulin-like growth factor-II and h19 in normal breast tissue and breast tumor. J Clin Endocrinol Metab 1996;81:1607–1612.

95. Nonomura N, Miki T, Nishimura K, Kanno N, Kojima Y, Okuyama A. Altered imprinting of the H19 and insulin-like growth factor II genes in testicular tumors. J Urol 1997;157:1977–1979.

96. Wu HK, Squire JA, Catzavelos CG, Weksberg R. Relaxation of imprinting of human insulin-like growth factor II gene, IGF2, in sporadic breast carcinomas. Biochem Biophys Res Commun 1997;235:123–129.

97. Chan JM, Stampfer MJ, Giovannucci E, Gann PH, Ma J, Wilkinson P, Hennekens CH, Pollak M. Plasma insulin-like growth factor-I and prostate cancer risk: a prospective study. Science 1998;279:563–565.

98. Hankinson SE, Willett WC, Colditz GA, Hunter DJ, Michaud DS, Deroo B, et al. Circulating concentrations of insulin-like growth factor-I and risk of breast cancer. Lancet 1998;351:1373–1375.

99. Cohen P. Serum insulin-like growth factor-I levels and prostate cancer risk: interpreting the evidence. J Natl Cancer Inst 1998;90:876–879.

100. Wolk A, Mantzoros CS, Andersson SO, Bergstrom R, Signorello LB, Lagiou P, Adami HO, Trichopoulos D. Insulin-like growth factor 1 and prostate cancer risk: a population-based; case-control study. J Natl Cancer Inst 1998;90:911–915.

101. Strohm O, Osterziel KJ, Dietz R. Insulin-like growth factor-I and risk of breast cancer. Lancet 1998;352:488,489.

102. Campagnoli C, Ambroggio S, Biglia N, Peris C, Sismondi P. Insulin-like growth factor-I and risk of breast cancer. Lancet 1998;352:488.

103. Florkowski C, Livesey J, Espiner E. Insulin-like growth factor-I and risk of breast cancer. Lancet 1998;352:489,490.

104. Hankinson SE, Willett WC, Speizer FE, Pollak M. Insulin-like growth factor-I and risk of breast cancer. Lancet 1998;352:488,489.

105. Janssen JAMJL, Lamberts SWJ. Insulin-like growth factor-I and risk of breast cancer. Lancet 1998;352:490.

106. Cohen P, Peehl DM, Lamson G, Rosenfeld RG. Insulin-like growth factors, IGF receptors, and IGF binding proteins in primary cultures of prostate epithelial cells. J Clin Endocrinol Metab 1991;73:401–407.

107. Plymate SR, Tennant M, Birnbaum RS, Thrasher JB, Chatta G, Ware JL. The effect of the insulin-like growth factor system human prostate epithelial cells of immortalization and transformation by simian virus-40 t antigen. J Clin Endocrinol Metab 1996;81:3709–3716.

108. Torring N, Vinter-Jensen L, Pederson SB, Sorenson FB, Flyvbjerg A, Nexo E. Systemic administration of insulin-like growth factor I (IGF-I) causes growth of rat prostate. J Urol 1997;158:222–227.

109. Huynh H, Seyam RM, Brock GB. Reduction of ventral prostate weight by finasteride is associated with suppression of insulin-like growth factor I (IGF-I) and IGF-I receptor genes wand with an increase in IGF binding protein 3. Cancer Res 1998;58:215–218.

110. Sporn MB, Roberts AB. Autocrine growth factors and cancer. Nature 1985;313:745–747.

111. Angelloz-Nicoud P, Binoux M. Autocrine regulation of cell proliferation by the insulin-like growth factor (IGF) and IGF binding protein-3 protease system in a human prostate carcinoma cell line (PC-3). Endocrinology 1995;136:5485–5492.

112. Connolly JM, Rose DP. Regulation of DU145 human prostate cancer cell proliferation by insulin-like growth factors and its interaction with the epidermal growth factor autocrine loop. Prostate 1994;24: 167–175.

113. Figueroa JA, Lee AV, Jackson JG, Yee D. Proliferation of cultured human prostate cancer cells is inhibited by insulin-like growth factor binding protein-1: evidence for an IGF-II autocrine loop. J Clin Endocrinol Metab 1995;80:3476–3482.

114. Huynh H, Pollak M, Zhang JC. Regulation of insulin-like growth factor (IGF) II and IGF binding protein 3 autocrine loop in human PC-3 prostate cancer cells by vitamin D metabolite 1;25(OH)2D3 and its analog EB1089. Int J Oncol 1998;13:137–143.

115. Iwamura M, Sluss PM, Casamento JB, Cockett ATK. Insulin-like growth factor-1: action and receptor characterization in human prostate cancer cell lines. Prostate 1993;22:243–252.

116. Matuo Y, Mishi N, Tanaka H, Sasaki I, Issacs JT, Wada F. Production of IGF-II-related peptide by an anaplastic cell line (AT-3) established from the Dunning prostate carcinoma of rats. In Vitro Dev Biol 1988;24:1053–1056.

117. Pietrzkowski Z, Wernicke D, Porcu P, Jameson BA, Baserga R. Inhibition of cellular proliferation by peptide analogues of insulin-like growth factor-1. Cancer Res 1992;52:6447–6451.

118. Pietrzkowski Z, Mulholland G, Gomella L, Jameson BA, Wernicke D, Baserga R. Inhibition of growth of prostatic cancer cell lines by peptide analogues of insulin-like growth factor-1. Cancer Res 1993; 53:1102–1106.

119. Damon SE, Maddison L, Ware JL, Plymate SR. Overexpression of an inhibitory insulin-like growth factor binding protein (IGFBP); IGFBP-4; delays onset of prostate tumor formation. Endocrinology 1998; 139:3456–3464.

120. Lamharzi N, Schally AV, Koppan M, Groot K. Growth hormone-releasing hormone antagonist MZ-5-156 inhibits growth of DU-145 human androgen-independent prostate carcinoma in nude mice and suppresses the levels and mRNA expression of insulin-like growth factor II in tumors. Proc Natl Acad Sci USA 1998;95:8864–8868.

121. Burfeind P, Chernicky CL, Rininsland F, Ilan J, Ilan J. Antisense RNA to the type I insulin-like growth factor receptor suppresses tumor growth and prevents invasion by rat prostate cancer cells in vivo. Proc Natl Acad Sci USA 1996;93:7263–7268.

122. Plymate SR, Bae VL, Maddison L, Quinn LS, Ware JL. Reexpression of the type 1 insulin-like growth factor receptor inhibits the malignant phenotype of simian virus 40 T antigen immortalized human prostate epithelial cells. Endocrinology 1997;138:1728–1735.

123. Tennant MK, Thrasher JB, Twomey PA, Drivdahl RH, Birnbaum RS, Plymate SR. Protein and messenger ribonucleic acid (mRNA) for the type 1 insulin-like growth factor (IGF) receptor is decreased and IGF-II mRNA is increased in human prostate carcinoma compared to benign prostate epithelium. J Clin Endocrinol Metab 1996;81:3774–3782.

124. Reinikainen P, Palvimo JJ, Janne OA. Effects of mitogens on androgen receptor-mediated transactivation. Endocrinology 1996;137:4351–4357.

125. Culig Z, Hobisch A, Cronauer MV, Radmayr C, Trapman J, Hittmair A, Bartsch G, Klocker H. Androgen receptor activation in prostatic tumor cell lines by insulin-like growth factor-I, keratinocyte growth factor, and epidermal growth factor. Cancer Res 1994;54:5474–5478.

126. Rechler MM. Growth inhibition by insulin-like growth factor (IGF) binding protein-3: what's IGF got to do with it? Endocrinology 1997;138:2645–2647.

127. Rajah R, Valentinis B, Cohen P. Insulin like growth factor (IGF)-binding protein-3 induces apoptosis and mediates the effects of transforming growth factor-beta 1 on programmed cell death through a p53- and IGF-independent mechanism. J Biol Chem 1997;272:12,181–12,188.

128. Lalou C, Lassarre C, Binoux M. A proteolytic fragment of insulin-like growth factor (IGF) binding protein-3 that fails to bind IGFs inhibits the mitogenic effects of IGF-I and insulin. Endocrinology 1996;137:3206–3212.

129. Zadeh SM, Binoux M. The 16-kDa proteolytic fragment of insulin-like growth factor (IGF) binding protein-3 inhibits the mitogenic action of fibroblast growth factor on mouse fibroblasts with a targeted disruption of the type 1 IGF receptor gene. Endocrinology 1997;138:3069–3072.

130. Cohen P, Graves HCB, Peehl DM, Kamarei M, Giudice LC, Rosenfeld RG. Prostate-specific antigen (PSA) is an insulin-like growth factor binding protein-3 protease found in seminal plasma. J Clin Endocrinol Metab 1992;75:1046–1053.

131. Fielder PJ, Rosenfeld RG, Graves HCB, Grandbois K, Maack CA, Sawamura S, et al. Biochemical analysis of prostate specific antigen-proteolyzed insulin-like growth factor binding protein-3. Growth Regul 1994;4:164–172.

132. Bonnet P, Reiter E, Bruyninx M, Sente B, Dombrowicz D, Deleval J, Closset J, Hennen G. Benign prostatic hyperplasia and normal prostate aging: differences in types I and II 5 alpha-reductase and steroid hormone receptor messenger ribonucleic acid (mRNA) levels, but not in insulin-like growth factor mRNA levels. J Clin Endocrinol Metab 1993;77:1203–1208.

133. Fiorelli G, De Bellis A, Longo A, Giannini S, Natali A, Costantini A, Vannelli GB, Serio M. Insulin-like growth factor-I receptors in human hyperplastic prostate tissue: characterization, tissue localization, and their modulation by chronic treatment with a gonadotropin-releasing hormone analog. J Clin Endocrinol Metab 1991;72:740–746.

134. Tennant MK, Thrasher JB, Twomey PA, Birnbaum RS, Plymate SR. Insulin-like growth factor-binding proteins (IGFBP)-4, -5, and -6 in the benign and malignant human prostate: IGFBP-5 messenger ribonucleic acid localization differs from IGFBP-5 protein localization. J Clin Endocrinol Metab 1996;81:3783–3792.

135. Tennant MK, Thrasher JB, Twomey PA, Birnbaum RS, Plymate SR. Insulin-like growth factor-binding protein-2 and -3 expression in benign human prostate epithelium, prostate intraepithelial neoplasia, and adenocarcinoma of the prostate. J Clin Endocrinol Metab 1996;81:411–420.

136. Li SL, Goko H, Xu ZD, Kimura G, Sun Y, Kawachi MH, et al. Expression of insulin-like growth factor (IGF)-II in human prostate, breast, bladder, and paraganglioma tumors. Cell Tissue Res 1998;291:469–479.

137. Monti S, DiSilverio F, Lanzara S, Varasano P, Martini C, TostiCroce C, Sciarra F. Insulin-like growth factor-I and -II in human benign prostatic hyperplasia: relationship with binding proteins 2 and 3 and androgens. Steroids 1998;63:362–366.

138. Cohen P, Peehl DM, Baker B, Liu F, Hintz RL, Rosenfeld RG. Insulin-like growth factor axis abnormalities in prostatic stromal cells from patients with benign prostatic hyperplasia. J Clin Endocrinol Metab 1994;79:1410–1415.

139. Karey KP, Sirbasku DA. Differential responsiveness of human breast cancer cell lines MCF-7 and T47D to growth factors and 17 beta-estradiol. Cancer Res 1988;48:4083–4092.

140. Umayahara Y, Kawamori R, Watada H, Imano E, Iwama N, Morishima T, et al. Estrogen regulation of the insulin-like growth factor I gene transcription involves an AP-1 enhancer. J Biol Chem 1994;269:16,433–16,442.

141. Osborne CK, Coronado EB, Kitten LJ, Arteaga CI, Fuqua SAW, Ramasharma K, Marshall M, Li CH. Insulin-like growth factor-II (IGF-II): a potential autocrine/paracrine growth factor for human breast cancer acting via the IGF-I receptor. Mol Endocrinol 1989;3:1701–1709.

142. Lee AV, Darbre P, King RJ. Processing of insulin-like growth factor-II (IGF-II) by human breast cancer cells. Mol Cell Endocrinol 1994;99:211–220.

143. Stewart A, Johnson MD, May FEB, Westley BR. Role of insulin-like growth factors and the type 1 insulin-like growth factor receptor in the estrogen-stimulated proliferation of human breast cancer cells. J Biol Chem 1990;265:21,172–21,178.

144. McGuire W Jr, Jackson JG, Figueroa JA, Shimasaki SA, Powell DR, Yee D. Regulation of insulin-like growth factor-binding protein (IGFBP) expression by breast cancer cells: use of IGFBP-1 as an inhibitor of insulin-like growth factor action. J Natl Cancer Inst 1992;84:1336–1341.

145. Stewart A, Westley B, May F. Modulation of the proliferative response of breast cancer cells to growth factors by oestrogen. Br J Cancer 1992;66:640–648.

146. Costantino A, Milazzo G, Giorgino F, Russo P, Goldfine ID, Vigneri R, Belfiore A. Insulin-resistant MDA-MB231 human breast cancer cells contain a tyrosine kinase inhibiting activity. Mol Endocrinol 1993;7:1667–1676.

147. Sepp-Lorenzino L, Rosen N, Lebwohl DE. Insulin and insulin-like growth factor signaling are defective in the MDA MB-468 human breast cancer cell line. Cell Growth Differ 1994;5:1077–1083.

148. Rubin R, Baserga R. Insulin-like growth factor-I receptor. Its role in cell proliferation, apoptosis, and tumorigenicity. Lab Invest 1995;73:311–331.

149. Gooch JL, Van Den Berg CL, Yee D. Insulin-like growth factor (IGF)-I rescues breast cancer cells from chemotherapy-induced cell death: proliferative and antiapoptotic effects. Breast Cancer Res Treat 1998;56:1–10.

150. Dunn SE, Hardman RA, Kari FW, Barrett JC. Insulin-like growth factor 1 (IGF-1) alters drug sensitivity of HBL100 human breast cancer cells by inhibition of apoptosis induced by diverse anticancer drugs. Cancer Res 1997;57:2687–2693.

151. Doerr ME, Jones JI. The roles of integrins and extracellular matrix proteins in the insulin-like growth factor I-stimulated chemotaxis of human breast cancer cells. J Biol Chem 1996;271:2443–2447.

152. Jones JI, Prevette T, Gockerman A, Clemmons DR. Ligand occupancy of the alpha-V-beta3 integrin is necessary for smooth muscle cells to migrate in response to insulin-like growth factor. Proc Natl Acad Sci USA 1996;93:2482–2487.

153. Dunn SE, Ehrlich M, Sharp NJ, Reiss K, Solomon G, Hawkins R, Baserga R, Barrett JC. A dominant negative mutant of the insulin-like growth factor-I receptor inhibits the adhesion, invasion, and metastasis of breast cancer. Cancer Res 1998;58:3353–3361.

154. Daly R, Harris W, Wang D, Darbre P. Autocrine production of insulin like growth factor-II using an inducible expression system results in reduced estrogen sensitivity of MCF-7 human breast cancer cells. Cell Growth Differ 1991;2:457–464.

155. Cullen K, Lippman M, Chow D, Hill S, Rosen N, Zwiebel J. Insulin-like growth factor-II over expression in MCF-7 cells induces phenotypic chances associated with malignant progression. Mol Endocrinol 1992;6:91–100.

156. Daws MR, Westley BR, May FE. Paradoxical effects of overexpression of the type I insulin-like growth factor (IGF) receptor on the responsiveness of human breast cancer cells to IGFs and estradiol. Endocrinology 1996;137:1177–1186.

157. Guvakova MA, Surmacz E. Overexpressed IGF-I receptors reduce estrogen growth requirements, enhance survival, and promote E-cadherin-mediated cell–cell adhesion in human breast cancer cells. Exp Cell Res 1997;231:149–162.

158. Nolan MK, Jankowska L, Prisco M, Xu S, Guvakova MA, Surmacz E. Differential roles of IRS-1 and SHC signaling pathways in breast cancer cells. Int J Cancer 1997;72:828–834.

159. Jackson JG, White MF, Yee D. Insulin receptor substrate-1 is the predominant signaling molecule activated by insulin-like growth factor-I, insulin, and interleukin-4 in estrogen receptor-positive human breast cancer cells. J Biol Chem 1998;273:9994–10,003.

160. Dufourny B, Alblas J, van Teeffelen HAAM, van Schaik FMA, van der Burg B, Steenbergh PH, Sussenbach JS. Mitogenic signaling of insulin-like growth factor I in MCF-7 human breast cancer cells requires phosphatidylinositol 3-kinase and is independent of mitogen-activated protein kinase. J Biol Chem 1997;272:31,163–31,171.

161. Katzenellenbogen B, Norman MJ. Multihormonal regulation of the progesterone receptor in MCF-7 human breast cancer cells: interrelationships among insulin/insulin-like growth factor-I, serum, and estrogen. Endocrinology 1990;126:891–898.

162. Cho H, Aronica S, Katzenellenbogen BS. Regulation of progesterone receptor gene expression in MCF-7 breast cancer cells: a comparison of the effects of cyclic adenosine 3'-5'-monophosphate, estradiol, insulin-like growth factor-I and serum factors. Endocrinology 1994;134:658–664.

163. Aronica SM, Katzenellenbogen BS. Stimulation of estrogen receptor-mediated transcription and alteration in the phosphorylation state of the rat uterine estrogen receptor by estrogen, cyclic adenosine monophosphate, and insulin-like growth factor-I. Mol Endocrinol 1993;7:743–752.

164. Kato S, Endoh H, Masuhiro Y, Kitamoto T, Uchiyama S, Sasaki H, et al. Activation of the estrogen receptor through phosphorylation by mitogen-activated protein kinase. Science 1995;270:1491–1494.

165. Bunone G, Briand PA, Miksicek RJ, Picard D. Activation of the unliganded estrogen receptor by EGF involves the MAP kinase pathway and direct phosphorylation. EMBO J 1996;15:2174–2183.

166. Lee AV, Weng CN, Jackson JG, Yee D. Activation of estrogen receptor-mediated gene transcription by IGF-I in human breast cancer cells. J Endocrinol 1997;152:39- 47.

167. Curtis SW, Washburn T, Sewall C, DiAugustine R, Lindzey J, Couse JF, Korach KS. Physiological coupling of growth factor and steroid receptor signaling pathways: estrogen receptor knockout mice lack estrogen-like response to epidermal growth factor. Proc Natl Acad Sci USA 1996;93:12,626–12,630.

168. Horwitz KB, Jackson TA, Bain DL, Richer JK, Takimoto GS, Tung L. Nuclear receptor coactivators and corepressors. Mol Endocrinol 1996;10:1167–1177.

169. Ahmed SR, Manni A, Gray G, Hammond JM. Characterisation and hormonal regulation of radioimmunoassayable IGF-I (insulin-like growth factor I) like activity and IGF-binding proteins secreted by human breast cancer cells. Anticancer Res 1990;10:1217–1223.

170. Yee D, Paik S, Levovic GS, Marcus RR, Favoni RE, Cullen KJ, Lippman ME, Rosen N. Analysis of insulin-like growth factor I gene expression in malignancy: evidence for a paracrine role in human breast cancer. Mol Endocrinol 1989;3:509–517.

171. Giani C, Cullen KJ, Campani D, Rasmussen A. IGF-II mRNA and protein are expressed in the stroma of invasive breast cancers: an in situ hybridization and immunohistochemistry study. Breast Cancer Res Treat 1996;41:43–50.

172. Paik S. Expression of IGF-I and IGF-II mRNA in breast tissue. Breast Cancer Res Treat 1992;22:31–38.

173. Toropainen EM, Lipponen PK, Syrjanen KJ. Expression of insulin-like growth factor II in human breast cancer as related to established prognostic factors and long-term prognosis. Anticancer Res 1995;15:2669–2674.

174. Cullen K, Yee D, Sly W, Perdue J, Hampton B, Lippman M, Rosen N. Insulin-like growth factor receptor expression and function in human breast cancer. Cancer Res 1990;50:48–53.

175. Singer C, Rasmussen A, Smith HS, Lippman ME, Lynch T, Cullen KJ. Malignant breast epithelium selects for insulin-like growth factor II expression in breast stroma: evidence for paracrine function. Cancer Res 1995;55:2448–2454.

176. Yang XF, Beamer WG, Huynh H, Pollak M. Reduced growth of human breast cancer xenografts in hosts homozygous for the lit mutation. Cancer Res 1996;56:1509–1511.

177. Pollak MN. Endocrine effects of IGF-I on normal and transformed breast epithelial cells: potential relevance to strategies for breast cancer treatment and prevention. Breast Cancer Res Treat 1998;47:209–217.

178. Westley BR, May FEB. Role of insulin-like growth factors in steroid modulated proliferation. J Steroid Biochem Mol Biol 1994;51:1–9.

179. Guvakova MA, Surmacz E. Tamoxifen interferes with the insulin-like growth factor I receptor (IGF-IR) signaling pathway in breast cancer cells. Cancer Res 1997;57:2606- 2610.

180. Milazzo G, Giorgino F, Damante G, Sung C, Stampfer M, Vigneri R, Goldfine I, Belfiore A. Insulin receptor expression and function in human breast cancer cell lines. Cancer Res 1992;52:3924–3930.

181. Peyrat J-P, Bonneterre J, Beuscart J, Dijane J, Demaille A. Insulin-like growth factor I receptors in human breast cancer and their relationship to estradiol and progesterone receptors. Cancer Res 1988;48: 6429–6433.

182. Turner BC, Haffty BG, Narayanan L, Yuan J, Havre PA, Gumbs AA, et al. Insulin-like growth factor-I receptor overexpression mediates cellular radioresistance and local breast cancer recurrence after lumpectomy and radiation. Cancer Res 1997;57:3079–3083.

183. Resnik JL, Reichart DB, Huey K, Webster NJ, Seely BL. Elevated insulin-like growth factor I receptor autophosphorylation and kinase activity in human breast cancer. Cancer Res 1998;58:1159–1164.

184. Yee D, Sharma J, Hilsenbeck SG. Prognostic significance of insulin-like growth factor-binding protein expression in axillary lymph node-negative breast cancer. J Natl Cancer Inst 1994;86:1785–1789.

185. Swisshelm K, Ryan K, Tsuchiya K, Sager R. Enhanced expression of an insulin growth factor-like binding protein (mac25) in senescent human mammary epithelial cells and induced expression with retinoic acid. Proc Natl Acad Sci USA 1995;92:4472–4476.

186. Burger AM, Zhang X, Li H, Ostrowski JL, Beatty B, Venanzoni M, Papas T, Seth A. Down-regulation of T1A12/mac25, a novel insulin-like growth factor binding protein related gene, is associated with disease progression in breast carcinomas. Oncogene 1998;16:2459–2467.

187. Yu H, Levesque MA, Khosravi MJ, Papanastasiou-Diamandi A, Clark GM, Diamandis EP. Associations between insulin-like growth factors and their binding proteins and other prognostic indicators in human breast cancer. Br J Cancer 1996;74:1242–1247.

188. Papa V, Gliozzo B, Clark G, McGuire W, Moore D, Fujita-Yamaguchi Y, et al. Insulin-like growth factor-I receptors are overexpressed and predict a low risk in human breast cancer. Cancer Res 1993; 53:3736–3740.

189. Bonneterre J, Peyrat JP, Beuscart R, Demaille A. Prognostic significance of insulin-like growth factor I receptors in human breast cancer. Cancer Res 1990;50:6931–6935.

190. Rocha RL, Hilsenbeck SG, Jackson JG, Van Den Berg CL, Weng C-N, Lee AV, Yee D. Insulin-like growth factor binding protein-3 and insulin receptor substrate-1 in breast cancer: correlation with clinical parameters and disease-free survival. Clin Cancer Res 1997;3:103–109.

191. Baserga R. Controlling IGF-receptor function: a possible strategy for tumor therapy. Trends Biotech 1996;14:150–152.

192. Baserga R. The insulin-like growth factor I receptor: a key to tumor growth? Cancer Res 1995;55: 249–252.

193. D'Ambrosio C, Ferber A, Resnicoff M, Baserga R. A soluble insulin-like growth factor I receptor that induces apoptosis of tumor cells in vivo and inhibits tumorigenesis. Cancer Res 1996;56:4013–4020.

194. Neuenschwander S, Roberts CT, Leroith D. Growth inhibition of human breast cancer cells by stable expression of an insulin-like growth factor I receptor antisense ribonucleic acid. Endocrinology 1995; 136:4298–4303.

195. Yee D, Jackson JG, Kozelsky TW, Figueroa JA. Insulin-like growth factor binding protein 1 expression inhibits insulin-like growth factor I action in MCF-7 cells. Cell Growth Differ 1994;5:73–77.

196. Arteaga CL, Osborne CK. Growth inhibition of human breast cancer cells *in vitro* with an antibody against the type I somatomedin receptor. Cancer Res 1989;49:6237- 6241.

197. Arteaga CL, Kitten LJ, Coronado EB, Jacobs S, Kull FC Jr, Allred DC, Osborne CK. Blockade of the type I somatomedin receptor inhibits growth of human breast cancer cells in athymic mice. J Clin Invest 1989;84:1418–1423.

198. Brunner N, Yee D, Kern FG, Spangthomsen M, Lippman ME, Cullen KJ. Effect of endocrine therapy on growth of T61 human breast cancer xenografts is directly correlated to a specific down-regulation of insulin-like growth factor-II (IGF-II). Eur J Cancer 1993;29A:562–569.

199. Ray BS, Pearson OH. Hypophysectomy in treatment of disseminated breast cancer. Surg Oncol Clin N Am 1962;12:419–433.

200. Di Leo A, Ferrari L, Bajetta E, Bartoli C, Vicario G, Moglia D, et al. Biological and clinical evaluation of lanreotide (BIM 23014), a somatostatin analogue, in the treatment of advanced breast cancer. A pilot study by the I.T.M.O. group. Italian Trials in Medical Oncology. Breast Cancer Res Treat 1995;34: 237–244.

201. Canobbio L, Cannata D, Miglietta L, Boccardo F. Somatuline (BIM 23014) and tamoxifen treatment of postmenopausal breast cancer patients: clinical activity and effect on insulin-like growth factor-I (IGF-I) levels. Anticancer Res 1995;15:2687–2690.

202. Weckbecker G, Tolcsvai L, Stolz B, Pollak M, Bruns C. Somatostatin analogue octreotide enhances the antineoplastic effects of tamoxifen and ovariectomy on 7,12-dimethylbenz(alpha)anthracene-induced rat mammary carcinomas. Cancer Res 1994;54:6334–6337.

203. Bontenbal M, Foekens JA, Lamberts SW, de Jong FH, van Putten WL, Braun HJ, et al. Feasibility, endocrine and anti-tumour effects of a triple endocrine therapy with tamoxifen, a somatostatin analogue and an antiprolactin in post-menopausal metastatic breast cancer: a randomized study with long-term follow-up. Br J Cancer 1998;77:115–122.

204. Baselga J, Tripathy D, Mendelsohn J, Baughman S, Benz CC, Dantis L, et al. Phase II study of weekly intravenous recombinant humanized anti-p185HER2 monoclonal antibody in patients with HER2/neu-overexpressing metastatic breast cancer. J Clin Oncol 1996;14:737–744.

205. Pegram MD, Lipton A, Hayes DF, Weber BL, Baselga JM, Tripathy D, et al. Phase II study of receptor-enhanced chemosensitivity using recombinant humanized anti-p185HER2/neu monoclonal antibody plus cisplatin in patients with HER2/neu-overexpressing metastatic breast cancer refractory to chemotherapy treatment. J Clin Oncol 1998;16:2659–2671.

206. Slamon DJ, Clark GM, Wong SG, Levin WJ, Ullrich A, McGuire WL. Human breast cancer: correlation of relapse and survival with amplification of the HER-2/neu oncogene. Science 1987;235:177–182.

11

Insulin-Like Growth Factor Binding Proteins in Endocrine-Related Neoplasia

Giuseppe Minniti, MD and Youngman Oh, PHD

CONTENTS

INTRODUCTION
IGFBPs: STRUCTURE AND FUNCTION
IGFBPs IN BC
PROSTATE CANCER
ENDOMETRIAL CANCER AND OC
CONCLUSION
REFERENCES

INTRODUCTION

The insulin-like growth factor binding proteins (IGFBPs) are components of the IGF signaling system, which is comprised additionally of the IGF-I, IGF-II, and insulin ligands, and a family of transmembrane receptors, including the insulin receptor (IR) and IGF-I and IGF-II receptors (IGF-IR and IGF-IIR) *(1–3)*. Six IGFBPs have been identified, cloned, and sequenced *(3–5)*. They share a high degree of similarity in their primary protein structure, particularly in their N- and C-terminal regions, which are separated by a variable midprotein segment of 55–95 amino acid residues *(5)*. IGFBPs bind IGF-I and IGF-II, but not insulin, with high affinity *(6)*, and are essential to transport IGFs, to prolong their half-lives, and to regulate the availability of free IGFs for interaction with IGFRs, thereby modulating the effects of IGFs on growth and differentiation *(6–10)*. Recent evidence indicates that some IGFBPs may themselves have direct receptor-mediated effects, independent of IGFs. A growing body of data has demonstrated that IGFBP-3 is an important growth-suppressing factor in various cell systems, through an IGF-independent mechanism *(11,12)*. In addition, the recent identification of proteins with significant similarity to IGFBPs in their N-terminal domains suggests the existence of other potential IGFBPs *(13)*. This has led to the concept of an IGFBP superfamily with high- and low-affinity members, capable of influencing cell growth and differentiation by both IGF-dependent and IGF-independent means (Fig. 1, *13–15*).

From: *Contemporary Endocrinology: Endocrine Oncology*
Edited by: S. P. Ethier © Humana Press Inc., Totowa, NJ

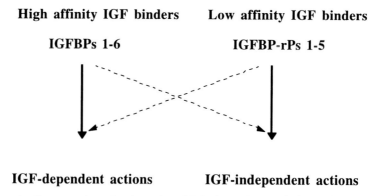

High affinity IGF binders   **Low affinity IGF binders**

IGFBPs 1-6   **IGFBP-rPs 1-5**

IGF-dependent actions   **IGF-independent actions**

Fig. 1. Schematic diagram of mechanisms for IGF-independent and -dependent antiproliferative actions of IGFBP superfamily.

Despite recent progress, several questions remain regarding the interaction of the IGFBPs with the IGFs and their receptors, the signaling pathways involved in IGF-independent action, and the role of some posttranslational modifications of IGFBPs that can alter their biological activity. In this chapter, the role of IGFBPs in human endocrine neoplasia is presented in the light of recent experimental and clinical evidence, especially IGF-independent antiproliferative action of IGFBP-3 and the role of the new low-affinity members of the IGFBP family.

IGFBPs: STRUCTURE AND FUNCTION

Structure

Six IGFBPs that bind IGFs with high affinity, designated IGFBP-1–6, have been well characterized *(3–6,13)*. They share a high degree of amino acid sequence similarity in their N- and C-terminal regions, including conserved cysteine (Cys) residues *(13)*. The N-terminal amino acid sequences of these proteins have an average of 58% similarity and contain 12 Cys; in IGFBP-1–5 these Cys are well conserved, and, in IGFBP-6, 10/12 are invariant. Within this region, a local motif, GCGCCXXC, is well conserved in IGFBP-1–5; in IGFBP-6, it is substituted with GCAEAEGC. The significance of this motif has not been elucidated. The C-terminal regions of the IGFBPs are also highly conserved and share a similarity of more than 30%, with six Cys strictly conserved. The N- and C-terminal regions are responsible for the high affinity binding to IGFs, and are separated by a variable midprotein region of 55–95 amino acids.

Recently, a group of Cys-rich proteins, with structural similarities to the IGFBPs and demonstrably lower affinity for IGFs, have been identified *(16–18)*, and it is proposed that these IGFBP-related proteins (IGFBP-rPs) and the classical IGFBPs constitute an IGFBP superfamily, as shown in (Table 1 *(14,15)*. Mac25 (renamed IGFBP-rP1) was originally cloned from leptomeninges *(19)*, and subsequently from human bladder carcinoma *(20)* and breast carcinoma cell lines *(21)*. The human connective tissue growth factor (IGFBP-rP2) *(22)*, nephroblastoma overexpression gene, NovH (IGFBP-rP3) *(23)*, and Cyr61 (provisional IGFBP-rP4) *(24)*, are members of the CCN family of proteins *(25)*. The CCN proteins are highly related, comprised of four protein domains, and share an overall similarity of 46% *(25)*. Within these four IGFBP-rPs, 11/12 Cys found in the

Table 1
Structural Characteristics of the Human IGFBP Superfamily

	Mol wt (kDa)[a]	No. of amino acids	No. of cysteines	N-linked glycosylation	Chromosomal location	mRNA size (kb)	Gene size (kb)
IGFBP: high-affinity IGF binder							
IGFBP-1	25.3	234	18	No	7p	1.6	5.2
IGFBP-2	31.4	289	18	No	2q	1.5	32
IGFBP-3	28.7	264	18	Yes	7p	2.4	10
IGFBP-4	26.0	237	20	Yes	17q	1.7	14
IGFBP-5	28.6	252	18	No	2q	1.7	33
IGFBP-6	22.8	216	16	No	12	1.1	?
IGFBP-related protein[b]: low-affinity IGF binder							
IGFBP-rP1	26.4	256	18	Yes	4q	1.1	>30
IGFBP-rP2	35.5	349 (pre)[c]	39	Yes	6q	2.4	?
IGFBP-rP3	36.0	357 (pre)	41	? (No)	8q	2.4	~7
IGFBP-rP4	39.5	381 (pre)	35	? (No)	1p	2.5	?
IGFBP-rP5	51.3	480 (pre)	16	?	?	2.3	?

[a] kDa, kiloDalton

[b] IGFBP-rP1, Mac25/TAF/PSF/IGFBP-7; IGFBP-rP2, CTGF; IGFBP-rP3, NovH; IGFBP-rP4, Cyr61; IGFBP-rP5, L56.

[c] pre = prepeptide.

N-terminus of the IGFBPs are conserved, as well as the GCGCCXXC motif *(13)*. Another related protein, L-56 (provisional IGFBP-rP5), shares 39% similarity with the IGFBP N-terminal domain, and retains all 12 conserved Cys in this region *(26)*.

With the discovery of these an Cys-rich proteins closely related to an IGFBPs, the concept of an IGFBP family is changing, and new nomenclature for the IGFBP superfamily has been proposed. IGFBPs, therefore, may be derived from an ancestor gene/protein that was involved in the regulation of cell growth and was capable of binding IGFs. In the course of evolution, some members evolved into high-affinity IGF binders (IGFBPs), and others into low-affinity binders (IGFBP-rPs), conferring to the IGF superfamily the ability to influence cell growth by both IGF-dependent and IGF-independent mechanisms.

Function

The current belief is that IGFBPs bind IGFs with high affinity to transport IGFs in circulation and modulate their availability to IGF receptors. The predominant IGFBP in humans is IGFBP-3. Most of the circulating IGF is sequestered by IGFBP-3 in a 150-kDa ternary complex, with a bound acid-labile subunit (ALS) *(27–29)*. When associated with the 150-kDa complex, the IGFs do not cross the capillary barrier *(29)*, and their half-life can be as long as 12 h; the half-life of free IGFs is less than 10 min *(30)*. However, IGFBPs are not simply carriers of IGFs, but also influence IGF function, either inhibiting or augmenting IGF action. Regulation of the interaction of IGFs with IGFRs by IGFBPs involves several factors: IGFBP affinity for IGFs, the association of the IGFBPs with proteins on the cell surface or in the extracellular matrix (ECM) *(5,6,9)*, and posttranslational modifications of IGFBPs, such as phosphorylation *(31–34)*, glycosylation *(6,9,35)*, and proteolysis *(36–47)*.

IGF-Dependent Action of the IGFBPs

IGFBP-1 appears to be involved in a variety of metabolic and reproductive processes *(9,10)*. Both insulin-dependent diabetes mellitus and fasting result in increased IGFBP-1 *(48,49)*. Inhibition of IGFBP-1 production by insulin and stimulation by glucocorticoids are responsible for much of the change in IGFBP-1 expression associated with catabolic processes *(49)*. IGFBP-1 is the predominant IGFBP in amniotic fluid *(50)*, suggesting involvement in gestational development, as well as in reproductive function, including the endometrial cycle and ovulation *(51,52)*. IGFBP-1 has been reported to inhibit IGF actions in various cell systems, including porcine aortic smooth muscle cells, fibroblasts, cultured human granulosa, and lutheal cells, as the result of the formation of IGF/IGFBP-1 complexes that cannot bind to the IGFR *(6,9)*.

IGFBP-2 is a nonglycosylated, nonphosphorylated IGFBP *(5)*, which is readily detectable in serum, as well as in cerebrospinal, follicular, endometrial, and seminal fluids *(9,10)*. In general, IGFBP-2 appears to inhibit IGF actions in some cell lines, such as chick embryo fibroblast *(53)* and human lung cancer cells *(54)*; however, in porcine aortic smooth cells, IGFBP-2 was shown to potentiate the response to IGF-1 *(55)*.

IGFBP-3 is the major form of binding protein present in human circulation, and exhibits a molecular mass of 38–43 kDa, depending on glycosylation status *(5,9)*. In circulation, IGFBP-3 is associated with IGFs and ALS to form a ternary complex of 150–200 kDa *(27–29)*. IGFBP-3 has also been found in several biological fluids, including urine, synovial fluid, milk, amniotic, and seminal fluids *(10)*. IGFBP-3 undergoes posttranslational modifications, including glycosylation *(35)*, phosphorylation *(33,34)*, and proteolysis *(36–47)*. There are no significant differences in affinity for IGF-1 between glycosylated and nonglycosylated IGFBP-3 (35), nor does direct mutagenesis of phosphorylated serines (Ser) affect IGF-binding characteristics (33). IGFBP-3 also has ability to bind proteoglycans on the ECM via heparin-binding motifs in the C-terminus. This ECM association of IGFBP-3 may contribute to the potentiation of IGF actions in some cell systems *(56)*.

IGFBP-4 is the smallest of the IGFBPs, and is present in biological fluids as a 24-kDa nonglycosylated form and a 28-kDa glycosylated species *(57,58)*. IGFBP-4 appears to be a potent inhibitor of IGF action in several human cell lines *(59–61)*, but there have been no reports to indicate a potentiation of IGF-stimulated cell proliferation.

IGFBP-5 is abundant in connective tissue, and is the predominant IGFBP in bone extracts, but is present at a very low concentration in serum *(62–64)*. There are heparin-binding motifs present in the C-terminus, and it has been demonstrated that IGFBP-5 adheres to the ECM and potentiates the effect of IGF-I on cell growth in bone *(65,66)*. When IGFBP-5 is associated with the ECM, its affinity for IGF-I is strongly reduced, explaining at least partially the ability of ECM-associated IGFBP-5 to potentiate IGF action. In contrast, IGFBP-5 exerts an inhibitory effect on follicle-stimulating hormone-stimulated steroidogenesis in granulosa cells, and also inhibits IGF-mediated cell maturation and proliferation, suggesting an important role in the process of follicular selection of the ovarian cycle *(67)*.

IGFBP-6 is a 30-kDa glycosylated protein present in serum and cerebrospinal and amniotic fluids *(10)*. Studies of IGFBP-6 in vivo and in vitro are limited; however, a recent paper *(68)* reports an antigonadotropic effect of IGFBP-6 in ovary, suggesting a possible role of this protein in female reproductive function.

IGF-dependent actions of IGFBP-rPs are not yet elucidated. The fact that these IGFBP-rPs exhibit significantly lower affinity for IGFs suggests that their primary function may not be regulating IGF action *(16–18)*.

IGF-Independent Action of IGFBPs

Recently, several experimental results have indicated that the IGFBPs might have their own biological actions beyond their ability to regulate IGF action. In addition to their structural and sequence similarity, some IGFBPs appear to possess unique characteristics. Ser phosphorylation occurs in IGFBP-1 *(32)*, and -3 *(33,34)*; IGFBP-1 and -2 contain the integrin receptor recognition sequence, Arg-Gly-Asp (RGD sequence) *(6,9)*; IGFBP-3, -5, and -6 contain heparin binding motifs *(6,9)*; and IGFBP-3 has a nuclear localization sequence, and can be translocated to the nucleus *(69,70)*.

The functional importance of specific binding of IGFBP-1 to the $\alpha5\beta1$-integrin receptor on the cell surface has been demonstrated in Chinese hamster ovary cells, in which IGFBP-1 treatment results in stimulation of cell migration in an IGF-independent manner *(71)*. IGFBP-2, which contains the RGD sequence, may also bind to integrins and exert IGF-independent action, although this has not yet been demonstrated.

The observation that IGFBP-3, -5, and -6 bind to heparin- or heparin-sulfate-containing proteoglycans in the ECM suggests IGF-dependent, as well as IGF-independent action of these IGFBPs. When IGFBP-5 is associated with ECM, its affinity for IGF-I is strongly reduced, explaining the ability of ECM-associated IGFBP-5 to potentiate IGF action *(65,66)*; however, the cell-surface association of IGFBP-5 could also mediate IGF-independent actions of IGFBP-5. Andress and Birbaum *(72)* have demonstrated that either a carboxyl-truncated form of IGFBP-5, derived from U2 osteosarcoma cells, or human recombinant carboxyl-truncated IGFBP-5[1-169] *(73)* can stimulate mitogenesis in osteoblasts, in absence of exogenous IGF-I, suggesting an IGF-independent mechanism.

IGFBP-3 is also a well-documented inhibitor of cell proliferation. Although restricting IGF access to the IGFRs appears to be an important mechanism by which IGFBP-3 inhibits cell growth, there is increasing evidence that IGFBP-3 by itself exerts an IGF-independent action through its own putative receptor *(74–81)*. This action seems to be important, especially in growth inhibition of some breast cancer (BC) and prostate cancer (PC) cell lines (*see* below).

The physiological functions of IGFBP-rPs, either in vitro or in vivo are not clear. IGFBP-rP1 has been detected in normal serum, urine, and amniotic, and cerebrospinal fluids, but its function is unknown *(21)*. IGFBP-rP1 mRNA has been detected in a wide range of normal tissues, including breast *(82)*, small intestine, colon, ovary, prostate, testes, heart, kidney, and pancreas *(16)*, and appears to be absent in various tumors, such as BC *(82)*, glioblastoma *(83)*, squamous cell carcinoma *(83)*, and in several cancer cell lines *(16)*, suggesting that IGFBP-rP1 may function as a growth-suppressing factor.

IGFBP-rP2 has been demonstrated in various human biological fluids, such as normal and pregnancy serum, and cerebrospinal, amniotic, follicular, and peritoneal fluids *(84)*. Some experimental evidence suggests that IGFBP-rP2 mediates the effects of transforming growth factor β (TGF-β) in some physiological and pathological processes, including wound repair *(85,86)* and atherosclerosis *(86)*.

IGFBP-rP3 has been recently identified in several human biological fluids, such as normal and pregnancy serum, and cerebrospinal, amniotic, and follicular fluids *(18)*. Moreover,

IGFBP-rP3 mRNA is widely distributed in several human tissues, especially prostate, testes, heart, brain, and pancreas, consistent with the hypothesis that IGFBP-rP3 may be involved in cell growth regulation. So far, its function is unknown *(18)*.

The provisional IGFBP-rP4, Cyr61, was identified in the mouse *(24)*, and the human counterpart has not yet been found *(86)*. In vitro, IGFBP-rP4 has no detectable mitogenic activity itself, but seems to potentiate the mitogenic effects of other growth factors, such as fibroblast growth factor, on fibroblasts and endothelial cells *(87)*.

Proteolysis of IGFBPs

Proteolysis has been shown for all IGFBPs. Several proteases have been identified in serum and other biological fluids, including the Ser proteases, plasmin, thrombin, and prostate-specific antigen (PSA); the acid protease, cathepsin, and the matrix, metallo-protease *(36–47)*.

IGFBP-3 can be specifically proteolyzed under various conditions, and an increase in proteolytic activity has been observed under different physiological and pathological circumstances *(8,44)*. Proteolysis reduces the affinity of IGFBP-3 for IGFs, and potentiates IGF-I action through a sustained release of free IGF-I available for the IGFR *(35,44)*. More recently, IGFBP-3 fragments, derived from in vitro plasmin digestion, have been shown to inhibit the mitogenic effects of IGF-I and insulin, including insulin-induced autophosphorylation of the IR, and subsequent IR substrate I phosphorylation in IR-over-expressing NIH-3T3 cells *(88,89)*, suggesting an IGF-independent biological activity of IGFBP-3 proteolytic fragments.

IGFBP-4 is cleaved by a specific protease that is activated in presence of IGF-I or IGF-II *(38,39,61)*. Proteolysis results in two fragments of 14 and 18 kDa, which appear to have very low or no IGF-binding capacity; as a consequence, proteolysis has been suggested as a mechanism whereby the inhibitory effect of IGFBP-4 can be relieved.

Proteolysis of IGFBP-5 results in fragments of approx 23, 20, and 17 kDa *(42,64)*; but the role of proteolysis is still unclear, because the fragments do not potentiate cell growth response to IGFs. However, the demonstration that the proteolytic 23-kDa IGFBP-5 fragment may stimulate mitogenesis in osteoblasts in the absence of exogenous IGF-I *(72,73)* suggests that IGFBP-5 proteolysis could be an important mechanism for regulating cell growth and proliferation, in an IGF-independent manner.

IGFBPs IN BC

Most neoplastic cells produce IGFBPs, which can regulate the biological activity of the IGFs in an autocrine and paracrine manner *(91)*. The expression pattern of IGFBPs is altered in cancer cells, compared with counterpart normal cells, again suggesting a specific role for IGFBPs in cancer. The direct biological function of IGFBPs has been extensively studied in endocrine-related neoplasia, such as BC, PC, ovaryian cancer (OC), and endometrial cancer.

The IGFs are important regulators of mammary epithelial cell (EC) growth, and play an important role in BC development *(90–94)*. Both IGF-I and IGF-II have been shown to be potent mitogens for a number of BC cell lines in vitro *(92)*, and IGF-I and IGF-II, as well as IGF-IR mRNA, are detectable in the majority of human breast tumor specimens *(93–95)*. The importance of the IGF system in the development of BC has been recently addressed by Hankinson et al. *(96)* in a large clinical case-control prospective study. In an investigation of the relationship of circulating IGF-I and IGFBP-3 plasma levels to the risk of BC, they found a positive correlation between IGF-I concentration and BC risk in premenopausal women. The risk of developing cancer dramatically increased in premenopausal women when plasma IGF-1 levels were adjusted for IGFBP-3 levels, suggesting a potential role for IGFBPs in the development of BC.

In BC, the predominant secreted IGFBP appears to correlate with the estrogen receptor status of the cells *(97,98)*. Estrogen-responsive cells secrete IGFBP-2 and IGFBP-4 as major species, and IGFBP-3 and IGFBP-5 as minor binding proteins; estrogen-non-responsive cells predominantly secrete IGFBP-3 and IGFBP-4, and, to a lesser extent, IGFBP-6. This clearly implies that IGF system is complex, and, depending on estrogen receptor status, the cellular response of IGFBPs to IGFs may be significantly different.

IGFBP-3 is the binding protein most extensively studied in BC. It appears to inhibit cell growth by modulating the biological action of IGFs, by regulating IGF availability to bind IGFRs (IGF-dependent action), or by exerting its own biological action directly in the target cells (IGF-independent action). In general, the binding affinity of IGFs for IGFBP-3 is higher than that of IGFRs, implying that IGFBP-3 can modulate IGF binding to its receptor, thereby blocking IGF's biological actions in the local environment. Co-incubation of cells with IGFBP-3 and IGFs results in an inhibition of the IGF-stimulated mitogenic effect in human BC cells in vitro *(99)*, suggesting that the paracrine or autocrine effects of IGFs can be modulated by IGFBP-3 produced by ECs and stromal fibroblasts.

In human BC cells, expression of IGFBP-3 is hormonally regulated: estrogens inhibit the expression of IGFBP-3 in estrogen-responsive MCF-7 human BC cells; antiestrogens, such as tamoxifen (TAM) and ICI182780, stimulate its production *(100)*. Proteolysis of IGFBP-3 may be an additional factor in this system, resulting in a lower affinity of IGFBP-3 for IGFs, thereby increasing the availability of IGFs to IGFRs. IGFBP-3 can be proteolyzed by proteases, such as cathepsin, PSA, and plasmin, all of which are detected in human BC cells *(41,44,101,102)*.

Restricting IGF access to the IGFR is an important mechanism by which IGFBP-3 inhibits mitogenic effects of IGF-I in human BC, recent data in estrogen-nonresponsive Hs578T and MDA-MB231 human BC cells suggest that IGFBP-3 inhibits cell growth by an IGF-independent mechanism, potentially mediated through an IGFBP-3 receptor *(75–78)*. In Hs578T cells, IGFs and their analogs, des-(1-3)-IGF-I and [QAYL-L]-IGF-II, which have high affinity for the IGF-IR and reduced affinity for IGFBPs, have no effect on Hs578T cell proliferation *(75)*. Since both IGFs and their analogs show no effect on Hs578T cells, the failure of IGFs to stimulate cell growth cannot be attributed to interference by endogenous IGFBPs. However, treatment with recombinant human IGFBP-3 shows a significant inhibitory effect on monolayer growth of Hs578T cells, and co-incubation of IGFBP-3 with [QAYL-L]-IGF-II did not result in attenuation of the IGFBP-3 inhibitory effect. In contrast, IGF-II, which binds with high affinity to IGFBP-3, is able to attenuate its inhibitory effect. Similar findings have been observed with IGF-I and IGF-I analogs, indicating that inhibitory action of IGFBP-3 cannot be attributed to blocking IGFs access to the IGFR. Taken together, these data suggest that IGFBP-3 can directly inhibit Hs578T cells, and that IGFs prevent the inhibitory effect by forming IGF–IGFBP-3 complexes. These observations provide the foundation for the concept of IGF-independent actions of IGFBP-3.

Affinity crosslinking of Hs578T monolayers and cell lysates with [^{125}I]-IGFBP-3 has been employed to investigate possible mechanisms for the cell surface interaction of

IGFBP-3 *(77)*. These studies revealed that IGFBP-3 interacts with a 25-kDa protein on the cell surface, and with 25-, 28-, and 55-kDa species in cell lysates. IGFBP-3 binding to these proteins appears to be specific, as demonstrated by a dose-dependent displacement of $[^{125}I]$-IGFBP-3 by unlabeled IGFBP-3; immunoprecipitation of IGFBP-3 with specific antibodies, but not with nonimmune serum; and Western ligand blots of cell lysates with $[^{125}I]$-IGFBP-3 reveals three proteins of the same size as those observed in cell lysate crosslinking experiments. More recently, some experimental evidence seems to indicate that the type V TGF-β receptor is the putative IGFBP-3 receptor *(103)*; however, further studies are needed to confirm this finding.

Other studies have confirmed that IGFBP-3, and possibly the IGFBP-3/IGFBP-3 receptor complex, functions as a major growth-suppressing factor in various cell systems. These studies have shown that the growth rate of fibroblast is significantly reduced in IGFBP-3-transfected cells, with a targeted disruption of the IGF-IR gene *(80)*; purified mouse IGFBP-3 binds to chick embryo fibroblasts cell surface and inhibits cell growth *(104)*; upregulation of IGFBP-3 expression is correlated with retinoic acid (RA)-induced cell growth inhibition in cervical ECs *(105)*; and the tumor suppressor, p53, induces IGFBP-3 expression, indicating that IGFBP-3 may be a mediator in p53 signaling *(81)*. Further studies have revealed that various growth-inhibiting factors, such as TGF-β, RA, and antiestrogens, stimulate the expression and secretion of IGFBP-3 in human BC cells *(78,79,100)*. Oh et al. *(78)* have reported that the potent antiproliferative factors, TGF-β and RA, stimulate the expression and secretion of IGFBP-3 in human BC cells, suggesting that it may act as a mediator of their antiproliferative effects. Treatment with either RA or TGF-β stimulated IGFBP-3 gene expression and protein expression 2–3-fold, with a concurrent inhibition of cell growth. IGFBP-3 antisense oligodeoxynucleotide (ODN) and IGF analogs have been employed to demonstrate that IGFBP-3 mediates RA and TGF-β antiproliferative action. Inhibition of IGFBP-3 gene expression, using an IGFBP-3 antisense ODN, blocks RA- and TGF-β-induced IGFBP-3 production by up to 90%, and inhibits their antiproliferative effect by 40–60%. Treatment with IGF-II analogs, which retain affinity for IGFBPs, but significantly reduced affinity for the IGF-IR also diminished TGF-β-inhibitory effects; in contrast, treatment with [QAYL-L]-IGF-II, which has a significantly reduced affinity for both IGFBPs and the IGF-IR, resulted in no change of TGF-β-inhibitory effect.

These findings suggest that TGF-β- or RA-induced IGFBP-3 inhibits cell growth in an IGF-independent manner, and that IGF can modulate its inhibitory effect by forming an IGF-IGFBP-3 complex, thereby preventing IGFBP-3 action. Similar observations have been reported in MDA-MB231 cells *(79)*. The direct antiproliferative effect of IGFBP-3 via an IGFBP-3/IGFBP-3 receptor system, on the basis of these experimental data, may be a major mechanism in the inhibitory actions of TGF-β and RA on these cells.

The potent growth inhibitory effect of antiestrogens is associated with increases in both IGFBP-3 mRNA and protein levels in MCF-7 human BC cells *(100)*. In addition, treatment with recombinant IGFBP-3 inhibits basal and estradiol (E_2)-stimulated MCF-7 cell proliferation, and the use of IGFBP-3 antisense ODNs can reverse antiestrogen-induced inhibition of cell proliferation *(100)*. Taken together, these data suggest that the antiproliferative action of antiestrogens could be mediated, at least in part, by upregulation of IGFBP-3. Similarly, it has been shown that IGFBP-3 expression may be induced by other growth inhibitory factors, such as tumor necrosis factor α (TNF-α) and vitamin D analogs *(106,107)*. In MCF-7 cells, TNF-α stimulates the expression and secretion of IGFBP-3, moreover, IGFBP-3 antisense ODN treatment antagonizes TNF-α-induced inhibition of cell proliferation and IGFBP-3 accumulation, implicating IGFBP-3 as downstream effector in the inhibitory action of TNF-α (106). The two vitamin D analogs, EB 1089 and CB 1093, enhance the production of IGFBP-3 in Hs578T and MCF-7 cells, suggesting a role for IGFBP-3 in the growth-inhibitory effects of vitamin D analogs in BC (107).

Some experimental data support the ability of IGFBP-3 to induce apoptosis (108,109). In MCF-7 cells, treatment with recombinant human IGFBP-3 for 72 h has been shown to increase apoptosis and to inhibit [^{3}H]-thymidine incorporation (108). In Hs578T human BC cells, IGFBP-3 results in no direct induction of apoptosis; however, Gill et al. (109) demonstrated that preincubation of the cells with IGFBP-3 caused a dose-dependent potentiation of apoptosis by ceramide, an apoptotic-inducing reagent, suggesting the involvement of an IGF-independent activity of IGFBP-3.

Less is known about the role of the other IGFBPs in BC. An inhibitory role for IGFBP-5 in BC has been addressed. In MCF-7 cells, the vitamin D_3 analog [1,25(OH)$_2D_3$], and two related compounds, stimulated production of IGFBP-5 and indirectly suppressed cell proliferation (110). Moreover, like IGFBP-3, IGFBP-5 seems to mediate the antiproliferative effects of the antiestrogen, ICI 182780 (111), but it is not clear whether the effect of IGFBP-5 on cell growth involves IGF peptides.

Some recent clinical studies have found that the combination of high IGF-I and low IGFBP-3 levels are associated with ductal carcinoma *in situ* (112), and with the early stage of breast carcinoma (113). Moreover, premenopausal women with high IGFBP-3 plasma levels had a decreased risk for ductal carcinoma, addressing the importance of alterations of IGFBPs, either in the progression or development of BC. These findings provide a novel rationale for the use of TAM and other drugs (antagonists of growth hormone-releasing hormine or growth hormone, somatostatin analogs) that can interfere with the IGF system as chemopreventive agents in BC; however, further large clinical trials are needed to address this point. Small-scale clinical studies have addressed the effect of treatment with the antiestrogens, TAM and droloxifene, on the IGF system in advanced BC (114,115). No significant effects on IGFBP-3 levels were found, but the decreased levels of IGF-I, and the consequent decrease IGF:IGFBP-3 ratio, may explain, at least in part, the antitumoral effects of antiestrogen treatment in BC. Treatment with antiestrogens increases the concentration of IGFBP-1, which may contribute to the inhibition of the suggested proliferative effect of IGF-I in BC.

A possible role in BC has been suggested for the new low-affinity members of the IGFBP family. IGFBP-rP1 is produced by Hs578T cells, and its expression is upregulated by TGF-β (12,116). In addition, treatment with IGFBP-rP1 resulted in inhibition of DNA synthesis and cell proliferation in a dose-dependent manner. It is clear that IGFBP-rP1 primarily functions as a modulator of cell growth in an IGF-independent manner, similar to the action observed with IGFBP-3; however, to date, no information exists about the specific mechanisms involved in IGFBP-rP1 inhibitory action. Burger et al. (117) have recently explored the expression of IGFBP-rP1 in vivo in sections of normal breast tissues, ductal carcinoma *in situ*, and infiltrating carcinoma. They found that the expression of IGFBP-rP1 is abrogated during BC progression, with concomitant loss of heterozygosity on chromosome 4q, indicating that this gene product may have a tumor-suppressor function.

Similarly, in a recent experiment (Minniti and Oh, unpublished data), IGFBP-rP2 has been demonstrated to be upregulated by TGF-β (84) and RA at both the mRNA and protein levels in various BC cell lines. Preliminary results indicate that treatment of Hs578T cells with IGFBP-rP2 results in inhibition of DNA synthesis, suggesting that IGFBP-rP2 could act as a downstream effector of TGF-β and RA in inhibiting cell proliferation in BC, as was observed for IGFBP-3 and IGFBP-rP1 (Minniti and Oh, unpublished data).

PROSTATE CANCER

The prostate is comprised of four glandular zones that differ in their histology and biology: the transitional zone, the periurethral zone, the peripheral zone, and the central zone *(118)*. The peripheral zone, which accounts for 70% of prostate mass, is the region most susceptible for malignant transformation, with about 70% of all PCs arising here *(118)*. In addition to this anatomical organization, the prostate is composed of ECs, which are the source of prostate carcinoma, and stromal cells, which are implicated in the development of benign prostatic hyperplasia *(118–120)*.

The IGF axis is involved in the control of prostate growth *(121–123)*. Normal prostate ECs express neither IGF-I nor IGF-II *(121)*; the stromal cells produce detectable levels of IGF-II, but not IGF-I *(122)*. However, the IGF-IR has been identified in both ECs and stromal cells, which respond to the mitogenic effect of IGFs *(123)*. Both prostate ECs and stromal cells are important sources of IGFBPs that modulate IGF action *(121,122,124)*. IGFBP-2 and IGFBP-4 are produced by ECs and stromal cells, and represent the majority of IGFBPs in seminal fluid. IGFBP-3 is synthesized by stromal and possibly ECs, and inhibits IGF-induced proliferation of normal prostate ECs in culture. IGFBP-5 and IGFBP-6 are produced by cultured prostatic cells, and have been shown in human prostate biopsies. IGFBP-1 has not been detected in either prostate ECs or stromal cells. Among the new low-affinity binding proteins, IGFBP-rP1 production has been demonstrated in normal ECs *(125)*; there are no data yet available for the other members of this family of proteins.

The importance of the IGF system, specially the role of plasma IGF-I and IGFBP-3 and the risk of developing PC, has been recently addressed. In a large prospective study *(126)*, IGF-I was significantly associated with PC risk, but IGF-II and IGFBP-3 were not. However, IGFBP-3 was inversely correlated with risk of PC after controlling for IGF-I levels. In addition, with further adjustment for IGFBP-3, men with high levels of IGF-I and low levels of IGFBP-3 had a fourfold increase of risk of PC compared to the reference control group.

Changes in the IGFBP profile have been shown in PC *(127–129)*, especially in secretion of IGFBP-2 and IGFBP-3. Tennant et al. *(128)*, comparing normal prostate ECs, prostate intraepithelial neoplasia, and prostatic carcinoma, found that both IGFBP-2 mRNA and protein levels increased with progressive malignancy, suggesting that the increased protein synthesis of IGFBP-2 is caused by increased gene expression. On the contrary, IGFBP-3 protein was significantly decreased in adenocarcinoma (AC) cells; IGFBP-3 mRNA labeling intensity in cancerous areas was no different from benign epithelium or prostate intraepithelial neoplasia. It therefore appears that IGFBP-3 protein may be regulated by pre- or posttranslational events, such as proteolysis.

PSA is a Ser protease that is secreted by prostate ECs and cleaves IGFBP-3. It is active in seminal fluid *(36)*, and presumably also in the prostate *(130)*. The development of PC is correlated with elevation in serum PSA *(131)* and decreased intact IGFBP-3 levels *(132)*. The significant negative association between PSA and IGFBP-3 in PC biopsies, by immunohistochemical analysis, supports the hypothesis that PSA affects IGFBP-3 proteolysis in malignant prostate tissue. Cathepsin D, another acid protease, has also been recognized in prostate carcinoma cells *(133)*. The impact of proteolysis on IGFBP-3 action in PC has been extensively studied in vitro, to investigate its relationship to cell proliferation and the IGF axis *(133,134)*. Angelloz-Nicoud and Binoux *(134)*, using PC-3 ECs derived from a human prostate AC, showed that the addition of a Ser protease inhibitor was able to block both cation-dependent and cation-independent proteases, and inhibited cell proliferation up to 80%. At the same time, immunoblotting and ligand blotting showed a reduction of proteolytic fragments and an increase of intact IGFBP-3. In addition, the stimulatory action of IGF-II was potentiated in the presence of larger proportions of proteolyzed IGFBP-3, and suppressed in the presence of intact IGFBP-3. Similarly, Nunn et al. *(133)* demonstrated that proteolysis by cathepsin D of IGFBP-3 and other IGFBPs, except IGFBP-6, resulted in proteolytic fragments with decreased affinity for IGFs. These results support the hypothesis that, in the prostate, the decreased levels of IGFBP-3 in cancer cells may allow for greater IGF action because of the loss of IGFBP-3 inhibition, resulting in abnormally high cell proliferation rates.

As in BC, the IGF-independent inhibitory action of IGFBP-3 in PC has been extensively studied. TGF-β and RA, both known to inhibit growth of prostate cells, positively regulate IGFBP-3 in a dose-dependent manner *(135,136)*. Using PC-3 cells, Hwa et al. *(135)* demonstrated an increase in IGFBP-3 protein levels in conditioned media of TGF-β- and RA-treated cells, which was correlated with enhanced steady-state levels of IGFBP-3 mRNA, suggesting that the increased protein synthesis of IGFBP-3 results from increased gene expression. In the prostate, the mechanism of TGF-β and RA effects on prostate cell growth are not known; however, the observation that these two factors upregulate IGFBP-3 expression suggests that IGFBP-3 may play an important role in the control of cell proliferation as a downstream effector of these growth-inhibitory factors.

Rajah et al. *(136)* recently demonstrated that addition of recombinant IGFBP-3 to PC-3 cells resulted in a dose-dependent induction of apoptosis, and that this action was mediated through an IGF–IGFR-independent pathway. In fact, in PC-3 cells, IGF-I only partially blocked IGFBP-3-induced apoptosis, even at fivefold higher molar concentration, supporting the notion that the pathway of IGFBP-3-induced apoptosis may be independent from IGF–IGFR interactions. In addition, the IGF analog, Long-R3-IGF-I, which binds to the IGFR and not to IGFBP-3, was unable to block IGFBP-3-induced apoptosis. These observations suggest, not only an IGF-independent role for IGFBP-3, but also that activation of the IGF-IR does not reverse IGFBP-3-induced apoptosis. Moreover, the authors demonstrated that IGFBP-3 mediates the growth-inhibitory effect of TGF-β by inducing apoptosis. In fact, the treatment of PC-3 cells with TGF-β caused a dramatic increase of IGFBP-3 protein within 12 h, and a significant effect of TGF-β on apoptosis was observed 18–24 h after treatment, suggesting that the TGF-β-induced elevation of IGFBP-3 is the signal of activation of apoptosis. Treatment with IGFBP-3 antisense ODNs inhibited TGF-β-induced apoptosis.

Changes in IGFBP-4 and -5 also occur in prostate carcinoma. Tennant et al. *(129)* found a significant increase in IGFBP-4 mRNA and protein levels in AC cells in comparison with benign ECs, but the observed changes were less than the changes observed for IGFBP-2 and IGFBP-3. Damon et al. *(137)* demonstrated that overexpression of IGFBP-4 could delay tumorogenesis in the M-12 PC cell line. In addition, IGFBP-4 was able to inhibit tumor development in athymic nude mice. Apoptosis was increased in cells overexpressing

IGFBP-4, explaining, at least in part, the slower rate of proliferation and tumor growth in these cells. Because des-(1-3)-IGF-I, an analog of IGF-I with high affinity for the IGF-IR, but low affinity for IGFBPs, was able to reverse the inhibiting action of IGFBP-4, the effect of IGFBP-4 overexpression is clearly caused by the inhibition of IGFs and not by an IGF-independent effect. IGFBP-5 protein levels were slightly increased in AC, but IGFBP-5 mRNA levels were no different when compared to normal epithelium. No changes were observed in IGFBP-6 protein and mRNA levels between normal and malignant epithelium.

The same pattern of IGFBPs changes seen in PC cell lines and primary culture occurs in the serum of patients with PC. The most dramatic alteration is the increase of IGFBP-2 *(132,138,139)*; however, IGFBP-2 does not have the sensitivity and the specificity of PSA as a screening tool in PC . The second most prominent alteration in serum IGFBPs in patients with PC is a decrease in IGFBP-3 levels *(132)*. Activation of a specific IGFBP-3 protease could be possible mechanism for this reduction.

Figuroa et al. *(140)*, using an RNase protection assay, examined the expression of IGFBPs in 23 paired benign and neoplastic prostate tissue samples obtained from prostatectomy. They found a significant difference in expression of IGFBP-2, IGFBP-3, and IGFBP-5 between tumors with high Gleason score, those with low score, and benign tissues. Expression of IGFBP-2 and IGFBP-5 was higher in high vs low Gleason score cancers; expression of IGFBP-3 was lower in high vs low Gleason score cancer specimens.

These results demonstrate that IGFBPs are significantly altered in the progression from benign to malignant tissue, and suggest that differential expression of these binding proteins in PC could be explored as a potential prognostic indicator in this disease. To date, no data are available on the role of the new low-affinity binding proteins in PC. Future studies will clarify whether these new low-affinity IGFBP-rPs could be responsible in part for transformation processes that occur in the development of PC.

ENDOMETRIAL CANCER AND OC

In uterine tissue, estrogen regulates various components of the IGF system. Induction of uterine IGFR expression by estrogen has been demonstrated in vivo in several species, including human endometrium *(141–143)*. The increased IGF-I and IGF-IR mRNA levels in the endometrium during the proliferative phase of the menstrual cycle suggests a role for IGF-I in estrogen-dependent endometrial proliferation *(142,143)*. IGFBPs are regulated by estrogens, and their expression changes during the menstrual cycle *(144)*. IGFBP-1 has been shown to be present in secretory, but not proliferative, endometrium. Endometrial cells synthesize and secrete IGFBP-2 and IGFBP-3, and their expression is upregulated by E_2 and progesterone. In addition, their expression is differentially regulated in secretory compared to proliferative-phase endometrium.

IGF-I is a potent stimulator of endometrial cancer cell growth *(145–147)*, and its action is modulated by IGFBP-3. In Ishikawa human endometrial cancer cells, Karas et al. *(148)* demonstrated that membrane-associated IGFBP-3 inhibits several components of the IGF-IR signal transduction pathway, such as receptor autophosphorylation, IR substrate-I tyrosine phosphorylation, c-Fos induction, and activating protein 1 activation.

In these cells, naturally expressing a high number of cell-surface-associated IGFBP-3, the IGF-I analog, des-(1-3)-IGF-I, is more potent than IGF-I in activating the IGF-IR response. This difference can be attributed to the attenuation of IGF-I-mediated IGF-IR signaling by membrane-associated IGFBP-3 in an IGF-dependent manner. In addition, an IGF-IR binding assay in Ishikawa cell membranes shows that [^{125}I]-IGF-I bound to cells could be completely displaced by IGF-I and IGF-II, but not by des-(1-3)-IGF-I, indicating that the majority of the binding sites for IGF-I on cell membranes are IGFBPs.

As in BC, estrogens are considered one of the most important factors in endometrial carcinoma (144,149). In endometrial cancer cell lines, E_2 upregulates IGFR levels and downregulates soluble IGFBP-3 levels, which results in more availability of IGFs for IGF-IR (149). The reduction of IGFBP-3 occurs at protein and mRNA levels, indicating an inhibition of IGFBP-3 gene expression by E_2. These results suggest that E_2-stimulated endometrial cancer cell growth could be mediated by the IGF system, upregulating IGF-IR levels and decreasing IGFBP-3 levels. In contrast to BC, in which TAM prevents estrogen-stimulated tumor growth, endometrial tumor growth is enhanced by TAM (150, 151), and the association between TAM treatment and development of endometrial carcinoma has been reported (152–154). Kleinman et al. (155) demonstrated that, in Ishikawa endometrial cancer cells, TAM and E_2, increased IGF-IR tyrosine phosphorylation, without affecting the number or affinity of IGF-IR, and reduced the levels of both soluble and membrane-associated IGFBPs. The decrease of IGFBP-3 levels makes IGF-I more available to its receptor, thus enhancing IGF activity. Huynh and Pollak (156) also found that, in the rat, the uterotropic action of TAM is associated with an inhibition of endometrial IGFBP-3 gene expression. These results indicate that the growth effects of TAM in endometrial cancer cells could be, at least partially, mediated by changes in IGF-I and IGFBP-3 levels.

Despite the volume of data, no convincing results address the role of the IGF system in endometrial cancer in vivo, and future studies will be fundamental to clarify the role IGFs and IGFBPs as risk factors in the development and progression of endometrial cancer.

Less data are available on the role of the IGF system in OC. IGF-I expression by normal human ovaries is well documented (157,158), and the mRNAs for both IGF-I and its receptor have been found in primary and metastatic epithelial OC and in several OC cell lines (159). OC cells express IGFBPs, predominantly IGFBP-2 and –3, which can modulate the mitogenic effect of IGF-I (160,161). Karasik et. al. (160) investigated the IGF system in patients with an ovarian epithelial cystic neoplasm, and found that, as in PC, the major alteration in IGFBPs is the dramatic rise of IGFBP-2 in cyst fluid and serum, in comparison to the control benign ovarian cysts. The analysis of OC specimens in malignant ovarian cyst fluid shows a significant increase in IGFBP-2 mRNA and protein levels, compared to benign neoplasia, suggesting that local production by the tumor is responsible for the increased IGFBP-2 in malignant cyst fluid (161). IGFBP-2 mRNA levels correlated with the aggressiveness of the tumor. In contrast, the level of IGFBP-3 was low in ovarian cyst fluid, as well as in sera from patients with OC, probably because of proteolytic degradation. Further studies in OC could clarify the significance of these changes in IGFBPs, as well as the potential clinical use of cyst fluid IGF-I/IGFBP measurements in the preoperative diagnosis and staging of OC.

CONCLUSION

In the past few years, the important role of IGFBPs in breast, prostate, endometrial, and ovarian neoplasia has been extensively investigated. IGFBP-3 in various experimental tumor models appears to be one of the most important factors in the regulation of cancer cell growth by both IGF-dependent and IGF-independent mechanisms. IGFBP-3, mediates the effects of the growth-inhibitory factors, TGF-β and RA, as well as the anti-proliferative effects of vitamin D analogs and the antiestrogen, TAM. If these results are confirmed, pharmacological and nutritional approaches to decreasing IGF-I and enhancing IGFBP-3 bioactivity could represent an important risk-reduction strategy in the development of cancer treatments. In addition, the discovery of the new low-affinity IGF binders (IGFBP-rPs) indicates a very complex system capable of modulating cancer growth, presumably in an IGF-independent manner.

A fuller understanding of the IGF-independent action of IGFBPs and IGFBP-rPs will allow understanding of how the growth of neoplastic cells can be modulated by an IGF/IGFBP system, and how other growth factors or pharmacological agents can interface with this system. Potentially, this will allow development of IGFBP agonists/antagonists as a new strategy for the endocrine therapy of endocrine-dependent neoplasia.

REFERENCES

1. Daughaday WH, Rotwein P. Insulin-like growth factors I and II: peptide messenger ribonucleic acid and gene structures serum and tissue concentrations. Endocr Rev 1989;10:68–91.
2. Werner H, Woloschak M, Stannard B, Shen-Orr Z, Roberts CT Jr, LeRoith D. Insulin-like growth factor receptor: molecular biology, heterogeneity and regulation. In LeRoith D, ed. Insulin-like Growth Factors: Molecular and Cellular Aspects. CRC, Boca Raton, 1991, pp. 17–47.
3. Baxter RC, Martin JL. Binding proteins for the insulin-like growth factors: structure, regulation and function. Prog Growth Factor Res 1989;1:49–68.
4. Rosenfeld RG, Lamson GL, Pham H, Oh Y, Conover C, DeLeon DD, et al. Insulin-like growth factor-binding proteins. Recent Progress Hormone Res 1991;46:99–159.
5. Shimasaki S, Ling N. Identification and molecular characterization of insulin-like growth factor binding proteins (IGFBP-1, -2, -3, -4, -5 and -6). Progress Growth Factor Res 1991;3:243–266.
6. Jones JI, Clemmons DR. Insulin-like growth factors and their binding proteins: biological actions. Endocr Rev 1995;16:3–34.
7. Lowe L. Biological actions of the insulin-like growth factors. In: LeRoith D, ed. Insulin-like Growth Factors: Molecular and Cellular Aspects. CRC, Boca Raton, 1991, pp. 49–85.
8. Oh Y, Muller HL, Neely EK, Lamson G, Rosenfeld RG. New concepts in insulin-like growth factor receptor physiology. Growth Regul 1993;3:113–123.
9. Kelley KM, Oh Y, Gargosky SE, Gucev Z, Matsumoto T, Hwa V, et al. Insulin-like growth factor-binding proteins (IGFBPs) and their regulatory dynamics. Int J Biochem Cell Biol 1995;28:619–637.
10. Rajaram S, Baylink DJ, Mohan S. Insulin-like growth factor-binding proteins in serum and other biological fluids: regulation and function. Endocr Rev 1997;18:801–831.
11. Oh Y. IGFBPs and neoplastic models: new concept for roles of IGFBPs in regulation of cancer cell growth. Endocrine 1997;7:111–113.
12. Oh Y. IGF-independent regulation of breast cancer growth by IGF binding proteins. Breast Cancer Res Treat 1998;47:283–293.
13. Hwa V, Oh Y, Rosenfeld RG. The insulin-like growth factor binding (IGFBP) superfamily. Acta Ped Scand 1999;428:37–45.
14. Baxter RC, Binoux M, Clemmons DR, Conover CA, Drop SLS, Holly JMP, et al. Recommendations for nomenclature for the insulin-like growth factor binding protein (IGFBP) superfamily. Endocrinology 1998;139:4036.
15. Baxter RC, Binoux MA, Clemmons DR, Conover CA, Drop SLS, Holly JMP, et al. Recommendations for nomenclature of the insulin-like growth factor-binding protein superfamily. J Clin Endocrinol Metab 1998;83:3213.
16. Oh Y, Nagalla SR, Yamanaka Y, Kim H-S, Wilson EM, Rosenfeld RG. Synthesis and characterization of insulin-like growth factor binding protein (IGFBP-7). J Biol Chem 1996;271:30,322–30,325.
17. Kim H-S, Nagalla SR, Oh Y, Wilson EM, Roberts CT Jr, Rosenfeld RG. Identification of a family of low-affinity insulin-like growth factor binding proteins (IGFBPs): characterization of connective tissue growth factor as a member of the IGFBP superfamily. Proc Natl Acad Sci USA 1997;94:12,981–12,986.

18. Burren CP, Wilson EM, Hwa V, Kim H-S, Oh Y, Rosenfeld RG. Binding properties and distribution of insulin-like growth factor binding protein-related protein 3 (IGFBP-rP3/NovH), an additional member of the IGFBP superfamily. J Clin Endocrinol Metab 1999;84:1096–1103.
19. Murphy M, Pykett MJ, Harnish P, Zang KD, George DL. Identification and characterization of genes differentially expressed in meningiomas. Cell Growth Differ 1993;4:715–722.
20. Akaogi K, Okabe Y, Funahashi K, Yoshitake Y, Nishikawa K, Yasunitsu H, Umeda M, Miyazaki M. Cell adhesion activity of a 30-kDa major secreted protein from human bladder carcinoma cells. Biochem Biophys Res Commun 1994;198:1046–1053.
21. Wilson EM, Oh Y, Rosenfeld RG. Generation and characterization of an IGFBP-7 antibody: identification of 31-kDa IGFBP-7 in human biological fluids and Hs578T human breast cancer conditioned media. J Clin Endocrinol Metab 1997;82:1301–1303.
22. Bradham DM, Igarashi A, Potter RL, Grotendorst GR. Connective tissue growth factor: a cysteine-rich mitogen secreted by human vascular endothelial cells is related to the SRC-induced immediate early gene product CEF-10. J Cell Biol 1991;114:1285–1294.
23. Joliot V, Martinerie C, Dambrine G, Plassiart G, Brisac M. Proviral rearrangements and overexpression of a new cellular gene (nov) in myeloblastosis-associated virus type I-induced nephroblastomas. Mol Cell Biol 1992;12:10–21.
24. O'Brien TP, Yang GP, Sanders L, Lau LF. Expression of cyr61, a growth factor-inducible immediate-early gene. Mol Cell Biol 1990;10:3569–3577.
25. Bork P. The modular architecture of a new family of growth regulators related to connective tissue growth factor. FEBS 1993;327:125–130.
26. Lenarcic B, Ritonja A, Strukelj B, Turk B, Turk V. Equistatin, a new inhibitor of cysteine proteinases from Actinia equina, is structurally related to thyroglobulin type-I domain. J Biol Chem 1997;272:13,899–13,903.
27. Baxter RC. Characterization of the acid-labile subunit of the growth hormone-dependent insulin-like growth factor-binding protein complex. J Clin Endocrinol Metab 1988;67:265–272.
28. Baxter RC. Circulating levels and molecular distribution of the acid-labile (alpha) subunit of the high molecular weight insulin-like growth factor-binding protein complex. J Clin Endocrinol Metab 1990;70:1347–1353.
29. Baxter RC Insulin-like growth factor-binding proteins in the human circulation, a review. Horm Res 1994;42:140–144.
30. Guler HP, Zapf J, Schimd C, Froesh ER. Insulin-like growth factor I and II in healthy man. Estimation of half-lives and production rates. Acta Endocrinol (Copenh) 1989;121:753–758.
31. Jones JI, D'Ercole AJ, Camacho-Hubner C, Clemmons DR. Phosphorylation of insulin-like growth factor binding proteins in cell culture and in vivo: effects on affinity for IGF-I. Proc Natl Acad Sci USA 1991;88:7481–7485.
32. Frost RA, Tseng L. Insulin-like growth factor-binding protein-1 is phosphorilated by cultured human endometrial stromal cells and multiple protein kinases in vitro. J Biol Chem 1991;266:18,082–18,088.
33. Hoeck WG, Mukku VR. Identification of the major sites of phosphorylation in IGF binding protein-3. J Cell Biochem 1994;56:262–273
34. Coverley J, Baxter RC. Regulation of insulin-like growth factor (IGF) binding protein-3 phosphorylation by IGF-I. Endocrinology 1995;136:5778–5781.
35. Conover CA. Glycosylation of insulin-like growth factor binding protein-3 (IGFBP-3) is not required for potentiation of IGF-I action, evidence for processing of cell-bound IGFBP-3. Endocrinology 1991;129:3259–3268.
36. Cohen P, Graves HCB, Peehl DM, Kamarei M, Giudice LC, Rosenfeld RG. Prostate-specific antigen (PSA) is an insulin-like growth factor binding protein-3 protease found in seminal plasma. J Clin Endocrinol Metab 1992;75:1046–1053.
37. Campbell PG, Novak JF, Yanosick TB, McMaster JH. Involvement of the plasmin system in dissociation of the insulin-like growth factor binding-protein complex. Endocrinology 1992;130:1401–1412.
38. Conover CA, Kiefer MC, Zapf J. Posttranslational regulation of insulin-like growth factor-binding protein-4 in normal and transformed human fibroblasts. J Clin Invest 1993;91:1129–1137.
39. Cheung PT, Wu J, Banach W, Chernausek SD. Glucocorticoid regulation of an insulin-like growth factor-binding protein-4 protease produced by a rat neuronal cell line. Endocrinology 1994;135:1328–1335.
40. Fowlkes JL, Enghild JJ, Suzuki K, Nagase H. Matrix metalloproteinases degrade the insulin-like growth factor binding protein-3 in dermal fibroblast cultures. J Biol Chem 1994;269:25,742–25,746.
41. Conover CA, De Leon DD. Acid-activated insulin-like growth factor-binding protein-3 proteolysis in normal and transformed cells. Role of cathepsin D. J Biol Chem 1994;269:7076–7080.

42. Nam TJ, Busby WH, Clemmons DR. Human fibroblasts secrete a serine protease that cleaves insulin-like growth factor-binding protein-5. Endocrinology 1994;135:1385–1391.

43. Giudice LC. IGF binding protein-3 proteases: how sweet it is. J Clin Endocrinol Metab 1995;80: 2279–2281.

44. Collett-Solberg PF, Cohen P. The role of insulin-like growth factor binding proteins and the IGFBP proteases in modulating IGF action. Endocrinol Metab Clin North Am 1996;25:591–614.

45. Both BA, Boes M, Bar RS. IGFBP-3 proteolysis by plasmin, thrombin, serum: heparin binding, IGF binding, and structure of fragments. Am J Physiol (Endocrinol Metab) 1996;34:E465–E470.

46. Irwin JC, Kirk D, Gwatkin RB, Navre M, Cannon P, Giudice LC. Human endometrial matrix metalloproteinase-2, a putative menstrual proteinase. Hormonal regulation in cultured stromal cells and messenger RNA expression during the menstrual cycle. J Clin Invest 1996;97:438–447.

47. Zumbrunn J, Trueb B. Primary structure of a putative serine protease specific for IGF-binding proteins. FEBS Lett 1996;398:187–192.

48. Lee PDK, Conover CA, Powell DA. Regulation and function of insulin-like growth factor-binding protein-1. Proc Soc Expl Biol Med 1993;204:4–29.

49. Thissen JP, Ketelslegers JM, Underwood LE. Nutritional regulation of the insulin-like growth factors. Endocr Rev 1994;15:80–101.

50. Wang HS, Chard T. Chromatografic characterization of insulin-like growth factor-binding proteins in human pregnancy serum. J Endocrinol 1992;133:149–159.

51. Giudice LC, Irwin JC, Dsupin BA, de las Fuentes L, Jin IH, Vu TH, Hoffman AR. Insulin-like growth factor (IGFs), IGF binding proteins (IGFBPs) and IGFBP proteases in human endometrium, their potential relevance to endometrial cyclic function and maternal-embryonic interactions. In: Baxter RC, Gluckman PD, Rosenfeld RG, eds. The Insulin-like Growth Factors and Their Regulatory Proteins. Elsevier, Amsterdam, 1994, pp. 351–361.

52. Adashi EY. Regulation of intrafollicular IGFBPs, possible relevance to ovarian follicular selection. In: Baxter RC, Gluckman PD, Rosenfeld RG, eds. The Insulin-like Growth Factors and Their Regulatory Proteins. Elsevier, Amsterdam, 1994, pp. 341–350.

53. Rechler MM, Nissley SP. Insulin-like growth factors. In: Sporn MB, Robert AB, eds. Peptide Growth Factors and Their Receptors. Springer Verlag, Berlin, 1990, pp. 263–367.

54. Reeve JG, Schwander J, Bleehen NM. IGFBP-2: an important regulator of insulin-like growth factor action in human lung tumors. Growth Regul 1993;3:82–84.

55. Bourner MJ, Busby WH, Seigel NR, Krivi GG, McCusker RH, Clemmons DR. Cloning and sequence determination of bovine insulin-like growth factor binding protein-2 (IGFBP-2): comparison of its structural and functional property with IGFBP-1. J Cell Biochem 1992;264:12,449–12,554.

56. Bar RS, Boes M, Dake BL, Moser DR, Erondu NE. Vascular endothelium, IGFs and IGF binding proteins. In: Baxter RC, Gluckman PD, Rosenfeld RG, eds. The Insulin-like Growth Factors and Their Regulatory Proteins. Elsevier, Amsterdam, 1994, pp. 237–244.

57. Ceda GP, Fielder PJ, Henzel WJ, Louie A, Donovan SM, Hoffman AR, Rosenfeld RG. Differential effects of insulin-like growth factor (IGF)-I and IGF-II on the expression of IGF binding proteins (IGFBPs) in a rat neuroblastoma cell line, isolation and characterization of two form of IGFBP-4. Endocrinology 1991;128:2574–2580.

58. Mohan S, Bautista CM, Wergedal J, Baylink DJ. Isolation of an inhibitory insulin-like growth factor (IGF) binding protein from bone cell-condioned medium: a potential local regulator of IGF action. Proc Natl Acad Sci USA 1989;86:8338–8342.

59. Cheung PT, Smith EP, Shimasaki S, Ling N, Chernausek SD. Characterization of insulin-like growth factor binding protein (IGFBP-4) produced by the B104 rat neuronal cell line, chemical and biological properties and differential synthesis by sublines. Endocrinology 1991;129:1006–1015.

60. Kiefer MC, Schmid C, Waldvogel M, Schlapfer I, Futo E, Masiarz FR, et al. Characterization of recombinant insulin-like growth factor-binding proteins 4,5, and 6 produced in yeast. J Biol Chem 1992;267:12,692–12,699.

61. Neely EK, Rosenfeld RG. Insulin-like growth factors (IGFs) reduce IGF-binding protein-4 (IGFBP-4) concentration and stimulate IGFBP-3 independently of IGF receptors in human fibroblasts and epidermal cells. Endocrinology 1992;131:985–993.

62. Bautista CM, Baylink DJ, Mohan S. Isolation of a novel insulin-like growth factor (IGF) binding protein from human bone, a potential candidate for fixing IGF-II in human bone. Biochem Biophys Res Commun 1991;176:756–763.

63. Mohan S. Insulin-like growth factor binding proteins in bone cells. Growth Regul 1993;3:67–70.
64. Mohan S, Strong DD, Linkhart TA, Baylink DJ. Regulation and action of insulin-like growth factor binding protein (IGFBP)-4 and IGFBP-5 in bone, physiological and clinical implications. In: Baxter RC, Gluckman PD, Rosenfeld RG, eds. The Insulin-like Growth Factors and Their Regulatory Proteins. Elsevier, Amsterdam, 1994, pp. 237–244.
65. Parker A, Clarke JB, Busby WHJ, Clemmons DR. Identification of the extracellular matrix binding sites for insulin-like growth factor-binding protein 5. J Biol Chem 1996;271:13,523–13,529.
66. Jones JI, Gockerman A, Busby WHJ, Camacho Hubner C, Clemmons DR. Extracellular matrix contains insulin-like growth factor-binding protein-5: potentiation of the effects of IGF-I. J Cell Biol 1993; 121:679–687.
67. Ling NC, Liu XJ, Malkowski M, Guo YL, Erickson GF, Shimasaki S. Structural and functional studies of insulin-like growth factor binding proteins in the ovary. Growth Regul 1993;3:70–74.
68. Rohan RM, Ricciarelli E, Kiefer MC, Resnick CE, Adashi EY. Rat insulin-like growth factor binding protein-6: a hormonally regulated theca-interstitial-selective species with limited antigonadotropic activity. Endocrinology 1993;132:2507–2512.
69. Li W, Fawcett J, Widmer HR, Fielder PJ, Rabkin R, Keller GA. Nuclear transport of insulin-like growth factor-I and insulin-like growth factor-binding protein-3 in opossum kidney cells. Endocrinology 1997;138:1763–1766.
70. Jaques G, Noll K, Wegmann B, Witten S, Kogan E, Radulescu RT, Havemann K. Nuclear localization of insulin-like growth factor-binding protein 3 in a lung cancer cell line. Endocrinology 1997;138: 1767–1770.
71. Jones JI, Gockeman A, Busby VH Jr, Wright G, Clemmons DR. Insulin-like growth factor binding protein 1 stimulates cell migration and binds to the $\alpha5\beta1$ integrin receptor by means of its Arg-Gly-Asp sequence. Proc Natl Acad Sci USA 1993;90:10,553–10,557.
72. Andress DL, Birbaum RS. Human osteoblast-derived insulin-like growth factor (IGF) binding protein-5 stimulates osteoblast mitogenesis and potentiates IGF action. J Biol Chem 1992;267:22,467–22,472.
73. Andress DL. Heparin modulates the binding of insulin-like growth factor (IGF) binding protein-5 to a membrane protein in osteoblast cells. J Biol Chem 1995;270:28,289–28,296
74. Liu L, Delbe J, Blat C, Zapf J, Harel L. Insulin-like growth factor binding protein (IGFBP-3), an inhibitor of serum growth factors other than IGF-I and II. J Cell Physiol 1992;153:15–21.
75. Oh Y, Muller HL, Lamson G, Rosenfeld RG. Insulin-like growth factor (IGF)-independent action of IGF-binding protein-3 in Hs578 human breast cancer cells. J Biol Chem 1993;268:14,964–14,971.
76. Cohen P, Lamson G, Okajima T, Rosenfeld RG. Transfection of the human insulin-like growth factor-binding protein-3 gene into Balb/c fibroblasts inhibits cellular growth. Mol Endocrinol 1993;7:380–386.
77. Oh Y, Muller HL, Pham HM, Rosenfeld RG. Demonstration of receptors for insulin-like binding protein-3 on Hs578T human breast cancer cells. J Biol Chem 1993;268:26,045–26,048.
78. Oh Y, Muller HL, Ng HM, Rosenfeld RG. Transforming growth factor-β induced cell growth inhibition in human breast cancer cells is mediated through IGFBP-3 action. J Biol Chem 1995;270:13,589–13,592.
79. Gucev ZS, Oh Y, Kelley KM, Rosenfeld RG. Insulin-like growth factor binding protein 3 mediates retinoic acid- and transforming growth factor $\beta2$-induced growth inhibition in human breast cancer cells. Cancer Res 1995;56:1545–1550.
80. Valentinis B, Bhala A, De Angelis T, Baserga R, Cohen P. The human insulin-like growth factor (IGF) binding protein-3 inhibits cell growth of fibroblasts with a target disruption of the IGF-I receptor gene. Mol Endocrinol 1995;9:361–367.
81. Buckbinder L, Talbott R, Velasco-Miguel S, Takenata I, Faha B, Seizinger BR, Kley N. Induction of the growth inhibitor IGF-binding protein 3 by p53. Nature 1995;377:646–649.
82. Swisshelm K, Ryan K, Tsuchiya K, Sager R. Enhanced expression of an insulin growth factor-like binding protein (mac 25) in senescent human mammary epithelial cells and induced expression with retinoic acid. Proc Natl Acad Sci USA 1996;92:4472–4476.
83. Akaogi K, Okabe Y, Sato J, Nagashima Y, Yasumitsu H, Sughara K, Miyazaki K. Specific accumulation of tumor-derived adhesion factor in tumor blood vessels and in capillary tube-like structures of cultured vascular endothelial cells. Proc Natl Acad Sci USA 1996;93:8384–8389.
84. Yang DH, Kim HS, Wilson EM, Rosenfeld RG, Oh Y. Identification of glycosylated 38-kDa connective tissue growth factor (IGFBP-related protein 2) and proteolytic fragments in human biological fluids, and up-regulation of IGFBP-rP2 expression by TGF-β in Hs578T human breast cancer cells. J Clin Endocrinol Metab 1998;83:2593–2596.

85. Igarashi A, Nashiro K, Kikuchi K, Sata S, Ihn H, Fujimoto M, Grotendorst GR, Takehara K. Connective tissue growth factor gene expression in tissue sections from localized scleroderma, keloid, and other fibrotic skin disorders. J Invest Dermatol 1996;106:729–733.

86. Oemar BS, Lusher TF. Connective tissue growth factor: friend or foe? Arterioscler Thromb Vasc Biol 1997;17:1483–1489.

87. Kireeva ML, Mo FE, Yang GP, Lau LF. Cyr61, a product of a growth factor-inducible immediate-early gene, promotes cell proliferation, migration, and adhesion. Mol Cell Biol 1996;16:1326–1334.

88. Lalou C, Lassarre C, Binoux M. A proteolytic fragments of insulin-like growth factor (IGF) binding protein-3 that fails to bind IGFs inhibits the mitogenic effects of IGF-I and insulin. Endocrinology 1996;137:3206–3212.

89. Yamanaka Y, Wilson EM, Rosenfeld RG, Ho Y. Inhibition of insulin receptor activation by insulin-like growth factor binding proteins. J Biol Chem 1997;272:30,729–30,734.

90. De Leon DD, Wilson DM, Powers M, Rosenfeld RG. Effects of insulin-like growth factors (IGFs) and IGF receptor antibodies on the proliferation of human breast cancer cells. Growth Factors 1992;6:327–336.

91. Werner H, LeRoith D. The role of the insulin-like growth factor system in human cancer. Advances Cancer Res 1996;68:183–223.

92. Yee D, Jackson JG, Weng CN, Gooch JL, Lee AV. The IGF system in breast cancer. In: Takano K, Hizuka N, Takahashi S-I, eds. Molecular Mechanisms to Regulate the Activities of Insulin-like Growth Factors. Elsevier, Amsterdam, 1998, pp. 319–325.

93. Yee D. The insulin-like growth factors and breast cancer-revisited. Breast Cancer Res Treat 1998;47:197–199.

94. Cullen KJ, Yee D, Sly WS, Perdue J, Hampton B, Lippman ME, Rosen N. Insulin-like growth factor receptor expression and function in human breast cancer. Cancer Res 1990;50:48–53.

95. Baserga R, Hongo A, Rubini M, Prisco M, Valentinis B. The IGF-I receptor in cell growth, transformation and apoptosis. Biochem Biophys Acta 1997;1332:F105–F126.

96. Hankinson SE, Willet WC, Coldits GA, Hunter DJ, Michaud DS, Deroo B, et al. Circulating concentrations of insulin-like growth factor-I and risk of breast cancer. Lancet 1998;351:1393–1396.

97. Pratt SE, Pollak MN. Estrogen and antiestrogen modulation of MCF-7 human breast cancer cell proliferation is associated with specific alterations in accumulation of insulin-like growth factor-binding proteins in conditioned media. Cancer Res 1993;53:5193–5198.

98. Figueroa JA, Jackson JG, McGuire WL, Krywicki RF, Yee D. Expression of insulin-like growth factor binding proteins in human breast cancer correlates with estrogen receptor status. J Cell Biochem 1993;52:196–205.

99. Martin JL, Coverley JA, Pattison ST, Baxter RC. Insulin-like growth factor-binding protein-3 production by MCF-7 breast cancer cells: stimulation by retinoic acid and cyclic adenosine monophosphate and differential effects of estradiol. Endocrinology 1995;136:1219–1226.

100. Huynh H, Yang X, Pollak M. Estradiol and antiestrogens regulate a growth inhibitory insulin like growth factor binding protein 3 autocrine loop in human breast cancer cells. J Biol Chem 1996;271:1016–1021.

101. Schmitt M, Goretzki L, Janicke F, Calvete, Eulitz M, Kobayashi H, Chucholowski N, Graeff H. Biological and clinical relevance of the urokinase-type plasminogen activator in breast cancer. Biomed Biofis Acta 1991;50:731–741.

102. Yu H, Diamandis EP, Sutherland DJA. Immunoreactive prostate-specific antigen levels in female and male breast tumors and its association with steroid hormone receptors and patient age. Clin Biochem 1994;27:75–79.

103. Leal SM, Liu Q, Huang SS, Huang JS. The type V transforming growth factor beta receptor is the putative insulin-like growth factor-binding protein 3 receptor. J Biol Chem 1997;272:20,572–20,576.

104. Delbe J, Blat C, Desauty G, Harel L. Presence of IDF45 (mIGFBP-3) binding sites on chick embryo fibroblasts. Biochem Biophys Res Commun 1991;179:495–501.

105. Andreatta-Van Leyen S, Hembree JR, Eckert RL. Regulation of insulin-like growth factor binding protein 3 levels by epidermal growth factor and retinoic acid in cervical epithelial cells. J Cell Physiol 1994;160:265–274.

106. Rozen F, Zhang J, Pollak M. Antiproliferative action of tumor necrosis factor-α on MCF-7 breast cancer cells is associated with increased insulin-like growth factor-binding protein-3 accumulation. Int J Oncol 1998;13:865–869.

107. Colston KW, Perks CM, Xie SP, Holly JM. Growth inhibition of both MCF-7 cells and Hs578T human breast cancer cell lines by vitamin D analogues is associated with increased expression of insulin-like growth factor-binding protein-3. J Mol Endocrinol 1998;20:157–162.

108. Nickerson T, Huynh H, Pollak M. Insulin-like growth factor binding protein-3 induces apoptosis in MCF7 breast cancer cells. Biochem Biophys Res Commun 1997;237:690–693.

109. Gill ZP, Perks CM, Newbcomb PVN, Holly JMP. Insulin-like growth factor binding protein-3 predisposes breast cancer cells to programmed cell death in a non-IGF dependent manner. J Biol Chem 1997; 272:25,602–25,606.

110. Rozen F, Yang XF, Huynh H, Pollak M. Antiproliferative action of vitamin D-related compounds and insulin-like growth factor-binding protein 5 accumulation. J Natl Cancer Inst 1997;89:652–656.

111. Huynh HT, Yang XF, Pollak M. A role for insulin-like growth factor-binding protein 5 in the antiproliferative action of the antiestrogen ICI 182780. Cell Growth Differ 1996;7:1501–1506.

112. Bohlke K, Cramer DW, Trichopulos D, Mantzoros CS. Insulin-like growth factor-I in relation to premenopausal ductal carcinoma *in situ* of the breast. Epidemiology 1998;9:570–573.

113. Bruning PF, Van Doorn J, Bonfrar JMG, Van Noord PAH, Korse CM, Linders TC, Hart AAM. Insulin-like growth-factor-binding protein 3 is decreased in early-stage operable pre-menopausal breast cancer. Int J Cancer 1995;62:266–270.

114. Helle SI, Holly JMP, Tally M, Hall K, Van Der Stappen J, Lφnning PE. Influence of treatment with tamoxifen and change in tumor burden on the IGF-system in breast cancer patients. Int J Cancer 1996; 69:335–339.

115. Helle SI, Anker GB, Tally M, Hall K, Lφnning PE. Influence of droloxifene on plasma levels of insulin-like growth factor (IGF)-I, pro-IGF-IIE, of insulin-like growth factor binding protein (IGFBP)-1 and IGFBP-3 in breast cancer patients. J Steroid Biochem Mol Biol 1996;57:167–171.

116. Oh Y, Wilson EM, Kim HS, Yang DH, Rutten MJ, Graham DL, et al. Regulation and biological action of IGFBP-7 in human breast cancer cells. Proc. 79th Annual Meeting Endocrine Soc 1997, p. 351.

117. Burger AM, Zhang X, Li H, Ostrowski JL, Beatty B, Venanzoni M, Papas T, Seth A. Down-regulation of T1A12/mac25, a novel insulin-like growth factor-binding protein related gene, is associated with disease progression in breast carcinomas. Oncogene 1998;16:2459–2467.

118. Mc Neal JE. Normal histology of the prostate. Am J Surg Pathol 1988;12:619–623.

119. Fiorelli G, De Bellis A, Longo A, Pioli P, Costantini A, Giannini S, Forti G, Serio M. Growth factor in the human prostate. J Steroid Biochem Mol Biol 1991;40:109–205.

120. Cunha GR, Donjacour AA, Cooke PS, Mee S, Bigbsy RM, Higgins SJ, Sugimura Y. The endocrinology and developmental biology of the prostate. Endocr Rev 1987;8:338–362.

121. Cohen P, Peehl DM, Lamson G, Rosenfeld RG. Insulin-like growth factor (IGFs), IGF receptors, and IGF-binding proteins in primary cultures of prostate epithelial cells. J Clin Endocrinol Metab 1991; 73:401–407.

122. Cohen P, Peehl DM, Baker B, Liu F, Hintz RL, Rosenfeld RG. Insulin-like growth factor axis abnormalities in prostatic stromal cells from patients with benign prostatic hyperplasia. J Clin Endocrinol Metab 1994;79:1410–1415.

123. Grimberg A, Rajah R, Zhao H, Cohen P. The prostatic IGF system: new levels of complexity. In: Takano K, Hizuka N, Takahashi S-I, eds. Molecular Mechanisms to Regulate the Activities of Insulin-like Growth Factors. Elsevier, Amsterdam, 1998, pp. 205–213.

124. Boudon C, Rodier G, Lechevallier E, Mottet N, Barenton B, Sultan CH. Secretion of insulin-like growth factors and their binding proteins in human normal and hyperplastic prostatic cells in primary culture. J Clin Endocrinol Metab 1996;81:612–617.

125. Hwa V, Tommasini-Sprenger C, Lopez Bermejo A, Rosenfeld RG, Plymate SR. Characterization of insulin-like growth factor-binding protein-related protein-1 in prostate cells. J Clin Endocrinol Metab 1998;83:4355–4362.

126. Chan JM, Stampfer MJ, Giovannucci E, Gann PH, Ma J, Wilkinson P, Hennekens, Pollak M. Insulin-like growth factor-I and prostate cancer risk: a prospective study. Science 1998;279:563–566.

127. Birnbaum RS, Ware JL, Playmate SR. Insulin-like growth factor binding protein-3 expression and secretion by cultures of human prostate epithelial cells and stromal fibroblasts. J Endocrinol 1994;141: 533–540.

128. Tennant MK, Thrasher JB, Twomey PA, Birnbaum RS, Plymate SR. Insulin-like growth factor-binding protein-2 and -3 expression in benign human prostate epithelium, prostate intraepithelial neoplasia, and adenocarcinoma of the prostate. J Clin Endocrinol Metab 1996;81:411–420.

129. Tennant MK, Thrasher JB, Twomey PA, Birnbaum RS, Plymate SR. Insulin-like growth factor-binding proteins (IGFBP)-4, -5, and -6 in the benign and malignant human prostate: IGFBP-5 messenger ribonucleic acid localization differs from IGFBP-5 protein localization. J Clin Endocrinol Metab 1996; 81:3783–3792.

130. Plymate SR, Rosen CJ, Paulsen CA, Ware JL, Chen J, Vessella RE, Birnbaum RS. Proteolysis of insulin-like growth factor binding protein-3 in the male reproductive tract. J Clin Endocrinol Metab 1995;81:618–624.

131. Stamey TA, Yang N, Hay AR, McNeal JE, Freiha FS, Redwine E. Prostate specific antigen is a serum marker for adenocarcinoma of the prostate. N Engl J Med 1987;317:909–918.

132. Kanety H, Madjar Y, Dagan Y, Levi J, Papa MZ, Pariente C, Goldwasser B, Karasik A. Serum insulin-like growth factor-binding protein-2 (IGFBP-2) is increased and IGFBP-3 is decreased in patients with prostate cancer: correlation with serum prostate-specific antigen. J Clin Endocrinol Metab 1993;7: 229–233.

133. Nunn SE, Peehl DM, Cohen P. Acid-activated insulin-like growth factor binding protein protease activity of cathepsin D in normal and malignant prostatic epithelial cells and seminal plasma. J Cell Physiol 1997;171:196–204.

134. Angelloz-Nicoud P, Binoux M. Autocrine regulation of cell proliferation by the insulin-like growth factor (IGF) and IGF binding protein-3 protease system in a human prostate carcinoma cell line (PC-3). Endocrinology 1995;136:5485–5492.

135. Hwa V, Oh Y, Rosenfeld RG. Insulin-like growth factor binding protein-3 and 5 are regulated by and transforming growth factor β and retinoic acid in the human prostate adenocarcinoma cell line PC-3. Endocrine 1997;6:235–242.

136. Rajah R, Valenyinis B, Pinchas C. Insulin-like growth factor binding protein-3 induces apoptosis and mediates the effect of transforming growth factor-β1 on programmed cell death through a p53- and IGF-independent mechanism. J Biol Chem 1997;272:12,181–12,188.

137. Damon SE, Maddison L, Ware JL, Plymate SR. Overexpression of an inhibitory insulin-like growth factor binding protein (IGFBP-4), delays onset of prostate tumor formation. Endocrinology 1998;130: 3456–3468.

138. Cohen P, Peehl DM, Stamey TA, Wilson KF, Clemmons DR, Rosenfeld RG. Elevated levels of insulin-like growth factor-binding protein-2 in the serum of prostate cancer patients. J Clin Endocrinol Metab 1993;76:1031–1035.

139. Ho PJ, Baxter RC. Insulin-like growth factor-binding protein-2 in patients with prostate carcinoma and benign prostatic hyperplasia. Clin Endocrinol 1997;46:333–342.

140. Figueroa JA, De Raad S, Tadlock L, Speights VO, Rinehart JJ. Differential expression of insulin-like growth factor binding proteins in high versus low gleason score prostate cancer. J Urol 1998;159: 1379–1383.

141. Murphy LJ, Murphy LC, Friesen HG. Estrogen induces insulin-like growth factor I expression in the rat uterus. Mol Endocrinol 1988;1:445–451.

142. Murphy LJ, Ghahary A. Uterine insulin-like growth factor I: regulation of expression and its role in estrogen-induced uterine proliferation. Endocr Rev 1990;11:443–453.

143. Boehm KD, Dalmon M, Gorodeski IG, Shelan LA, Utian VH, Ilan J. Expression of insulin-like and platelet-derived growth factor genes in human uterine tissues. Mol Reprod Dev 1990;27:93–97.

144. Giudice LC, Milkowski DA, Lamson G, Rosenfeld RG, Irwin JC. Insulin-like growth factor binding proteins in human endometrium: steroid-dependent messenger ribonucleic acid expression and protein synthesis. J Clin Endocrinol Metab 1991;72:779–787.

145. Kleinman D, Roberts CT Jr, LeRoith D, Schally AV, Levy J, Sharoni Y. Growth regulation of endometrial cancer cells by insulin-like growth factors and by luteinizing hormone-releasing hormone antagonist SB-75. Regul Pept 1993;48:91–98.

146. Talavera F, Reynolds RK, Roberts JA, Menon KMJ. Insulin-like growth factor I receptors in normal and neoplastic human endometrium. Cancer Res 1990;50:3019–3024.

147. Naganami M, Stuart CA, Dunhardt PA, Doherty MG. Specific binding sites for insulin and insulin-like growth factor-I in human endometrial cancer. Am J Obstet Gynecol 1991;165:1865–1871.

148. Karas M, Danilenko M, Fishman D, LeRoith D, Levy J, Sharoni Y. Membrane-associated insulin-like growth-factor binding protein-3 inhibits insulin-like growth factor-I-induced insulin-like growth factor-I receptor signaling in Ishikawa endometrial cancer cells. J Biol Chem 1996;272:16,514–16,520.

149. Kleinman D, Karas M, Roberts CT Jr, LeRoith D, Phillip M, Segev Y, Levy J, Sharoni Y. Modulation of insulin-like growth factor I (IGF-I) receptor and membrane-associated IGF-binding proteins in endometrial cancer cell by estradiol. Endocrinology 1995;136:2531–2537.

150. Gottardis MM, Robinson SP, Satyaswaroop PG, Jordan VC. Contrasting actions of tamoxifen on endometrial and breast tumor growth in the athymic mouse. Cancer Res 1993;48:812–815.

151. Marshall E. Tamoxifen: hanging in the balance. Science 1994;264:1526,1527.

152. Magriples U, Naftolin F, Schwartz PE, Carcangiu ML. High-grade endometrial carcinoma in tamoxifen-treated breast cancer patients. J Clin Oncol 1993;11:485–490.

153. Fisher B, Costantino JP, Redmond CK, Fisher ER, Wickermam DL, Cronin WM. Endometrial cancer in tamoxifen-treated breast cancer patients: findings from the National Surgical Adjuvant Breast and Bowel Project (NSABP) B-14. J Natl Cancer Inst 1994;86:527–537.

154. Van Leeuwen F, Benraadt J, Coebergh JW, Kiemeney LA, Gimbrere CH, Otter R, et al. Risk of endometrial cancer after tamoxifen treatment of breast cancer. Lancet 1994;343:448–452.

155. Kleinman D, Karas M, Danilenko M, Arbeli A, Roberts CT Jr, LeRoith D, Levy J, Sharoni Y. Stimulation of endometrial cancer cell growth by tamoxifen is associated with increased insulin-like growth factor (IGF)-I induced tyrosine phosphorylation and reduction in IGF binding proteins. Endocrinology 1996;137:1089–1095.

156. Huyhn H, Pollak M. Uterotrophic actions of estradiol and tamoxifen are associated with inhibition of uterine insulin-like growth factor binding protein 3 gene expression. Cancer Res 1994;54:3115–3159.

157. Adashi EY, Resnick CE, Hernandez, Svoboda ME, Van Wyk JJ. Potential relevance of insulin-like growth factor I to ovarian physiology: from basic science to clinical application. Semin Reprod Endocrinol 1989;7:94–99.

158. Geisthovel F, Moretti-Rojas I, Rojas FJ, Asch RH. Insulin-like growth factors and thecal-granulosa cell function. Hum Reprod 1990;5:785–799.

159. Yee D, Morales FR, Hamilton TC, Von Hoff DD. Expression of insulin-like growth factor I, its binding proteins, and its receptor in ovarian cancer. Cancer Res 1991;51:5107–5112.

160. Karasik A, Menczer J, Pariente C, Kanety H. Insulin-like growth factor-I (IGF-I) and IGF-binding protein-2 are increased in cyst fluids of epithelial ovarian cancer. J Clin Endocrinol Metab 1994;78:271–276.

161. Kanety H, Kattan M, Goldberg I, Kopolovic J, Ravia J, Menczer J, Karasik A. Increased insulin-like growth factor binding protein-2 (IGFBP-2) gene expression and protein production lead to high IGFBP-2 content in malignant ovarian cyst fluid. Br J Cancer 1996;73:1069–1073.

12

Fibroblast Growth Factors and Their Receptors in Breast and Prostate Cancer

*R. C. Coombes, MD, PHD, S. Marsh, FRCS, MD,
J. Gomm, PHD, and C. Johnston, PHD*

CONTENTS

INTRODUCTION

Fibroblast Growth Factors

The fibroblast growth factor (FGF) family has emerged as perhaps the largest group of polypeptide growth factors to be involved in cellular growth and differentiation. It presently comprises more than 20 published members that share a varying degree of homology, and, with the exception of FGF7 and FGF10, which specifically act on epithelial cells (ECs), have a similar broad mitogenic spectrum, i.e., they promote the proliferation of a variety of cells, including those of mesodermal origin, and are angiogenic. With the exception of FGF8, their genes have similar organization and, in some cases, map to comparable regions on human and mouse chromosomes. Their pattern of expression is very different, ranging from restricted expression in some stages of development, e.g., FGF3, FGF4, and FGF5, to rather ubiquitous expression in a variety of tissues and organs, in the cases of FGF1 and FGF2. They all appear to bind heparin and heparan sulphate proteoglycans (HSPG) in the extracellular matrix, which originally led to their alternative grouping, as the heparin-binding growth factors *(1)*.

Three other members of the family (K-FGF/HST, FGF5, INT2) were originally identified as oncogenes *(2–4)*; FGF6 and KGF/FGF7 were isolated by sequence homology or factor purification and cloning *(5,6)*. FGF8 was discovered as an androgen-induced factor in a hormone-sensitive mouse mammary tumor cell line. FGF9 was identified as

From: *Contemporary Endocrinology: Endocrine Oncology*
Edited by: S. P. Ethier © Humana Press Inc., Totowa, NJ

a glial-activating factor *(7)*, and FGF-10 was identified from rat embryos, using homology-based polymerase chain reaction (PCR) *(8)*. Further complexity arises because some of the members of the family exist in multiple forms arising from the initiation of translation at alternative codons. Although it is clear that some of the FGFs can act as potent oncogenes in model systems, their involvement in human development and physiology, pathology and malignant disease, remains to be clarified.

FGF1, -2, and -9 lack a classical signal sequence; although FGF9 does have an N terminal sequence that may be involved with secretion, it is not a signal peptide. Both FGF1 and FGF2 can, however, still be detected in conditioned media in culture, showing that they can be secreted by viable cells, and are able to gain access to the cell surface receptors by a novel secretory mechanism *(9)*. For example, cultured cells that have been transfected to express FGF1 or FGF2 demonstrate an autocrine growth loop *(10,11)*. Other FGFs (e.g., FGF3, -4, -5, -6, and -8, all of which have oncogenic potential, along with FGF7) have a secretory signal sequence, and can follow the classical secretory pathway of packaging into Golgi-associated secretory granules, fusion with the plasma membrane, and release to the extracellular environment, on receipt of the specific signal. The FGFs can then act locally, either on the producing cell in an autocrine fashion, or on adjacent cells in a juxacrine fashion, or on neighboring cells via a paracrine mechanism. In all cases, the FGF must bind to its cognate receptor to produce a physiological effect.

FGF Receptors

The FGFs act through two distinct types of receptors. First, there is a family of high-affinity tyrosine kinase (TK) receptors (the FGFRs), and second, the low-affinity HSPGs. Although the latter were originally thought to serve only a storage and release function and the former to act as the true signaling receptor, it is probable that both are required to produce a balanced cellular response in vivo *(12)*, although the situation remains to be clarified.

The intracellular signaling of the FGFs is mediated by a group of high-affinity TK receptors. Four distinct genes have been discovered, each coding for a different receptor, designated FGFR1–4. The first FGFR to be identified was cloned by its homology to the *fms* proto-oncogene, and termed the *flg* receptor *(13)*. When the amino acid sequence of an affinity-purified receptor for FGF-1 was obtained, it became apparent that *flg* was a transmembrane receptor for FGF1, and became known as FGFR1 *(14)*. All four FGFRs share a similar structure. The extracellular portion consists of a signal sequence and three immunoglobulin (Ig)-like domains. There is a group of acidic amino acids between the first and second Ig domains, which is unique to the FGFRs. There follows a transmembrane region leading to the cytoplasmic section, consisting of a TK domain that is split in two by a 14-amino-acid kinase insert, and ends in a C-terminal tail. The intracytoplasmic regions of the FGFRs share 55–70% sequence homology, being most highly conserved in the kinase domain. A characteristic of the FGFRs is that the exon structure of the genes allows several different forms of the receptors to be generated by alternative RNA splicing. Multiple variants of FGFR1, in addition to the full-length form, have been described. They are classified according to whether the variations are extracellular or intracellular, or whether the receptor variants exist as secreted forms *(15–17)*.

Other than the full-length form, the most common variant is that with the first Ig-like loop deleted. Of those isoforms with intracellular alterations, many still contain sufficient structural information for ligand binding, but are not able to initiate signal transduction, because of a nonfunctional TK domain. By undergoing dimerization with fully functional receptors, these variants can act to decrease the signaling potential of a particular ligand. Secreted forms include one form that consists of only the first Ig-like loop and a short amino acid tail, and another possesses all three loops with a slightly longer tail. In common with FGFR2 and FGFR3, the exon structure allows for two alternative forms for the third Ig-like loop, designated IIIb and IIIc *(15,17)*. FGFR1-IIIc is the most common form, and is found in many tissues, but not in the liver. FGFR1-IIIb is found mostly in the skin. As well as the IIIb/IIIc variants, FGFR2 exhibits a similar complexity to FGFR1 regarding other isoforms that exist. The variation in the third Ig-like loop, seen in FGFR1, -2, and −3, is not seen in FGFR4, in which, so far, no splice variants have been detected *(18)*. Only parts of the second and third Ig-like loops are required for ligand binding *(19,20)*, but, despite the fact that the first loop has no independent ligand-binding activity, it does interact with loops 2 and 3 to lower the affinity for the same FGF *(21)*. Association of the ligand with heparin results in ligand binding, which, in turn, leads to receptor dimerization *(22)*; autophosphorylation of the receptor at specific tyrosine residues follows, leading to activation of the kinase domain and phosphorylation of intracellular signaling molecules *(23)*.

The FGFs display differential affinity for the different FGFRs. The genes for FGFR1, -2, and -3 possess two variable exons in the region coding for the C-terminal half of the third Ig loop, and the exon that is expressed is chiefly responsible for the ligand-binding specificity *(20)*. Exon IIIb appears to specify preference for FGF1, and, in FGFR2, for FGF7. The IIIb form of FGFR2 has been designated the FGF7 (KGF) receptor *(15,19)*; FGFR1, -2, and -3 containing the IIIc loop, will bind FGF1 and FGF2. These studies of the different isoforms of the FGFRs, along with evidence from mutagenesis and peptide antagonists, suggests that the ligand-binding site must be formed by the second and third Ig loops *(24)*. It is likely that these differences in isoform expression coupled with the different ligand binding affinities lead to the varying cellular responses that can occur with the different receptors. It is possible that the different isoforms act to modulate the activity of the receptors.

FGF AND THEIR RECEPTORS IN BREAST CANCER

FGF1 In Breast Cancer

FGF1 is found in both normal development of the mammary gland and in tumorigenesis. In the normal virgin mouse mammary gland, high levels of FGF1 mRNA were found in ECs, with little expression found in the stroma *(25)*. In humans, a similar situation is found, with FGF1 mRNA and protein detected in normal ECs, but not in stromal cells *(26,27)*. On malignant transformation, there appears to be a decrease in the expression of FGF1, although, using sensitive methods, FGF1 can be detected in most breast cancer (BC) tissues analyzed *(28,29)*. Significantly lower levels of mRNA were detected in BC tissues, compared to normal breast tissue $(P = 0.001)$ *(26–30)*. FGF1 protein levels were also lower in BC tissues, as shown by Western blot and immunohistochemistry (IHC) *(26)*. A more extensive IHC study of FGF1 expression in breast tissues showed that FGF1 was present in the ECs of normal breast tissue, and was present at much lower levels, or not detectable in the ECs of malignant breast samples *(31)*. However, incubation of sections at 37°C in the presence of protease inhibitors revealed FGF1 in the stroma of all BC tissues analyzed, particularly around malignant cells, but not in the stroma of nonmalignant breast tissues *(31)*. The authors postulated that a protease specific to malignant breast tissue may be releasing FGF1 from sites where it is sequestered within the stroma. The presence of FGF1 in the stroma of cancer tissues explains the source of released FGF1 detected in the conditioned medium of BC tissues *(32)*.

The receptors to which FGF1 binds are present on BC cells, implying that the presence of stromally released FGF1 may effect the behavior of BC cells *(31,33,34)*. FGF1 has been shown to have a stimulatory effect on the growth of mouse mammary ECs cultured in collagen gels *(35)* and on the growth of human mammary ECs *(33,36,37)*. Transfection experiments have demonstrated an increased malignant phenotype of MCF-7 cells overexpressing FGF1, suggesting that this growth factor may have a role in BC progression. Empty-vector-transfected MCF-7 cells remain estrogen-dependent in vivo, forming only small tumors in ovariectomised mice; FGF1-transfected MCF-7 cells form large, progressively growing tumors in ovariectomized mice *(36)*. Overexpression of FGF1 also increases growth in soft agar, in media deleted of estrogens and resistance to the antiestregen ICI 182,780 and aromatase inhibitors *(39)*. The effects of FGF1 overexpression on MCF-7 growth in ovariectomized mice are likely to result from a paracrine, as well as an autocrine component, since the expression of a dominant-negative FGFR in the MCF-7 cells failed to inhibit tumor growth *(38)*. One possible paracrine role for FGF1 is the promotion of angiogenesis, allowing more rapid tumor proliferation *(40)*.

Tumor invasion and metastasis are important in the outcome of BC, and it is possible that FGF1 may have a role in this. FGF1 is able to promote a membrane-ruffling response in BC cell lines, and such behavior has been linked to increased cell motility *(33)*. Micrometastases have been detected at high frequency in the lungs and lymph nodes of mice bearing tumors containing FGF1 transfected cells, at least partially because of increased neoangiogenesis *(38)*.

FGF2 in Normal and Neoplastic Breast Cells

Studies by Li and Shipley *(41)* showed that HBL100 cells and SV40 transformed cell line derived from normal breast cells possessing FGF2 mRNA. The authors were uncertain as to the origin of HBL100, because they display some myoepithelial characteristics, and subsequently FGF2 expression was studied in purified breast epithelial, myoepithelial and fibroblasts. These studies showed that mRNA for FGF2 was only present in the myo-ECs, despite the presence of immunocytochemical staining for FGF2 in both cell types. FGF2 had no effect on proliferation of myo-ECs, but it maintained the survival of separated ECs in low serum, and stimulated their growth in 5 and 10% fetal calf serum. Low-affinity binding sites for FGF2 were synthesized by ECs and myo-ECs, but myo-ECs possess a greater proportion of higher-affinity HSPGs. These results suggested that myo-EC-derived FGF2 may be an important paracrine factor controling ECs survival and growth in the normal human breast *(42)*.

A further role for FGF2 in differentiation is in branching morphogenesis. Although FGF2 has not been shown to play a role in branching in mammary cells, the authors' studies have shown that the presence of myo-ECs is a requisite for luminal epithelial branching morphogenesis *(42)*, suggesting that a combination of integrin ligation (specific to myoepithelial contact) and paracrine FGF2 from myo-ECs could play an important role in luminal epithelial morphogenesis. FGF2 could also modulate integrin function *(43)*. The net effect of FGF2 on these pleitrophic responses will determine the ultimate phenotype observed in BC cells.

Studies *(29,30)* in human breast tissue have shown high levels of FGF2 mRNA in nonmalignant breast tissue, with reduced FGF2 mRNA levels in neoplastic breast tissue. However, both studies indicated that a small proportion of breast carcinomas expressed FGF2 mRNA at levels similar to those found in benign tissue. In contrast to the normal breast, in which myo-ECs are the principal source of FGF2, myo-ECs are generally absent from BCs containing FGF2 mRNA. The authors' previous IHC studies, using paraffin sections, showed that FGF2 is predominantly in myo-ECs and basement membrane of the benign breast *(44)*. Subsequent studies of the prognostic impact of FGF2 in BC found that tumors displaying a higher level of FGF2 mRNA were associated with improved overall disease-free survival *(42)*. Univariant log-rank analysis showed that this difference was significant, even taking into account all other prognostic parameters, particularly regarding to disease-free survival. The reduction in mRNA is mirrored by a reduction in the protein level, using Western blotting. IHC of BC sections showed some FGF2 staining of the nucleus and cytoplasm of a proportion of BC cells. FGF2 causes proliferation of some breast carcinoma cells lines (41.37), but inhibits proliferation of other cell lines, e.g., MCF-7 *(46)*. The reported effects of FGF2 on MCF-7 cells are conflicting, however, with some reports indicating a stimulation of proliferation *(47)*. Stewart et al. *(48)* reported that estradiol was required for FGF2 growth stimulation of MCF-7 cells.

The mechanisms by which FGF2 cells modulate BC cell proliferation remain uncertain. In MCF 7 cells, FGF2 treatment, although resulting in an upregulation of growth-inhibitory proteins responsible for mitogenic events, such as cyclin D1 and cyclin-dependent kinase 4, also decreases cyclin A and increases p21, which results in an inactivation of cyclin-dependent kinase 2 and dephosphorylation of Rb. This leads to a net decrease in cell proliferation *(46)*. Concomitantly, FGF2 leads to an increase in ERK1 and -2 activation in a dose-and-time-dependent manner *(49)*.

The role of FGF2 in other breast carcinoma cells is unclear, but some studies have been done *(50)* in which MCF-7 breast carcinoma cells were retrovirally transduced with 18-kDa or 18-kDa, together with the 22- and 24-kDa, basic FGF, showed that these constructs grew more slowly than control cells. Cells transduced with 18-kDa FGF2 showed upregulation of p21, WAF1/CIP1, and cells transduced all forms of FGF2 failed to reveal either an upregulation of p21 or FGF1 autophosphorylation or MAP kinase (MAPK) activation. In contrast, cells transduced with the 18-kDa form showed an increase in FGFR1 and MAPK phosphorylation.

The authors' results (Coombes, R. C. et al, submitted), in which it is shown that MCF-7 cells transduced with the FGF2 gene also grow more slowly, also disclose that FGF2 overexpression results in branching morphogenesis and suppression of tumorigenicity in nude mice.

The inhibitory effect of FGF2 predominated over the growth stimulatory effect of 17-β estradiol, insulin, or epidermal growth factor. The authors found an activation in P42 MAPK and P44 MAPK. Their observations also suggest that FGF2 is a pleiotrophic biological activator capable of inducing mutually exclusive cellular functions (i.e., proliferation and antiproliferative effect) under different conditions, because some MCF-7 cell lines can be inhibited by FGF2 when cultured in standard media, but proliferate when stimulated by basic FGF, and by FGF2 under serum and hormone deprivation. A clearer picture of the role of FGF2 has emerged in other tumor types, in which the growth factor appears to result in enhanced tumorigenicity, by either enhancing angiogenesis or metastatic potential examples are in melanoma, in which cells, infected with an Epstein-Barr virus-based mammalian expression vector, containing antisense FGF2, showed complete growth arrest *(51)*. Tumors regress as a result of inhibition of endothelial cell proliferation. This also seems to be the mechanism by which endometrial cells, transfected with an FGF2 expression vector, showed an upregulation of urokinase-type plasminogen activator. In renal cell carcinoma, introduction of FGF2 results in enhanced metastatic potential *(52)*.

Other roles of FGF2 in breast carcinoma cells are, as yet, ill defined. FGF2 has inhibitory properties on some carcinoma cells (*see* above), but is also capable of *rac* activation, which results in membrane ruffling *(33)*. FGF2 can also activate plasminogen activator synthesis, which can play a role in invasion and metastases *(53)*.

FGF7 and Its Receptor, FGFR2-IIIb, in Breast Cells

FGF7 and FGF10 are unusual, in that they have a stromal origin and appear to act specifically on ECs, and are therefore exclusively paracine growth factors *(54,55)*. FGF7 activates a splice variant of the FGFR2 *(56)*. Alternative splicing of the carboxy terminal half of the third Ig-like domain changes the ligand-binding properties for FGFR2, leading to FGFR2-IIIb binding to FGF1 and FGF7, and FGFR2-IIIc binding to FGF1 and FGF2 *(57)*. Whereas ECs express FGFR2-IIIb, cells of mesenchymal origin express FGFR2-IIIc *(58,59)*, and this is found to be the case in most epithelial organs, including the breast *(60)*.

Previously published reports have indicated the importance of FGF7 in controling the growth of mammary epithelium, including the report of Imagawa *(35)*, who showed, in murine mammary epithelium, that FGF7 induced the growth of mammary ECs in a collagen gel matrix, in a heparin-independent manner, and the studies of Ulich *(61)*, which demonstrated that parenteral administration of FGF7 resulted in hyperplastic mammary ductal epithelium and excess new duct formation in rats. Histologically, these changes in female rats arose from the growth of new ducts lined by a mitotically active epithelium, and resulted in hyperplasia, which was so excessive that the lumina were often occluded. Transgenic mice, in which FGF7 has been targeted to the breast, under the control of the mouse mammary tumor virus (MMTV) long terminal repeat, were generated by Kitsberg and Leder *(62)*. These mice showed high levels of FGF7 transgene expression during pregnancy and lactation, and developed hyperproliferation of the end buds and adenocarcinomas, with high frequency. FGF7 stimulates the proliferation of both luminal ECs and myo-ECs and the growth of whole breast organoids within a Matrigel matrix.

Using IHC, the authors have demonstrated FGF7 to be located predominantly in a stromal location, both inter- and intralobular stroma (Roberts-Clarke, D. et al., submitted). The source of FGF7 in the normal breast appears to be a subset of fibroblasts, which are responsible for FGF7 synthesis and secretion. The proportion of fibroblasts positive for FGF7 increases with FGF1 and FGF2 treatment. Occurrence of the KGF/FGF7 receptor, FGFR2, was also demonstrated, homogeneously distributed in the membrane and cytoplasm of normal and neoplastic ECs. It was shown that breast fibroblast conditioned medium contains FGF7, and that the conditioned medium-induced growth-promoting effect on ECs is abolished by an FGF7 neutralizing antibody (Ab).

Variations in FGFR2-IIIb Structure and Expression in Cancers

The authors' group has studied the expression of mRNA encoding both the FGFR2-IIIc and KGFR forms of FGFR2. In BC, the level of either variant was not related to prognosis or clinical status in patients with BC, except that patients with larger tumors appeared to have a higher FGFR-2IIIc:-IIIb ratio ($P = 0.01$). Ten BC cell lines were also studied and eight expressed predominantly FGF2-IIIb (KGFR); two had both FGFR2-IIIc and FGFR2-IIIb (60). Others (63) have described two forms of KGFR: one form, with a short C-terminus lacking the putative (PLC) γ association site (tyrosine 769), and the other with a full-length carboxy terminus, with this site intact. They found that the form of the receptor with the short C-terminus displayed a greater transforming activity than did the full-length receptor. The shortened receptor was less autophosphorylated in NIH 3T3 cells, but, the cells transfected with the shortened version showed a stronger mitogenic response to KGF than the full-length transfectants.

In addition, these cells showed no response when cultured in a differentiation-inducing medium; the cells transfected with the full-length differentiated appropriately. These results suggest that the receptor may be similar to the c-ErbB-2 protein, which is regulated negatively by its major autophosphorylation site, tyrosine 1248, at the C-terminus domain. These observations were corroborated by another group (64), who also demonstrated the importance of the C-terminal domain in regulating receptor activity, and suggested that the isoforms of FGFR with C-terminal alterations had enhanced growth-promoting activity. The group also examined the different receptor subtypes in a variety of human BC cell lines. Their studies also showed that overexpression of FGFR2 isoforms for truncated C-terminal domains could, in part, enhance growth properties without an overall increase in receptor content. They therefore carried out Northern blots, as well as in vitro kinase studies to examine the activity of FGFR2-IIIb. MDA-MB415 BC cell lines expressed the receptor at high levels as both protein and mRNA. MCF-7 cells, however, showed exaggerated phosphorylation, despite possessing very low levels of full-length FGFR2-IIIb protein, suggesting that receptor is highly phosphorylated.

FGF8 in Normal and Neoplastic Breast Cells

FGF8 was originally isolated from the conditioned medium of an androgen-dependent mouse mammary carcinoma line (SC-3) as an androgen-induced growth factor, and was later assigned as a member of the FGF family, on the basis of structural similarity (65). FGF8 appears to have an important role in embryogenesis. It is expressed in several areas of the developing mouse, and may play a critical role in the development of the face, limb, and central nervous system (66–69). Little expression of FGF8 is found in adult mouse tissues, with comparatively low amounts detected only in the ovaries and testes (70,71). FGF8 was identified as an oncogene on the basis of overexpression of FGF8 in NIH3T3 cells, leading to focus formation, growth in soft agar, and tumor formation in nude mice (72). FGF8 was subsequently found to act as a proto-oncogene co-operating with *Wnt-1* in mouse mammary tumorigenesis (70).

The structure of the FGF8 gene is more complex than the other members of this family. Most FGFs are encoded by three exons, but, in the case of FGF8, there are at least four exons corresponding to the usual first exon of the other genes. Alternative splicing potentially gives rise to eight different protein isoforms in the mouse, differing at the amino terminus, but remaining identical at the carboxyl end (66,67). In humans, only four of these forms will be possible, because of a stop codon in exon 1B (73). The biological significance of these forms is, as yet, unknown, but there is already evidence that they possess different transforming potentials with FGF8b having the highest transforming activity and widest receptor-binding properties (67,74,75).

The interaction of several splice variants of FGF8 with high-affinity receptors has been investigated (67): FGF8c activates FGFR3-IIIc and FGFR4; FGF8b activates FGFR2-IIIc, as well as FGFR3-IIIc and FGFR4. There is some debate as to whether FGFR1 may be a receptor for FGF8, since a splice variant of FGFR1 has been shown to bind FGF8 (72).

Several experiments have linked FGF8 expression to BC. Insertion of MMTV adjacent to FGF8 has been shown to induce BC in transgenic mice expressing wnt-1 (70). Northern analysis showed that 50% of tumors from these mice showed increased FGF8 transcription, making it the preferred activation in mice with a wnt-1 background (76). Further experiments showed that MMTV-FGF8 transgenic mice developed mammary and salivary gland neoplasia, as well as ovarian stromal hyperplasia (77). FGF8 is the first member of the FGF family whose expression is increased in BC, leading to the possibility that it plays a role in the initiation or maintenance of aspects of the malignant phenotype. FGF8 mRNA expression has been studied in human breast, and is found to be present in more malignant human breast tissues, compared to nonmalignant breast tissues $(P = 0.019)$ and at higher levels $(P = 0.031)$ (78). Analysis of BC cell lines and purified populations of normal breast cell populations showed that the highest levels of FGF8 mRNA expression were found in malignant ECs, and this has been confirmed using in situ hybridization (78). IHC staining of breast tissues for FGF8 also found that FGF8 was present in both normal and malignant human breast tissues (79). Of the receptors to which FGF8 binds, FGFR2-IIIc is expressed in cells of mesenchymal origin, and is not present in breast ECs, although it is present in breast fibroblasts (80). Similarly, FGFR3-IIIc is not found in breast ECs (the authors' observations). However, FGFR-4 and FGFR-1 have been detected in BC cells, opening the possibility of an autocrine loop in breast ECs. If there are a proportion of BCs that are driven by such a loop, then interrupting this cycle could lead to the development of novel therapies.

FGFR in Normal Breast and Breast Disease

The majority of surveys (e.g., see refs. 81 and 82) showed that FGFRs are present in nearly all tissues, particularly in early embryonic development. Initial studies from this group (29), in which mRNA for FGFR1 and FGFR2 was examined in breast tissue and BC cell lines, showed that both FGFR1 and -2 were present in the majority of normal breast tissues, and also in BC samples. The authors' early observations also suggested that there was considerable variation, particularly in the expression of FGFR2, in BC cell lines. Some of this variation could result from amplification or deletion of FGFR genes, especially because FGF3, FGF4, and KGF are co-localized in band 11q13, and FGFR1 and FGFR2 are localized in band 8p12 and 10q26, respectively (83–85). A large proportion of tumors possessing amplification of 11q13 also show amplification of FGFR1. The FGFR1 gene is amplified in BC and ovarian cancer (14.5 and 7.8%, respectively) (86), and, in many cases, FGFR1 gene amplification was associated with overexpression. The same group studied the expression of FGFR1 in human breast carcinoma cells (87), and found increased copy number for FGFR1 in 9% of carcinomas. Amplification and overexpression were approximately correlated, but did not strictly overlap. This group, as did the authors' group (88), showed that FGFR1 mRNA originated from the breast ECs. FGFRs have been found to be expressed in the mammary gland (84), using binding studies, and they are expressed immunohistochemically (90). FGFR1, FGFR2, and FGFR4 are expressed at high levels in 22, 4, and 32%, respectively, of breast carcinomas in another study (28).

The exon-deleted forms of FGFR1 have also been studied in the human breast *(88)*. Carcinomas were found to express FGFR1 at the protein level (135 kDa and 115 kDa), compared to FGFR1α and FGFR1β (lacking external Ig domain). The predominant FGFR isoform appeared to be FGFR1β, which was demonstrated, by microdisection, to be in carcinoma cells. In this study, the authors found that the predominant form of cancer-associated FGFR1 was FGFR1β; FGFR1α predominated in normal breast ECs.

In order to determine the localization of FGFRs, the authors have raised specific antibodies to FGFR1-4 *(33)*, and have also studied their involvement in membrane ruffling. Essentially, the findings indicate that different FGFRs gave different staining patterns, indicating that they occupied different sites within the cell. Abs against FGFR1 showed localization in cytoplasmic areas, but Abs against FGFR2 and -4 showed staining consistent with plasma membrane localization, with vesicular staining in the cytoplasm. For each of FGFR2 and -4, higher levels of staining were seen in BC cells, compared with normal breast ECs studied. Unexpectedly, the Ab against FGFR3 showed a nuclear staining pattern, and it was found that nuclear staining resulted from spliced variant of FGFR3, which lacks exons 7 and 8. This resulted in a translation of FGFR3 lacking the transmembrane domain, with an intact kinase domain, which could be a soluble intra-cellular receptor *(33)*.

Although all four receptors appear to be present in BC cells, the authors' studies indicated that the different receptors had different roles. A ruffling response, for example, was only seen when cells were transiently transfected with FGFR4, but not with FGFR1, -2, or -3 *(33)*. The authors' studies also showed that membrane ruffling was more pronounced in carcinoma cells, since normal breast cells showed very little ruffling in response to FGF1 and FGF2. Subsequently, the localization of FGFRs in normal breast ECs, myo-ECs, and stromal cells was examined, using a system in which these cell types can be separated and purified. These studies show that luminal ECs, myo-ECs, and stromal cells all possess FGFR1 transcripts; the FGFR2-IIIc isoform is absent from these three cell types. In contrast, FGFR2-IIIb is expressed in both ECs and myo-ECs, but absent from stromal cells. FGFR3 was only found in ECs, and FGFR4 was expressed in all three cells types *(36)*.

Although the high-affinity FGFR phenotype (in terms of FGFR1 and -4) did not appear to differ among ECs, myo-ECs, and stromal cells, low-affinity receptors for FGF2 differed significantly among the cell types. The HSPG synthesized by the myo-ECs has a far greater proportion of high-affinity FGF2-binding molecules than those from either epithelial cultures or breast cell lines, both in the conditioned medium and in the cell layer fraction *(36)*.

Subsequently, the authors have studied distribution of FGFR1 in BCs, using immuno-staining, as have others *(91)*. The authors' studies *(31)* disclosed that all BCs stained showed extensive localization of FGFR1 to principally the ECs in all breast carcinomas examined. However, normal breast also expresses this receptor. More recent results *(45)* have shown that the 115-kDa β-form of FGFR1 was the predominant isoform expressed in breast tissues. Probing with an Ab against the ligand binding domain of FGFR1, a 106-kDa band was visualized in benign cells, and, in particular, in myo-ECs. The 106-kDa form, unlike the 135- and 115-kDa forms, was difficult to detect in malignant tissues where there is loss of myo-ECs. Table 1 summarizes the published studies concerning FGFR expression in BC cell lines.

Four elements of FGFR function have recently been reported, which are relevant to FGFR function in breast cells. These are the intracellular localization of FGFR1 and its

Table 1
Summary of FGFR Expression in Breast Cell Lines

	No. (%) positive	
	Breast carcinoma	Nonneoplastic breast cells
FGFR 1		
Both/either variant	17/23 (74)	0/2 (0)
IIIb variant	0/5 (0)	3/3 (100)
IIIc variant	3/5 (60)	1/2 (50)
FGFR2		
Both/either variant	10/22 (45)	1/4 (25)
IIIb variant	6/10 (60)	0/2 (0)
IIIc variant	8/10 (80)	2/4 (50)
FGFR3		
Both/either variant	5/17 (29)	0/2 (0)
IIIb variant	1/5 (20)	2/2 (100)
IIIc variant	2/5 (40)	2/2 (100)
FGFR4	20/22 (91)	4/4 (100)

function in nuclear trafficking, effects of FGFR1 in the acquisition of mesenchymal phenotype, the effect of FGFR1 in chemotaxis, and the interaction between FGFRs and estrogen responsiveness. The nuclear trafficking function has also been studied (92). Those workers studied the trafficking of FGFR1 to the perinuclear locale. The understanding of nuclear traffic is important, because FGF1, -2, and -3 are frequently located in the nucleus. They showed that FGFR1β (the form lacking the external third Ig domain) induces morphological changes, upon stimulation of L6 myoblast cells with FGF1. In contrast, FGFR1α transfection failed to induce any change in morphology in the transfected cells. However, FGFR1α was the only form that was able to mediate the nuclear localization of FGF1. Those workers also showed that it was exclusively the FGFR1α that was in a nuclear localization, suggesting that the first Ig loop contains the structural information requisite for perinuclear trafficking. Glycosylation may well be important for nuclear trafficking, since tunicamycin reduces the level of the high-mol wt forms of FGFR in the nucleus.

In Madin-Darby canine kidney ECs, overexpression of FGFR1 resulted in the acquisition of a fibroblast-like morphology as a result of FGF1 stimulation. This transformation was also accompanied by changes in actin cellular distribution (93).

Studies using site-directed mutagenesis have disclosed that a mutant FGFR1, lacking the 63 C-terminal amino acid residues, failed to mediate chemotaxis (94). Because this mutant was truncated from amino acid 759, and Y766 is the site for the PLC γ-1 docking site, they also studied whether the defect in PLC γ-1 docking was responsible for that. However, cells expressing the mutant Y766F FGFR1 migrated as efficiently as the wild-type receptor. The PI-3-kinase inhibitor, wortmannin, suppressed wild-type FGFR1 mediated migration. The exact molecules mediating migration through the C-terminus of FGFR1 have not yet been defined.

The role of FGF signaling in estrogen responsiveness and proliferation of MCF-7 cells has also been studied (95): Johnston et al. (1998) group studied the crosstalk between FGF signaling and estrogen-response pathways in breast ECs, and confirmed that FGF signaling is growth-inhibitory for MCF-7 cells, and that it can downregulate estrogen response, despite activating the MAPK pathway. In MCF-7 cells treatment with FGF4 reduced estrogen receptor (ER) transcriptional activity around 2.5-fold, compared with estrogen alone. These results were mirrored in NIH3T3 cells transfected with an ER expression plasmid and an ERE-CAT reporter construct, which suggested that FGF could have a repressive effect on estrogen-stimulated ERE-CAT, particularly, since FGF treatment also inhibited progesterone receptor induction. The inhibitory effect of FGF was independent of MAPK phosphorylation of Serine 118, because it occurred in a mutant, (S118A)ER. Since STAT activation in response to EGF has been shown to be associated with growth inhibition, Johnston et al. (1998) determined whether FGF treatment activated the STAT pathway, and found that FGF treatment induced a STAT1 phosphorylation. Recent findings also suggest that the signaling by mutant FGFR3 can induce STAT1 activation, leading to p21 induction *(96)*. It may be, therefore, that STAT1-induced gene expression is responsible for the FGF induction of inhibition of proliferation in MCF-7 cells.

Table 1 summarizes the current situation regarding receptor expression in normal (non-neoplastic) breast cell lines. There is general agreement that FGFR4 is expressed in the vast majority (24/26) of cell lines tested. Next in frequency is FGFR1 (20/26). Most cell lines lack FGFR1-IIIb expression, and only a minority appear to express FGFR2-IIIb and FGFR3-IIIb.

The comparison with normal cell lines is difficult, because these comprise HBL100 (an SV40-transformed probable myo-EC line), H578TBst, and normal cell lines prepared from a reduction mammoplasty. Arguably, the latter is most representative of the normal luminal epithelial phenotype, since these cells are purified from contaminating myoepithelial, stromal, and other cell types *(36)*. These cells express the FGFR2-IIIb receptor: the authors have never found the FGFR2-IIIc receptor in any sample tested so far.

These results suggest that a characteristic of some BCs may be to use exons generally used in mesenchymal cells, particularly since some breast carcinomas express both iso-forms *(60)*. This exon-switching has also been observed in prostatic ECs *(97)*, and correlates with androgen insensitivity *(98)*.

FGFs AND THEIR RECEPTORS IN PROSTATE CANCER

Several characterized members of the FGF family have been shown to be expressed in human prostate cells. These include FGF1, FGF2 *(99)*, FGF7 *(54)*, and FGF8 *(65)*. In general, the roles of FGF2 and FGF7 have been studied in most depth. Other groups have shown that prostatic fibroblast and ECs are both stimulated by FGF2, and that transfection of prostate ECs with FGF2 causes an increase in proliferation rate and also a conversion to anchorage-independent growth *(100)*. Proliferation was inhibited by FGF2-neutralizing Abs. In contrast to BC, therefore, FGF2 appears to have an active role in proliferation of these cells.

There is less known about the expression of FGFRs in prostate cancer (PC) cells, compared with BC cells. Variable expression of FGFR1observed in PC3DU145 and LnCaP cells by Northern blotting and in rat prostate both FGFR1 and FGF2 are expressed in the nor-mal organ. FGFR1 is expressed by cultured prostate stromal cells, but not by ECs; FGFR2 is expressed by both stromal and ECs *(101)*.

The expression of a variety of ligands and receptors has been studied in the prostate, and only FGF7 was expressed in amounts detectable by Northern blotting *(102)*. FGF2 was also expressed, but no FGF1 or FGF8 was found to be expressed unless PCR was used, in which case the authors found a small level of FGF1 mRNA.

Those authors *(102)* also carried out Northern hybridization to quantitate FGFRs in human prostatic tissue. They failed to find FGFR4, but FGFR1, -2, and -3 were present. In terms of the isoforms expressed, FGFR1-IIIc, expressed in prostate, epithelial, and stromal cells, as was FGFR2-IIIc and FGFR2-IIIb. FGFR2-IIIb was found in total prostate cells and cultured ECs, but not in stromal cells, as is the case in breast cells. FGFR3 was found in the IIIc form, and was found in both stromal cells and ECs. No FGFR3-IIIb form was found.

Various groups have studied the effects of FGF1 and -2 on growth of prostate ECs. A mitogenic response to FGF2 and FGF1 has been reported *(103,104)*. However, FGF1 and -2 are not actively secreted, and it is uncertain as to the role of these two factors.

Both FGF8 and FGF7 have secretory peptides, and it is the occurrence of these ligands, with their respective receptors, that this review now focuses on.

FGF8 in Prostatic Tissue

FGF8 is expressed by PC cell lines *(79,105)*. Three forms of FGF8 mRNA encoding FGF8a, FGF8b, and FGF8e, were found to be expressed in a prostatic carcinoma cell line. Although northern analysis failed to detect FGF8 mRNA in adult human tissues, including prostate, reverse transcription (RT)-PCR could detect FGF8b mRNA in adult prostate tissue *(74)*. Nested RT-PCR was also able to detect FGF8 mRNA in normal adult rat prostate, and also in the human prostate tumor cell lines, LNCaP and DU145 *(105)*. An involvement in malignant prostate disease has been demonstrated, since FGF8 is detected in PCs, but not in benign prostatic hypertrophy *(106)*. IHC staining of human benign and malignant prostate tissues revealed that FGF8 was frequently expressed in human PCs (93%); normal and prostatic hyperplasia specimens showed no staining for FGF8 *(107)*.

FGF7 and its Receptor in Normal Prostate and PC

FGF7 (KGF) is expressed in the prostate, and mediates androgen action in androgen-dependant epithelial organs, such as prostate and seminal vesicles *(91,100)*. Other studies carried out on in vitro organ culture systems of the prostate have shown that KGF is a potent growth factor in the system, as well.*(109)*. In addition, testosterone can induce KGF release in this system *(102)*. Targeted overexpression results in mice developing hyperplasia of the male genital tract, including the seminal vesicle vas deferens and the prostate. Hyperplasia of the ventral and dorsolateral prostate were seen *(62)*.

The expression and cellular localization of KGF and its receptor have been carried out by immunocytochemistry and *in situ* hybridization *(110)*. Those studies show that, in benign prostatic hypertrophic tissues, KGF mRNA was abundant, and appeared to be predominantly expressed in the stromal cells; the receptor was mostly localized in the prostatic epithelium. KGF was determined by immunocytochemistry, and was also found to be present by histochemistry *(111)*. This mitogen was present in the stroma throughout the prostate, regardless of the functional region. To determine the effects of androgen removal on the pattern of KGF expression, those authors obtained prostatic biopsies at 0, 4, 7, and 21 d postcastration. By d 4, immunoreactivity for KGF was greatly reduced in the stroma. After involution, KGF immunoreactivity returned. However, after androgen replacement, no change in stromal KGF staining was seen, but KGF staining was observed in the epithelium after this time. These results suggest that a regulation of KGF expression is highly complex. An androgen-inducible element in the KGF promoter has been described, but KGF synthesis is also affected by glucocorticoids *(112,113)*. This report was unusual, in that KGF staining in ECs was seen, but further work needs to be done to elucidate this possible redistribution of expression.

The alternative splicing of FGFR2 in human PC has been studied *(98)*. The LnCaP cell line and two xenografts (DUKAP 1 and DUKAP 2) were characterized as androgen-sensitive; two other cell lines (DU145 and PC-3 and the xenograft, DU9479) were shown to be androgen-independent. Those authors examined FGFR2-IIIb expression, and showed that the loss of FGFR2 IIIb correlated with androgen insensitivity; indeed, DU9479 consisted almost entirely of FGFR2 transcript containing exon IIIc (97%). PC3 contained no detectable FGFR2. Because FGFR2 is located on chromosome 10q26, and this chromosome is disrupted in these cells, it may be that translocational deletion of the gene for FGFR2 has occurred.

This work is substantiated by other groups (114,115). Those authors have studied the Dunning R3327 PAP rat prostate cell line, which originally was androgen sensitive, but, after castration, an aggressive-androgen insensitive line, R338T3, was generated. These cells consist of a heterogenous group of cells, all of which possessed FGFR1, but a sub-population possessed FGFR2, with both IIIb and IIIc isoforms, and others possessed the FGFR2-IIIc isoform only. This subline showed no influence on proliferation with the addition of FGF1, -2, or -7. In contrast, the cell line, AT3R1 (expressing FGFR1), showed stimulation of proliferation by FGF1 and FGF2, but no effect of FGF7, since FGFR2-IIIb was absent. Initial studies by that group *(115)* showed that expression of the FGFR1 kinase in premalignant type 1 tumor ECs by transfection rapidly accelerated progression to a malignant phenotype. Indeed, after 6 mo, the cells transfected with FGFR1-β1 were 10× the weight of control cells. In contrast, transfection of FGFR2-IIIb resulted in a dramatically reduced growth rate of derived tumors, and co-inoculation of transfected AT3 cells with stromal cells derived from the differentiated tumor dramatically depressed the growth rate of the resultant tumors. In addition, AT3 cells, transfected with FGFR2-IIIb, gave rise to tumors that were less aggressive and exhibited more cell–cell contacts. There was some appearance of gland-like structures, and, in addition, the reappearance of cytokeratins was observed in these tumors *(116)*.

The same group *(114)* transfected cells with either the wild-type FGFR2 IIIb kinase or an artificial chimeric construct (FGFR2-IIIb/R1) composed of the FGFR2-IIIb ectodomain and the FGFR1 kinase domain. Both of these bind only FGF7, in contrast to untransfected tumor cells, and FGF7 was found to result in a dose-dependent net inhibition of population growth rates of cells expressing the full-length FGFR2-IIIb construct.

Thus, in contrast to the nonmalignant parent cells, in which 100% of ECs express exclusively the FGFR2-IIIb spliced variant, but no FGFR1, these cell lines express an FGFR1 that these authors observe as normally restricted to stromal cells *(114)*. When the FGFR2-IIIb ectodomain was fused to the FGFR1 kinase, no effect was seen, suggesting that the FGFR1 and -2 kinases are different, and do not elicit identical signals. The FGFR2-IIIb kinase may be acting as a dominant-negative inhibitor of dimerization and activation of the FGFR1 kinase. These studies *(114)* confirmed that the FGFR2 kinase has a net growth-controling role in ECs, in addition to a role in stimulating cell proliferation, which is distinct from the FGFR1 kinase in the context of prostate ECs.

REFERENCES

1. Burgess WH, Macaig T. The heparin-binding (fibroblast) growth factor family of proteins. Ann Rev Biochem 1989;58:575–606.
2. Delli Bovi P, Curatoia AM, Kern FG, Greco A, Ittmann M, Basilico C. An oncogene isolated by transfection of Kaposi's sarcoma DNA encodes a growth factor that is a member of the FGF family. Cell 1987;50:729–737.
3. Zhan X, Bates B, Hu X, Goldfarb M. The human FGF-5 oncogene encodes a novel protein related to fibroblast growth factor. Mol Cell Biol 1988;8:3487–3495.
4. Partanen J, Vainikka S, Akitako K. Structural and functional specificity of FGF receptors. Phil Trans R Soc Lond 1993;340:297–303.
5. Marics L, Adelaide J, Raybaud F, Mattei M-G, Coulier F, Planche J, de Lapeyriere O, Birnbaum D. Characterisation of the HST-related FGF6 gene, a new member of the fibroblast growth factor gene family. Oncogene 1989;4:335–340.
6. Finch PW, Rubin JS, Miki R, Ron D, Aaronson SA. Human KGF is FGF-related with properties of a paracine effector of epithelial cell growth. Science 1989;245:752–755.
7. Hecht D, Zimmerman N, Bedford N, Avivi A, Yayon A. Identification of fibroblast growth factor 9 (FGF9) as a high affinity, heparin dependent ligand for FGF receptors 3 and 2 but not for FGF receptors 1 and 4. Growth Factors 1995;12:223–233.
8. Yamasaki M, Miyake A, Tagashire S, Itoh N. Structure and expression of the rat mRNA encoding a novel member of the fibroblast growth factor family. J Biol Chem 1996;271:15,918–15,921.
9. Mignatti P, Morimoto T, Rifkin DB. Basic fibroblast growth factor, a protein devoid of secretory signal sequence, is released by cells via a pathway independent of the endoplasmic reticulum-Golgi complex. J Cell Physiol 1992;151:81–93.
10. Joaunneau J, Gavrilovic J, Caruelle D, Jaye M, Moens G, Caruells JP, Thiery JP. Secreted or nonsecreted forms of acidic fibroblast growth factor produced by transfected epithelial cells influence cell morphology, motility, and invasive potential. Proc Natl Acad Sci USA 1991;88:2893–2897.
11. Chao HH, Yang VC, Chen JK. Acidic FGF and EGF are involved in the autocrine growth stimulation of a human nasopharyngeal carcinoma cell line and sub-line cells. Int J Cancer 1993;54:807–812.
12. Klagsbrun M, Baird A. Dual receptor system is required for basic fibroblast growth factor activity. Cell 1991;67:229–231.
13. Ruta M, Howk R, Ricca G, Drohan W, Zabelshansky M, Laureys G, et al. Novel protein tyrosine kinase gene whose expression is modulated during endothelial cell differentiation. Oncogene 1988;3:9–15.
14. Lee PL, Johnson DE, Cousens LS, Fried VA, Williams LT. Purification and complementary DNA cloning of a receptor for basic fibroblast growth factor. Science 1989;245:57–60.
15. Johnson DE, Lu J, Chen H, Werner S, Williams LT. The human fibroblast growth factor receptor genes: a common structural arrangement underlies the mechanism for generating receptor forms that differ in their third immunoglobulin domain. Mol Cell Biol 1991;11:4627–4634.
16. Hou JZ, Kan MK, McKeehan K, McBride G, McKeehan WL. Fibroblast growth factor receptors from liver vary in three structural domains. Science 1991;251:665–668.
17. Jaye M, Schlessinger J, Dionne CA. Fibroblast growth factor receptor tyrosine kinases: molecular analysis and signal transduction. Biochim Biophys Acta 1992;1135:185–199.
18. Vainikka S, Partanen S, Bellosta P, Coulier C, Basilico C, Jaye M, Alitalo K. Fibroblast growth factor receptor-4 shows novel features in genome structure, ligand binding, and signal transduction. EMBO J 1992;11:4273–4280.
19. Zimmer Y, Givol D, Yayon A. Multiple structural elements determine ligand binding of fibroblast growth factor receptors. J Biol Chem 1993;268:7899–7903.
20. Wang F, Kan M, Xu J, Yan G, McKeehan WL. Ligand-specific structural domains in the fibroblast growth factor receptor. J Biol Chem 1995;270:10,222–10,230.
21. Wang F, Kan M, McKeehan K, Feng S, McKeehan WL. A homeointeraction sequence in the ectodomain of the fibroblast growth factor receptor. J Biol Chem 1997;272:23,887–23,895.
22. Heldin CH. Dimerization of cell surface receptors in signal transduction. Cell 1995;80:213–223.
23. Fantl WJ, Johnson DE, William LT. Signalling by receptor tyrosine kinases. Ann Rev Biochem 1993; 62:453–481.
24. Hou JZ, Kan MK, McKeehan K, McBride G, McKeehan WL. Fibroblast growth factor receptors from liver vary in three structural domains. Science 1991;251:665–668.
25. Coleman-Krnaick S, Rosen JM. Differential temporal and spatial gene expression of fibroblast growth factor family members during mouse mammary gland development. Mol Endocrinol 1994;8:218–229.

26. Bansal GS, Yiangou C, Coope RC, Gomm JJ, Luqmani YA, Coombes RC, Johnston CL. Expression of fibroblast growth factor 1 is lower in breast cancer than in the normal human breast. Br J Cancer 1995;72:1420–1426.

27. Renaud F, El Yazidi I, Boilly-Marer Y, Cortois Y, Laurent M. Expression and regulation by serum of multiple FGF1 mRNA in normal transformed, and malignant human mammary epithelial cells. Biochem Biophys Res Commun1996;219:679–685.

28. Penault-Llorca F, Bertucci F, Adelaide J, Parc RC, Coulier F, Jacquemier J, Birnbaum D, Delapeyrier O. Expression of FGF and FGF receptors in human breast cancer. Int J Cancer 1995;61:170–176.

29. Lugmani YA, Graham M, Coombes RC. Expression of basic fibroblast growth factor, FGFR1 and FGFR2 in normal and malignant human breast, and comparison with other normal tissues. Br J Cancer 1992; 66:273–280.

30. Anandappa SY, Winstanley JHR, Leinster S, Green B, Rudland PS, Barraclough R. Comparative expression of fibroblast growth factor mRNAs in benign and malignant breast disease. Br J Cancer 1994;69:772–776.

31. Coope RC, Browne PJ, Yiangou C, Bansal GS, Walters J, Groome N, et al. The location of acidic fibroblast growth factor in the breast is dependent on the activity of proteases present in breast cancer tissue. Br J Cancer 1997;75:1621–1630.

32. Smith J, Yelland A, Baillie R, Coombes RC. Acidic and basic fibroblast growth factors in human breast tissue. Eur J Cancer 1994;30A:496–503.

33. Johnston CL, Cox HC, Gomm JJ, Coombes RC. Fibroblast growth factor receptors localise in different cellular compartments. J Biol Chem 1995;270:1–8.

34. McLeskey SW, Ding IYF, Lippman ME, Kern HG. MDA-MB-134 breast carcinoma cells overexpress fibroblast growth factor (FGF) receptors and are growth-inhibited by FGF ligands. Cancer Res 1994; 54:523–530.

35. Imagawa W, Cunha GR, Young P, Nandi S. Keratinocyte growth factor and acidic fibroblast growth factor are mitogens for primary cultures of mammary epithelium. Biochem Biophys Res Commun 1994; 204:1165–1169.

36. Gomm JJ, Browne PJ, Coope RC, Bansal GS, Yiangou C, Johnston CL, Mason R, Coombes RC. A paracrine role for myoepithelial cell-derived FGF2 in the normal human breast. Exp Cell Res 1997; 234:165–173.

37. Souttou B, Gamby C, Crepin M, Hamelin R. Tumoral progression of human breast epithelial cells secreting FGF2 and FGF4. Int J Cancer 1996;68:675–681.

38. Zhang L, Kharbanda S, Chen D, Bullocks J, Miller DL, Ding I, et al. MCF-7 breast carcinoma cells overexpressing FGF-1 from vascularised, metastatic tumors in ovariectomised or tamoxifen-treated nude mice. Oncogene 1997;15:2093–2108.

39. McLeskey SW, Zhang L, El-Ashey D, Trock BJ, Lopez CA, Kharbanda S, et al. Tamoxifen-resistant fibroblast growth factor-transfected MCF-7 cells are cross-resistant in vivo to the antiestrogen ICI 182,780 and two aromatase inhibitors. Clin Cancer Res 1998;4:697–711.

40. Jouanneau J, Moens G, Montesano R, Thiery J-P. FGF-1 but not FGF-4 secreted by carcinoma cells Promotes in vitro and in vivo angiogenesis and rapid tumour proliferation. Growth Factors 1995;12: 37–47.

41. Li S, Shipey GD. Expression of multiple species of basic fibroblast growth factor mRNA and protein in normal and tumor-derived mammary epithelial cells in culture. Cell Growth Differ 1991;2:195–202.

42. Gomm JJ, Browne PJ, Coope RC, Bansal GS, Yiangou C, Johnston CL, Mason R, Coombes RC. A paracrine role for myoepithelial cell-derived FGF2 in the normal human breast. Exp Cell Res 1997;234: 165–173.

43. Plopper GE, McNamee PH, Dike LE, Bojanowski K, Ignber DE. Convergence of intergrin and growth factor receptor signalling pathways within the focal adhesion complex. Mol Biol Cell 1995;6:1349–1365.

44. Gomm JJ, Smith J, Ryall GK, Baillie R, Turnbull L, Coombes RC. Localisation of basic fibroblast growth factor and transforming growth factor beta 1 in the human mammary gland. Cancer Res 1991; 51:4685–4692.

45. Yiangou C, Johnston CL, Gomm JJ, Coope RC, Luqmani YA, Shousha S, Coombes RC. Fibroblast growth factor 2 in breast cancer: occurrence and prognostic significance. Br J Cancer 1997;75:38–33.

46. Wang H, Rubin M, Fenig E, DeBlasio A, Mendelson J, Yahalom J. Basic fibroblast growth factor causes growth arrest in MCF-7 human breast cancer cells while inducing both mitogenic and inhibitory G1 events. Cancer Res 1977;57:1750–1757.

47. Karey KP, Sirbasku DA. Differential responsiveness of human breast cancer cell lines MCF-7 and T47D to growth factors and 17β-estradiol. Cancer Res 1988;38:4083–4092.

48. Stewart AJ, Westly BR, May FE. Modulation of the proliferative response of breast cancer cells to growth factors by oestrogen. Br J Cancer 1992;66:640–648.

49. Fenig E, Wider R, Paglin S, Wang H, Persaud R, Haimovitz-Friedman A, Fuks Z, Yahalom J. Basic fibroblast growth factor confers growth inhibition and ERK activation in human breast cancer cells. Clin Cancer Res 1997;3:135–142.

50. Weider R, Wang H, Shirke S, Wang O, Menzel T, Feirt N, Jakubowksi AA, Gabrilove JL. Low level expression of basic FGF upregulates Bcl-2 and delays apoptosis, but high intracellular levels are required to induce transformation in NIH 3T3 cells. Growth Factors 1997;15:41–60.

51. Wang Y, Beck D. Antisense targeting of basic fibroblast growth factor and fibroblast growth factor receptor-1 in human melanomas blocks intratumoral angiogenesis and tumor growth. Nat Med 1997;3: 887–893.

52. Miyake H, Hara I, Yoshimura K, Eto H, Arakaw S, Wada S, Chihara K, Kamidono S. Introduction of basic fibroblast growth factor gene into mouse renal cell carcinoma cell line enhances its metastatic potential. Cancer Res 1996;56:2440–2445.

53. Rusnati M, Dell'Era P, Urbinati C, Tanghetti E, Massardi ML, Nagamine Y, Monti E, Presta M. Distinct basic fibroblast growth factor (FGF-2)?FGF receptor interaction distinguishes urokinase-type plasminogen activator induction from mitogenicity in endothelial cells. Mol Biol Cell 1996;7:369–381.

54. Rubin JS, Osada H, Finch PW, Taylor GW, Rudikoff S, Aaaronson SA. Purification and character-isation of a newly identified growth factor specific for epithelial cells. Proc Natl Acad Sci USA 1989; 86:802–806.

55. Emoto H, Tagashira S, Mattei MG, Yamasaki M, Hashimoto G, Katsumata T, et al. Structure and expression of human fibroblast factor 10. J Biol Chem 1997;272:23,191–23,194.

56. Miki T, Fleming TP, Bottaro DP, Rubib JS, Ron D, Aaronson SA. Expression cDNA cloning of the KGF receptor by reaction of a transforming autocrine loop. Science 1991;251:27–75.

57. Yayon A, Zimmer Y, Guo-Hong S. Avivi A, Yosef Y, Givol D. A confined variable region confer ligand specificity on fibroblast growth factor receptors: implications for the origin of the immunoglo-bulin fold. EMBO J 1992;11:1885–1890

58. Pekonen F, Nyman T, Rutanen EM, Differential expression of keratinocyte growth factor and its recep-tor in the human uterus. Mol Cell Endocrinol 1993;95:43–49.

59. Savagner P, Valles AM, Jouanneau J, Yamada KM, Thiery JP. Alternative splicing in fibroblast growth factor receptor 2 is associated with induced epithelial-mesenchymal transition in rat bladder carci-noma. Mol Cell Biol 1994;5:851–862.

60. Luqmani YA, Bansal GS, Mortimer C, Buluwela L, Coombes RC. Expression of FGFR2 BEK and K-SAM mRNA variants in normal and malignant human breast. Eur J Cancer 1996;32A:518–524.

61. Ulich TR, Yi ES, Cardiff R, Yin S, Bikhazi N, Biltz R, Morris CF, Pierce GF. Keratinocyte growth factor is a growth factor for mammary epithelium. In vivo. Am J Pathol 1994;144:862–868.

62. Kitsberg DI, Leder P. Keratinocyte growth factor induces mammary and prostatic hyperplasia and mammary adenocarcinoma in transgenic mice. Oncogene 1996;13:2507–2515.

63. Ishii H, Yoshida T, Oh H, Yoshida S, Terada M. A Truncated K-sam product lacking the distal car-boxyl-terminal portion provides a reduced level of autophosphorylation and greater resistance against induction of differentiation. Mol Cell Biol 1995;15:3664–3671.

64. Lorenzi MV, Castagnino P, Chen Q, Chedid M, Miki T. Ligand-independent activation of fibroblast growth factor receptor-2 by carboxyl terminal alterations. Oncogene 1997;15:817–826.

65. Tanaka A, Miyamoto K, Minamino N, Takeda M, Sato B, Matsuo H, Matsumoto K. Cloning and char-acterization of an androgen-induced growth factor essential for the androgen-dependent growth of mouse mammary-carcinoma cells. Proc Natl Acad Sci USA 1992;89:8928–8932.

66. Crossley PH, Martin GR. The mouse Fgf8 gene encodes a family of polypeptides and is expressed in regions that direct outgrowth and patterning in the developing embryo. Development (Camb) 1995;121: 439–451.

67. MacArthur CA, Lawshe A, Xu J, Santos-Ocampo S, Heikinheimo M, Chellaiah AT, Ornitz DM. FGF8 isoforms activate receptor splice forms that are expressed in mesenchymal regions of mouse develop-ment. Development (Camb) 1995;121:3603–3613.

68. Crossley PH, Martinez S, Martin GR. Midbrain development induced by FGF8 in the chick embryo. Nature (Lond) 1996;380:66–68.

69. Crossley PH, Minowada G, MacArthur CA, Martin GR. Roles for FGF8 in the induction, initiation and maintenance of chick limb development. Cell 1996;84:127–136.

70. MacArthur CA, Shankar DB, Shackleford GM. FGF-8, activated by proviral insertion, cooperates with the Wnt-1 transgene in murine mammary tumourigenesis. J Virol 1995;69:2501–2507.

71. Lorenzi MV, Long JE, Miki T, Aaronson SA. Expression cloning, developmental expression and chromosomal localization of fibroblast growth factor-8. Oncogene 1995;10:2051–2055.
72. Kouhara H, Koga M, Kasayama S, Tanaka A, Kishimoto T, Sato B. Transforming activity of a newly cloned androgen-induced growth factor. Oncogene 1994;9:455–462.
73. Gemel J, Gorry M, Enruch GD. Structure and sequence of human FGF8. Genomics 1996;35:253–257.
74. Ghosh AK, Shankar DB, Shackleford GM, Wu K, T'Ang A, Miller GJ, Zheng J, Roy-Burman P. Molecular cloning and characterisation of human FGF8 alternative messenger RNA forms. Cell Growth Differ 1996;7:1425–1434.
75. MacArthur CA, Lawshe A, Shankar DB, Heikinheimo M, Shackleford GM. FGF-8 isoforms differ in NIH3T3 cell transforming potential. Cell Growth Differ 1995;6:817–825.
76. Kapoun AM, Shackleford GM. Preferential activation of Fgf8 by proviral insertion in mammary tumors of Wnt1 transgenic mice. Oncogene 1997;14:2985–2989.
77. Daphna-Iken D, Shankar DB, Lawshe A, Ornitz DM, Shackleford GM, MacArthur CA. MMTV-Fgf8 transgenic mice develop mammary and salivary gland neoplasia and ovarian stromal hyperplasia. Oncogene 1998;17:2711–2717.
78. Marsh SK, Bansal GS, Zammit C, Barnard R, Coope R, Roberts-Clarke D, et al. Increased expression of fibroblast growth factor 8 in human breast cancer. Oncogene 1999;18:1052–1060.
79. Tanaka A, Miyamoto K, Matsuo H, Matsumoto K, Yoshida H. Human androgen-induced growth factor in prostate and breast cancer cells: its molecular cloning and growth properties. FEBS Lett 1995;363:226–230.
80. Bansal GS, Cox HC, Marsh S, Gomm JJ, Yiangou C, Luqmani Y, Coombes RC, Johnston CL. Expression of keratinocyte growth factor and its receptor in human breast cancer. Br J Cancer 1997;75:1567–1574.
81. Kornbluth S, Paulson KS, Hanafusa H. Novel tyrosine kinase identified by phosphotyrosine antibody screening. Mol Cell Biol 1988;8:5541.
82. Reid HH, Wilks AF, Bernard O. Two forms of the basic fibroblast growth factor receptor-like mRNA are expressed in the developing mouse brain. Proc Natl Acad Sci USA 1990;87:1596.
83. Ruta M, Burgess W, Givol D, Epstein J, Neiger N, Kaploy J, et al. Receptor for acidid fibroblast growth factor is related to tyrosine kinase encoded by the fms-like gene (FLG). Proc Natl Acad Sci USA 1989;86:8722–8726.
84. Mattei MG. Moreau A, Gesnel MC, Houssaint E, Breatnach R. Assignment by in situ hydridisation of a fibroblast growth factor receptor gene to human chomosome band 10q26. Hum Genet 1991;87:84–86.
85. Dionne C, Modi W, Crumley G, O'Brien S, Schlessinger J, Jaye M. BEK, a receptor for multiple members of the fibroblast growth factor (FGF) family, maps to human chromosome 10q25.3-q26. Cytogenet Cell Genet 1992;60:34–36.
86. Theillet C, Adelaide J, Louason G, Bonnet-Doriun F, Jacquemier J, Adnane J, et al. FGFR1 and Plat genes and DNA amplification at 8p12 in breast and ovarian cancers. Genes Chromosomes Cancer 1993;7:219–226.
87. Jacquemier J, Adelaide J, Parc P, Penault-Llorca F, Planche J, DeLapeyiere O, Birnbaum D. Expression of the FGFR1 gene in human breast carcinoma cells. Int J Cancer 1994;59:373–378.
88. Luqmani Y, Mortimer C, Yiangou C, Johnston CL, Bansal GS, Sinnett D, Law M, Coombes RC. Expression of 2 variant forms of fibroblast growth factor receptor 1 in human breast. Int J Cancer 1995;64:274–279.
89. Peyrat JP, Bonneterre J, Hondermarck H, Hecquet B, Adenis A, Louchez MM, et al. Basic fibroblast growth factor (bFGF): mitogenic activity and binding sites in human breast cancer. J Steroid Biochem Mol Biol 1992;43:87–94.
90. Hughes SE, Hall PA. Immunolocalization of fibroblast growth factor receptor 1 and its ligands in human tissues. Lab Invest 1993;69:173–182.
91. Morikawa Y, Ishihara Y, Tohya K, Kakudo K, Kurokawa M, Matsuura N. Expression of the fibroblast growth factor receptor-1 in human normal tissues and tumours determined by a new monoclonal antibody. Arch Pathol Lab Med 1996;120:490–496.
92. Prudovsky IA, Savion N, LaVallee TM, Maciag T. The nuclear trafficking of extracellular fibroblast growth factor (FGF)-1 Correlates with the perinuclear association of the FGF receptor-1α isoforms but not the FGF receptor-1β isoforms. J Biol Chem 1996;271:14,198–14,205.
93. Migdal M, Soker S, Yarden Y, Neufeld G. Activation of a transfected FGFR-1 receptor in Madin-Darby epithelial cells results in a reversible loss of epithelial properties. J Cell Physiol 1995;162:266–276.
94. Langren E, Klint P, Yokote K, Claesson-Welsh L. Fibroblast growth factor receptor 1 mediates chemotaxis independently of direct SH-2-domain protein binding. Oncogene 1998;17:283–291.

95. Johnston MR, Valentine C, Basilico C, Mansukhani A. FGF signaling activates STAT1 and p21 and inhibits the estrogen response and proliferation of MCF-7 cells. Oncogene 1998;16:2647–2656.

96. Su WC, Kitagawa M, Xue N, Xie B, Garofalo S, Cho J, et al. Activation of Stat1 by mutant fibroblast growth-factor receptor in thanatopheric dysplasia in type II dwarfism. Nature 1997;386:288–292.

97. Yan G, Fukabori Y, McBride G, Nikolaropolous SM, McKeehan WL. Exon switching and activation of stromal and embryonic fibroblast growth factor (FGF)-FGF receptor genes in prostate epithelial cells accompany stromal independence and malignancy. Mol Cell Biol 1993;13:4513–4522.

98. Carstens RP, Eaton JV, Krigman HR, Walther PJ, Garcia-Blanco MA. Alternative splicing of fibroblast growth factor receptor 2 (FGF-R2) in human prostate cancer. Oncogene 1997;15:3059–3065.

99. Storey MT, Hopp KA, Molter M, Meier DA. Characteristics of FGF-receptors expressed by stromal and epithelial cells cultured from normal and hyperplastic prostates. Growth Factors 1994;10:269–280.

100. Ropiquet F, Berthon P, Villette J-M, Le Brun G. Maitland NJ, Cussenot O, Fiet J. Constitutive expression of FGF2/bFGF in non-tumorigenic human prostatic epithelial cells results in the acquisition of a partial neoplastic phenotype. Int J Cancer 1997;72:532–547.

101. Nakamota T, Chang CS, Li AK, Chodak GW. Basic fibroblast growth factor in human prostate-cancer cells. Cancer Res 1992;52:571–577.

102. Ittman M, Mansukhani A. Expression of fibroblast growth factors (FGFs) and FGF receptors in human prostate. J Urol 1997;157:351–356.

103. Sherwood E, Fong C, Lee C, Kozlowski J. Basic fibroblast growth factor: a potential mediator of stromal growth in the human prostate. Endocrinology 1992;130:2955.

104. Story MT. Regulation of prostate growth by fibroblast growth factors. World J Urol 1995;13:297–305.

105. Schmitt JF, Hearn MTW, Risbridger GP. Expression of fibroblast growth factor 8 in adult rat tissues and human prostate carcinoma cells. J Steroid Biochem Mol Biol 1996;57:173–178.

106. Leung HY, Dickson C, Robson CN, Neal DE. Over-expression of fibroblast growth factor-8 in human prostate cancer. Oncogene 1996;12:1833–1835.

107. Tanaka A, Furuya A, Yamasaki M, Hanai N, Kuriki K, Kamiakito T, et al. High frequency fibroblast growth factor (FGF) 8 expression in clinical prostate cancers and breast tissues, immunohistochemically demonstrated by a newly established neutralizing monoclonal antibody against FGF8. Cancer Res 1998;58:2053–2056.

108. Cunha GR, Role of mesenchymal-epithelial interactions in normal and abnormal development of the mammary gland and prostate. Cancer 1994;74:1030–1044.

109. Rubin JS, Bottaro DP, Chedid M, Miki T, Ron D, Cheon G, et al. Keratinocyte growth factor. Cell Biol Int 1995;19:339–411.

110. De Bellis A, Crescioli C, Grappone C, Milani S, Ghiandi P, Forti G, Serio M. Expression and cellular localization of keratinocyte growth factor and its receptor in human hyperplastic prostate tissue. J Clin Endocrinol Metab 1998;83:2186–2191.

111. Nemeth JA, Zelner DJ, Lang S, Lee C. Keratinocyte growth factor in the rat ventral prostate androgen-independent expression. J Endocrinol 1998;156:115–125.

112. Fasciana C, Van-Der-Made AC, Faber PW, Trapman J. Androgen regulation of the rat keratinocyte growth factor (KGF/FGF7) promoter. Biochem Biophys Res Commun 1996;220:858–863.

113. Chedid M. Rubin JS, Csaky KG, Aaronson SA. Regulation of keratinocyte growth factor gene expression by interleukin 1. J Biol Chem 1994;269:10,753–10,757.

114. Feng S, Wang F, Matsubara A, Kan M, McKeehan WL. Fibroblast growth factor receptor 2 limits and receptor 1 accelerated tumorigenicity of prostate epithelial cells. Cancer Res 1997;57:5369–5378.

115. Matsubara A, Kan M, Feng S, McKeehan WL. Inhibition of growth of malignant rat prostate tumor cells by restoration of fibroblast growth factor receptor 2. Cancer Res 1998;58:1509–1514.

13

Steroid Receptors in Prostate Cancer Development and Progression

Marco Marcelli, MD, Nancy L. Weigel, PHD, and Dolores J. Lamb, PHD

INTRODUCTION

The steroid receptor superfamily plays an important role in the development and maintenance of differentiated function in the prostate. Notably, androgens are required for the development of the prostate, the normal function of the prostate in the adult, and may play a role in the development of prostate cancer (PC) and progression of the disease. Nevertheless, other steroid receptors have also been implicated in the development and progression of PC.

There is considerable homology between members of the steroid receptor superfamily (reviewed in ref. *1*). There are three major regions of conserved amino acids. The most highly conserved region is in the DNA-binding domain. In this region, there are nine conserved cysteine residues with α-helices that recognize the steroid-responsive elements required for DNA specific binding *(2–4)*. Conserved regions II and III, consisting of approx 220–250 amino acids, are found within the C-terminal portion of the molecule, and are found within the steroid-binding domain of the protein. The N-terminal domain is more immunogenic, and contains the regions required for transactivation. In addition to the classical receptors (such as androgen, estrogen [ER], progesterone [PR], glucocorticoid [GR], mineralocorticoid), and receptors such as the thyroid hormone receptor, vitamin D receptor, and retinoic acid (RA) receptors, there are a series of orphan receptors with structural homology to the classical receptors. At least some of these gene-regulatory transcription factors are known to be required for development, although the ligand for most has not yet been identified. At least one of these orphan receptors, TR3, is expressed in prostate. Because a number of these receptors are expressed in normal prostate, and play a role in the normal development and maintenance of differentiated

From: *Contemporary Endocrinology: Endocrine Oncology*
Edited by: S. P. Ethier © Humana Press Inc., Totowa, NJ

function in the adult, it is perhaps not surprising to learn that they also play an important role in PC. The following review focuses on the role of several members of the steroid receptor superfamily in the regulation of PC development and progression.

PC: Lack of Cure for Advanced Disease

PC remains the second leading cause of cancer deaths in American men. The number of new cases of PC predicted in the United States for 1999 was 179,300. There may be 37,000 PC-related deaths in 1999, accounting for 13% of all cancer deaths among American men *(10)*. Radical prostatectomy is the chief curative treatment for men with organ-confined disease. Most men with nonorgan-confined disease will undergo palliation with radiation or androgen ablation *(11)*. Androgen ablation successfully shrinks primary and metastatic lesions by inducing apoptosis of androgen-dependent PC cells *(12)*. Unfortunately, nonorgan-confined PC is a heterogeneous lesion, and at the time of diagnosis contains foci of both androgen-dependent and -independent cells *(13)*. Androgen-independent cells escape apoptosis induced by androgen ablation *(14)*, and by many cytotoxic drugs. They continue to proliferate and metastasize, despite profound changes of the surrounding hormonal milieu, and represent the most direct threat to patient survival. To develop new successful forms of treatment for nonorgan-confined PC, it is important that there is understanding of the molecular basis of hormone-refractory disease.

Androgens play an essential role in regulating the development, growth, and differentiation of the normal prostate. The intracellular mediator of androgen action is the androgen receptor (AR), a member of a superfamily of ligand-activated nuclear transcription factors *(1)*. Abnormal androgen production or loss of function of the AR are associated with various phenotypic abnormalities of the prostate. The ensuing clinical picture depends on whether the defect developed in utero, before puberty, or after puberty. Typically, the prostate is absent or rudimentary in 46,XY patients, with prenatal abnormalities of androgen biosynthesis or in the AR. Although prepubertal dysfunction of androgen biosynthesis is associated with a small, not fully matured gland, postpubertal abnormalities are usually associated with involutional changes. A hormonal etiology involving androgen action has been hypothesized for PC *(5,6)*. There is anecdotal evidence suggesting that the risk of developing PC and benign prostatic hyperplasia is decreased in men with anomalies of androgen biosynthesis or the AR, and is increased in hypogonadal men treated with androgens *(7–9)*. Therefore, normal androgen biosynthesis and/or AR signaling pathway play at least a permissive role in the development of these two diseases.

MOLECULAR BASIS OF HORMONAL INSENSITIVITY IN PC

Androgen Receptor

There is evidence that AR is expressed in all stages of PC evolution, including prostatic intraepithelial neoplasia *(15)*, primary *(16,17)*, and metastatic *(18,19)* disease, before and after androgen ablation therapy. Only a minority of cancers are AR-negative *(20)*, and thus, even hormone-refractory tumors are AR-positive. In view of this, investigators have proposed the following AR-related mechanisms to explain progression to androgen-independent growth:

1. Amplification of the AR gene, which would facilitate tumor growth at very low concentrations of the ligand.

2. Point mutations of the AR gene.
3. Changes in the number of glutamines in the aminoterminal polyglutamine repeats, which may increase the response of AR to stimulation with androgens.
4. Androgen-independent activation of AR.
5. Activation of growth-stimulating signaling pathways with the ability to bypass AR-regulated growth and differentiation.
6. Increased local bioavailability of androgens to activate AR.
7. Alternative co-activator-mediated mechanisms activating androgen signaling.

AMPLIFICATION OF THE AR GENE

Using comparative genomic hybridization for genome-wide screening of genetic aberrations, Visakorpi et al. *(21)* identified a common DNA-amplification site in recurrent, hormone-refractory PCs in Xq11-q13, the site of the AR gene. High-level amplification of the AR gene was subsequently identified in 30% of these specimens by fluorescence *in situ* hybridization, using an AR-specific probe *(22,23)*. Amplification of AR was not observed before implementation of androgen-ablative treatment, suggesting that this phenomenon is not involved in the genesis of PC, and occurred as a result of selection during androgen-deprivation therapy. Additionally, molecular analysis of the AR in 13 cases showed only one point mutation (G-A) at codon 674. Because this mutation did not change the transactivational properties of the receptor, those authors concluded that AR amplification promotes a hormone-refractory phenotype, independent of point mutations, by sustaining cell growth, even in the presence of substantially reduced concentrations of androgens.

POINT MUTATIONS OF AR

The possibility that point mutations in the AR may account for progression from androgen-dependent to androgen-independent growth has been a popular theory ever since the AR cDNA was cloned *(23–28)*. Numerous investigators have used polymerase chain reaction (PCR) single-stranded conformational polymorphism of DNA extracted from foci of PC to search for AR variants. A review of data published in the literature shows that there is still considerable controversy in the field. As shown in Table 1, 581 cases of PC have been analyzed at the molecular level for the presence of AR mutations. A total of 47 mutations (frequency 8%) causing amino acid changes or additions have been detected. Twenty-two of these mutations (46% of total) were reported by three groups, from a total of 59 patients (frequency of mutations in these 59 patients, 37%) *(29–31)*. The remaining 25 mutations were detected in 522 patients (frequency, 4.7%). To understand the reason for these discrepancies in the relative frequency of AR mutations among different groups, the authors have correlated the prevalence of AR mutations to differences in patient sampling or to methodological variables. There is uniform agreement that early PC (i.e., stage A or B disease) is rarely associated with mutations of AR (five mutations in 231 cases [2.1%]) *(32–42)*. Primary lesions from patients with more advanced PC (stage C and D) are more likely to contain mutations of AR; however, the overall incidence is not high (29/238 cases [12%]) *(21,22,29,31–34,36–39,41–44)*. Finally, the data available show that the prevalence of AR mutations is more substantial in metastatic PC (7/26 cases [22%] *(30,33,42,45,46)*. This indicates that mutations of AR are not early events leading to neoplastic degeneration of prostatic tissue, but late developments that may affect biologic behavior and/or response to conventional treatments.

Table 1
Summary of Mutations
Detected in Patients with Clinically Diagnosed PC

	No. of cases[a]	No. of mutations[b]	% of mutations
Total (18, 19, 29, 46, 114)	581	47	8
Stage A-B (32–41)	231	5	2.1
Stage C-D (Primary lesion) (18, 19, 29, 31–34, 36–39, 41, 42, 44, 115)	238	29	12
Metastatic tissue (33, 41, 45, 46)	59	13	22

[a] The sum of cases with stage A-B, C-D, and metastatic tissue is lower than the total number of patients, because it was not always possible to assign a disease stage to each patient reported. In addition 11 cases were analyzed both at the primary and metastatic site *(19,30)*.

[b] Only mutations resulting in amino acid residue changes or additions have been inserted in the list.

Methodological variables correlating positively with increased prevalence of AR mutations are the analysis of tumor-enriched DNA after microdissection of the sample, and the analysis of exon 1. This was shown by Tilley et al. *(29)*, who performed careful microdissection of the tissue, and detected 11 mutations in 25 patients tested. Five of 11 mutations were localized to the first exon, which constitutes about 50% of the coding region. Another potential methodological variable is the quality of DNA extracted from paraffin embedded tissue, which, according to some reports, is not optimal, and may account for an increased frequency of PCR infidelity *(47)*.

FUNCTIONAL CONSEQUENCES OF AR MUTATIONS

Functional analysis of AR mutants detected in PC have identified a number of different phenotypes. In some cases, the mutation is of the gain-of-function type, and the resulting AR molecule is stimulated by ligands that cannot ordinarily activate the normal AR *(43,48–50)*. Other mutations are associated with the creation of a superactive AR, in which a supraphysiologic activation of the molecule is observed in response to physiologic concentrations of ligand *(51)*. In other cases, the mutation results in the loss of function. In this case, the resulting AR is transcriptionally impaired and cannot be activated. Finally, polymorphisms in the number of the poly-Q or poly-G repeats of the AR have been described in the general population and in rare cases of PC, and are asso-ciated with differences in the transcriptional activity of the resulting receptor, and in the epidemiological risk of developing PC *(35,52–57)*.

Mutations Causing Gain of Function. AR carrying gain-of-function mutations have also been promiscuous receptors *(58)*. Historically, the first mutation associated with gain of function of the AR was described in the PC cell line, LNCaP *(59)*, and resulted in the replacement of T877 with A. Transfection studies with this receptor showed increased binding affinities for progestens and estradiol (E_2). In addition, these ligands activated transcription at concentrations that were not sufficient for activation of the wild-type (WT) receptor. The T877A AR mutant was also activated by antiandrogens such as hydroxyflutamide, nilutamide, and cyproterone acetate, but not bicalutamide *(60)*. Subsequently, functional analysis of other AR mutations detected in PC identified a subset of AR molecules with a phenotype similar to the T877A variant. These mutant AR molecules were transcriptionally activated to a larger degree than WT AR by the antiandrogens, hydroxyflutamide *(48–50)* and nilutamide *(50)* (but not bicalutamide), and by weak agonists, such as the adrenal precursors, dehydroepiandrosterone *(43,48,49)* and androstenedione *(48)*, or the androgen metabolites, androsterone and androstanediol *(48)*.

A final interesting group of superactive mutants was identified by Tilley et al. *(51)*. These receptors (I670T and S780N) produced a 2–3-fold increase in transcriptional activity, compared to the WT AR, upon stimulation with dihydrotestosterone (DHT), and may therefore be activated by low circulating level of androgens, and be responsible for stimulation of growth in patients previously treated with conventional androgen ablation. The functional characteristics of these mutations have several implications and the potential to explain some of the molecular aspects of hormone refractoriness in patients with PC. Since most patients undergo procedures that remove testicular, but not adrenal, androgens, or receive potentially agonistic antiandrogens, PCs carrying mutations of the gain-of-function type can continue to sustain growth of the tumor. A clinical correlate to the observation that hydroxyflutamide can activate AR under certain conditions is the so-called "flutamide withdrawal syndrome," which was described in patients with advanced disease experiencing an unexpected decrease of PSA following withdrawal of antiandrogen treatment *(61)*.

An extension to this initial observation has recently been formulated by the group of Balk et al. *(46)*. These authors observed that a larger number of AR mutations (5/16) occurred in micrometastases obtained from patients undergoing treatment with androgen ablation and flutamide, compared to patients treated with androgen-ablation monotherapy (1/17). The mutations of the first group were all localized to codon 877 (T877A or T877S), and were strongly stimulated by hydroxyflutamide, but the mutation of the second group (D890N) was not stimulated by hydroxyflutamide. When these patients were switched to bicalutamide (which does not activate the T877A AR), a distinct decrease in PSA was observed in each of them. Many gain-of-function mutations may be the result of selective pressure from an AR antagonist. Thus, AR mutations may contribute to maintain AR stimulation, and maybe tumor growth, in patients treated with flutamide. The molecular significance of the more recently described Casodex *(62)*, diethylstilbestrol *(63)* and medroxyprogesterone acetate (MPA) *(64)* withdrawal syndromes is not clear, but could similarly be associated with AR variants that are activated by these drugs.

These observations point to the fact that the use of antiandrogens is not associated with an antiandrogenic effect in every circumstance. In addition, Miyamoto et al. *(65)* have recently observed that the testicular precursor of testosterone 5α-androstenediol is an AR agonist in its own right, and that its ability to transactivate AR is not blocked by the antiandrogens, hydroxyflutamide and bicalutamide. In view of this, the effectiveness of these chemicals in the treatment of PC should be re-evaluated.

Mutations Causing Loss of Function. Mutations causing a loss of AR function have been described by the authors' group in genomic DNA microdissected from metastatic lymph nodes of patients affected by stage D PC. Functional analysis of these mutations is significant for a complete loss of transcriptional activation in co-transfection experiments, using the mutated AR and a reporter plasmid driven by an androgen-inducible promoter.

One such mutant, C619Y, was fused to a green fluorescent protein and analyzed by high-resolution light and electron microscopy. The WT receptor undergoes immediate nuclear redistribution following addition of androgens, but the C619Y variant formed large, hollow cytoplasmic aggregates immediately following hormone addition, and underwent a gradual redistribution to the nucleus within minutes. These aggregates interacted and appeared to sequester most of the transfected SRC-1 from the cell. These results indicated that inactivating mutations of AR can have far-reaching effects on cell metabolism and function, in part resulting from AR inactivation itself, and in part because of sequestration/inactivation of molecules regulating other critical activities within the cell.

Inactivating AR mutations are associated with PC. Activation of AR has traditionally been considered necessary to sustain growth of prostatic epithelium. However, evidence for a pure growth stimulatory role of AR in prostatic epithelium is controversial, and loss of AR function may be associated with progressive loss of differentiated functions and with a faster replication rate of the cell. At least four observations illustrate these concepts:

1. The cell line, LNCaP, the most widely diffused PC cell line with a functioning AR, shows a typical biphasic response to androgens. At subsaturating concentrations of DHT (10-10 M), LNCaP cells growth is stimulated. However, concentrations of 10-9 M or higher inhibit growth *(66,67)*, and this effect is associated with induction of differentiated functions, i.e., induction of secretory proteins such as PSA *(67)*.
2. The growth of PC-3 cells, stably transfected with a WT *(68)* or truncated *(69)* AR cDNA, is also inhibited. Additionally, differentiated functions, such as PSA production, have been detected in an AR-transfected PC-3 cell line *(70)*.
3. Two LNCaP variants (LNCaP 104R1 and R2), grown for more than 100 passages in steroid-depleted medium, were inhibited by androgens, both in vitro *(71,72)* and in vivo *(71)*. These variants were growth-stimulated by the 5α-reductase inhibitor, finasteride, in vivo *(71)*.
4. Also, the AR-positive PC cell line, AR CaP, derived from the ascitic fluid of a patient who failed castration therapy, and showed an androgen-repressed phenotype, both in vitro and in vivo *(73)*.

These findings, and the presence of inactivating mutations in some PC specimens, raise the possibility that disrupted androgen-mediated regulation of prostate cell differentiation may allow for unchecked tumor cell proliferation.

The presence of a loss-of-function mutation in patients who eventually succumbed to the disease may represent a novel mechanism by which the AR plays an important role in PC, by allowing for a less-differentiated and more-invasive phenotype. AR contains two microsatellites, consisting of poly-Q and poly-G repeats in exon 1. The length of these two repeats is highly polymorphic in the general population *(74)*. Transcriptional activity of AR is affected by the size of the poly-Q tract. Investigators agree that an expanded poly-Q tract is associated with reduced transcriptional activity *(75–79)*. For instance, the AR of patients with Kennedy's disease *(80)* contains more than 41 glutamine residues. This abnormality is associated with decreased transcriptional activity, but normal ^{3}H-DHT-binding capacity *(75)*. This initial observation generated studies in which differences in the size of the poly-Q repeat were correlated to the transcriptional activity of AR. Some *(76,77,79)*, but not all *(78)*, authors have concluded that there is an inverse correlation between poly-Q size and transcriptional activity, and that the poly-Q tract exerts an inhibitory effect on transcription, either directly *(76,77)*, or indirectly, by affecting AR mRNA stability *(79)*. Somatic changes in the size of the poly-Q stretch have been found in specimens of PC, but they are infrequent *(35,55)*.

Because of the relatively low frequency of AR mutations in PC *(55)*, some authors have postulated that the role of androgen in PC must be mediated by the normal, WT AR. Thus, data have been generated in which the number of Q repeats were compared to the incidence of PC in the general population. This analysis has generated interesting conclusions, and has provided an association between an increased risk of developing the disease and a shorter poly-Q tract *(45,53,54,56)*. In addition, some studies have also detected an association between a shorter poly-Q repeat and the presence of metastatic disease *(45,54)*, high histologic grade *(54)*, and younger age of onset *(52)*. A correlation between the shorter median number of Qs *(74)* and the increased incidence, higher mortality, and more aggressive nature of PC in the African-American population *(81,82)* has been detected in two studies *(55,83)*. On the contrary, ethnic groups with lower epidemiological risk of developing PC (Asian) have an increased median number of Q repeats *(83)*. A correlation between a shorter poly-G repeat and PC risk has also been identified in two studies *(53,55)*. However, since AR with a reduced poly-G tract has reduced transcriptional activity *(78)*, it is not clear how such receptors may predispose to PC.

LIGAND-INDEPENDENT ACTIVATION OF AR

Phosphorylation of steroid receptors is an important posttranslational event that is thought to affect transcriptional activity *(84)*. Members of the steroid family of receptors can be transcripitonally activated by molecules that directly or indirectly increase intracellular kinase activity or decrease phosphatase activity *(85–89)*. Examples of these compounds include 8-bromo-cyclic adenosine monophosphate, forskolin, okadaic acid, growth factors such as insulin-like growth factor I (IGF-I), epidermal growth factor (EGF), and keratocyte growth factor (KGF), and the neurotransmitter, dopamine.

Ligand-independent activation of AR has far-reaching implications. Because the current systemic treatment for metastatic PC removes circulating androgen, but leaves AR in place, it is conceivable that circulating molecules other than androgen can activate the AR signaling pathway, and stimulate growth of the residual AR-positive tumor. That the AR signaling pathway can be stimulated by molecules other than androgen has been demonstrated in vitro using IGF-1, EGF, KGF *(90–92)*, forskolin *(91)*, and interleukin-6 *(92)*. Stimulation of the AR signaling pathway by these nonandrogenic compounds was counteracted by the AR antagonists, bicalutamide *(90–92)* and, in the case of forskolin, flutamide *(91)*. The clinical implications of these observations are still uncertain. There is evidence that some of these molecules (i.e., IGF-I) promote growth of prostatic epithelial cells (EC) in vitro *(93,94)*. In addition, plasma level of IGF-I is elevated in patients with PC *(95)*, an observation suggesting an independent role of the IGF axis in promoting PC. Nevertheless, it is conceivable that IGF-I may also contribute to transactivation of AR, and to inducing growth of residual PC cells in the androgen-depleted environment of men who underwent androgen ablation.

The concept of a growth-supporting role for some of the other molecules that activate AR in a ligand-independent fashion is still controversial. For instance, available data demonstrate clearly that interleukin-6 transactivates AR *(92)*, but there is no uniform consensus on the role of this cytokine in regulating growth of PC cell lines.

DEVELOPMENT OF PATHWAYS BYPASSING AR REGULATION

Clones of PC cells survive in the androgen-deprived endocrine milieu of patients who underwent androgen ablation, presumably because they have developed growth mechanisms that are independent from AR signaling. An experimental model describing such a possibility was described by Voeller et al. in 1991 *(96)*. Those authors stably transfected the cell line, LNCaP, with cadmium-inducible plasmid containing the cDNA of the proto-oncogene v-*rasH*. Clones of LNCaP cells overexpressing v-*rasH* were obtained after addition of Cd^{2+} to the medium. Their growth rate was comparable to that induced by addition of DHT to native LNCaP cells. Although mutated *ras* genes have not been detected at high frequency in Caucasian men *(97–99)*, this molecular abnormality is detected with higher frequency in Japanese men (100-103), and could facilitate the development of hormone-independent disease in this ethnic group, by sustaining growth of prostatic epithelium in an androgen-independent way. The experiment of Voeller et al. was pivotal in creating a theory *(96)*. Based on this theory, progression to hormone-independence could occur following overexpression or activating mutations of molecules that can sustain growth of prostatic epithelium in an androgen-independent way. No molecule with these characteristics was identified until the description of the role played by caveolin-1 in PC *(104,105)*.

Caveolin-1 was found to be overexpressed in metastatic PC cell lines (and metastatic specimens obtained from patients) relative to their primary tumor counterparts *(104)*. Further experiments with this model have produced information that could help in understanding the molecular basis of androgen-independence in PC *(105)*. Those authors found that suppression of caveolin expression with an antisense vector converted androgen-insensitive PC cell lines to an androgen-sensitive phenotype *(105)*. The mechanism by which caveolin (over) expression prevents androgen sensitivity is not known at this time. However, this observation has the potential to represent a groundbreaking development, and links the development of androgen resistance to the development of the metastatic phenotype.

INCREASED LOCAL BIOAVAILABILITY OF ANDROGENS TO ACTIVATE AR

The prostate contains high concentrations of the enzyme steroid 5α-reductase type II (SRD5A2), that catalyzes the conversion of testosterone into its more bioactive metabolite 5α-DHT, the prevalent androgen binding to the AR in the prostate *(106)*. Population-based analysis for mutations of the SRD5A2 was performed to explore the hypothesis that differences in the efficiency of the reaction catalyzed by SRD5A2 could be associated with differences in the risk of developing PC. This investigation has identified two variants with broad potential implications in patients with PC *(107)*. The first variant (V89L) was relatively common among Asians, the ethnic group with the lowest incidence of PC, and accounted for the genotype of 22% of Chinese and Japanese men *(108)*. On the contrary, this variant was found only in a minority of the ethnic groups with a higher prevalence of PC (4% of whites and 3% of African-Americans). V89L correlated with lower circulating levels of androstanediol glycuronide, an index of in vivo 5α-reductase activity that was predicted to have ~33% lower activity than the WT enzyme *(108)*. Thus, this variant was believed to have a protective effect for the development of PC.

Another significant SRD5A2 variant was A49T *(107)*. Although very uncommon in healthy men, this mutation was associated with nearly 10% of all advanced PCs in African-American and Latino men. In vitro functional analysis of the A49T variants indicated a fivefold higher V_{max} for testosterone conversion than the normal enzyme *(107)*, suggesting that a more efficient intraprostatic production of DHT may increase the risk of developing PC. Although the clinical significance of these observations is still uncertain, one can argue that differences in the way testosterone is converted to DHT in the prostate may account for differences in the local bioavailability of androgens to activate AR. This, in turn, could translate into an increased/decreased risk to develop PC, or in an increased resistance to androgen ablation in the different ethnic groups.

ALTERNATIVE MECHANISMS ACTIVATING ANDROGEN SIGNALING

AR interacts with a large number of accessory proteins when binding to DNA and activating transcription. Co-activators, such as ARA-70 *(109)*, SRC-1 *(107)*, and RAC3 *(111)*, have the ability to amplify the transcriptional activity of AR *(112)*. One such co-activator, ARA-70, thought to be relatively specific for AR, stimulates AR activity in vitro, not only in the response to androgens, but also in response to E_2 *(112)* and to antiandrogens, such as bicalutamide, hydroxyflutamide, and cyproterone acetate *(113)*. These results argue that local expression of co-activators, such as ARA-70 or others, may play a role in determining the response of AR to molecules that, under normal circumstances, have an inhibitory effect (such as the antiandrogens), or no effect at all (E_2).

Progesterone Receptors

There are conflicting reports in the literature regarding the presence and significance of PRs in PC. PRs are present both in normal prostatic tissue and some prostatic adenocarcinomas. Early-binding assays using radiolabeled [^{3}H]-R5020 demonstrated the presence of an 8S form of the PR in prostate adenocarcinoma, which could be specifically competed with excess unlabeled R5020 *(116,117)*. Although the steroid receptor profile of primary prostatic carcinoma (early-stage disease) resembled that of normal prostate, cytosol PR levels and ER levels were reduced in metastases, compared to the primary tumor *(118,119)*. Some authors found a total absence of immunoreactivity in advanced metastatic lesions *(120)*. Others, using immunohistochemical techniques, found that the PR was present only in the nuclei of the stromal cells, but sparse in the ECs of the prostate *(121,122)*. In another study, PR immunoreactivity in stromal cells was higher than in the carcinoma cells. Again, as the disease advanced, fewer cells stained positively for PR *(123)*.

In contrast, prostatic stromal sarcomas, a much less commonly found histologic type of PC, showed only an occasional sample with ER present (1/7 samples), but 6/7 samples were positive for PR *(124)*. Similarly, Sak et al. *(125)* found diffuse and strong staining of a carcinosarcoma specimen, but the adenocarcinoma specimen was negative for PR.

The role of the PR in the regulation of prostate function and tumor growth is not clearly understood. Lin et al. *(126)* observed growth inhibition of PC-3 cell tumors in a xenograft model using the nude mouse. They reported a 20% inhibition of tumor cell growth with progesterone treatment, and mifepristone (RU486) elicited more than a 60% inhibition over a 16-d exposure period. Whether this steroid antagonist was acting through the PR or GR is not known. In vitro studies using the PC-3 cell line have demonstrated that high-dose (10 μ*M*) progestogen administration (MPA) to PC-3 cells results in a cytotoxic action *(127)*. Uptake studies suggested that the action of this progestin might have been directly on the cell membrane to influence ion transport and membrane permeability. In some cell types, such as sperm, a nonnuclear PR has been identified.

Estrogen Receptors

The ER is found in normal prostate and some PC specimens *(119,128–131)*. ER-positive nuclei have been detected only in stromal cell nuclei in carcinomatous prostates *(121)*, and occasionally in some normal ECs of normal prostate tissue and benign prostate hypertrophy (BPH) specimens *(121)*. Again, similar to the studies of the PR, ER content in the metastatic tissue was significantly lower than that observed in primary prostatic carcinoma obtained in the early stages of the disease *(118,119)*.

Hiramatsu et al. *(123)* reported that immunoreactive ER was expressed exclusively in the stromal cells of 23% of 26 patients with PC, but none of those with BPH. Lack of ER expression in BPH has been noted by others *(131)* as well, and yet others *(117)* found ER present in 85% of BPH cases studied. When ER expression was studied after androgen ablation therapy or estrogen therapy, despite the atrophic changes to the prostate, intense ER expression (immunoreactivity) was noted in stromal cells surrounding the prostatic glands, and some ECs also stained positive for ER expression. This was in contrast to untreated patients, who were predominantly ER-negative *(131)*. In at least one study *(116)*, the ER could not be detected in the prostate gland, perhaps because the patient was treated with high doses of diethylstilbestrol diphosphate prior to surgery.

ER status has also been correlated with tumor grade. Nativ et al. *(132)* suggested that there was an inverse correlation between ER values and histologic or pathologic stage.

Recently, a new ER, named ERβ, was found to be present in prostate tissue. In the rat, Couse et al. *(133)* and Prins et al. *(134)* have shown that ERβ is found in the prostatic ECs (in contrast to the stromal localization of ERα), and its expression is developmentally regulated. The gene structure is similar to the ER, with a high degree of conservation in the DNA-binding domain and significant homology in the ligand binding domain *(135)*. The gene is composed of a 1590-bp open reading frame, and GST pull-down assays and immunoprecipitation assays suggest that the ERβ and ERα may interact in vivo *(136)*. In support of this hypothesis, ER knockout mice had slightly reduced levels of ERβ mRNA in the prostate, suggesting again that some functions of ERβ may require the presence of ERα *(133)*. At least five isoforms of the gene exist in the human *(137)*.

The function of E_2 in human PC is unclear. In a study of 89 men who underwent prostatic biopsy because of suspicion of neoplastic change, the presence of cytoplasmic ERs correlated positively with time to progression on hormone therapy. Receptor status (androgen and estrogen, nuclear or cytoplasmic) did not influence disease survival *(129)*. E_2 administration to PC-3 human PC cells in vitro resulted in significant growth inhibition *(138)*. The absolute level of ER expressed in PC3 cells is lower than in LNCaP cells, but, in the LNCaP cells, estrogen administration stimulates cell proliferation. This biological response can be blocked by administration of the antiestrogen, ICI 182, 780-128. Nevertheless, because there is a mutation in the ligand-binding domain of the AR, causing estrogen to be an agonist for the AR, it is possible that some of this growth stimulation may occur through the action of this steroid on the AR. In fact, Hobisch et al. *(139)* examined both ER and PR expression in LNCaP, PC-3, and DU-145 cells, using reverse transcriptase-PCR, ligand-binding assays, and immunohistochemistry, and found no ER or PR. In addition, PCs metastatic to lymph nodes from 21 patients were negative for ERs or PRs.

Markaverich and Alejandro *(140)* showed that naturally occurring bioflavonoids and related compounds (known to interact with the type II ER, which is not a steroid receptor), decreased mouse prostate weight, and had a direct effect on LNCaP and PC-3 cell proliferation. This resulted in a cytostatic inhibition of cell proliferation and an accumulation in cells in G2/M- and S-phase, through a block in mitosis. Although this type II receptor has not yet been cloned, it may offer an additional pathway for pharmacologic inhibition of PC growth in vivo.

GLUCOCORTICOID RECEPTORS

Glucocorticoids (GC) have been used in the treatment of advanced PC after androgen ablation therapy has failed *(141–150)*. Hydrocortisone, prednisone, medroxyprogesterone, and cortisone have been administered to patients after flutamide withdrawal or failure of androgen ablation. The positive effect of these steroids may in part result from the suppression of adrenal steroid production *(151–153)*, because agents such as ketoconazole, which inhibit adrenal and testicular steroidogenesis, may also prove effective *(154–157)*. Scher et al. *(158)* observed that analysis of the clinical studies in the literature of GC action in refractory PC is complicated by the variety of treatment regimens preceding the GC trials and by variations in patient classification.

GRs are present in several cell lines derived from rat prostate tumors, and steroid treatment inhibited cell proliferation in some of these studies *(159–163)*. This inhibitory action of GCs may be through the protein kinase C pathway *(164)*. Additional basic research studies are required to clarify the effect of GCs and their mechanism of action on PC cell proliferation.

Vitamin D and PC

Low levels of vitamin D have been implicated as a potential risk factor for PC, and there is evidence that the active metabolite of vitamin D, 1,25-dihydroxyvitamin D_3 (calcitriol), or a less calcemic analog, may be of benefit in treating PC. Calcitriol acts through binding to the vitamin D receptor (VDR) *(167)*, a member of the superfamily of ligand-activated nuclear receptors, and this results in induction or repression of target genes. In contrast to the classical steroid receptors, which act as homodimers, the VDR forms heterodimers with retinoid X receptors (RXR) *(168)*, so that the activity of the VDR can also be modulated by 9-*cis* RA, the RXR ligand. Although the actions of VDR in bone and mineral metabolism have been the focus of VDR studies *(167,169)*, more recent studies have shown that VDR is expressed in a wide variety of tissues, and may play a role in differentiation *(170–173)*. VDR is expressed in virtually all PC lines examined *(174–176)*, and Peehl et al. *(187)* have shown that normal prostate stromal and ECs, as well as primary cultures of human prostate tumors, express VDR.

Although Americans obtain some vitamin D through dietary sources, much vitamin D is synthesized in the skin by a ultraviolet catalyzed reaction *(177)*. Vitamin D is hydroxylated in the liver, then in the kidney, to produce the active metabolite, calcitriol *(177)*. Studies of the relationship between vitamin D metabolite levels and PC risk have yielded mixed results. One study *(179)* showed that men who subsequently developed PC had lower serum levels of calcitriol than did a matched control population; other studies *(180,181)* have failed to find any relationship between vitamin D levels and PC incidence. However, several of the risk factors (age, race, and geographic location) associated with PC may also be correlated with lower levels of vitamin D. For example, older men convert dehydrocholesterol to vitamin D less efficiently than younger men, and typically are exposed to less sunlight than are younger men *(182,183)*. African-American men have a higher incidence of PC than Caucasian men: Melanin pigment in the skin reduces the efficiency of conversion of dehydrocholesterol *(184)*. Finally, men from geographical areas that receive higher levels of sunlight, or where fish oil (a dietary source of vitamin D) is a major component of the diet, are less likely to die from PC than men from regions that receive lower levels of sunlight *(185,186)*.

Additional studies indicate that VDR agonists may be useful in reducing tumor growth. A number of investigators *(176,187,188)* have shown that calcitriol inhibits the growth of PC cell lines and primary PC cell cultures in vitro. That this is a VDR-mediated response has been shown by Hedlund et al. *(189)*, who have demonstrated that JCA-1 cells, which are unresponsive to calcitriol and do not express receptor, are growth-inhibited when stably transfected with an expression plasmid for VDR. Similarly, Alva 31 cells lose responsiveness to calcitriol when treated with antisense VDR to reduce VDR expression *(190)*. To date, studies of responses in animal models have been limited. One study *(191)* demonstrated tumor growth inhibition in a Dunning rat model of PC, but the levels of calcitriol required to achieve these results cause hypercalcemia. However, Schwartz et al. *(192)* were able to reduce PC3 cell tumor cell growth in a nude mouse model, with-out elevation of calcium levels, by using an analog, 1,25-dihydroxy-16-ene-23-yne vitamin D_3.

Several polymorphisms have been identified in the gene that encodes the VDR *(193, 194)*, and some of these have been associated with altered levels of vitamin D and altered bone mineral density. A number of studies have been performed to determine whether these alleles alter PC risk. The alleles can be identified by the presence or absence of characteristic restriction enzyme sites, or by the length of the poly-A microsatellite in the 3'-flanking region (L ≥ 18 As or S ≤ 17 As) *(194)*. The restriction sites examined include a polymorphism in intron 8, which forms a BsmI site (B = no site; b = BsmI site), and an alteration in exon 9, which generates a TaqI site (T = no site; t = Taq site). These polymorphisms do not alter the coding sequence of VDR. Ingles et al. *(194)* found that PC risk was increased in nonhispanic whites with the presence of at least one L allele. In contrast, Ingles et al. *(195)* reported that the BL haplotype was associated with increased risk in African-Americans and the bL haplotype with decreased risk. Finally, Kibel et al. *(196)* failed to find a correlation with the length of the poly-A microsatellite repeat and the risk of lethal PC. Collectively, these studies suggest that there may be another, as yet unidentified, alteration in or near the VDR gene that may contribute to PC risk.

Orphan Receptors

Investigations of orphan receptor members of the steroid receptor superfamily and PC are still at an early stage. Chang et al. *(165)* first cloned TR3 from a human prostate library. The gene was later shown to be an immediate early gene expressed rapidly after androgen administration, and is also known as *nur77* and *NGF1B*. Expression of this gene is also induced in the regressing prostate after androgen ablation. Recent studies *(166)* suggest that TR3 may modulate the cellular response to agents that induce apoptosis. It is clear that studies of TR3, as well as other orphan receptors expressed in the prostate, will be of great importance to understanding the role of these genes in regulating prostate growth, development, and cancer progression.

SUMMARY

Understanding the molecular mechanisms responsible for the transition of PC to androgen independence is the initial step toward the development of new and effective way to treat hormone-independent disease. Although the evidence supports a permissive role of androgen and of AR in the development of this disease, it is not yet clear what the mechanism is for development of androgen independence. The available evidence is controversial. Point mutations causing the development of promiscuous receptors have been described in a minority of cases. Although the concept of a receptor that is activated by molecules other than androgen is fascinating, there is no evidence that such mutations play a role in the development of PC. However, they provide a theoretical explanation for the maintenance of tumor growth in patients who underwent androgen ablation.

Inactivating point mutations of AR have also been described. PCs carrying these mutations have probably developed androgen-independent mechanisms to sustain their growth. Nevertheless, because the overall incidence of AR mutations is low, other mechanisms should be considered. Some authors have postulated that progression of PC occurs through activation of the WT AR through alternative pathways. These could involve amplification of the AR gene, changes in the size of the poly-Q repeat, or differences in the local bioavailability of androgens, nonandrogenic ligands, or co-activators.

Many interesting observations have increased understanding of the molecular mechanisms leading to androgen independence in PC. Although none of these has offered a comprehensive explanation of this phenomenon, continuing research in the field may generate useful information to guide the development of new effective therapeutic approaches.

REFERENCES

1. O'Malley BO. Steroid receptor superfamily: more excitement predicted for the future. Mol Endocrinol 1990;4:363–369.
2. Evans RM. The steroid and thyroid hormone receptor superfamily. Science 1988;240:889–895.
3. Chang CS, Kokontis J, Liao ST. Molecular cloning of human and rat complementary DNA encoding androgen receptor. Science 1988;240:324–326.
4. Lubahn DB, Joseph DR, Sar M, et al. Cloning of human androgen receptor complementary DNA and localization of the X chromosome. Science 1988;240:327–330.
5. Wilding G. The importance of steroid hormones in prostate cancer. Cancer Surv 1992;14:113–130.
6. Nomura AM, Kolonel LN. Prostate cancer: a current perspective. Epidemiol Rev 1991;13:200–227.
7. Schroeder F. Does testosterone treatment increase the risk or induction of progression of occult cancer of the prostate? In: Bhasin S, Gabelnick H, Spieler J, Swerdloff R, Wang C, eds. Pharmacology, Biology, and Clinical Applications of Androgens. Wiley-Liss, New York, 1996, pp. 137–141.
8. Cunningham G. Overview of androgens on the normal and abnormal prostate. In: Bhasin S, Gabelnick H, Spieler J, Swerdloff R, Wang C, eds. Pharmacology, Biology, and Clinical Applications of Androgens. Wiley-Liss, New York, 1996, pp. 79–93.
9. Geller J. Androgen inhibition and BPH. Bhasin S, Gabelnick H, Spieler J, Swerdloff R, Wang C, eds. Pharmacology, Biology, and Clinical Applications of Androgens. Wiley-Liss, New York, 1996, pp. 103–110.
10. Landis S, Murray T, Bolden S, Wingo P. Cancer statistics 1999. CA Cancer J Clin 1999;49:8–31.
11. Santen RJ. Endocrine treatment of prostate cancer. J Clin Endocrinol Metab 1992;75:685–689.
12. Kyprianou N, English H, Isaacs J. Programmed cell death during regression of PC-82 human prostate cancer following androgen ablation. Cancer Res 1990;50:3748–3753.
13. Isaacs J, Coffey D. Adaptation vs. selection as the mechanism responsible for the relapse of prostatic cancer to androgen ablation as studied in the Dunning R-3327 H adenocarcinoma. Cancer Res 1981; 41:5070–5075.
14. Isaacs J, Lundmo P, Berges R, Martikainen P, Kyprianou N, English H. Androgen regulation of programmed cell death of normal and malignant prostatic cells. J Androl 1992;13:457–464.
15. Van-der-Kwast T, Tetu B. Androgen receptors in untreated and treated prostatic intraepithelial neoplasia. Eur Urol 1996;30:265–268.
16. Sadi MV, Walsh PC, Barrack ER. Immunohistochemical study of androgen receptors in metastatic prostate cancer. Cancer 1991;67:30,547–30,557.
17. Tilley WD, Lim-Tio SS, Horsfall DJ, Aspinall JO, Marshall VR, Skinner JM. Detection of discrete androgen receptor epitopes in prostate cancer by immuno-staining: measurement by color video image analysis. Cancer Res 1994;54:4096–4102.

18. Hobisch A, Culig Z, Radmayr C, Bartsch G, Klocker H, Hittmair A. Androgen receptor status of lymph node metastases from prostate cancer. Prostate 1996;28:129–135.

19. Hobisch A, Culig Z, Radmayr C, Bartsch G, Klocker H, Hittmair A. Distant metastases from prostatic carcinoma express androgen receptor protein. Cancer Res 1995;55:3068–3072.

20. Van-der-Kwast TH, Schalken J, Ruizeveld-de-Winter JA, Van-Vroonhoven CCJ, Mulder E, Boersma W, Trapman J. Androgen receptors in endocrine-therapy resistant human prostate cancer. Int J Can 1991;48:189–193.

21. Visakorpi T, Hyytinen E, Koivisto P, Tanner M, Keinanen R, Palmberg C, et al. In vivo amplification of the androgen receptor gene and progression of human prostate cancer. Nat Genet 1995;9:401–406.

22. Koivisto P, Kononen J, Palmberg C, Tammela T, Hyytinen E, Isola J, et al. Androgen receptor gene amplification: a possible molecular mechanism for androgen deprivation therapy failure in prostate cancer. Cancer Res 1997;57:314–319.

23. Chang CS, Kokontis J, Liao ST. Structural analysis of complementary DNA and amino acid sequences of human and rat androgen receptors. Proc Natl Acad Sci USA 1988;85:7211–7215.

24. Chang CS, Kokontis J, Liao ST. Molecular cloning of human and rat complementary DNA encoding androgen receptors. Science 1988;240:324–326.

25. Lubahn DB, Joseph DR, Sullivan PM, Willard HF, French FS, Wilson EM. Cloning of human androgen receptor complementary DNA and localization to the X chromosome. Science 1988;240:327–330.

26. Lubahn DB, Joseph DR, Sar M, Tan J, Higgs HN, Larson RE, French FS, Wilson EM. The human androgen receptor: complementary deoxyribonucleic acid cloning, sequence analysis and gene expression in the prostate. Mol Endocrinol 1988;2:1265–1275.

27. Trapman J, Klaassen P, Kuiper GG, van der Korput JA, Faber PW, van Rooij HC, et al. Cloning, structure and expression of a cDNA encoding the human androgen receptor. Biochem Biophys Res Commun 1988;153:241–248.

28. Tilley WD, Marcelli M, Wilson JD, McPhaul JM. Characterization and cloning of a cDNA encoding the human androgen receptor. Proc Natl Acad Sci USA 1989;86:327–331.

29. Tilley W, Buchanan G, Hickey T, Bentel J. Mutations of the androgen receptor gene are associated with progression of human prostate cancer to androgen independence. Clin Cancer Res 1996;2:277–285.

30. Taplin ME, Bubley GJ, Shuster T, Frantz M, Spooner A, Ogata G, Keer H, Balk S. Mutation of the androgen-receptor gene in metastatic androgen-independent prostate cancer. N Engl J Med 1995;332:1393–1398.

31. Gaddipati JP, McLeod DG, Heidenberg HB, Sesterhenn IA, Finger MJ, Moul JW, Srivastava S. Frequent detection of codon 877 mutation in the androgen receptor gene in advanced prostate cancers. Cancer Res 1994;54:2861–2864.

32. Newmark JR, Hardy DO, Tonb DC, Carter BS, Epstein JI, Isaacs WB, Brown TR, Barrack ER. Androgen receptor gene mutations in human prostate cancer. Proc Natl Acad Sci USA 1992;89:6319–6323.

33. Suzuki H, Sato N, Watabe Y, Masai M, Seino S, Shimazaki J. Androgen receptor gene mutations in human prostate cancer. J Steroid Biochem Mol Biol 1993;46:759–765.

34. Castagnaro M, Yandell DW, Dockhorn-Dworniczak B, Wolfe HJ, Poremba C. [Androgen receptor gene mutations and p53 gene analysis in advanced prostate cancer]. Verh Dtsch Ges Pathol 1993;77:119–123.

35. Shoenberg MP, Hakimi JM, Wang SP, Bova GS, Fischbeck KH, Isaacs WB, Walsh PC, Barrack ER. Microsatellite mutation (Cag(24->18)) in the androgen receptor gene in human prostate cancer. Biochem Biophys Res Commun 1994;198:74–80.

36. Ruizeveld-de-Winter JA, Janssen PJA, Sleddens HMEB, Verleun-Moojman MCT, Trapman J, Brinkmann AO, et al. Androgen receptor status in localized and locally progressive hormone refractory human prostate cancer. Am J Pathol 1994;144:735–746.

37. Elo JP, Kvist L, Leinonen K, Isomaa V, Henttu P, Lukkarinen O, Vihko P. Mutated human androgen receptor gene detected in a prostatic cancer patient is also activated by estradiol. J Clin Endocrinol Metab 1995;80:3494–3500.

38. Suzuki H, Akakura K, Komiya A, Aida S, Akimoto S, Shimazaki J. Codon 877 mutation in the androgen receptor gene in advanced prostate cancer: relation to antiandrogen withdrawal syndrome. Prostate 1996;29:153–158.

39. Evans BA, Harper ME, Daniels CE, Watts CE, Matenhelia S, Green J, Griffiths K. Low incidence of androgen receptor gene mutations in human prostatic tumors using single strand conformation polymorphism analysis. Prostate 1996;28:162–171.

40. Paz A, Lindner A, Zisman A, Siegel Y. A genetic sequence change in the 3'-noncoding region of the androgen receptor gene in prostate carcinoma. Eur Urol 1997;31:209–215.

41. Watanabe M, Ushijima T, Shiraishi T, Yatani R, Shimazaki J, Kotake T, Sugimura T, Nagao M. Genetic alterations of androgen receptor gene in Japanese human prostate cancer. Jpn J Clin Oncol 1997;27: 389–393.

42. Wang C, Uchida T. [Androgen receptor gene mutations in prostate cancer]. Nippon Hinyokika Gakkai Zasshi 1997;88:550–556.

43. Culig Z, Hobisch A, Cronauer MV, Cato ACB, Hittmair A, Radmayr C, et al. Mutant androgen receptor detected in an advanced stage prostatic carcinoma is activated by adrenal androgens and progesterone. Mol Endocrinol 1993;7:1541–1550.

44. de Vere White R, Meyers F, Chi SG, Chamberlain S, Siders D, Lee F, Stewart S, Gumerlock PH. Human androgen receptor expression in prostate cancer following androgen ablation. Eur Urol 1997;31: 1–6.

45. Hakimi J, Ahmed R, Isaacs W, Bova W, Barrack E. Mutational analysis of the androgen receptor gene in hormone refractory metastases of prostate cancer. Eighty-ninth Annual Meeting of the American Association for Cancer Research. New Orleans, 1998, pp. 3754.

46. Taplin ME, Rajeshkumar B, Small E, Bubley G, Ko Y-K, Upton M, Balk S. Selection for androgen receptor mutations specifically in prostate cancers treated with flutamide. In: New Research Approaches in the Prevention and Cure of Prostate Cancer. Indian Wells, CA, 1998, pp. A–33.

47. Shiao YH, Buzard G, Weghorst C, Rice J. DNA template as a source of artifact in the detection of p53 gene mutations using archived tissue. Bio-Techniques 1997;22:608–612.

48. Peterziel H, Culig Z, Stober J, Hobisch A, Radmayr C, Bartsch G, Klocker H, Cato AC. Mutant androgen receptors in prostatic tumors distinguish between amino-acid-sequence requirements for transactivation and ligand binding. Int J Cancer 1995;63:544–550.

49. Tan J, Sharief Y, Hamil KG, Gregory CW, Zang DY, Sar M, et al. Dehydroepiandrosterone activates mutant androgen receptors expressed in the androgen-dependent human prostate cancer xenograft CWR22 and LNCaP cells. Mol Endocrinol 1997;11:450–459.

50. Fenton MA, Shuster TD, Fertig AM, Taplin ME, Kolvenbag G, Bubley GJ, Balk SP. Functional characterization of mutant androgen receptors from androgen-independent prostate cancer. Clin Cancer Res 1997;3:1383–1388.

51. Tilley W, Pickering M, Buchanan G, Freeman N, Holds D, Bentel J, Marshall V. Functional analysis of androgen receptor gene mutations in human prostate cancer. Eighty-ninth Annual Meeting of the American Association for Cancer Research. New Orleans, LA, 1998, p. 84.

52. Hardy DO, Scher HI, Bogenreider T, Sabbatini P, Zhang ZF, Nanus DM, Catterall JF. Androgen receptor CAG repeat lengths in prostate cancer: correlation with age of onset. J Clin Endocrinol Metab 1996;81:4400–4405.

53. Stanford JL, Just JJ, Gibbs M, Wicklund KG, Neal CL, Blumenstein BA, Ostrander EA. Polymorphic repeats in the androgen receptor gene: molecular markers of prostate cancer risk. Cancer Res 1997;57: 1194–1198.

54. Giovannucci E, Stampfer MJ, Krithivas K, Brown M, Dahl D, Brufsky A, et al. The CAG repeat within the androgen receptor gene and its relationship to prostate cancer [published erratum appears in Proc Natl Acad Sci USA 1997;94:8272], Proc Natl Acad Sci USA 1997;94:3320–3323.

55. Hakimi JM, Schoenberg MP, Rondinelli RH, Piantadosi S, Barrack ER. Androgen receptor variants with short glutamine or glycine repeats may identify unique sub-populations of men with prostate cancer. Clin Cancer Res 1997;3:1599–1608.

56. Irvine RA, Yu MC, Ross RK, Coetzee GA. The CAG and GGC microsatellites of the androgen receptor gene are in linkage disequilibrium in men with prostate cancer. Cancer Res 1995;55:1937–1940.

57. Ingles SA, Ross RK, Yu MC, Irvine RA, La Pera G, Haile RW, Coetzee GA. Association of prostate cancer risk with genetic polymorphisms in vitamin D receptor and androgen receptor. J Natl Cancer Inst 1997;89:166–170.

58. Wilson J. The promiscuous receptor. Prostate cancer comes of age. New Engl J Med 1995;332: 1440,1441.

59. Veldscholte J, Ris-Stalpers C, Kuiper GGJM, Jentser G, Berrevoets C, Claassen E, et al. A mutation in the ligand binding domain of the androgen receptor of LnCAP cells affects steroid binding characteristics and response to anti-androgens. Biochem Biophys Res Commun 1990;173:534–540.

60. Veldscholte J, Berrevoets CA, Brinkmann AO, Grootegoed JA, Mulder E. Anti-androgens and the mutated androgen receptor of LNCaP cells: differential effects on binding affinity, heat-shock protein interaction, and transcription activation. Biochemistry 1992;31:2393–2399.

61. Scher H, Kelly W. Flutamide withdrawal syndrome: its impact on clinical trials in hormone-refractory prostate cancer. J Clin Oncol 1993;11:1566–1572.

62. Small EJ, Carroll PR. Prostate-specific antigen decline after casodex withdrawal: evidence for an anti androgen withdrawal syndrome. Urology 1994;43:408–410.

63. Bissada NK, Kaczmarek AT. Complete remission of hormone refractory adenocarcinoma of the prostate in response to withdrawal of diethylstilbestrol. J Urol 1995;153:1944,1945.

64. Dawson NA, McLeod DG. Dramatic prostate specific antigen decrease in response to discontinuation of megestrol acetate in advanced prostate cancer: expansion of the anti androgen withdrawal syndrome. J Urol 1995;153:1946,1947.

65. Miyamoto H, Yeh S, Lardy H, Messing E, Chang C. Delta5-androstenediol is a natural hormone with androgenic activity inhuman prostate cancer cells. Proc Natl Acad Sci USA 1998;95:11,083–11,088.

66. Sonnenschein C, Olea N, Pasanen M, Soto A. Negative controls of cell proliferation: human prostate cancers and androgens. Cancer Res 1989;49:3474–3481.

67. Lee C, Sutkowski D, Sensibar J, Zelner D, Kim I, Amsel I, et al. Regulation of proliferation and production of prostate specific antigen in androgen-sensitive prostate cancer cells, LNCaP, by dihydrotestosterone. Endocrinology 1995;136:796–803.

68. Yuan S, Trachtenberg J, Mills G, Brown T, Xu F, Keating A. Androgen-induced inhibition of cell proliferation in an androgen-insensitive prostate cancer cell line (PC-3) transfected with a human androgen receptor complementary DNA. Cancer Res 1993;53:1304–1311.

69. Marcelli M, Haidecher SJ, Plymate SR, Birnbaum RS. Altered growth and insulin-like growth factor binding protein-3 (IGFBP-3) production in PC3 prostate carcinoma cells stably transfected with a constitutively active androgen receptor cDNA. Endocrinology 1995;136:1040–1048.

70. Dai JL, Maiorino CA, Gkonos PJ, Burnstein KL. Androgenic up-regulation of androgen receptor cDNA expression in androgen-independent prostate cancer cells. Steroids 1996;61:531–539.

71. Umekita Y, Hiipakka R, Kokontis J, Liao S. Human prostate tumor growth in athymic mice: inhibition by androgens and stimulation by finasteride. Proc Natl Acad Sci USA 1996;93:11,802–11,807.

72. Kokontis JM, Hay N, Liao S. Progression of LNCaP prostate tumor cells during androgen deprivation: hormone-independent growth, repression of proliferation by androgen, and role for p27Kip1 in androgen-induced cell cycle arrest. Mol Endocrinol 1998;12:941–953.

73. Zhau H, Chang S-M, Chen B-Q, Wang Y, Zhang H, Kao C, et al. Androgen-repressed phenotype in human prostate cancer. Proc Natl Acad Sci USA 1996;93:15,152–15,157.

74. Edwards A, Hammond HA, Jin L, Caskey CT, Chakraborty R. Genetic variation at five trimeric and tetrameric tandem repeat loci in four human population groups. Genomics 1992;12:241–253.

75. Mhatre AN, Trifiro MA, Kaufman M, Kazemi-Esfarjani P, Figlewicz D, Rouleau G, Pinsky L. Reduced transcriptional regulatory competence of the androgen receptor in X-linked spinal and bulbar muscular atrophy [published erratum appears in Nat Genet 1994;6:214]. Nat Genet 1993;5:184–188.

76. Kazemi-Esfarjani P, Trifiro MA, Pinsky L. Evidence for a repressive function of the long polyglutamine tract in the human androgen receptor: possible pathogenetic relevance for the (CAG)n-expanded neuronopathies. Hum Mol Genet 1995;4:523–527.

77. Chamberlain NL, Driver ED, Miesfeld RL. The length and location of CAG trinucleotide repeats in the androgen receptor N-terminal domain affect transactivation function. Nucleic Acids Res 1994;22: 3181–3186.

78. Gao T, Marcelli M, McPhaul M. Transcriptional activation and transient expression of the human androgen receptor. J Steroid Biochem Mol Biol 1996;59:9–20.

79. Choong CS, Kemppainen JA, Zhou ZX, Wilson EM. Reduced androgen receptor gene expression with first exon CAG repeat expansion. Mol Endocrinol 1996;10:1527–1535.

80. La Spada AR, Wilson EM, Lubahn DB, Harding AE, Fischbeck KH. Androgen receptor gene mutations in X-linked spinal and bulbar muscular atrophy. Nature 1991;352:77–79.

81. Ross RK, Paganini-Hill A, Henderson BE. The etiology of prostate cancer: what does the epidemiology suggest? Prostate 1983;4:333–444.

82. Morton RA Jr. Racial differences in adenocarcinoma of the prostate in North American men. Urology 1994;44:637–645.

83. Coetzee GA, Ross RK. Re: Prostate cancer and the androgen receptor [letter]. J Natl Cancer Inst 1994; 86:872,873.

84. Orti E, Bodwell JE, Munck A. Phosphorylation of steroid hormone receptors. Endocr Rev 1992;13: 105–128.

85. Denner LA, Weigel NL, Maxwell BL, Schrader WT, O'Malley BW. Regulation of progesterone receptor-mediated transcription by phosphorylation. Science 1990;250:1740–1743.

86. Power RF, Mani SK, Codina J, Conneely OM, O'Malley BW. Dopaminergic and ligand-independent activation of steroid hormone receptors. Science 1991;254:1636–1639.

87. Zhang Y, Bai W, Allgood VE, Weigel NL. Multiple signaling pathways activate the chicken proges-terone receptor. Mol Endocrinol 1994;8:577–584.

88. Ignar-Trowbridge DM, Nelson KG, Bidwell MC, Curtis SW, Washburn TF, McLachlan JA, Korach KS. Coupling of dual signaling pathways: epidermal growth factor action involves the estrogen recep-tor. Proc Natl Acad Sci USA 1992;89:4658–4662.

89. Smith CL, Conneely OM, O'Malley BW. Modulation of the ligand-independent activation of the human estrogen receptor by hormone and antihormone. Proc Natl Acad Sci USA 1993;90:6120–6124.

90. Culig Z, Hobish A, Cronauer MV, Radmayr C, Trapman J, Hittmair A, Bartsch G, Klocker H. Andro-gen receptor activation in prostatic tumor cell lines by insulin-like growth factor I: keratinocyte growth factor, and epidermal growth factor. Cancer Res 1994;54:5474–5478.

91. Nazareth L, Weigel N. Activation of the human androgen receptor through a proteinase A signaling pathway. J Biol Chem 1996;271:19,900–19,907.

92. Hobisch A, Eder IE, Putz T, Horninger W, Bartsch G, Klocker H, Culig Z. Interleukin-6 regulates prostate-specific protein expression in prostate carcinoma cells by activation of the androgen receptor. Cancer Res 1998;58:4640–4645.

93. Cohen P, Peehl D, Lamson G, Rosenfeld RR. Insulin-like growth factors, IGF receptors and IGF-bind-ing proteins in primary cultures of prostate epithelial cells. J Clin Endocrinol Metab 1991;73:401–407.

94. Iwamura M, Sluss PM, Casamento JB, Cockett AT. Insulin-like growth factor, I, action and receptor characterization in human prostate cancer cell lines. Prostate 1993;22:243–252.

95. Chan JM, Stampfer MJ, Giovannucci E, Gann PH, Ma J, Wilkinson P, Hennekens CH, Pollak M. Plasma insulin-like growth factor-I and prostate cancer risk: a prospective study. Science 1998;279:563–566.

96. Voeller H, Wilding G, Gelmann E. v-rasH expression confers hormone-independent in-vitro growth to LnCAP prostate carcinoma cells. Mol Endocrinol 1991;5:209–216.

97. Carter BS, Epstein JI, Isaacs WB. ras gene mutations in human prostate cancer. Cancer Res 1990; 50:6830–6832.

98. Gumerlock PH, Poonamallee UR, Meyers FJ, deVereWhite RW. Activated as alleles in human carci-noma of the prostate are rare. Cancer Res 1991;51:1632–1637.

99. Moul JW, Friedrichs PA, Lance RS, Theune SM, Chang EH. Infrequent RAS oncogene mutations in human prostate cancer. Prostate 1992;20:327–338.

100. Konishi N, Enomoto T, Buzard G, Ohshima M, Ward JM, Rice JM. K-ras activation and ras p21 expression in latent prostatic carcinoma in Japanese men. Cancer 1992;69:2293–2299.

101. Anwar K, Nakakuki K, Shiraishi T, Naiki H, Yatani R, Inuzuka M. Presence of ras oncogene mutations and human papillomavirus DNA in human prostate carcinomas. Cancer Res 1992;52:5991–5996.

102. Konishi N, Hiasa Y, Tsuzuki T, Tao M, Enomoto T, Miller GJ. Comparison of ras activation in prostate carcinoma in Japanese and American men. Prostate 1997;30:53–57.

103. Shiraishi T, Muneyuki T, Fukutome K, Ito H, Kotake T, Watanabe M, Yatani R. Mutations of ras genes are relatively frequent in Japanese prostate cancers: pointing to genetic differences between popula-tions. Anticancer Res 1998;18:2789–2792.

104. Yang G, Truong LD, Timme TL, Ren C, Wheeler TM, Park SH, et al. Elevated expression of caveolin is associated with prostate and breast cancer. Clin Cancer Res 1998;4:1873–1880.

105. Nasu Y, Timme T, Yang G, Bangma C, Li L, Ren C, et al. Suppression of caveolin expression induces androgen sensitivity in metastatic androgen-insensitive mouse prostate cancer. Nature Med 1998;4: 1062–1064.

106. Bruchovsky N, Wilson JD. The intranuclear binding of testosterone and 5-alpha-androstan-17-beta-ol-3-one by rat prostate. J Biol Chem 1968;243:5953–5960.

107. Ross RK, Pike MC, Coetzee GA, Reichardt JK, Yu MC, Feigelson H, et al. Androgen metabolism and prostate cancer: establishing a model of genetic susceptibility. Cancer Res 1998;58:4497–4504.

108. Makridakis N, Ross RK, Pike MC, Chang L, Stanczyk FZ, Kolonel LN, et al. A prevalent missense sub-stitution that modulates activity of prostatic steroid 5alpha-reductase. Cancer Res 1997;57:1020–1022.

109. Yeh S, Chang C. Cloning and characterization of a specific coactivator, ARA70, for the androgen receptor in human prostate cells. Proc Natl Acad Sci USA 1996;93:5517–5521.

110. Onate SA, Tsai SY, Tsai MJ, O'Malley BW. Sequence and characterization of a coactivator for the steroid hormone receptor superfamily. Science 1995;270:1354–1357.

111. Chen H, Lin RJ, Schiltz RL, Chakravarti D, Nash A, Nagy L, et al. Nuclear receptor coactivator ACTR is a novel histone acetyl transferase and forms a multimeric activation complex with P/CAF and CBP/ p300. Cell 1997;90:569–580.

112. Yeh S, Miyamoto H, Shima H, Chang C. From estrogen to androgen receptor: a new pathway for sex hormones in prostate. Proc Natl Acad Sci USA 1998;95:5527–5532.

113. Miyamoto H, Yeh S, Wilding G, Chang C. Promotion of agonist activity of anti androgens by the androgen receptor coactivator, ARA70, in human prostate cancer DU145 cells. Proc Natl Acad Sci USA 1998;95: 7379–7384.

114. Takahashi H, Furusato M, Allsbrook WC Jr, Nishii H, Wakui S, Barrett JC, Boyd J. Prevalence of androgen receptor gene mutations in latent prostatic carcinomas from Japanese men. Cancer Res 1995; 55:1621–1624.

115. Culig Z, Klocker H, Eberle J, Kaspar F, Hobisch A, Cronauer MV, Bartsch G. DNA sequence of the androgen receptor in prostatic tumor cell lines and tissue specimens assessed by means of the polymerase chain reaction. Prostate 1993;22:11–22.

116. Bashirelahi N, Felder CC, Young JD. Characterization and stabilization of progesterone receptors in human benign prostatic hypertrophy. J Steroid Biochem 1983;18:801–809.

117. Kumar VL, Wadhwa SN, Kumar V, Farooq A. Androgen estrogen and progesterone receptor contents and serum hormone profiles in patients with benign hypertrophy and carcinoma of the prostate. J Surg Oncol 1990;44:122–128.

118. Ekman P, Brolin J. Steroid receptor profile in human prostate cancer metastases as compared with primary prostatic carcinoma. Prostate 1991;18:147–153.

119. Mobbs BG, Johnson IE, Liu Y. Quantitation of cytosolic and nuclear estrogen and progesterone receptor in benign, untreated, and treated malignant human prostatic tissue by radio ligand binding and enzyme-immunoassays. Prostate 1990;16:235–244.

120. Hobisch A. Metastatic lesions from prostate cancer do not express oestrogen and progesterone receptors. J Pathol 1997;182:356–361.

121. Brolin J, Skoog L, Ekman P. Immunohistochemistry and biochemistry in detection of androgen, progesterone, and estrogen receptors in benign and malignant human prostatic tissue. Prostate 1992; 20:281–295.

122. Mobbs BG, Liu Y. Immunohistochemical localization of progesterone receptor in benign and malignant human prostate. Prostate 1990;16:245–251.

123. Hiramatsu M, Maehara I, Orikasa S, Sasano H. Immunolocalization of estrogen and progesterone receptors in prostatic hyperplasia and carcinoma. Histopathology 1996;28:163–168.

124. Gaudin PB, Rosai J, Epstein JI. Sarcomas and related proliferative lesions of specialized prostatic stroma: a clinico pathologic study of 22 cases. Am J Surg Pathol 1998;22:148–162.

125. Sak SD, Orhan D, Yaman O, Tulunay O, Ozdiler E. Carcino sarcoma of the prostate. A case report and a possible evidence on the role of hormonal therapy. Urol Int 1997;59:50–52.

126. Lin MF, Kawachi MH, Stallcup MR, Grunberg SM, Lin FF. Growth inhibition of androgen-insensitive human prostate carcinoma cells by a 19-norsteroid derivative agent, mifepristone. Prostate 1995;26: 194–204.

127. Widmark A, Grankvist K, Bergh A, Henriksson R, Damber JE. Effects of estrogens and progestogens on the membrane permeability and growth of human prostatic carcinoma cells (PC-3) in vitro. Prostate 1995;26:5–11.

128. Castagnetta LA, Carruba G. Human prostate cancer: a direct role for oestrogens. Ciba Found Symp 1995;191:269–286.

129. Emtage LA, Dunn PJ, Rowse AD. Androgen and oestrogen receptor status in benign and neoplastic prostate disease. Study of prevalence and influence on time to progression and survival in prostate cancer treated by hormone manipulation. Br J Urol 1989;63:627–633.

130. Konishi N, Nakaoka S, Hiasa Y, et al. Immunohistochemical evaluation of estrogen receptor status in benign prostatic hypertrophy and in prostate carcinoma and the relationship to efficacy of endocrine therapy. Oncology 1993;50:259–263.

131. Kruithof-Dekker IG, Tetu B, Janssen PJ, Van der Kwast TH. Elevated estrogen receptor expression in human prostatic stromal cells by androgen ablation therapy. J Urol 1996;156:1194–1197.

132. Nativ O, Umehara T, Colvard DS, et al. Relationship between DNA ploidy and functional estrogen receptors in operable prostate cancer. Eur Urol 1997;32:96–99.

133. Couse JF, Lindzey J, Grandien K, Gustafsson JA, Korach KS. Tissue distribution and quantitative analysis of estrogen receptor-alpha (ERalpha) and estrogen receptor-beta (ERbeta) messenger ribonucleic acid in the wild-type and ERalpha-knockout mouse. Endocrinology 1997;138:4613–4621.

134. Prins GS, Marmer M, Woodham C, et al. Estrogen receptor-beta messenger ribonucleic acid ontogeny in the prostate of normal and neonatally estrogenized rats. Endocrinology 1998;139:874–883.

135. Mosselman S, Polman J, Dijkema R. ER beta: identification and characterization of a novel human estrogen receptor. FEBS Lett 1996;392:49–53.

136. Ogawa S, Inoue S, Watanabe T, et al. The complete primary structure of human estrogen receptor beta (hER beta) and its heterodimerization with ER alpha in vivo and in vitro. Biochem Biophys Res Commun 1998;243:122–126.
137. Moore JT, McKee DD, Slentz-Kesler K, et al. Cloning and characterization of human estrogen receptor beta isoforms. Biochem Biophys Res Commun 1998;247:75–78.
138. Carruba G, Pfeffer U, Fecarotta E, et al. Estradiol inhibits growth of hormone-nonresponsive PC3 human prostate cancer cells. Cancer Res 1994;54:1190–1193.
139. Hobisch A, Hittmair A, Daxenbichler G, et al. Metastatic lesions from prostate cancer do not express oestrogen and progesterone receptors. J Pathol 1997;182:356–361.
140. Markaverich BM, Alejandro MA. Type II [^{3}H] estradiol binding site antagonists: inhibition of normal and malignant prostate cell growth and proliferation. Int J Oncol 1998;12:1127–1135.
141. Bezwoda WR. Treatment of stage D2 prostatic cancer refractory to or relapsed following castration plus oestrogens. Comparison of aminoglutethimide plus hydrocortisone with medroxy progesterone acetate plus hydrocortisone. Br J Urol 1990;66:196–201.
142. Chang AY, Bennett JM, Pandya KJ, Asbury R, McCune C. A study of amino glutethemide and hydrocortisone in patients with advanced and refractory prostate carcinoma. Am J Clin Oncol 1989;12:358–360.
143. Dowsett M, Shearer RJ, Ponder BA, Malone P, Jeffcoate SL. The effects of aminoglutethimide and hydrocortisone alone and combined, on androgen levels in postorchiectomy prostatic cancer patients. Br J Cancer 1988;57:190–192.
144. Figg WD, Kroog G, Duray P, et al. Flutamide withdrawal plus hydrocortisone resulted in clinical complete response in a patient with prostate carcinoma. Cancer 1997;79:1964–1968.
145. Harland SJ, Duchesne GM. Suramin and prostate cancer: the role of hydrocortisone [letter]. Eur J Cancer 1992;28A:1295.
146. Kelly WK, Curley T, Leibretz C, Dnistrian A, Schwartz M, Scher HI. Prospective evaluation of hydrocortisone and suramin in patients with androgen-independent prostate cancer. J Clin Oncol 1995;13:2208–2213.
147. Kelly WK, Scher HI, Mazumdar M, et al. Suramin and hydrocortisone: determining drug efficacy in androgen-independent prostate cancer. J Clin Oncol 1995;13:2214–2222.
148. Labrie F, Dupont A, Belanger A, et al. Anti-hormone treatment for prostate cancer relapsing after treatment with flutamide and castration. Addition of aminoglutethimide and low dose hydrocortisone to combination therapy. Br J Urol 1989;63:634–638.
149. Plowman PN, Perry LA, Chard T. Androgen suppression by hydrocortisone without aminoglutethimide in orchiectomised men with prostatic cancer. Br J Urol 1987;59:255–257.
150. Small EJ, Baron A, Bok R. Simultaneous antiandrogen withdrawal and treatment with ketoconazole and hydrocortisone in patients with advanced prostate carcinoma. Cancer 1997;80:1755–1759.
151. Brendler H. Adrenalectomy and hypophysectomy for prostatic cancer. Urology 1973;2:99–102.
152. Schoonees R, Schalch DS, Reynoso G, Murphy GP. Bilateral adrenalectomy for advanced prostatic carcinoma. J Urol 1972;108:123–125.
153. Sogani PC, Fair WR. Treatment of advanced prostatic cancer. Urol Clin North Am 1987;14:353–371.
154. Gerber GS, Chodak GW. Prostate specific antigen for assessing response to ketoconazole and prednisone in patients with hormone refractory metastatic prostate cancer. J Urol 1990;144:1177–1179.
155. Mahler C, Verhelst J, Denis L. Ketoconazole and liarozole in the treatment of advanced prostatic cancer. Cancer 1993;71:1068–1073.
156. Small EJ, Baron AD, Fippin L, Apodaca D. Ketoconazole retains activity in advanced prostate cancer patients with progression despite flutamide withdrawal. J Urol 1997;157:1204–1207.
157. Trachtenberg J, Zadra J. Steroid synthesis inhibition by ketoconazole: sites of action. Clin Invest Med 1988;11:1–5.
158. Scher HI, Steineck G, Kelly WK. Hormone-refractory (D3) prostate cancer: refining the concept. Urology 1995;46:142–148.
159. Peehl DM, Stamey TA. Growth responses of normal, benign hyperplastic, and malignant human prostatic epithelial cells in vitro to cholera toxin, pituitary extract, and hydrocortisone. Prostate 1986;8:51–61.
160. Chan SY. Androgen and glucocorticoid receptors in the Pollard prostate adenocarcinoma cell lines. Prostate 1980;1:53–60.
161. Koutsilieris M, Grondin F, Lehoux JG. The expression of mRNA for glucocorticoid receptor gene and functional glucocorticoid receptors detected in PA-III rat prostate adenocarcinoma cells. Anticancer Res 1992;12:899–904.

162. Reyes-Moreno C, Frenette G, Boulanger J, Lavergne E, Govindan MV, Koutsilieris M. Mediation of glucocorticoid receptor function by transforming growth factor beta I expression in human PC-3 prostate cancer cells. Prostate 1995;26:260–269.

163. Smith RG, Syms AJ, Nag A, Lerner S, Norris JS. Mechanism of the glucocorticoid regulation of growth of the androgen-sensitive prostate-derived R3327H-G8-A1 tumor cell line. J Biol Chem 1985; 260:12,454–12,463.

164. Sosnowski J, Stetter-Neel C, Cole D, Durham JP, Mawhinney MG. Protein kinase C mediated anti-proliferative glucocorticoid-sphinganine synergism in cultured Pollard III prostate tumor cells. J Urol 1997;158:269–274.

165. Chang C, Kokontis J, Liao SS, Chang Y. Isolation and characterization of human TR3 receptor: a member of steroid receptor superfamily. J Steroid Biochem 1989;34:391–395.

166. Uemura H, Chang C. Antisense TR3 orphan receptor can increase prostate cancer cell viability with etoposide treatment. Endocrinology 1998;139:2329–2334.

167. Haussler MR, Mangelsdorf DJ, Komm BS, Terpening CM, Yamazaki K, Allegretto EA, et al. Molecular biology of the vitamin D hormone. In: Anonymous, ed. Recent Progress in Hormone Research. Academic, New York, 1988, pp. 263–305.

168. Haussler MR, Jurutka PW, Hsieh J-C, Thompson PD, Selznick SH, Haussler CA, Whitfield GK. New understanding of the molecular mechanism of receptor-mediated genomic actions of the vitamin D hormone. Bone 1995;17:33S–38S.

169. Anderson JJB, Toverud SU. Diet and vitamin D: a review with an emphasis on human function. J Nutr Biochem 1994;5:58–65.

170. Walters MR. Newly identified actions of the vitamin D endocrine system. Endocr Rev 1992;13:719–764.

171. Fife RS, Sledge GW, Proctor C. Effects of vitamin D_3 on proliferation of cancer cells in vitro. Cancer Lett 1997;120:65–69.

172. Colston KW, James SY, Ofori-Kuragu EA, Binderup L, Grant AG. Vitamin D receptors and anti-proliferative effects of vitamin D derivatives in human pancreatic carcinoma cells in vivo and in vitro. Br J Cancer 1997;76:1017–1020.

173. Colston KW, Colston JM, Feldman D. 1,25-Dihydroxyvitamin D_3 and malignant melanoma: the presence of receptors and inhibition of cell growth in culture. Endocrinology 1981;108:1083–1086.

174. Miller GJ, Stapleton GE, Ferrara JA, Lucia MS, Pfister S, Hedlund TE, Upadhya P. Human prostatic carcinoma cell line LNCaP expresses biologically active, specific receptors for 1 alpha, 25-dihydroxyvitamin D_3. Cancer Res 1992;52:515–520.

175. Miller GJ, Stapleton GE, Hedlund TE, Moffat KA. Vitamin D receptor expression, 24-hydroxylase activity, and inhibition of growth by 1,25-dihydroxyvitamin D_3 in seven human prostatic carcinoma cell lines. Clin Cancer Res 1995;1:997–1003.

176. Skowronski RJ, Peehl DM, Feldman D. Vitamin D and prostate cancer: 1,25-dihydroxyvitamin D_3 receptors and actions in human prostate cancer cell lines. Endocrinology 1993;132:1952–1960.

177. Holick MF. The photobiology of vitamin D3 in man. In: Kumar R, ed. Vitamin D: Basic and Clinical Aspects. Martinus Nijhoff, Boston, 1984, pp. 197–216.

178. Studzinski GP, Moore DC. Sunlight—can it prevent as well as cause cancer? Cancer Res 1995;55: 4014–4022.

179. Corder EH, Guess HA, Hulka BS, Friedman GD, Sadler M, Vollmer RT, et al. Vitamin D and prostate cancer: a prediagnostic study with stored sera. Cancer Epidemiol Biomarkers Prev 1993;2:467–472.

180. Braun MM, Helzlsouer KJ, Hollis BW, Comstock GW. Prostate cancer and prediagnostic levels of serum vitamin D metabolites. Cancer Causes Control 1995;6:235–239.

181. Gann PH, Ma J, Hennekens CH, Hollis BW, Haddad JG, Stampfer MJ. Circulating vitamin D metabolites in relation to subsequent development of prostate cancer. Cancer Epidemiol Biomarkers Prev 1996; 5:121–126.

182. Baker MR, Peacock M, Nordin BE. The decline in vitamin D status with age. Age Ageing 1980;9: 249–252.

183. Lawson DE, Paul AA, Black AE, Cole TJ, Mandal AR, Davie M. Relative contributions of diet and sunlight to vitamin D state in the elderly. Br Med J 1979;2:303–305.

184. Matusoka LY, Wortsman J, Haddad JG, Kolm P, Hollis BW. Racial pigmentation and the cutaneous synthesis of vitamin D. Arch Dermatol 1991;127:536–538.

185. Haenszel W, Kurihara M. Studies of Japanese migrants. I. Mortality from cancer and other diseases among Japanese in the United States. J Natl Cancer Inst 1968;40:43–68.

186. Hanchette CL, Schwartz GG. Geographic patterns of prostate cancer mortality. Evidence for a protective effect of ultraviolet radiation. Cancer 1992;70:2861–2869.

187. Peehl DM, Skowronski RJ, Leung GK, Wong ST, Stamey TA, Feldman D. Antiproliferative effects of 1,25-dihydroxyvitamin D_3 on primary cultures of human prostatic cells. Cancer Res 1994;54:805–810.

188. Blutt SE, Allegretto EA, Pike JW, Weigel NL. 1,25-dihydroxyvitamin D_3 and 9-*cis*-retinoic acid act synergistically to inhibit the growth of LNCaP prostate cells and cause accumulation of cells in G_1. Endocrinology 1997;138:1491–1497.

189. Hedlund TE, Moffat KA, Miller GJ. Stable expression of the nuclear vitamin D receptor in the human prostatic carcinoma cell line JCA-1: evidence that the antiproliferative effects of 1α, 25-dihydroxyvitamin D_3 are mediated exclusively through the genomic signaling pathway. Endocrinology 1996;137:1554–1561.

190. Hedlund TE, Moffatt KA, Miller GJ. Vitamin D receptor expression is required for growth modulation by 1a, 25-dihydroxyvitamin D_3 in the human prostatic carcinoma cell line ALVA-31. J Steroid Biochem 1996;58:277–288.

191. Getzenberg RH, Light BW, Lapco PE, Konety BR, Nangia AK, Acierno JS, et al. Vitamin D inhibition of prostate adenocarcinoma growth and metastasis in the Dunning rat prostate model system. Urology 1998;50:999–1006.

192. Schwartz GG, Hill CC, Oeler TA, Becich MJ, Bahnson RR. 1,24-dihydroxy-16-ene-23-yne-vitamin D_3 and prostate cancer cell proliferation *in vivo*. Urology 1995;46:365–369.

193. Taylor JA, Hirvonen A, Watson M, Pittman G, Mohler JL, Bell DA. Association of prostate cancer with vitamin D receptor gene polymorphism. Cancer Res 1996;56:4108–4110.

194. Ingles SA, Ross RK, Yu MC, Irvine RA, Lapera G, Haile RW, Coetzee GA. Association of prostate cancer risk with genetic polymorphisms in vitamin D receptor and androgen receptor. J Natl Cancer Inst 1997;89:166–170.

195. Ingles SA, Coetzee GA, Ross RK, Henderson BE, Kolonel LN, Crocitto L, Wang W, Haile RW. Association of prostate cancer with vitamin D receptor haplotypes in African-Americans. Cancer Res 1998;58:1620–1623.

196. Kibel AS, Isaacs SD, Isaacs WB, Bova GS. Vitamin D receptor polymorphisms and lethal prostate cancer. J Urol 1998;160:1405–1409.

197. Schwartz GG, Hulka BS. Is vitamin D deficiency a risk factor for prostate cancer? (hypothesis). Anticancer Res 1990;10:1307–1312.

14

Type I Family Growth Factor Receptors and Their Ligands in Prostate Cancer

K. E. Leverton, PhD and W. J. Gullick, PhD

INTRODUCTION

Cancer cells characteristically grow in an apparently unregulated manner, and it is reasonable to hypothesize that this is a consequence of some derangement in their natural growth regulatory systems. Many experiments have been carried out to test this hypothesis, and there is much evidence to support the concept. The family of receptors and ligands most manifestly implicated, and in some cases proven, to be involved in cell transformation is the type I family, which consists of four receptors, epidermal growth factor receptor (EGFR), c-erbB-2, c-erbB-3, and c-erbB-4 (also known as HER1–4). A plethora of ligands has been identified, currently totaling nine separate genes, but several of these are produced as very complex sets of splice variants. Indeed, c-erbB-4 has recently also been shown to be subject to splicing to produce four alternative full-length transcripts, and EGFR, c-erbB-2, and c-erbB-3 are all produced as alternatively spliced extracellular domain truncated proteins.

Despite the complexity of this family and their multiple interactions, some practical knowledge has emerged on their role in human cancers. EGFR is commonly overexpressed in squamous cancers, and is mutated in gliomas, and c-erbB-2 is overexpressed

From: *Contemporary Endocrinology: Endocrine Oncology*
Edited by: S. P. Ethier © Humana Press Inc., Totowa, NJ

in many types of adenocarcinoma. c-erbB-3 and c-erbB-4 have been less well studied, but there is a suggestion that, although they may be important co-receptors, they are not themselves involved in cell transformation, and may indeed be more influential in cell differentiation.

In some cancer types, the structure and pattern of expression of these receptors and ligands has been studied in detail. Indeed, in breast cancer, there is even a consensus as to the prevalence and mechanism of their activation, which has identified them as targets for new drug development. This is not yet the case in an equally important disease, prostate cancer (PC). The purpose of this review is to draw together what information there is on this family, and, as will become apparent, to criticize it, with the intention of identifying deficiencies in knowledge and priorities for new experiments.

PC is the second leading cause of cancer death in men in the Western world. The incidence of the disease increases with age, and, by 80 yr up to 80% of men have evidence of malignant cells at autopsy (1). However, it is currently difficult to predict the behavior of individual PCs, because localized tumors may remain latent or progress to clinical significance, but other, apparently localized tumors, may already have developed unde-tectable metastatic disease. There is currently a pressing need to develop markers that can be used to predict the behavior of individual tumors, which would be greatly aided by an improvement in the knowledge of the molecular changes that occur during initiation and development of the disease. In addition, more understanding of the molecular biology of the disease may identify targets for new drug development.

The glandular composition of the prostate comprises two layers of epithelial cells (ECs): secretory (luminal) and basal (thought to be stem cells for secretory epithelia), interspersed with neuroendocrine cells, and separated by the basement membrane from the stroma (a mixture of smooth muscle cells, fibroblasts, blood vessels, neuromuscular tissue, and extracellular matrix). Benign prostate hyperplasia (BPH), which is usually already present when prostate carcinoma occurs, is a condition that increases in prev-alence with age, but is thought not to be a precursor of malignancy. BPH frequently accompanies prostatic intraepithelial neoplasia (PIN), which is characterized by prolifer-ation of secretory ECs and eventual loss of the basal cell layer. PIN, classified as grade I, II, or III, is found in greater than 85% of prostatic adenocarcinoma (PCA) specimens, and is thought to be the most likely precursor of this malignancy. However, the molecular mechanisms underlying the initiation and progression of PC are currently unclear. Andro-gens, acting through the androgen receptor (AR), are important in hormonal control in the normal prostate, and may be involved in the development of malignancy. Treatment for PC often includes androgen ablation (deprivation) therapy, but, although tumors are usually initially responsive, many eventually progress to androgen independence. The mechanisms by which this occurs are not well characterized, but may include amplifica-tion of the AR gene during acquired resistance to treatment, expression of mutated forms of the protein, and eventual decrease and loss of AR expression in metastatic disease (1).

The establishment of PC cells in culture has proved difficult and there are currently only three principal human PCA cell lines (2,3). LNCaP cells, derived from the lymph node of a patient with hormone-refractory PCA, express a mutated form of the AR, are hormone-responsive, but not metastatic in animals. The hormonally unresponsive PC3 cell line was derived from a bone marrow metastasis, is metastatic, and does not appear to express the AR. DU145 cells, derived from a central nervous system metastasis, are also hormone-unresponsive, and the majority of reports suggest that they are AR-negative.

Knowledge of the involvement of type I growth factor (GF) receptors and their ligands in prostate malignancy is currently incomplete. Many studies have looked for changes in levels and/or patterns of expression of these receptors that could result in alterations in cellular signaling pathways. Normal and hyperplastic prostate tissues, PCAs, PCA cell lines, and xenografts have all been examined. These studies have used a number of different methods, including protein expression by immunohistochemistry (IHC), Western blot, and ligand-binding assays; mRNA expression by Northern/dot blot, reverse transcriptase-polymerase chain reaction (RT-PCR) and RNase protection assays; and genomic DNA analysis by PCR and Southern blot.

Experimental studies have also been carried out to ascertain the effects of altering expression levels of GFs and receptors in prostate-derived cell lines in vitro and prostate tissues in vivo. However, contrary to the frequently observed dramatic overexpression of EGFR in squamous cell carcinomas and c-erbB-2 in adenocarcinomas, similar changes have not been identified in prostate malignancy. In fact, the levels of these molecules in normal and malignant prostate tissues are not high, compared to many other normal or tumor tissues. Thus, most studies face the technical challenge of attempting to quantify small changes in expression levels. Another potentially confounding factor is that PCAs are heterogeneous in cellular composition. Indeed IHC studies have shown that tumor cells may infiltrate surrounding benign prostate, and the ratio of stroma to PCA to benign epithelium may vary considerably between specimens, making interpretation of quantitative assays difficult. Thus, in some assays, reports of increased or overexpression of a particular molecule may actually result from an increase in the proportion of tumor cells in the tissue being analyzed, rather than specific increases in expression levels in the cancer cells. It is, nonetheless, possible that signal transduction mediated by these GF receptors and their ligands, rather than gross changes in expression levels, may be important in their role in prostate malignancy.

EGFR, EGF, AND TRANSFORMING GROWTH FACTOR α

Many studies have investigated, in parallel, the expression of the EGFR and two of its ligands, EGF and transforming growth factor α (TGF-α), in PC, and, thus, these molecules are reviewed together. Other ligands, about which there is generally less information, are discussed later.

Quantitative Analyses of Protein Expression

Attempts to determine differences in EGFR levels in benign and malignant prostate tissues, using quantitative methods of analysis on whole tissues, have yielded conflicting results, probably because tissue samples being analyzed are generally very heterogeneous, and also because there are no major changes in protein expression levels. ^{125}I-EGF ligand-binding studies *(4,5)* showed a statistically significant increase in EGF-binding by extracts of PCA tissues and cell lines, compared with benign prostate tissue, levels increased with increasing tumor grade. Another study, using fluorescence-activated cell sorting analysis, determined that the DU-145 and PC-3 cell lines express relatively high levels of EGFR (approx 10^5 receptors/cell); the androgen-responsive LNCaP cell line expresses lower levels (approx 10^4/cell) of surface receptor *(6)*. These levels do not, however, approach those found in the squamoucarcinoma cell lines, A431 and MDA-MB468 (2×10^6 receptors/cell) or HN5 (1.5×10^7 receptors/cell), which result from

amplification of the EGFR gene. One study *(7)* found that BPH tissues bound approx 2.5×
as much EGF as PCA tissues, and that there was a propensity for poorly differentiated
tumors to express less EGFR than well-differentiated tumors. Interpretation of competi-
tive ligand-binding assays is, however, complicated by the presence of endogenous,
unlabeled ligands in the tissue being analyzed, which may reduce the apparent number
of binding sites, and also by the presence of more than one receptor type within a cell/
tissue to which each ligand may bind with varying affinity. At the time most of these
experiments were performed, few of the new ligands for EGFR had been identified.
Clearly, the presence of these factors could confound such measurements, and should
be taken into account when assessing ligand-binding data. Western blot analyses, which
would be unaffected by these factors, have shown that EGFR is expressed in an immortalized, nontransformed prostate EC line, MLC-SV40, a PCA xenograft, CWR22 *(8)*,
and also the PCA cells lines, LNCaP, DU145, and PC-3 *(8,9)*. Levels of EGFR expression
and activation are higher in PC3 and DU145 than in normal prostate epithelium or LNCaP
(which is in agreement with ligand-binding studies), and are not altered in LNCaP by
androgen stimulation, implying that this receptor does not appear to have a functional
role in androgen-stimulated growth of LNCaP in vitro *(9)*. Other prostate-derived tumorigenic sublines have been shown by Western blot analysis to have decreased EGFR expression, although TGF-α levels are increased, suggesting the presence of an EGFR/TGF-α
autocrine network in these cells *(10)*.

Western blot analyses have also demonstrated the presence of EGF and TGF-α in
hyperplastic human prostate tissue *(11)*. Levels of these ligands, as determined by radioimmunoassay, are reportedly unchanged between benign (hyperplastic) and malignant
(PCA) prostate tissues, with a TGF-α-EGF ratio of approx 2:1, although an increase in
TGF-α and EGF levels, with increasing tumor grade, was observed *(12)*.

Immunohistochemistry

IHC methods are more appropriate for the assessment of heterogeneous tissue samples,
because the analysis provides information about specific cellular localization, as well as
levels of expression. In recent years, a number of studies, by IHC analysis, of frozen or
fixed tissue specimens, and of PCA cell lines and xenografts, have attempted to assess
possible changes in expression levels and/or localization of EGFR, and some of its
ligands during the development and progression of prostate malignancy. It is, however,
difficult to correlate the results of different analyses, because the methods employed and
the conditions chosen for the measurement vary considerably: For example, the use of
different antibodies (Abs), incubation conditions, differences in the number of samples
analyzed, different methods of tissue preparation and preservation, and individual variations in assessment of tumor grade all can affect results. Bearing this in mind, the observations published to date tend to suggest that there are no gross changes in expression
levels of EGFR and/or its ligands. However, it is possible that the receptor may still be
involved in the development of PC by more subtle changes. For instance, there may be
a shift toward autocrine rather than paracrine regulation in tumor cells, and perhaps also
increased activation and/or decreased downregulation of receptors.

A number of studies have used IHC to assess the expression of EGFR, EGF, and TGF-α
in normal and hyperplastic prostate tissues. The majority of reports suggest that staining
for EGFR is strong in basal ECs of normal and hyperplastic prostate, but low or absent
in secretory ECs, and absent in the stroma *(13–20)*. An investigation of EGFR expression

during development of the human prostate *(21)* revealed that, in fetal/neonatal and pre-pubertal human prostate tissue, EGFR expression was detected in basal ECs, but, in adult and hyperplastic tissues, expression was also noted in the lateral membranes of secretory cells, with staining more intense in hyperplastic than in normal tissue. Reports of TGF-α expression in normal and hyperplastic prostate are more inconsistent. Some investigators *(18,20,22,23)* have claimed that there is very little or no TGF-α in normal or hyperplastic cells, although this is contradicted by others *(24)*, who have observed weak staining of adult human prostatic glandular cells, using a TGF-α monoclonal antibody (mAb) on frozen tissue sections, or stromal staining in frozen BPH tissues *(19)*. Analysis of TGF-α expression during development of the human prostate *(21)* indicated expression at all stages in stromal smooth muscle; staining in basal and secretory epithelia was only detected in fetal tissues. Neonatal and prepubertal tissues showed a low level of staining in secretory epithelia, but this was absent in normal and hyperplastic adult tissues. IHC analysis of the developing rat prostate *(25)* revealed co-expression of TGF-α and EGFR in ECs, but not stromal cells, of the ventral, but not the dorsal, prostate, although another group reported TGF-α staining in the lateral and dorsal, but not ventral, rat prostate *(26)*. It has also been reported *(27)* that TGF-α expression varies in different regions of the post-pubertal rat prostate, with cells being either androgen-sensitive or –insensitive, and those authors suggest that the contradictions contained in previous reports may be explained in part as a consequence of the specific region of the prostate sampled. Information on EGF expression in benign prostate tissue is also inconsistent. Some reports *(23,28)* have suggested that there is no positive staining for EGF in normal or hyperplastic human and normal rat prostate cells, but others *(18)* have observed staining for EGF in basal epithelia of normal and hyperplastic glands, and in smooth muscle of hyperplastic cells, although the authors themselves suggest that the staining may be nonspecific. In the normal rat prostate, expression of EGF has been reported to occur mostly in secretory acini in the dorsal lobe, with low expression in the lateral lobe, and virtually none in ventral lobe, and once again, no stromal staining was detected *(26,29)*.

Thus, in the light of these somewhat conflicting observations, it is difficult to draw conclusions regarding obvious changes in expression of EGFR and ligands in premalignant and malignant prostate. If anything, investigators have tended to report a general decrease in the percentage of cells staining positive for EGFR from benign tissue, through low-grade PIN (discontinuous staining in basal layer, with gaps corresponding to disruption of basal layer), high-grade PIN, and increasing grades of PCA, with staining becoming more diffuse and less intense, although variable between and within different specimens *(15–19,23,30,31)*. One group reported that EGFR-positive tumors were generally of a higher grade than those that were negative, and that these patients had a worse 10-yr survival, although this was not significant in a multivariate analysis *(17)*. Recent studies *(20,21)* describe the localization of EGFR in PIN/PCA to the membranes of proliferating (secretory) cells, and co-expression in these cells of TGF-α, which suggests the presence of an autocrine regulatory system. Furthermore, it has been suggested that regulation via EGFR/TGF-α in the normal and hyperplastic adult prostate is paracrine, and that the situation in malignancy is similar to that during development of the prostate, in which autocrine regulation occurs *(18,21)*. High levels of TGF-α expression have been observed in PCAs, with a tendency toward increasing expression with more poorly differentiated tumors *(18,20,22)*, although, contrary to this, it has also been reported that TGF-α staining is absent in low- and high-grade PIN and most tumors. Staining for EGF has been observed in malignant epithelial tissues and in smooth muscle of malignant prostates *(18, 32)*, although this could well be nonspecific, because others have reported weak or absent staining for EGF in low- and high-grade PIN and most tumors *(23)*.

Immunocytochemical analysis of cultured PC cell lines indicated positive staining for EGFR in basolateral cell membranes of DU145 cells. More diffuse, cytoplasmic, staining was detected in PC-3 cells *(33)*, and a highly metastatic, androgen-repressed human PCA cell line, ARCaP, stained intensely for EGFR *(34)*. PCA cell lines have also been shown to secrete EGF and TGF-α *(35–38)*.

Analysis of mRNA Expression

As with protein analyses, different methods of mRNA detection may provide information about the levels of expression and/or the site of mRNA synthesis. Whole-tissue analyses, such as Northern blots, RNase protection, and RT-PCR, are complicated by the heterogeneity of the specimen being analyzed; *in situ* hybridization (ISH) provides more specific information about the location of mRNA expression within specific cells, but is more difficult to quantify. In both types of analyses, tissue preparation methods cause variations in observed expression levels, because RNA is particularly labile to degradation during handling and storage of samples. Additionally, methods based on amplification from small quantities of target mRNA may be difficult to quantify, and may also be sensitive to contamination.

As with studies of protein expression, reports of mRNA expression and localization for EGFR and its ligands in benign and malignant prostate tissues vary. Using mRNA ISH EGFR, EGF, and TGF-α mRNA were all localized to the epithelial compartment of hyperplastic human prostate tissues *(11)*. In another study *(23)* using this method, normal and hyperplastic prostate tissues and PIN showed weak or absent expression of EGFR mRNA, but strong expression was seen in prostate tumors, although, in the same study, a corresponding upregulation of EGFR protein was not observed. Others *(20)* have reported strong EGFR mRNA expression by ISH in basal ECs of benign and malignant prostate tissues; TGF-α mRNA was detected in secretory cells, and expression appeared to correlate more directly with the protein. High levels of EGFR mRNA expression have also been detected by ISH in the PC-3 cell line, and in variants with different metastatic potentials *(39)*.

EGF mRNA has been detected in normal pig prostate, using RNase protection assay *(40)*. Northern blot analyses of total RNA from normal prostates of male human postmortems were positive for EGFR in all cases *(41)*. However, a study of hyperplastic human prostate tissues detected no expression of EGFR, EGF, or TGF-α by Northern blot analysis *(11)*. In a study of benign and malignant prostate tissues, as well as the PCA cell lines, DU145 and PC-3, all samples were positive for EGFR and TGF-α mRNA by Northern blot, with no significant differences in levels between benign and malignant samples, and no detectable expression of EGF in any of the tissues or cell lines analyzed. However, previous analyses by Northern blot, RNA dot blot, and RNase protection assay found that PCA tissues express higher levels of EGFR *(42)*, EGF, and TGF-α *(43)* mRNA than hyperplastic prostate tissues, with the highest levels detected in PCA cell lines (EGF greatest in LNCaP; TGF-α and EGFR were higher in DU145 and PC-3).

RT-PCR analyses of mouse and rat tissues, and tissue recombination systems have indicated that EGFR, EGF, and TGF-α are all expressed in both epithelial and, to a lesser extent, mesenchymal tissues, with EGFR levels varying during development and adult-hood; TGF-α expression is reported to remain more constant *(44–47)*. EGFR mRNA has also been detected in the normal human prostate by RT-PCR, with apparently increased levels in hyperplastic tissues *(48)*. Another study detected expression of EGFR, EGF, and TGF-α mRNA in hyperplastic human prostate tissues by RT-PCR, although the same samples were negative by Northern blot analysis *(11)*. In studies to establish tyrosine kinase (TK) expression profiles for benign and malignant prostate tissues and cell lines, EGFR expression was observed by RT-PCR analysis in all samples tested *(49,50)*. The results of an RT-PCR analysis of three transformed (LNCaP, DU145, PC-3) and one immortalized, nontransformed (MLC-SV40) human prostate cell lines, for EGF and TGF-α mRNA expression *(8)*, indicated that all the cell lines expressed TGF-α mRNA, but only the transformed cell lines were positive for EGF mRNA.

Gene Analysis

In contrast to the frequently observed amplification of EGFR and c-erbB-2 observed in other cancers, there have been no reports of such changes in prostate malignancy. The few studies that appear to have addressed this question report an absence of amplification or gene rearrangements in hyperplastic prostate or PC cell lines, compared with normal human prostate *(43,48)*, and it is probable that the small number of reports reflects the lack of positive findings by investigators. Only one study *(51)* has reported EGFR gene ampli-fication (approx 10× normal) in an immortalized, nontransformed, prostate-derived cell line, PNT1B, with a concomitant increase in EGFR mRNA expression and EGF-binding sites, but no structural alterations of the gene were detected. Amplification and mutation of the AR gene, however, is frequently reported during the development of prostate carci-noma, suggesting that such changes can take place, and indicating that any alterations that may occur in the EGFR gene are not selected for in this malignancy.

Models of EGFR Function in PC

Experimental observations in tumors have, despite not identifying gross alterations in expression levels, suggested an involvement of EGFR and its ligands in normal and malig-nant prostate, and laboratory experiments support these findings. Androgens, acting through the AR, a member of the nuclear receptor superfamily of transcription factors, play a significant role in controling the growth and differentiation of prostatic cells, and many prostatic cancers show an initial androgen dependence. The actions of androgen have been shown to influence the expression of locally produced GFs and studies have been carried out to assess the role that the AR may play in the expression of EGFR and its ligands. A number of studies *(44,47,52–54)* have reported that androgen negatively regulates EGFR expression, but does not directly regulate TGF-α expression in the mouse and rat, although stimulation of mRNA synthesis, for either EGFR/TGF-α or EGFR alone, has been reported upon treatment of androgen-sensitive human prostate tumor cell lines, ALVA101 *(55)* and PC3-hAR *(56)*, respectively, with androgen in vitro. Exoge-nous ligands have been used to assess the response of various models to receptor activa-tion. A number of studies *(8,35–37,57)* have shown that TGF-α and/or EGF are mitogenic in DU145 and LNCaP cells. An equally valid experimental approach, to determine the role of these molecules, is to assess the contribution of endogenous ligand expression. One way to assess this is to use Abs that prevent ligand binding. An anti-EGFR mAb,

C225, has been shown to inhibit the growth of PC3 and DU145 xenografts in nude mice, as well as the ability of EGF to induce EGFR phosphorylation in PC3, DU145, and LNCaP cells *(6)*, and it has been suggested that DU145 and PC-3 require EGFR activation for continued progression in a tumor environment. It is likely that the activity of the EGFR is also moderated by other molecules within the cell, for instance, it has been reported that human prostatic acid phosphatase (PAcP) selectively dephosphorlylates EGFR, and is associated with a reduction in TK activity of the receptor *(58)*.

c-erbB-2

Whereas the combined evidence for expression of the EGFR suggests that loss of expression is associated with increasing malignancy in PCs, overexpression of c-erbB-2 has been reported. Because gene amplification has not been found, the range of expression is apparently much less than in breast cancer. Again, therefore, the method of measurement and the care taken in its analysis have tended to lead to some variation in the conclusions of studies on the expression of this receptor.

Immunohistochemistry

Some studies have reported a failure to detect expression of c-erbB-2 by IHC analysis of fixed tissues *(17,59,60)*, although others *(61)* have reported that the polyclonal Ab used (Ab-1) is not reactive in fixed tissues, calling into question the validity of these results. Lack of expression in benign prostate tissues has also been reported, using different Abs and/or frozen tissue sections *(60,62)*; however, other researchers *(15,31,61, 63–65)* have reported IHC detection of c-erbB-2 in normal and hyperplastic benign prostate tissues localized to basal ECs, with low/absent expression in luminal cells, and none in the stroma *(64,65)*.

The majority of studies *(31,59–62,64)* using IHC have reported increased expression of c-erbB-2 in PIN and PCA. One group *(64)* observed that, in PIN, staining for c-erbB-2 is moderate to strong in basal and luminal ECs in both the membrane and cytoplasm. Similar patterns were seen in the majority of cells in localized PCA, in high-grade PCAs and matching metastatic lesions. The authors, therefore, suggest that the change in expression pattern is an early event in PCA, which remains stable throughout progression to high-grade PCA and metastasis. Another study *(31)* has shown a significant association between c-erbB-2 expression and poor survival in PCA, but there was no association between EGFR and survival. Others *(15,65)* have reported no difference in c-erbB-2 expression between benign and malignant prostate tissue, or even no detectable expression of c-erbB-2 in prostate carcinomas *(66)*. IHC analyses of PCA cell lines (LNCaP, DU145, PC-3, ARCaP) have indicated that all express c-erbB-2 *(34,62,65)*.

Quantitative Protein Analysis

Using Western blotting to analyze c-erbB-2 expression in prostate tissues and cell lines, investigators *(8,62)* have reported no detectable c-erbB-2 in normal/hyperplastic tissue; 60–80% of PCAs were positive, as were the PCA cell lines LNCaP, DU145 and PC-3, and the immortalized, nontransformed, prostate-derived cell line, MLC-SV40. Others *(67)* have shown that the level of c-erbB-2 phosphorylation in LNCaP cells is inversely correlated with the expression of PAcP, and note that c-erbB-2 is highly phosphorylated in PC-3 and DU145 cell lines, which do not express PAcP.

Analysis of mRNA Expression

There have been few descriptions of c-erbB-2 mRNA expression levels in normal and malignant prostate tissues. It has been reported *(48)*, using RT-PCR analysis, that the receptor is overexpressed in some cases of BPH, compared to normal prostate, although RT-PCR relies on amplification from small amounts of template, and the results were not confirmed by other methods. A similar study, also by RT-PCR, of hyperplastic and malignant prostate tissues, a PCA xenograft (CWR22), and PCA cell lines (LNCaP, DU145, PC-3), showed that all except one tumor sample were positive for c-erbB-2.

Gene Analysis

To date, there are no reports of amplification or abnormalities of the c-*erb*B-2 gene in PC. Analyses by PCR and Southern blot of benign and malignant prostate tissues and PCA cell lines have shown no amplification of c-*erb*B-2 in prostate hyperplasia or malignancy *(48,59,62,68,69)*.

Models of c-erbB-2 Function in PC

Experimental studies have shown that an activated form of the rat c-erbB-2 receptor, Neu, is transforming when transfected into rat prostatic ECs in culture *(70)*, and when expressed in rat prostate ECs injected into nude mice *(71)*. It has also been reported that c-erbB-2 is necessary for interleukin-6 signaling in LNCaP cells, where treatment with interleukin-6-induced phosphorylation of c-erbB-2 and c-erbB-3, but not EGFR *(72)*. As yet, however, other reports have not confirmed these findings. Since no ligand is known to bind directly to c-erbB-2, it cannot be selectively activated. However, c-erbB-2 acts as a powerful co-receptor with all the other receptors in the family, and thus its presence appreciably affects the response of cells to ligand addition. Reduction of c-erbB-2 signaling and its effect on malignant cells, has not been reported, but, with the development of Abs and selective TK inhibitors, such experiments are becoming feasible. At present, therefore, there is no compelling evidence that c-erbB-2 is a transforming influence in this disease, nor that it is a target for treatment. Further experiments may, however, put its role more clearly in context.

c-erbB-3

The c-erbB-3 receptor, unusual among the erbB family because it has a greatly reduced TK activity, has been identified as a receptor for the neuregulins NDFs, or heregulins, and appears to be involved in the development of the peripheral nervous system, in particular, in the growth and development of Schwann cells *(73)*. Preliminary studies have identified variable levels of c-erbB-3 expression in a range of human tumors *(74)*, although gene amplification has not been observed. There have been few reports regarding c-erbB-3 expression in prostate tissues, but the studies published to date suggest that patterns of expression may be similar to those of c-erbB-2, with increased expression detected in malignant, compared with benign, prostate.

Analysis of Protein Expression

Just as for c-erbB-2, some authors *(75,76)* have reported a failure to detect expression of c-erbB-3 in benign prostate glandular tissue, using IHC, although others *(64,65)* have reported positive staining in basal ECs of normal and hyperplastic prostate, and possible low levels of staining in luminal ECs. IHC studies of c-erbB-3 expression in prostate tumors have shown increased expression, compared with benign prostate tissues *(64,75, 76)*, although a statistical analysis showed no correlation with tumor grade *(76)*. Localization of the receptor is described within the membrane and cytoplasm of basal ECs in PIN, with a similar moderate-to-strong pattern of expression in the majority of PCA cells *(64)*. IHC analyses have also demonstrated c-erbB-3 expression in LNCaP, DU145, and PC-3 cells *(65)*, and an androgen-repressed cell line, ARCaP *(34)*. Expression of c-erbB-3 in human PCA cell lines (LNCaP, DU145, PC-3), as well as an immortalized, nontransformed cell line (MLC-SV40) and a xenograft (CWR22), has also been demonstrated by Western blot analyses, with the highest levels detected in the AR-positive cell line, LNCaP, and the xenograft, CWR22 *(8)*.

mRNA Expression and Gene Analysis

An analysis of the expression of mRNAs encoding a range of TKs, by RT-PCR, in benign and malignant human prostate tissues and cell lines, indicated expression of c-erbB-3 mRNA in hyperplastic prostate tissues, as well as 7/8 PCAs, a PCA xenograft (CWR22), and PCA cell lines (LNCaP, DU145, and PC-3) *(50)*. There have been no reports of mutations in, or amplification of, the c-*erb*B-3 gene in prostate malignancy.

c-erbB-4

Studies of the c-erbB-4 receptor are in their infancy. The protein shows greatest homology to c-erbB-3, is also a receptor for the NDFs, and appears to be important in cardiac muscle and neural development *(77)*. Analysis of c-erbB-4 mRNA and protein expression in human tumors has shown loss of expression in most tumors *(65,78)*, with a few tumors showing overexpression *(78,79)*, although the occurrence of gene amplification and/or rearrangement have not been examined. Analysis of prostate tissues for c-erbB-4, by IHC, has shown strong expression of the protein in basal and luminal ECs, but not the stroma, of benign tissues, with expression significantly less in PIN and PCA *(65)*. In the same study, PCA cell lines (LNCaP, DU145, and PC-3) were all negative for c-erbB-4. Another IHC study *(78)* showed moderate and weak immunoreactivity with adult human prostatic epithelium and smooth muscle cells, respectively, again with reduced expression in the majority (7/10) of PCAs analyzed, and overexpression in a small number (2/10). Analyses of c-erbB-4 mRNA expression, by RT-PCR, have failed to detect expression in PCA specimens, xenografts, or tumor cell lines *(8)*.

HB-EGF, BETACELLULIN, AND EPIREGULIN

Heparin-binding EGF-like growth factor (HB-EGF), a ligand for EGFR and c-erbB-4, is a potent smooth muscle cell GF. HB-EGF mRNA has been detected in adult pig prostate by RT-PCR, although Northern blot analysis was negative, suggesting that expression levels were low *(80)*. Expression was, however, detected by Northern blot analysis of adult human prostate tissues *(81)*. IHC of hyperplastic and malignant human prostate specimens showed staining for HB-EGF mostly in interstitial and vascular smooth muscle cells of the fibromuscular stroma, but no staining in normal glandular epithelium or carcinoma cells, and with no evidence of increased expression in malignant, compared with hyperplastic, specimens *(81)*. Analysis of LNCaP cells revealed low levels of HB-EGF mRNA (positive by RT-PCR, negative by Northern blot analysis); however, the ligand is mitogenic for these cells in culture, inducing phosphorylation of EGFR and c-erbB-3, and it has been suggested that HB-EGF may have a specific role in PCA as a stromal mediator of tumor cell growth *(81)*.

Betacellulin, a ligand for EGFR and c-erbB-4, is expressed predominantly in the pancreas and small intestine. Weak expression has been detected in the normal human prostate by Northern blot analysis *(82)*, but analysis of expression in malignant prostate tissues has not been reported.

Epiregulin is apparently a relatively low-affinity ligand for several of the type I GF receptors *(83)*. Expression of the mRNA for this ligand in human tissues has been described, predominantly in the placenta and peripheral blood leukocytes (by Northern blot analysis) *(84)*. High levels of expression have also been described in some carcinomas, but there have been no reports of analysis of prostate tumors.

NEUREGULINS

The neuregulins (NRGs, also known as NDFs or heregulins) are now known to be a family of three separate genes, NRG1, -2, and -3, which encode a number of alternatively spliced transcripts, most of which encode integral membrane proteins containing an extracellular EGF-like domain. A limited number of studies to date *(85,86)* suggest that neuregulins are both growth and differentiation factors, which are expressed in normal epithelia and in some cancers.

IHC analysis of human prostate specimens with mAbs against NRG1α and NRG1β isoforms *(65)* revealed strong expression in the stroma and in basal ECs, and moderate expression in luminal ECs of normal and hyperplastic tissues, with very low levels in PIN and PCA, and no detectable expression in PCA cell lines. Conversely, another IHC study *(76)*, using a polyclonal Ab against NRG1α, showed no detectable expression in hyperplastic prostate, but expression in the epithelium, but not stroma of approx 70% of PCAs. Western blot analysis of prostatic cell lines (LNCaP, DU145, PC-3, MLC-SV40) and a PCA xenograft (CWR22), revealed that only the nontransformed cell line, MLC-SV40, expressed NRG1 *(8)* and others *(72)* have also reported that NRG1 is not detected in LNCaP cells. Northern blot analyses have shown that NRG3 is highly expressed in normal brain, but undetectable in other tissues *(87)*. mRNA ISH on whole, paraffin-embedded mouse embryos and tissues showed a similar pattern, but prostate tissues were not specifically investigated *(87)*. NRG1 mRNA has been detected in PCA cell lines (LNCaP, DU145, and PC-3) by RT-PCR, but NRG1 protein was not detected in these cells by IHC *(65)*. Models of NRG function in prostate tumor cells have shown that addition of NRG1β to LNCaP cells in culture inhibits growth *(8,65)*, and induces epithelial differentiation *(8)*, although growth inhibitory effects were not seen in DU145 or PC-3 cells *(65)*.

SUMMARY

Gene amplification and concomitant gross overexpression of EGFR and c-erbB-2 are now well established, both in clinical studies and in laboratory experiments, to be one of the events causing the development of several types of cancer. These do not occur in PC. However, a subset of the receptors and ligands of this highly interactive family are expressed both in normal prostate and in intermediate stages, up to and including metastatic cancers. The relatively modest levels of expression require rigorous, careful, measurement to assess if meaningful changes occur in expression. Such studies will generate hypotheses that can be tested experimentally. In addition, it may be worth exploring the relative production of GFs by cancer cells and surrounding stromal cells, and any changes that occur in this balance during transformation. Such studies may possibly identify pathways that could be targeted by the new generation of signal transduction inhibitors currently being evaluated as treatments for other tumor types.

REFERENCES

1. Lalani E-L, Laniado ME, Abel PD. Molecular and cellular biology of prostate cancer. Cancer Metastasis Rev 1997;16:29–66.
2. Leong SS, Horoszewicz JS. In vitro models for human prostatic cancer: cell lines of human prostatic carcinoma. In: Webber MM, Sekely LI, eds. In Vitro Models for Cancer Research. Carcinoma of the Prostate and Testis, Vol. 5. CRC, Boca Raton, FL, 1988, pp. 127–137.
3. Webber MM, Bello D, Quader S. Immortalized and tumorigenic adult human prostate epithelial cell lines: characteristics and applications, part 2. Tumorigenic cell lines. Prostate 1997;30:58–64.
4. Davies P, Eaton CL, France TD, Phillips MEA. Growth factor receptors and oncogene expression in prostate cells. Am J Clin Oncol 1988;11(Suppl 2):S1–S7.
5. Eaton CL, Davies P, Phillips MEA. Growth factor involvement and oncogene expression in prostatic tumours. J Steroid Biochem 1988;30:341–345.
6. Prewett M, Rockwell P, Rockwell RF, Giorgio NA, Mendelsohn J, Scher HI, Goldstein NI. The biologic effects of C225, a chimeric monoclonal antibody to the EGFR, on human prostate carcinoma. J Immunother 1997;19:419–427.
7. Maddy SQ, Chisholm GD, Busuttil A, Habib FK. Epidermal growth factor receptors in human prostate cancer: correlation with histological differentiation of the tumour. Br J Cancer 1989;60:41–44.
8. Grasso AW, Duanzhi W, Miller CM, Rhim JS, Pretlow TG, Kung H-J. ErbB kinases and NDF signalling in human prostate cancer cells. Oncogene 1997;15:2705–2716.
9. Sherwood ER, Van Dongen JL, Wood CG, Liao S, Kozlowski JM, Lee C. Epidermal growth factor receptor activation in androgen-independent but not androgen-stimulated growth of human prostatic carcinoma cells. Br J Cancer 1998;77:855–861.
10. Bae VL, Jackson-Cook CK, Brothman AR, Maygarden SJ, Ware JL. Tumorigenicity of SV40 T antigen immortalized human prostate epithelial cells: association with decreased epidermal growth factor receptor (EGFR) expression. Int J Cancer 1994;58:721–729.
11. de Bellis A, Ghiandi P, Comerci A, Fiorelli G, Grappone C, Milani S, et al. Epidermal growth factor, epidermal growth factor receptor, and transforming growth factor-α in human hyperplastic prostate tissue: expression and cellular localization. J Clin Endocrinol Metab 1996;81:4148–4154.
12. Yang Y, Chisholm GD, Habib FK. Epidermal growth factor and transforming growth factor α concentrations in BPH and cancer of the prostate: their relationships with tissue androgen levels. Br J Cancer 1993;67:152–155.
13. Damjanov I, Mildner B, Knowles BB. Immunohistochemical localization of the epidermal growth factor receptor in normal human tissues. Lab Invest 1986;55:588–592.
14. Maddy SQ, Chisholm GD, Hawkins RA, Habib FK. Localization of epidermal growth factor receptors in the human prostate by biochemical and immunocytochemical methods. J Endocrinol 1987;112:147–153.
15. Mellon K, Thompson S, Charlton RG, Marsh C, Robinson M, Lane DP, et al. p53, c-erbB-2 and the epidermal growth factor receptor in the benign and malignant prostate. J Urol 1992;147:496–499.
16. Maygarden SJ, Strom S, Ware JL. Localization of epidermal growth factor receptor by immunohistochemical methods in human prostatic carcinoma, prostatic intraepithelial neoplasia, and benign hyperplasia. Arch Pathol Lab Med 1992;116:269–273.
17. Visakorpi T, Kallioniemi OP, Koivula T, Harvey J, Isola J. Expression of epidermal growth factor receptor and ERBB2 (HER-2/Neu) oncoprotein in prostatic carcinomas. Modern Pathol 1992;5:643–648.
18. Myers RB, Kudlow JE, Grizzle WE. Expression of transforming growth factor-α, epidermal growth factor and the epidermal growth factor receptor in adenocarcinoma of the prostate and benign prostatic hyperplasia. Modern Pathol 1993;6:733–737.
19. Robertson CN, Robertson KM, Herzberg AJ, Kerns B-JM, Dodge RK, Paulson DF. Differential immunoreactivity of transforming growth factor alpha in benign, dysplastic and malignant prostatic tissues. Surg Oncol 1994;3:237–242.

20. Glynne-Jones E, Goddard L, Harper ME. Comparative analysis of mRNA and protein expression for epidermal growth factor receptor and ligands relative to the proliferative index in human prostate tissue. Hum Pathol 1996;27:688–694.
21. Leav I, NcNeal JE, Ziar J, Alroy J. The localization of transforming growth factor-α and epidermal growth factor receptor in stromal and epithelial compartments of developing human prostate and hyperplastic, dysplastic, and carcinomatous lesions. Hum Pathol 1998;29:668–675.
22. Harper ME, Goddard L, Glynne-Jones E, Wilson DW, Price-Thomas M, Peeling WB, Griffiths K. An immunocytochemical analysis of TGFα expression in benign and malignant prostate tumors. Prostate 1993;23:9–23.
23. Turkeri LN, Sakr WA, Wykes SM, Grignon DJ, Pontes JE, Macoska JA. Comparative analysis of epidermal growth factor receptor gene expression and protein product in benign, premalignant, and malignant prostate tissue. Prostate 1994;25:199–205.
24. Yasui W, Ji Z-Q, Kuniyasu H, Ayhan A, Yokozaki H, Ito H, Tahara E. Expression of transforming growth factor alpha in human tissues: immunohistochemical study and Northern blot analysis. Virchows Archiv A Pathol Anat 1992;421:513–519.
25. Taylor TB, Ramsdell JS. Transforming growth factor-α and its receptor are expressed in the epithelium of the rat prostate gland. Endocrinology 1993;133:1306–1311.
26. Wu HH, Kawamata H, Kawai K, Lee C, Oyasu R. Immunohistochemical localization of epidermal growth factor and transforming growth factor alpha in the male rat accessory sex organs. J Urol 1993;150:990–993.
27. Banerjee S, Banerjee PP, Zirkin BR, Brown TR. Regional expression of transforming growth factor-α in rat ventral prostate during postnatal development, after androgen ablation, and after androgen replacement. Endocrinology 1998;139:3005–3013.
28. Poulsen SS, Nexo E, Olsen PS, Hess J, Kirkegaard P. Immunohistochemical localization of epidermal growth factor in rat and man. Biochemistry 1986;85:389–394.
29. Torring N, Jorgensen PE, Poulsen SS, Nexo E. Epidermal growth factor in the rat prostate: production, tissue content and molecular forms in the different prostatic lobes. Prostate 1998;35:35–42.
30. Ibrahim GK, Kerns B-JM, MacDonald JA, Ibrahim SN, Kinney RB, Humprey PA, Robertson CN. Differential immunoreactivity of epidermal growth factor receptor in benign, dysplastic and malignant prostatic tissues. J Urol 1993;149:170–173.
31. Fox SB, Persad RA, Coleman N, Day CA, Silcocks PB, Collins CC. Prognostic value of c-erbB-2 and epidermal growth factor receptor in stage A1 (T1a) prostatic adenocarcinoma. Br J Urol 1994;74:214–220.
32. Fowler JE, Lau JL, Ghosh L, Mills SE, Mounzer A. Epidermal growth factor and prostatic carcinoma: an immunohistochemical study. J Urol 1988;139:857–861.
33. Jones HE, Dutkowski CM, Barrow D, Harper ME, Wakeling AE, Nicholson RI. New EGF-R selective tyrosine kinase inhibitor reveals variable growth responses in prostate carcinoma cell lines PC-3 and DU-145. Int J Cancer 1997;71:1010–1018.
34. Zhau HYE, Chang S-M, Chen B-Q, Wang Y, Zhang H, Kao C, et al. Androgen-repressed phenotype in human prostate cancer. Proc Natl Acad Sci USA 1996;93:15,152–15,157.
35. Connolly JM, Rose DP. Secretion of epidermal growth factor and related polypeptides by the DU 145 human prostate cancer cell line. Prostate 1989;15:177–186.
36. Wilding G, Valverius E, Knabbe C, Gelmann EP. Role of transforming growth factor-alpha in human prostate cancer cell growth. Prostate 1989;15:1–12.
37. Connolly JM, Rose DP. Production of epidermal growth factor and transforming growth factor-alpha by the androgen-responsive LNCaP human prostate cancer cell line. Prostate 1990;16:209–218.
38. Hofer DR, Sherwood ER, Bromberg WD, Mendelsohn J, Lee C, Kozlowski JM. Autonomous growth of androgen-independent human prostatic carcinoma cells: role of transforming growth factor alpha. Cancer Res 1991;51:2780–2785.
39. Greene GF, Kitadai Y, Pettaway CA, von Eschenbach AC, Bucana CD, Fidler IJ. Correlation of metastasis-related gene expression with metastatic potential in human prostate carcinoma cells implanted in nude mice using an in situ messenger RNA hybridisation technique. Am J Pathol 1997;150:1571–1581.
40. Vaughan TJ, Pascall JC, James PS, Brown KD. Expression of epidermal growth factor and its mRNA in pig kidney, pancreas and other tissues. Biochem J 1991;279:315–318.
41. Kumar VL, Majumder PK, Murty OP, Kumar V. Detection of receptor transcripts for androgen, epidermal growth factor and basic fibroblast growth factor in human prostate postmortem. Int Urol Nephrol 1998;30:301–304.
42. Morris GL, Dodd JG. Epidermal growth factor receptor mRNA levels in human prostatic tumors and cell lines. J Urol 1990;143:1272–1274.

43. Ching KZ, Ramsey E, Pettigrew N, Cunha RD, Jason M, Dodd JG. Expression of mRNA for epidermal growth factor, transforming growth factor-alpha and their receptor in human prostate tissue and cell lines. Mol Cell Biochem 1993;126:151–158.

44. Thomson AA, Foster BA, Cunha GR. Analysis of growth factor and receptor mRNA levels during development of the rat seminal vesicle and prostate. Development 1997;124:2431–2439.

45. Haughney PC, Hayward SW, Dahiya R, Cunha GR. Species-specific detection of growth factor gene expression in developing murine prostatic tissue. Biol Reprod 1998;59:93–99.

46. Hayward SW, Haughney PC, Rosen MA, Greulich KM, Weier H-UG, Dahiya R, Cunha GR. Interactions between adult human prostatic epithelium and rat urogenital sinus mesenchyme in a tissue recombination model. Differentiation 1998;63:131–140.

47. Itoh N, Patel U, Skinner MK. Developmental and hormonal regulation of transforming growth factor-α and epidermal growth factor receptor gene expression in isolated prostatic epithelial and stromal cells. Endocrinology 1998;139:1369–1377.

48. Schwartz S, Caceres C, Morote J, de Torres I, Rodriguez-Vallejo JM, Gonzalez J, Reventos J. Overexpression of epidermal growth factor receptor and c-erbB2/neu but not of int-2 genes in benign prostatic hyperplasia by means of semi-quantitative PCR. Int J Cancer 1998;76:464–467.

49. Wainstein MA, He F, Robinson D, Kung HJ, Schwartz S, Giaconia JM, et al. CWR22: androgen-dependent xenograft model derived from a primary human prostatic carcinoma. Cancer Res 1994;54:6049–6052.

50. Robinson D, He F, Pretlow T, Kung H-J. A tyrosine kinase profile of prostate carcinoma. Proc Natl Acad Sci USA 1996;93:5958–5962.

51. Degeorges A, Hoffschir F, Cussenot O, Gauville C, Le Duc A, Dutrillaux B, Calvo F. Recurrent cytogenetic alterations of prostate carcinoma and amplification of c-myc or epidermal growth factor receptor in subclones of immortalized PNT1 human prostate epithelial cell line. Int J Cancer 1995;62:724–731.

52. Traish AM, Wotiz HH. Prostatic epidermal growth factor receptors and their regulation by androgens. Endocrinology 1987;121:1461–1467.

53. Hiramatsu M, Kashimata M, Minami N, Sato A, Murayama M, Minami N. Androgenic regulation of epidermal growth factor in the mouse ventral prostate. Biochem Int 1988;17:311–317.

54. St-Arnaud R, Poyet P, Walker P, Labrie F. Androgens modulate epidermal growth factor receptor levels in the rat ventral prostate. Mol Cell Endocrinol 1988;56:21–27.

55. Liu X-H, Wiley HS, Meikle AW. Androgens regulate proliferation of human prostate cancer cells in culture by increasing transforming growth factor-α (TGF-α) and epidermal growth factor (EGF)/TGF-α receptor. J Clin Endocrinol Metab 1993;77:1472–1478.

56. Brass AL, Barnard J, Patai BL, Salvi D, Rukstalis DB. Androgen upregulates epidermal growth factor receptor expression and binding affinity in PC3 cell lines expressing the human androgen receptor. Cancer Res 1995;55:3197–3203.

57. Jones HE, Eaton CL, Barrow D, Dutkowski CM, Gee JMW, Griffiths K. Comparative studies of the mitogenic effects of epidermal growth factor and transforming growth factor-α and the expression of various growth factors in neoplastic and non-neoplastic prostatic cell lines. Prostate 1997;30:219–231.

58. Lin MF, Clinton GM. The epidermal growth factor receptor from prostate cells is dephosphorylated by a prostate-specific phosphotyrosyl phosphatase. Mol Cell Biol 1988;8:5477–5485.

59. Kuhn EJ, Kurnot RA, Sesterhenn IA, Chang EH, Moul JW. Expression of the c-erbB-2 (HER-2/neu) oncoprotein in human prostatic carcinoma. J Urol 1993;150:1427–1433.

60. Sadasivan R, Morgan R, Jennings S, Austenfeld M, van Veldhuizen P, Stephens R, Noble M. Overexpression of HER-2/NEU may be an indicator of poor prognosis in prostate cancer. J Urol 1993;150:126–131.

61. Ware JL, Maygarden SJ, Koontz WW, Strom SC. Immunohistochemical detection of c-erbB-2 protein in human benign and neoplastic prostate. Hum Pathol 1991;22:254–258.

62. Zhau HE, Wan DS, Zhou J, Miller GJ, von Eschenbach AC. Expression of c-erbB-2/neu proto-oncogene in human prostatic cancer tissues and cell lines. Mol Carcinogen 1992;5:320–327.

63. Giri DK, Wadhwa SN, Upadhaya SN, Talwar GP. Expression of NEU/HER-2 in prostate tumours: and immunohistochemical study. Prostate 1993;23:329–336.

64. Myers RB, Srivastava S, Oelschlager DK, Grizzle WE. Expression of p160[erbB-3] and p185[erbB-2] in prostatic intraepithelial neoplasia and prostatic adenocarcinoma. J Natl Cancer Inst 1994;86:1140–1145.

65. Lyne JC, Melhem MF, Finley GG, Wen D, Liu N, Deng DH, Salup R. Tissue expression of neu differentiation factor/heregulin and its receptor complex in prostate cancer and its biologic effects on prostate cancer cells in vitro. Cancer J Sci Am 1997;3:21–30.

66. McCann A, Dervan PA, Johnston PA, Gullick WJ, Carney DN. c-erbB-2 oncoprotein expression in primary human tumors. Cancer 1990;65:88–92.

67. Meng T-C, Lin M-F. Tyrosine phosphorylation of c-erbB-2 is regulated by the cellular form of prostatic acid phosphatase in human prostate cancer cells. J Biol Chem 1998;273:22,096–22,104.

68. Latil A, Baron JC, Cussenot O, Fournier F, Boccon-Gibod L, Le Duc A, Lidereau R. Oncogene amplifications in early-stage human prostate carcinomas. Int J Cancer 1994;59:637,638.

69. Fournier G, Latil A, Amet Y, Abalain JH, Volant A, Mangin P, Floch HH, Lidereau R. Gene amplifications in advanced-stage human prostate cancer. Urol Res 1995;22:343–347.

70. Sikes RA, Chung LWK. Acquisition of a tumorigenic phenotype by a rat ventral prostate epithelial cell line expressing a transfected activated *neu* oncogene. Cancer Res 1992;52:3174–3181.

71. Marengo SR, Sikes RA, Anezinis P, Chang S-M, Chung LWK. Metastasis induced by overexpression of p185neu-T after orthotopic injection into a prostatic epithelial cell line (NbE). Mol Carcinogen 1997;19:165–175.

72. Qiu Y, Ravi L, Kung H-J. Requirement of ErbB2 for signalling by interleukin-6 in prostate carcinoma cells. Nature 1998;393:83–85.

73. Riethmacher D, Sonnenberg-Riethmacher E, Brinkmann V, Yamaai T, Lewin G.R, Birchmeier C. Severe neuropathies in mice with targeted mutations in the ErbB3 receptor. Nature 1997;389:725–730.

74. Gullick WJ. The c-erbB3/HER3 receptor in human cancer. Cancer Surveys 1997;27:339–349.

75. Poller DN, Spendlove I, Baker C, Church R, Ellis IO, Plowman GD, Mayer RJ. Production and characterization of a polyclonal antibody to the c-*erb*B-3 protein: examination of c-*erb*B-3 protein expression in adenocarcinomas. J Pathol 1992;168:275–280.

76. Leung HY, Weston J, Gullick WJ, Williams G. A potential autocrine loop between heregulin-alpha and erbB-3 receptor in human prostatic adenocarcinoma. Br J Urol 1997;79:212–216.

77. Gassmann M, Casagranda F, Orioli D, Simon H, Lai C, Klein R, Lemke G. Aberrant neural and cardiac development in mice lacking the ErbB4 neuregulin receptor. Nature 1995;378:390–394.

78. Srinivasan R, Poulsom R, Hurst HC, Gullick WJ. Expression of the c-erbB-4/HER4 protein and mRNA in normal human fetal and adult tissues and in a survey of nine solid tumour types. J Pathol 1998;185: 236–245.

79. Faksvag-Haugen DR, Akslen LA, Varhaug JE, Lillehaug JR. Expression of c-erbB-3 and c-erbB-4 proteins in papillary thyroid carcinomas. Cancer Res 1996;56:1184–1188.

80. Vaughan TJ, Pascall JC, Brown KD. Tissue distribution of mRNA for heparin-binding epidermal growth factor. Biochem J 1992;287:681–684.

81. Freeman MR, Paul S, Kaefer M, Ishikawa M, Adam RM, Renshaw AA, Elenius K, Klagsbrun M. Heparin-binding EGF-like growth factor in the human prostate: synthesis predominantly by interstitial and vascular smooth muscle cells and action as a carcinoma cell mitogen. J Cell Biochem 1998;68:328–338.

82. Seno M, Tada H, Kosaka M, Sasada R, Igarashi K, Shing Y, et al. Human betacellulin, a member of the EGF family dominantly expressed in pancreas and small intestine, is fully active in a monomeric form. Growth Factors 1996;13:1–11.

83. Shelly M, Pinkas-Kramarski R, Guarino BC, Waterman H, Wang L-M, Lyass L, et al. Epiregulin is a potent pan-erbB ligand that preferentially activates heterodimeric receptor complexes. J Biol Chem 1998;273:10,496–10,505.

84. Toyoda H, Komurasaki T, Uchida D, Morimoto S. Distribution of mRNA for human epiregulin, a differentially expressed member of the epidermal growth factor family. Biochem J 1997;326:69–75.

85. Salomon DS, Brandt R, Ciardiello F, Normanno N. Epidermal growth factor-related peptides and their receptors in human malignancies. Crit Rev Oncol/Hematol 1995;19:183–232.

86. Alroy I, Yarden Y. The ErbB signaling network in embryogenesis and oncogenesis: signal diversification through combinatorial ligand-receptor interactions. FEBS Lett 1997; 410:83–86.

87. Zhang D, Sliwkowski MX, Mark M, Frantz G, Akita R, Sun Y, et al. Neuregulin-3 (NRG3): A novel neural tissue-enriched protein that binds and activates ErbB4. Proc Natl Acad Sci USA 1997;94: 9562–9567.

15 Hormonal Manipulation of Prostate Cancer

Jeffrey M. Kamradt, MD,
and Kenneth J. Pienta, MD

Contents

INTRODUCTION

Prostate cancer (PC) is a hormonally responsive disease. Testosterone (T) is required for the development of early PC and the disease retains this dependence through most of its natural history. The reliance of most PC cells on T offers an opportunity for clinical intervention in patients with this disease. That is, if the level of T can be diminished, the prostate cancer should respond with a reduction in size, which should bring about an improvement in clinical symptoms. Hormonal manipulations of PC all share one ultimate goal: Decrease the physiologic effect of T.

The majority of a male's T production is from the Leydig cells of the testis, in response to leutinizing hormone (LH) released from the anterior pituitary (pit). This mechanism of production is regulated by a negative feedback mechanism. That is, increased levels of T suppress gonadotropin-releasing hormone (GnRH) release from the hypothalamus, with subsequent decreases in LH levels. However, approx 5–10% of T is produced from the conversion of adrenal androgens to T. Regardless of the site of production, T enters the PC cell and is converted to dihydrotestosterone (DHT), a more potent physiologic form. This conversion is mediated by the enzyme, 5α-reductase. DHT then binds the androgen receptor (AR), and this complex enters the nucleus, binds to androgen-responsive elements, and DNA transcription is effected.

The suppression of T can be accomplished through a variety of mechanisms (Fig. 1). T production can be curtailed through surgical orchiectomy or with the use on GnRH analogs. Likewise, a decrease in adrenal androgen synthesis (ketoconazole, aminoglutethimide

From: *Contemporary Endocrinology: Endocrine Oncology*
Edited by: S. P. Ethier © Humana Press Inc., Totowa, NJ

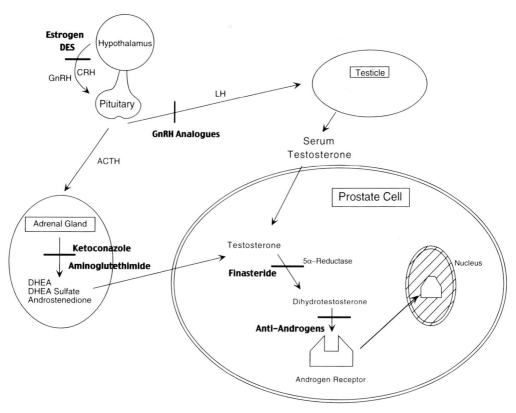

Fig. 1. Regulation of T and adrenal androgen synthesis. Sites of activity for clinically useful agents are represented by thick hash marks.

[AG]) will lead to a diminished overall T activity. Also, the conversion of T to DHT can be inhibited through clinical suppression (finasteride). The interaction of DHT with the AR can also be inhibited (nonsteroidal antiandrogens). Also, suppression of native GnRH levels can be accomplished by capitalizing on the inherent negative feedback mechanism between certain hormones and the hypothalamus (estrogen therapy, diethylstilbestrol [DES]).

All of the previously mentioned mechanisms have been used to treat PC. Traditionally, hormonal therapy had been reserved for patients with advanced disease. However, hormonal therapy has recently been investigated for patients with earlier stages of disease.

HORMONAL THERAPY OF ADVANCED DISEASE

Primary Therapy

ORCHIECTOMY

Huggins et al., in the early 1940s, demonstrated the responsiveness of PC to hormonal manipulation *(1–3)*. They examined the effect orchiectomy and estrogen therapy had on patients with advanced, symptomatic prostate cancer. They presented a case series of 21 patients treated with bilateral orchiectomy *(2)*. They described a clinical effect that was manifested by shrinkage of the primary prostate lesion, declines in serum phosphatases (an indication of the level of bone damage), improvement in performance status with weight gain, improved anemia, pain relief, decreased sexual desire with loss of erectile function, and hot flashes. These studies established orchiectomy as one the first effective and simple means of relieving the symptoms of advanced PC. These conclusions have not changed over the intervening 50 yr, and orchiectomy remains an effective and definitive treatment option. Serum T levels are reduced quickly and reliably. However, many patients are bothered by the stigma associated with surgical castration, and therefore orchiectomy remains an underutilized treatment option.

Estrogen Therapies

In one of his seminal papers on the treatment of PC, Huggins (3) proposed several possible explanations for the mechanism of action of estrogen: "a direct action on prostatic epithelium, inactivation of the androgens, depression of the gonadotropic agents of the anterior pituitary, and depression of interstitial cells of the testis." His suppositions were correct; the primary mode of action is feedback on the pit with suppression of gonadatropin secretion, with a subsequent decrease of Leydig cell T production (4). DES, the estrogen with the largest clinical experience, decreases serum LH levels and suppresses serum T. A dose of 5 mg/d DES has been shown to reliably suppress serum T into the castrate range; some patients on a dose of 1 mg/d broke through (5,6). Also, when given for longer than 3 yr, DES may be withdrawn with no increase in T levels, indicating irreversible damage to the Leydig cells (7).

In 1967, the Veterans Administration Cooperative Urological Cooperative Research Group (VACURG) published the results of their first study of PC in 2316 patients (8). Patients were divided into two clinical groups, those with disease confined to the prostate (stages 1 and 2) and those with more advanced disease (stages 3 and 4). Patients with stage 1 or 2 disease were randomized to receive prostatectomy with either adjuvant DES (5 mg/d) or placebo. Patients with stage 3 or 4 disease were randomized to one of four treatment groups: estrogen therapy alone (DES 5 mg/d), orchiectomy alone, orchiectomy plus estrogen therapy or placebo. If a patient progressed on a particular therapy, he was given further treatment, but was still considered in the analysis of results to belong to his original treatment groups (i.e., "intention to treat" analysis). The study demonstrated that not only was there no survival advantage for stage 1 and 2 patients who received DES, but that these patients actually had a poorer survival. For patients with stage 3 disease, the results were similar: Patients treated with DES had significantly lower survivals than those not receiving this therapy. For stage 4 patients, those receiving placebo had lower survival than estrogen-treated patients (although this did not reach statistical significance). When the cause of death was analyzed, it was found that patients receiving DES had a lower death rate from PC, but had a larger noncancer mortality that was mostly cardiovascular in etiology. The recommendations arising from this study were: delaying hormonal therapy does not compromise outcome; DES at 5 mg/d is associated with excessive cardiovascular mortality; and combination therapy with DES and orchiectomy offers no advantage over orchiectomy alone.

The second VACURG study enrolled 508 patients, and divided them into the same clinical categories as the earlier trial (9,10). Patients with stage 1 or 2 disease were randomized to either placebo or prostatectomy plus placebo. Results from this study did not find a benefit to prostatectomy, although the authors believed a limited interpretation was required because of small sample size and lack of thorough preoperative staging (11). Patients with stage 3 or 4 disease were randomized to one of the following treatment arms: placebo, 0.2 mg DES, 1.0 mg DES, or 5.0 mg DES. This study was stopped early because

Table 1
Results of VACURG Studies

1. 5.0 mg DES is associated with prohibitive cardiac morbidity.
2. The combination of DES and orchiectomy is no more effective than either treatment alone.
3. 1.0 mg DES is as effective at controling PC as higher doses.
4. 1.0 mg DES is associated with less toxicity than higher doses.
5. Other forms of estrogen therapy are no more effective than DES.
6. Young patients and those with high-grade disease are candidates for early hormonal therapy.

DES, diethylstilbestrol.

of excessive cardiac mortality of the 5 mg DES patients. The conclusions from VACURG II were that 1.0 mg DES is as effective as 5.0 mg at preventing progression of disease; treatment with 1.0 mg of DES, beginning at diagnosis, increased overall survival (OS) in stage 3 and 4 patients, compared to placebo; and immediate estrogen therapy for young patients and those with high-grade tumors is preferred *(12)*.

The third VACURG trial enrolled 1112 patients from 1969 to 1975. Patients with stage 3 or 4 disease were randomized to one of the following treatments: 2.5 mg Premarin, 30 mg Provera, 30 mg Provera plus 1.0 mg DES, or 1.0 mg DES alone. The DES-alone arm was more effective than the other treatments, leading the investigators to conclude that the other endocrine treatments were no better than 1.0 mg DES *(12)*. Subgroup analysis revealed that there was higher morbidity associated with the DES treatments in patients older than 75 yr.

The VACURG investigators published a summary of their findings of the three trials *(12)*. They drew six main conclusions from the studies (Table 1).

The VACURG studies established estrogen therapy as the chief treatment modality of advanced PC. The indications and toxicities were established in several large trials. This therapy was used for many years, until supplanted by the development of GnRH agonists.

GnRH ANALOGS

The toxicity of estrogen-based therapy and the psychological impact of castration led investigators to continue to look for alternative forms of hormonal therapy for PC. Out of this work came the GnRH analogs. When administered at a constant and sustained level, rather than the normal pulsatile manner of release of GnRH from the hypothalamus, these compounds initially stimulate LH and T release to about 1.5× basal levels within several days. This is followed by downregulation of the GnRH receptors in the pit, and castrate levels of T by 1 mo *(13)*. This initial increase in T can serve as a growth stimulus to the tumor, and produce a flare reaction, with an increase in disease-related symptoms. In one trial, 5–10% of patients treated with an GnRH analog alone exhibited worsening urinary symptoms *(14)*. This tumor flare can be prevented by pretreatment with an antiandrogen.

Several trials have compared GnRH analogs to the previous standard therapies of DES *(14–16)* or orchiectomy *(15,17–19)*, and found similar response rates and duration. The trials with DES all used 3.0 mg/d, in order to guarantee testicular suppression. Therapy with DES was associated with more adverse effects, such as gynecomastia, nausea, edema, and thromboembolism. Also, the time to respond was shorter in the GnRH analog patients. In the largest trial comparing treatment to DES, the GnRH analog, leuprolide, produced a response rate of 86%, and DES had a similar response rate of 85%; time to progression, as well as survival at 1 yr, were equivalent *(14)*. One trial of the GnRH analog, goserelin, vs orchiectomy found similar rates of objective response (82 vs 77%), median times to disease progression (52 vs 53 wk), and survival (119 vs 136 wks) *(17)*. Adverse effects were similar in both treatment arms, with the main toxicities being pain, hot flashes, and lower urinary tract symptoms.

The results of these and other trials established treatment with an GnRH as the favored treatment of advanced PC. Currently, the two most widely used agents are leuprolide and goserelin. Both come in 1-mo and multiple-month depot preparations.

ANTIANDROGEN MONOTHERAPY

Flutamide (FLU) and bicalutamide are the two most widely used nonsteroid antiandrogens in PC. They compete with androgens for binding to the AR, and, when bound, have an antagonistic action *(13)*. In peripheral tissues, they block cellular binding of androgens, and, centrally, they oppose the negative feedback of T on the pit. Both of these agents have been compared to standard hormonal therapy in randomized trials of patients with metastatic PC.

The Eastern Cooperative Oncology Groups conducted a trial comparing 3 mg/d DES and 750 mg/d FLU *(20)*. The overall response rates were similar between the two groups: 62% for DES and 50% for FLU ($P = 0.36$). However, DES produced both a significantly longer time to treatment failure (26 vs 10 mo) and longer OS than Flu (43 vs 29 mo). This improvement in survival was significant, despite increased cardiovascular and thrombotic toxicity in the DES-treated patients. The authors concluded that monotherapy with FLU was not as effective as traditional treatment with DES.

Bicalutamide has been studied in randomized trials in comparison to castration as initial treatment for either locally advanced or metastatic PC. In the first trial, 50 mg/d bicalutamide was compared to castration (surgical or medical) in a three-group, open, randomized design with over 1000 patients, conducted in the United States and Europe *(21)*. This study found that monotherapy with bicalutamide produces a shorter time to treatment failure, time to progression, and OS, compared with castration. Quality of life analysis revealed higher sexual function and interest in the bicalutamide arm. Also, overall health and well being was higher in the bicalutamide group at the first month; however, by 3–6 mo, this advantage reversed, with the castration patients scoring higher on quality of life scales. A second multinational study compared 150 mg/d bicalutamide with castration (medical or surgical) *(22)*. This study also demonstrated an advantage for castration, compared to bicalutamide, in patients with metastatic disease at time of entry into the study; the hazard ratio for time to death was 1.3 for bicalutamide to castration. The data for patients with locally advanced disease was immature, and further analysis was planned. Quality of life analysis once again demonstrated an advantage for bicalutamide monotherapy relative to castration.

It appears that monotherapy with either FLU or bicalutamide is associated with regression of disease in patients with advanced PC. However, this response is associated with a shortened time to disease progression and OS, compared to castration. Sexual interest and function are better-preserved with this treatment modality. Antiandrogen monotherapy could be considered as a second-best option for the treatment of advanced PC in patients for whom castration is unacceptable.

COMBINED ANDROGEN BLOCKADE

Combined androgen blockade, the combined suppression of both testicular and adrenal androgens, as a modality to treat advanced PC, reemerged as a therapeutic strategy secondary to the realization of two clinical observations and the development of readily available nonsteroidal antiandrogens. The first observation was that certain patients escaped the effects of testicular androgen suppression alone, as a result of T produced from the conversion of adrenal precursors. Second, elevated intracellular levels of DHT were demonstrated in a subset of patients, despite a castrate level of serum T while on therapy *(23)*. Combined androgen blockade had been attempted in the past, in a different manner: Patients who had failed bilateral orchiectomy underwent adrenalectomy *(24)*. Early experiences with this procedure were associated with substantial mortality *(25)*; however, modern postoperative endocrine management with cortisone allowed the procedure to be less dangerous, and a number of trials were performed, which demonstrated occasional responses. However, the development that initiated the modern use of combined androgen blockade was the discovery of oral nonsteroidal antiandrogens. These compounds are better tolerated than steroidal agents, because of decreased progestational adverse effects.

In an early phase II trial, the combination of a GnRH analog and an antiandrogen produced a response rate of 97% in a series of previously untreated patients *(26)*. This trial and other similar trials suffered from being nonrandomized studies of a small number of patients with varying definitions of response. A large, randomized, and blinded multicenter trial was performed to see if the initial encouraging results of combined androgen blockade could be verified *(27;* Table 2). This study enrolled 603 patients with previously untreated metastatic PC (stage D2), and randomly assigned them to treatment with the GnRH analog, leuprolide, and either the antiandrogen, FLU, or placebo. Patients treated with combined androgen blockade demonstrated both significantly longer time to progression (16.5 vs 13.9 mo; $P = 0.039$) and median survival time (35.6 vs 28.3 mo; $P = 0.035$). Subgroup analysis revealed this difference to be more evident for patients with minimal disease and good performance status. Also, symptomatic improvement for combined androgen blockade was greatest in the first 12 wk; however, this is when leuprolide monotherapy is known to produce a flare response (i.e., the exacerbation of symptoms secondary to the initial surge in LH seen with GnRH monotherapy). Other large studies have found an advantage to combined androgen blockade, compared to testicular suppression. A European trial of combined androgen blockade with goserelin and FLU vs orchiectomy in 320 patients found increased time to progression and a survival advantage for the combined androgen blockade arm *(28)*. Another trial of 457 patients found a prolonged time to disease progression in patients treated with orchiectomy and nilutamide, compared to those who received orchiectomy and placebo *(29)*. However, not all the trials of combined androgen blockade have found an advantage for the combined modality *(30)*. Most trials have enrolled small numbers of patients. A number of meta-analyses have been performed in an attempt to overcome this shortcoming. Unfortunately, some of these studies used only published patient results, instead of obtaining actual data from the original investigators. These studies have shown an advantage for combined androgen blockade *(31)*. A meta-analysis using original data from 22/25 published trials of combined androgen blockade did not find a survival advantage for combined therapy *(32)*.

A large trial, comparing treatment with orchiectomy and either placebo or flutamide in 1387 patients with advanced PC, failed to demonstrate any difference in progression-free survival (18.6 vs 20.4 mo; $P = 0.26$) or improvement in survival (29.9 vs 33.5; $P = 0.16$) between placebo and FLU-treated patients *(33)*. This trial was conducted by

Table 2
Select Trials of Combined Androgen Blockage

	Year	N	Treatment	Progression-free survival (mo)		Median survival (mo)		Benefit for CAB
				Signal-agent androgen blockade	Combined androgen blockade	Single-agent androgen blockade	Combined androgen blockade	
Crawford (27)	1989	603	Leuprolide vs leuprolide/flutamide	13.9	16.5	28.3	35.6	Yes
Denis (28)	1993	320	Orchiectomy vs goserelin/flutamide	11.5	17.75	27.1	34.4	Yes
Janknegt (29)	1993	457	Orchiectomy vs orchiectomy/nilutamide	14.9	20.8	29.8	37.1	Yes
Crawford (30)	1998	1387	Orchiectomy vs orchiectomy/flutamide	18.6	20.4	29.9	33.5	No
						5-yr survival (%)		
						Single-agent androgen blockade	Combined androgen blockade	
PCTCP meta-analysis	1995	5710	Single-agent vs combined androgen blockade			22.8	26.2	No

PCTCP, Prostate Cancer Trialists' Collaborative Group.

the same investigators who had originally demonstrated an advantage with combined androgen blockade *(27)*. An explanation for these differences may be the flare reaction that occurs with GnRH analog therapy, which can be blocked by treatment with an anti-androgen *(34)*. In the original study, the improved time to progression may be a result of the flare suppression by the antiandrogen. The more recent trial removes the confounding effect of flare, by using orchiectomy instead of medical castration. The authors conclude that the benefit of combined androgen blockade in advanced PC is negligible.

Currently, the authors' practice is to initially pretreat patients with an antiandrogen, when initiating therapy with a GnRH analog. The antiandrogen is then discontinued after 1–3 mo and the patient is maintained only on the GnRH agonist. Patients who choose orchiectomy for hormonal therapy do not require antiandrogen therapy.

INTERMITTENT ANDROGEN DEPRIVATION

Intermittent androgen deprivation entails the withdrawal of androgenic stimuli from a tumor until a maximum level of response is achieved, followed by the reintroduction of androgen. The early preclinical work was performed on the androgen-dependent Shionogi mouse mammary carcinoma *(35,36)*. Implanted tumors were allowed to progress to a predetermined size, at which time the host animals were castrated. Predictably, the tumors would regress by approx 90%, then progress in an androgen-independent fashion after approx 50 d. The strategy of cyclic androgen deprivation entailed taking tumor after regression and before secondary proliferation, and implanting into an intact mouse. The tumor cells would proliferate in the new host, and, when the predetermined size was achieved, the host would be castrated. The tumor would again regress, demonstrating androgen responsiveness. This cycle was repeated until the tumor failed to demonstrate androgen responsiveness, which occurred after the fifth transplantation. The mean time to progression to an androgen-independent phenotype was 150 d in the intermittent deprivation group and 50 d in the continuous androgen deprivation group. One possible theoretical explanation for this phenomena would be activation of previously androgen-repressed genes *(37)*. That is, the androgen-sensitive cells, through some undetermined mechanism, suppress the growth of the androgen independent clone.

A number of studies investigating intermittent androgen deprivation in a variety of clinical situations have been reported. Two trials *(38,39)* treated patients both with localized disease and with a biochemical failure (i.e., rising prostate specific antigen [PSA] values in asymptomatic patients), following initial radical therapy. These patients were initially treated with combined androgen blockade for 6–9 mo. Treatment was then withheld until the PSA value reached a predetermined value, at which point, treatment was reinitiated. It took between 3.5 and 5 mo to reach the initial PSA nadir. The average amount of time that patients were able to be off therapy was 38–45% of the observation period. While off treatment, patients reported less symptomatology associated with androgen blockade. It took about 8 wk for T to return to baseline levels following cessation of therapy. In a subset of 14 patients with metastatic PC, seven progressed during the study period; the median time to progression was 128 wk *(38)*. In a study of 16 patients with metastatic disease, 10 patients demonstrated a stable hormone response following the first cycle of androgen suppression, and were given a treatment holiday *(40)*. The duration of response ranged from 2 to 8 mo, and all patients demonstrated a response following reinitiation of therapy. Another trial examined the utility of intermittent androgen deprivation in patients with clinically localized PC *(41)*. This trial also found the mean nadir time to be 4 mo. Patients were able to spend 47% of time off study.

Intermittent androgen deprivation appears to be a viable, although still experimental, option for certain patients with PC. The optimal patient population for treatment with this modality has yet to be determined. Also, the durability and advantages of intermittent androgen deprivation, compared to traditional continuous therapy, are unknown. The Southwest Oncology Group is conducting a randomized trial of intermittent androgen deprivation vs continuous therapy. The results from this trial should answer some of these unresolved questions.

SEQUENTIAL ANDROGEN BLOCKADE

Combined androgen blockade with a GnRH agonist and an antiandrogen is accompanied by the physiological effects of a decreased level of T. These adverse effects include hot flashes, gynecomastia, impotence, breast tenderness, weight gain, and possible osteoporosis. The ideal treatment for PC would have the anticancer properties of combined androgen blockade, but not the adverse events. The combination of finasteride and an antiandrogen has been investigated as a mechanism to treat PC without suppressing T. Finasteride works by inhibiting 5α-reductase, the enzyme responsible for the intracellular conversion of T to DHT. Both finasteride and FLU have been examined as single agents in treatment of PC, and have been shown to be not as effective as castration *(20,42)*. Studies of the drug combination have included patients with locally advanced PC (disease that had spread outside of the prostate capsule or to regional lymph nodes without evidence of distant metastasis) or patients with an asymptomatic rise in PSA following either prostatectomy or radiation therapy (RT) *(43–48)*. An early study of 22 patients with locally advanced PC, treated with finasteride and FLU, revealed a PSA decrease from a pretreatment average of 43 ng/mL to a nadir of 2.8 ng/mL at 9 mo *(45)*. This was accompanied by an increase in T by 46% from baseline. The majority of men (86%) maintained sexual potency. A trial of 20 patients examined the sequential administration of FLU until a PSA nadir was achieved, followed by finasteride *(43)*. PSA declined 87% from baseline following single-agent FLU therapy and 94% from baseline with the combination of FLU and finasteride. The significance of this additional decrease in PSA is uncertain. A third trial examined initial treatment with finasteride until a PSA nadir, followed by FLU *(44)*. Treatment with single-agent finasteride did not lower PSA or suppress T; however, DHT decreased by 74%. The addition of FLU produced a 91% decrease in PSA, as well as a 56% increase in T, with no further change in DHT.

The combination of finasteride and FLU appears to have achieved the goal of anticancer activity, while maintaining circulating T and minimizing adverse effects. However, the PSA declines seen with this combined approach are not as complete as those of patients on combined androgen blockade. The significance of this is not known. Currently, trials comparing the combination of finasteride and FLU to combined androgen blockade are maturing. The appropriate patient population to receive this therapy is not yet determined. Most patients in the trials had locally advanced disease or asymptomatic rises in PSA following initial radical treatment. Other potential patient groups would include older patients who did not desire radical treatments for early disease and those with advanced disease who wished to remain potent. Further study will be required to resolve these unanswered issues.

EARLY VS DELAYED THERAPY

Because the initial demonstration by Huggins and Hodges *(1,2)* that PC is a hormonally responsive disease, investigators have been attempting to determine the optimal timing of this therapeutic intervention. Early retrospective studies in the 1940s and 1950s, comparing the survival rate between patients treated with androgen deprivation and historic controls, found a survival advantage to hormonal therapy *(49,50)*. These studies provided the scientific basis for early initiation of hormonal therapy in patients with advanced PC through the 1960s.

Several studies produced results that questioned the concept of early therapy for advanced PC. For example, the findings of the first VACURG study called into question the early initiation of hormonal therapy. Although the death rate from PC was less in those treated with early therapy, the increased cardiovascular mortality in the treatment group caused the overall death rates to be similar. The authors wrote, "What estrogen treatment wins from the cancer, it more than loses to other causes of death" *(8)*. The study also demonstrated that patients who had treatment deferred received relief of symptoms when treatment was initiated later. The investigators concluded that therapy should be withheld until symptoms warrant treatment.

Published in 1973, the second VACURG study, using lower doses of DES, confirmed these findings *(9)*. Finally, a proportional hazards model was used to compare the outcomes of 100 historic nonhormonal-treated patients treated between 1937 and 1940 with 100 patients who received hormonal therapy beginning in 1942 *(51)*. The most significant variable was found to be date of diagnosis, rather than administration of hormonal therapy. These findings combined to form the rationale for the decision to defer initiation of hormonal therapy until patients exhibit symptoms requiring treatment *(52)*.

Further analysis of the VACURG outcomes has produced the recommendation that patients with higher-grade tumors and young patients most likely would benefit from early initiation of hormonal therapy *(12)*. The authors offer the caveat that these studies were not designed to determine if early hormonal therapy is advantageous to a deferred approach. Several studies have examined the question of early hormonal therapy in the context of stage D1 PC (i.e., cancer that has spread to lymph nodes without evidence of distant disease) *(53–56)*. These small single-institution retrospective studies suggest an advantage for early therapy in this clinical situation. For example, in one study, the time to death from diagnosis was 90 mo in the delayed group and 150 mo in the immediate-treatment group *(53)*. These findings await validation in a more rigorous, controlled prospective manner.

The Medical Research Council conducted a trial specifically designed to assess the difference between early and delayed hormonal therapy (Table 3; *57*). This study enrolled 938 patients with either locally advanced or asymptomatic metastatic PC. Hormonal therapy was either orchiectomy or monotherapy with a GnRH agonist. Data was analyzed on an intention-to-treat basis. Overall, 11% of patients in the deferred arm died of unrelated causes before treatment was required; however, only 3.8% of patients younger than 70 yr at randomization did not require therapy. In the deferred arm, 91% of patients with metastatic, and 75% with locally advanced, disease required treatment. Notably, treatment was started as frequently for symptoms related to local progression as for the development of metastatic disease. Progression to metastatic disease or death from PC in the patients with localized disease was 37.5% in the early treatment arm and 59% in the deferred treatment arm ($P < 0.001$). Also, spinal cord compression, pathologic fractures, and extraskeletal metastases occurred more commonly in deferred treatment patients. Overall, 67% of the patient deaths during the study were attributed to PC. Considering all patients, more patients in the deferred treatment group died, relative to the

Table 3
Summary of Medical Research Council Study of Early vs Deferred Hormonal Therapy

	Localized disease (%)		Metastatic disease (%)	
	Early therapy	Delayed therapy	Early therapy	Delayed therapy
Progression to metastatic disease or death from PC	38[a]	59	NA	NA
Intervention for local progression	25[a]	58	NA	NA
Development of cord compression	1	1	4[b]	11
Overall survival	41[c]	30	14	14
Percent of deaths from PC	54[a]	70	76	80

NA, Not available.
[a] = p < 0.001.
[b] = p < 0.05.
[c] = p < 0.01 for immediate vs delayed treatment; otherwise, no significant difference.

immediate therapy arm from all causes (77.6 vs 69.9%, $P = 0.02$) and from PC (71 vs 62%, $P = 0.0001$). Analyzing the stratification variable of disease stage, the survival differences were not significant for patients with metastatic disease at randomization, but were significant for those with locally advanced disease, both in terms of OS and survival from PC.

Several key findings come out of this randomized trial. First, the majority of patients younger than 70 yr old in the deferred-treatment arm eventually required therapy. Also, the death rate from PC in this study was higher (67%) than that of the VACURG trial (41%) *(9)*, reflecting the improved life expectancy for men achieved since the two trials were undertaken. For patients with localized disease, there is improved survival associated with early initiation of hormonal therapy. This finding validates the results of the earlier trials in patients with stage D1 PC *(53–56)*. Although this does not hold true for patients with metastatic disease, there was a lower incidence of the catastrophic complications of cord compression and pathologic fracture.

The findings of this study provide support for the early initiation of hormonal therapy in patients with locally advanced or asymptomatic metastatic disease. This finding, however, may not apply to all patients with PC. For example, many patients present with a rising PSA following prostatectomy or RT. At this time, it is not known whether early hormonal treatment is beneficial for this group.

Secondary Therapy

ANTIANDROGEN WITHDRAWAL

Antiandrogen withdrawal syndrome refers to a significant decline in PSA, occurring in patients after withdrawal of antiandrogen therapy. The first patients demonstrating a sustained decline in PSA following the discontinuation of the antiandrogen FLU, were described in 1993 *(58)*. Three studies, including an extension of the original series, have looked at series of patients undergoing antiandrogen withdrawal (Table 4; *59–61*). These trials have evaluated 139 patients and demonstrated greater than 50% decline in baseline PSA in 15–33% of cases. The duration of this response varied from 3.5 to 5 mo. Besides declines in PSA, patients also experienced relief of symptoms. Five of eight

Table 4
Summary of Trials
Addressing Antiandrogen Withdrawal

Study	No. of patients	Response	Duration (mo)
Scher (59)	36	10/35 (29%)	5+
Figg (60)	21	7/21 (33%)	3.7+
Small (61)	82	12/82 (15%)	3.5

patients (62%) with symptoms in one trial experienced relief (61). In all three series, the median duration of FLU therapy was longer in the responders (range, 18–28 mo) than in the nonresponders (range, 12–18 mo).

The response to FLU withdrawal may be explained by the presence of functionally altered ARs, which recognized FLU as an androgen agonist, or by the unmasking of the agnostic property of FLU. An antiandrogen withdrawal response, with a decline in PSA, has also been reported with bicalutamide (62), megesterol acetate (63), and DES (64). It is recommended that, on disease progression during antiandrogen therapy, a trial of observation occur for any evidence of antiandrogen withdrawal effect, before the evaluation of any subsequent interventions are made.

ANTIADRENAL THERAPY

There are two distinct pathways of androgen production (13). The great majority of male androgens are produced by the testes. The remaining 5–10% are produced by the adrenal glands. Corticotrophin-releasing hormone from the hypothalamus signals the release of adrenocorticotrophic hormone from the pit gland. This in turn stimulates the release of adrenal androgens: androstenedione, dehydroepiandrosterone (DHEA) and DHEA sulfate. DHEA is then sequentially converted into T and DHT.

This adrenal source of androgen production is not suppressed by either orchiectomy or treatment with a GnRH agonist. In the past, adrenalectomy was used to treat patients with progressive disease, and produced occasional responses (24). Treatment with AG, which inhibits 20–24 desmolase, and therefore decreases adrenal androgen production, replaced the surgical approach. Besides suppressing adrenal androgen production, AG also decreases the synthesis of glucocorticoids and mineralocorticoids. Therefore, patients receiving therapy were also treated with hydrocortisone, to prevent clinical adrenal insufficiency. This concurrent use of hydrocortisone, which has demonstrated activity against hormone-refractory PC as a single agent, limits interpretation of the activity of AG (65). Early trials of the combination of AG and hydrocortisone, performed before the emergence of PSA monitoring of PC, demonstrated mild subjective therapeutic activity, with occasional objective responses (66–68).

Recently, studies have examined treatment of patients with hormone-refractory PC with AG, in relation to antiandrogen withdrawal. A trail of 29 patients, who progressed after initial combined hormonal therapy and treatment with suramin, were treated with simultaneous FLU withdrawal and initiation of AG, and demonstrated PSA declines of greater than 80% in 48% of patients (69). This response rate is greater than would be expected with antiandrogen withdrawal alone. Other investigators examined the role of FLU withdrawal in patients who were already receiving therapy, some with AG and hydrocortisone, and found significant PSA declines in greater than 70% of patients (70). It appears that some patients with hormone refractory PC will benefit from suppression of adrenal androgens. However, the exact relationship between treatment with AG and anti-androgen withdrawal needs further investigation.

Ketoconazole is an antifungal agent and imidazole that interferes with gonadal and adrenal androgen production, as well as the synthesis of cholesterol *(13)*. These effects are dose-dependent and reversible. Also, ketoconazole has demonstrated suppression of the growth of human PC cell lines in an in vitro clonogenic tumor assay *(71)*. This raises the possibility of a cytotoxic antitumor effect independent of hormonal suppression. In a trial conducted before both the routine use of PSA and antiandrogens, 14% of 36 patients with soft tissue disease experienced a partial response when treated with 1200 mg/d ketoconazole *(72)*. A trial of ketoconazole in 50 patients with progressive disease following antiandrogen withdrawal established a PSA response rate of 63% *(73)*. There was no difference in response rates between patients who exhibited a response to anti-androgen withdrawal (40%) and those who did not (65%). Although certain responses were more durable, the median response duration was 3.5 mo. A second trial examined simultaneous antiandrogen withdrawal and initiation of ketoconazole *(74)*. A PSA response rate of 55% was seen in 20 patients. However, the median duration of response was 8.5 mo. Further investigation into the optimal timing of antiandrogen withdrawal and treatment with ketoconazole is required.

HIGH-DOSE BICALUTAMIDE

Bicalutamide is a nonsteroidal antiandrogen used in combination therapy with medical castration for the treatment of advanced PC. The drug has been extensively investigated in a variety of clinical settings for the treatment of PC *(75)*. Bicalutamide differs from FLU, the first antiandrogen with wide clinical experience, in a number of ways. Bicalutamide's affinity for the AR is 4× greater than the active metabolite of FLU *(76)*. Also, a longer half-life allows once-daily dosing, and the drug is better-tolerated clinically with less-adverse events, leading to discontinuation of therapy. In the hormone-sensitive PC cell line, LNCaP, bicalutamide functions as an antagonist and FLU functions as an agonist *(77,78)*. These differences raise the possibility that crossresistance to antiandrogens may not be present in all patients with hormone-refractory PC.

Two trials have examined this question of crossresistance. Patients who had documented disease progression while on FLU were treated with bicalutamide. Investigators at Memorial Sloan-Kettering treated 51 patients with hormone refractory PC with high-dose single-agent bicalutamide (200 mg/d) *(79)*. These androgen-independent patients were divided into three categories: patients who had progressed after orchiectomy or monotherapy with a GnRH agonist, patients who had progressed after combined androgen blockade with FLU, and patients who had progressed after two or more hormonal therapies. Overall, 12 patients experienced a 50% or greater decline in PSA from pretreatment values (this degree of PSA decline has been associated with increased survival in patients treated with cytotoxic chemotherapy *[80]*). However, none of the 16 patients with soft tissue disease demonstrated a response in this parameter. None of the 12 patients who had received two or more prior hormonal therapies had a PSA decline. Fifteen percent (2/13) of patients who had failed orchiectomy or GnRH monotherapy, and 38% (10/26) of patients with prior exposure to FLU, had a PSA response. There was no difference in response rates in the FLU treatment group between patients who demonstrated a FLU withdrawal response and those who did not.

A second trial of high-dose bicalutamide found a difference in response rates between patients with prior FLU exposure and those without *(81)*. In this trial, 31 patients with hormone-refractory PC, who had failed orchiectomy or androgen blockade, received high-dose bicalutamide (150 mg/d). Seven patients (23%) demonstrated a PSA decline of greater than 50% from pretreatment values; six of these patients had been treated previously with FLU. Examining the data from the perspective of prior FLU therapy demonstrates this to be a significant variable in predicting response. Six/14 (43%) of patients with prior exposure to FLU experienced a response to high-dose bicalutamide. However, only 1/17 (6%) of patients with no prior FLU treatment demonstrated a response to high-dose bicalutamide.

Low-dose DES

DES has played a historic role as an initial treatment for advanced PC. However, the use of GnRH agonists has eclipsed DES as the primary endocrine treatment for PC. The tumor-inhibiting effects of DES have been attributed to the suppression of androgens via an estrogen-mediated mechanism. However, some patients with metastatic disease demonstrate disease regression without maximal suppression of plasma T *(52)*. Recent laboratory evidence demonstrates that DES has direct cytotoxic effects against PC cells, independent of its estrogen effect *(82)*. This effect was seen in both androgen-sensitive (LNCaP) and androgen-independent cell lines (DU145 and PC-3). Cells were incubated with DES at a concentration that is cytotoxic to one-half of the cells. Flow cytometry of the remaining androgen-insensitive cells demonstrated increased hypodiploid cell number, a decrease in G1- and S-phase fractions, and an accumulation of cells at the G2/M-phase. The microtubule apparatus of PC-3 cells appeared to remain intact when examined by immunohistochemistry. Androgen-sensitive cells revealed a reverse pattern; a lower percentage of hypodiploid cells and no accumulation of cells at the G2/M-phase of the cell cycle. These effects were affected by the presence of the estrogen receptor. Estrogen-receptor-positive and -negative cells responded similarly. These results demonstrate that DES has cytotoxic effects in PC that are independent of the estrogen receptor, and involve cell cycle arrest and apoptosis, but are independent of microtubule disruption.

DES has been investigated as a second-line hormonal therapy for patients with PC who have failed initial androgen blockade *(83)*. Twenty-one asymptomatic patients with rising PSA were enrolled in a phase II study of DES at a dose of 1 mg/d. The treatment was tolerated well, with the main side effect being nipple tenderness. Only one patient experienced a thrombotic event (a deep venous thrombosis) while on study. Nine patients (43%) experienced PSA decline of greater than 50% from pretreatment values. None of the patients had soft tissue lesions that could be assessed for response. Similar to the trend seen in metastatic breast cancer patients treated with hormonal therapy, the fewer the number of prior hormonal therapies, the more likely the patient was to respond to DES. Eight/13 patients (62%) who had failed only one prior hormonal manipulation demonstrated a PSA response; only 1/8 (13%) who had received two or more prior manipulations responded.

HORMONAL THERAPY OF EARLY DISEASE

Adjuvant GnRH Therapy with RT for Locally Advanced Disease

Patients with cancer that has spread outside of the prostate gland, but has not spread to a distant site, are no longer candidates for surgical resection. These patients with locally advanced disease may be treated with external beam RT, which has about a 25% OS, at 15 yr rate *(84)*. The subgroup of patients with local control, who do not demonstrate a local relapse, have substantially longer survival than those with local recurrence *(85)*. Hormonal therapy has been investigated as a means of improving the local control rate, and perhaps increasing survival in this group of patients.

A trial of 277 patients with locally advanced disease randomized patients to one of three treatment arms: orchiectomy alone, radiotherapy alone, or the combination of orchiectomy and RT *(86)*. This study found no differences between the three arms in terms of local recurrence. A Radiation Therapy Oncology Group (RTOG) study randomizing 471 patients to either combined androgen blockade with goserelin and FLU, beginning 2 mo prior to radiation and ending with RT, or observation, found an improvement in disease progression rates at 5 yr for the hormonally treated patients (71 vs 46%; $P < 0.001$) *(87)*. This study failed to detect a survival advantage for this particular hormonal regimen.

Another RTOG study evaluated adjuvant goserelin treatment added to standard RT *(88)*. This trial randomized 977 patients to RT followed by either immediate goserelin treatment (continued until disease progression) or observation with initiation of goserelin at the time of disease progression. Patients treated with adjuvant hormonal therapy at 5 yr had better local control (84 vs 71%; $P < 0.0001$), freedom from distant metastasis (83 vs 70%; $P < 0.001$), and disease-free survival (60 vs 44%; $P < 0.0001$). However, this improved disease control did not translate into improved survival; the survival rates at 5 yr for the adjuvant and observation groups were 75 and 71%, respectively. Subgroup analysis did demonstrate increased survival for those patients with a higher-grade tumor (Gleason 8–10).

A third trial randomized 415 patients with locally advanced disease to either RT alone or RT with immediate treatment with goserelin for 3 yr *(89)*. This trial confirmed the improved disease progression rate for patients treated with hormonal therapy in the RTOG study (85 vs 48%; $P < 0.001$). Most noteworthy, however, was an increase in OS seen at 5 yr for the patients who received goserelin (79 vs 62%; $P = 0.001$).

Based on the results of these randomized trials, the use of an adjuvant GnRH analog is becoming the standard of care for patients with locally advanced PC.

Neoadjuvant Hormonal Therapy Prior to Prostatectomy

With the growing awareness of the importance of PC screening, the number of patients being diagnosed with early PC is increasing. A large number of these cases are potentially curable with surgery. Involvement of the surgical margin at the time of resection is a risk factor for local recurrence, metastatic disease, and death from PC *(90)*. For example, 5-yr progression rates are about 50% for margin-positive disease and 20% for margin-negative disease *(90)*. Hormonal therapy (generally with GnRH agonist monotherapy) prior to surgery (i.e., neoadjuvant) has been considered as a means of decreasing both tumor size and the incidence of involvement of the margins.

Several nonrandomized phase II trials have shown a decrease in prostate volume, PSA values, and the rate of positive margins in patients treated with neoadjuvant hormonal therapy. To follow-up these promising results, several randomized phase III trials of neoadjuvant hormonal therapy have been performed *(91–93)*. These trials have consistently demonstrated a decreased rate of positive-margin disease. However, involvement of both the seminal vesicles and regional lymph nodes have not been decreased with neoadjuvant therapy. Most importantly, longer follow-up from these and other trials has failed to demonstrate a difference in disease progression rates *(94)*. Also, neoadjuvant therapy can induce a fibrous reaction and increase the complexity of the surgery.

Neoadjuvant therapy, although able to decrease the rate of surgical margin involvement, has not demonstrated any benefit in terms of slowing disease progression.

CONCLUSION

The role for hormonal manipulation of PC is expanding. Treatment plans for localized disease, which rely on some form of hormonal suppression, are emerging as options for patients previously not considered candidates for hormonal therapy. Also, new strategies in the hormonal treatment of advanced PC are being explored. These approaches may increase the hormonally responsive time and minimize the toxicity of treatment for patients with advanced PC.

REFERENCES

1. Huggins C, Hodges C. Studies on prostatic cancer. I: The effect of castration, of estrogen and of androgen injection on serum phosphotases in metastatic carcinoma of the prostate. Cancer Res 1941;1:293–297.
2. Huggins C, Stevens RE, Hodges C. Studies on prostatic cancer. II: The effects of castration on advanced carcinoma of the prostate gland. Arch Surg 1941;43:209–223.
3. Huggins C, Scott WW, Hodges CV. Studies on prostatic cancer III. The effects of fever, of deoxycorticosterone and of estrogen on clinical patients with metastatic carcinoma of the prostate. J Urol 1941;46:997–1001.
4. Cox RL, Crawford ED. Estrogens in the treatment of prostate cancer. J Urol 1995;154:1991–1998.
5. Kent JR, Bischoff AJ, Arduino LJ, et al. Estrogen dosage and suppression of testosterone levels in patients with prostatic carcinoma. J Urol 1973;109:858–862.
6. Beck PH, McAninch JW, Goebel JL, Stutzman RE. Plasma testosterone in patients receiving diethylstilbestrol. Urology 1978;11:157–160.
7. Baker HW, Burger HG, DeKretser DM, Hudson B, Straffon WG. Effects of synthetic oral oestrogens in normal men and patients with prostatic carcinoma: lack of gonadotrophin suppression by chlorotrianisene. Clin Endocrinol 1973;2:297–301.
8. The Veteran's Administration Cooperative Urological Research Group. Carcinoma of the prostate: treatment comparisons. J Urol 1967;98:516–522.
9. Byar DP. Veterans Administration Cooperative Urological Research Group's studies of cancer of the prostate. Cancer 1973;32:1126–1130.
10. Bailar III JC, Byar DP. Veterans Administration Cooperative Urological Research Group. Estrogen treatment for cancer of the prostate: early results with three doses of diethylstilbestrol and placebo. Cancer 1970;26:257–261.
11. Byar DP, Corle DK. Veterans Administration Cooperative Urological Research Group randomized trial of radical prostatectomy for stages I and II prostate cancer. Urology 1981;17(Suppl):7–11.
12. Byar DP, Corle DK. Hormone therapy for prostate cancer: results of the Veteran's Administration Cooperative Urological Research Group Studies. Natl Cancer Inst Monogr 1988;7:165–170.
13. Galbraith SM, Duchesne GM. Androgens and prostate cancer: biology, pathology and hormonal therapy. Eur J Cancer 1997;33:545–554.
14. Leuprolide Study Group. Leuprolide versus diethylstilbestrol for metastatic prostate cancer. N Engl J Med 1984;311:1281–1286.
15. Peeling WB. Phase III studies to compare goserelin (Zoladex) with orchiectomy and with diethylstilbestrol in treatment of prostatic carcinoma. Urology 1989;33(Suppl 5):45–52.
16. Waymont B, Lynch TH, Dunn JA, et al. Phase III randomised study of Zoladex versus stilbestrol in the treatment of advanced prostate cancer. Br J Urol 1992;69:614–620.
17. Vogelzang NJ, Chodak GW, Soloway MS, et al. Goserelin versus orchiectomy in the treatment of advanced prostate cancer: final results of a randomized trial. Urology 1995;46:220–226.
18. Kaisary AV, Tyrrell CJ, Peeling WB, Griffiths K. Comparison of LHRH analogue (Zoladex) with orchiectomy in patients with metastatic prostatic carcinoma. Br J Urol 1991;67:502–508.

19. Parmar H, Edwards L, Phillips RH, Allen L, Lightman SL. Orchiectomy versus long acting D-Trp-6-LHRH in advanced prostate cancer. Br J Urol 1987;59:248–254.

20. Chang A, Yeap B, Davis T, et al. Double-blind, randomized study of primary hormonal treatment of stage D2 prostate carcinoma: flutamide versus diethylstilbesterol. J Clin Oncol 1996;14:2250–2257.

21. Bales GT, Chodak GW. A controlled trial of bicalutamide versus castration in patients with advanced prostate cancer. Urology 1996;47(Suppl 1A):38–43.

22. Tyrrell CJ, Kaisary AV, Iversen P, et al. A randomised comparison of 'Casodex' (bicalutamide) 150 mg monotherapy versus castration in the treatment of metastatic and locally advanced prostate cancer. Eur Urol 1998;33:447–456.

23. Geller J, de la Vega DJ, Albert JD, Nachtsheim DA. Tissue dihydrotestosterone levels and clinical response to hormonal therapy in patients with advanced prostate cancer. J Clin Endocrinol Metab 1984;58:36–40.

24. Brendler H. Adrenalectomy and hypophysectomy for prostatic cancer. Urology 1973;2:99–102.

25. Huggins C, Scot WW. Bilateral adrenalectomy in prostatic cancer. Ann Surg 1945;122:1031–1041.

26. Labrie F, Dupont A, Belanger A, et al. New approach in the treatment of prostate cancer: complete instead of partial withdrawal of androgens. Prostate 1983;4:579–594.

27. Crawford ED, Eisenberger MA, McLeod DG, et al. A controlled trial of leuprolide with and without flutamide in prostatic carcinoma. N Engl J Med 1989;321:419–424.

28. Denis L, Whelan P, Carneiro de Moura JL, et al. Goserelin acetate and flutamide versus bilateral orchiectomy: a phase III EORTC trial (30853). Urology 1993;42:119–130.

29. Janknegt RA, Abbou CC, Bartoletti R, et al. Orchiectomy and nilutamide or placebo as treatment of metastatic prostatic cancer in a multinational double–blind randomized trial. J Urol 1993;149:77–83.

30. Denis L, Murphy GP. Overview of phase III trials on combined androgen treatment in patients with metastatic prostate cancer. Cancer 1993;72(Suppl):3888–3895.

31. Caubet J, Tosteson TD, Dong EW, et al. Maximum androgen blockade in advanced prostate cancer: a meta-analysis of published randomized controlled trials using nonsteroidal antiandrogens. Urology 1997;49:71–78.

32. Prostate Cancer Trialists' Collaborative Group. Maximum androgen blockade in advanced prostate cancer: an overview of 22 randomised trials with 3283 deaths in 5710 patients. Lancet 1995;346:265–269.

33. Eisenberger MA, Blumenstein BA, Crawford ED, et al. Bilateral Orchiectomy with or without flutamide for metastatic prostate cancer. N Engl J Med 1998;339:1036–1042.

34. Kuhn J, Billebaud T, Navrath H, et al. Prevention of the transient adverse effects of a gonadatropin-releasing hormone analogue (buserelin) in metastatic prostate carcinoma by administration of an anti-androgen (nilutamide). N Engl J Med 1989;321:413–418.

35. Akakura K, Bruchovsky N, Goldenberg SL, Rennie PS, Buckley AR, Sullivan LD. Effects of intermittent androgen suppression on androgen-independent tumors. Cancer 1993;71:2782–2790.

36. Bruchovsky N, Rennie PS, Goldman AJ, Goldenberg SL, To M, Lawson D. Effects of androgen withdrawal on the stem cell composition of the Shionogi carcinoma. Cancer Res 1990;50:2275–2282.

37. Tunn UW. Intermittent endocrine therapy of prostate cancer. Eur Urol 1996;30(Suppl 1):22–25.

38. Goldenberg SL, Bruchovsky N, Gleave ME, Sullivan LD, Akakura K. Intermittent androgen suppression in the treatment of prostate cancer: a preliminary report. Urology 1995;45:839–844.

39. Higano CS, Ellis W, Russell K, Lange PH. Intermittent androgen suppression with leuprolide and flutamide for prostate cancer: a pilot study. Urology 1996;48:800–804.

40. Horwich A, Huddart RA, Gadd J, et al. A pilot study of intermittent androgen deprivation in advanced prostate cancer. Br J Urol 1998;81:96–99.

41. Grossfeld GD, Small EJ, Carroll PR. Intermittent androgen deprivation for clinically localized prostate cancer: initial experience. Urology 1998;51:137–144.

42. Presti JC, Fair WR, Andriole G, et al. Multicenter, randomized, double-blind, placebo controlled study to investigate the effect of finasteride (MK-906) on stage D prostate cancer. J Urol 1992;148:1201–1204.

43. Brufsky A, Fontaine-Roth P, Berlane K, et al. Finasteride and flutamide as potency-sparing androgen-ablative therapy for advanced adenocarcinoma of the prostate. Urology 1997;49:913–920.

44. Ornstein DK, Rao GS, Johnson B, Charlton ET, Andriole GL. Combined finasteride and flutamide therapy in men with advanced prostate cancer. Urology 1996;48:901–905.

45. Fleshner NE, Trachtenberg J. Combination finasteride and flutamide in advanced carcinoma of the prostate: effective therapy with minimal side effects. J Urol 1995;154:1642–1646.

46. Fleshner NE, Fair WR. Anti-androgenic effects of combination finasteride plus flutamide in patients with prostatic carcinoma. Br J Urol 1996;78:907–910.

47. Fleshner NE, Trachtenberg J. Treatment of advanced prostate cancer with the combination of finasteride plus flutamide: early results. Eur Urol 1993;24(Suppl 2):106–112.
48. Staiman VR, Lowe FC. Tamoxifen for flutamide/finasteride induced gynecomastia. Urology 1997;50: 929–933.
49. Vest SA, Frazier TH. Survival following castration for prostatic cancer. J Urol 1946;56:97–102.
50. Nesbit RM, Baum WC. Endocrine control of prostatic carcinoma: clinical and statistical survey of 1,818 cases. J Am Med Assoc 1950;143:1317–1320.
51. Lepor H, Ross A, Walsh PC. The influence of hormonal therapy on survival of men with advanced prostatic cancer. J Urol 1982;128:335–340.
52. Scott WW, Menon M, Walsh PC. Hormonal therapy of prostatic cancer. Cancer 1980;45:1929–1936.
53. Kramolowsky EV. The value of testosterone deprivation in stage D1 carcinoma of the prostate. J Urol 1988;139:1242–1244.
54. van Aubel OGJM, Hoekstra WJ, Schroder FH. Early orchiectomy for patients with stage D1 prostatic carcinoma. J Urol 1985;134:292–294.
55. Zincke H. Extended experience with surgical treatment of stage D1 adenocarcinoma of prostate: significant influences of immediate adjuvant hormonal treatment (orchiectomy) on outcome. Urology 1989; 33(Suppl 5):27–36.
56. Myers RP, Zincke H, Fleming TR, Farrow GM, Furlow WL, Utz DC. Hormonal treatment at time of radical retropubic prostatectomy for stage D1 prostate cancer. J Urol 1983;130:99–101.
57. Medical Research Council Prostate Cancer Working Party Investigators Group. Immediate versus deferred treatment for advanced prostatic cancer: initial results of the Medical Research Council trial. Br J Urol 1997;79:235–246.
58. Kelly WK, Scher HI. Prostate specific antigen decline after antiandrogen withdrawal: the flutamide withdrawal syndrome. J Urol 1993;149:607–609.
59. Scher HI, Kelly WK. Flutamide withdrawal syndrome: its impact on clinical trials in hormone-refractory prostate cancer. J Clin Oncol 1993;11:1566–1572.
60. Figg WD, Sartor O, Cooper MR, et al. Prostate specific antigen decline following the discontinuation of flutamide in patients with stage D2 prostate cancer. Am J Med 1995;98:412–415.
61. Small EJ, Srinivas S. The antiandrogen withdrawal syndrome. Experience in a large cohort of unselected patients with advanced prostate cancer. Cancer 1995;76:1428–1434.
62. Small EJ, Carroll PR. Prostate-specific antigen decline after Casodex withdrawal: evidence for an antiandrogen withdrawal syndrome. Urology 1994;43:408–410.
63. Dawson NA, McLeod DG. Dramatic prostate specific antigen decrease in response to discontinuation of megesterol acetate in advanced prostate cancer: expansion of the antiandrogen withdrawal syndrome. J Urol 1995;153:1946–1949.
64. Bissada NK, Kaczmarek AT. Complete remission of hormone refractory adenocarcinoma of the prostate in response to withdrawal of diethylstilbestrol. J Urol 1995;153:1944,1945.
65. Kelly WK, Curley T, Leibretz C, Dnistrian A, Schwartz M, Scher HI. Prospective evaluation of hydrocortisone and suramin in patients with androgen-independent prostate cancer. J Clin Oncol 1995;13:2208–2213.
66. Drago JR, Santen RJ, Lipton A, et al. Clinical effect of aminoglutethimide, medical adrenalectomy, in treatment of 43 patients with advanced prostatic carcinoma. Cancer 1984;53:1447–1450.
67. Elomaa I, Taube T, Blomqvist C, Rissanen P, Rannikko S, Alfthan O. Aminoglutethimide for advanced prostatic cancer resistant to conventional hormonal therapy. Eur Urol 1988;14:104–106.
68. Chang AYC, Bennett JM, Pandya KJ, Asbury R, McCune C. A study of aminoglutethimide and hydrocortisone in patients with advanced and refractory prostate carcinoma. Am J Clin Oncol 1989;12:358–360.
69. Sartor O, Cooper M, Weinberger M, et al. Surprising activity of flutamide withdrawal, when combined with aminoglutethimide in treatment of "hormone refractory" prostate cancer. J Natl Cancer Inst 1994;86: 222–227.
70. Dupont A, Gomez J, Cusan L, Koutsiliers M, Labrie F. Response to flutamide withdrawal in advanced prostate cancer in progression under combination therapy. J Urol 1993;150:908–913.
71. Eichenberger T, Trachtenberg J, Toor P, Keating A. Ketoconazole: a possible direct cytotoxic effects on prostate carcinoma cells. J Urol 1989;141:190–191.
72. Trump DL, Havlin KH, Messing EM, Cummings KB, Lange PH, Jordan VC. High-dose ketoconazole in advanced hormone-refractory prostate cancer: endocrinologic and clinical effects. J Clin Oncol 1989; 7:1093–1098.
73. Small EJ, Baron AD, Fippin L, Apodaca D. Ketoconazole retains activity in advanced prostate cancer patients with progression despite flutamide withdrawal. J Urol 1997;157:1204–1207.

74. Small EJ, Baron A, Bok R. Simultaneous antiandrogen withdrawal and treatment with ketoconazole and hydrocortisone in patients with advanced prostate carcinoma. Cancer 1997;80:1755–1759.

75. Kolvenberg GJCM, Blackledge GRP, Gotting-Smith K. Bicalutamide (Casodex) in the treatment of prostate cancer: history of clinical development. Prostate 1998;34:61–72.

76. Furr BJA. Casodex: preclinical studies. Eur Urol 1990;18(Suppl 3):22–25.

77. Figg WD, McNall NA, Reed E, et al. The in vitro response of four antisteroid receptor agents on the hormone responsive prostate cancer cell line LNCaP. Oncol Rep 1995;2:295–298.

78. Wilding G, Chen M, Gelman EP. Aberrant response in vitro of hormone responsive prostate cancer cells to anti-androgens. Prostate 1989;14:103–115.

79. Scher HI, Liebertz C, Kelly WK, et al. Bicalutamide for advanced prostate cancer: the natural versus treated history of disease. J Clin Oncol 1997;15:2928–2938.

80. Smith DC, Dunn RL, Strawderman MS, Pienta KJ. Change in serum prostate-specific antigen as a marker of response to cytotoxic therapy for hormone refractory prostate cancer. J Clin Oncol 1998;16: 1835–1843.

81. Joyce R, Fenton MA, Rose P, et al. High dose bicalutamide for androgen independent prostate cancer: effect of prior hormonal therapy. J Urol 1998;159:149–153.

82. Robertson CN, Roberson KM, Padilla GM, et al. Induction of apoptosis by diethylstilbestrol in hormone-insensitive prostate cancer cells. J Natl Cancer Inst 1996;88:908–917.

83. Smith DC, Redman BG, Flaherty LE, Li L, Strawderman M, Pienta KJ. Phase II trial of oral diethylstilbesterol as a second line hormonal agent in advanced prostate cancer. Urology 1998;52:257–260.

84. Hanks GE, Corn BW, Lee WR, Hunt M, Hanlon A, Schultheiss TE. External beam irradiation of prostate cancer: conformal treatment techniques and outcomes for the 1990s. Cancer 1995;75:1972–1977.

85. Leibel SA, Fuks Z, Zelefsky MJ, Whitmore WF. The effects of local and regional treatment on the metastatic outcome in prostatic carcinoma with pelvic lymph node involvement. Int J Radiat Oncol Biol Phys 1994;28:7–16.

86. Fellows GJ, Clark PB, Beynon LL, et al. Treatment of advanced localised prostatic cancer by orchiectomy, radiotherapy or combined treatment: a Medical Research Council study. Br J Urol 1992;70:304–309.

87. Pilepich MV, Suase WT, Shipley WU, et al. Androgen deprivation with radiation therapy compared with radiation therapy alone for locally advanced prostatic carcinoma: a randomized comparative trial of the Radiation Therapy Oncology Group. Urology 1995;45:616–623.

88. Pilepich MV, Caplan R, Byhardt RW, et al. Phase III trial of androgen suppression using goserelin in unfavorable-prognosis carcinoma of the prostate treated with definitive radiotherapy: report of Radiation Therapy Oncology Group protocol 85–31. J Clin Oncol 1997;15:1013–1021.

89. Bolla M, Gonzalez D, Warde P, et al. Improved survival in patients with locally advanced prostate cancer treated with radiotherapy and goserelin. N Engl J Med 1997;337:295–300.

90. Walsh PC, Partin AW, Epstein JI. Cancer control and quality of life following anatomical radical prostatectomy: results at ten years. J Urol 1994;152:1831–1836.

91. Soloway MS, Sharifi R, Wajsman Z, et al. Randomized prospective study comparing radical prostatectomy alone versus radical prostatectomy preceded by androgen blockade in clinical stage B2 (T2bNxM0) prostate cancer. J Urol 1995;154:424–428.

92. Van Poppel H, de Ridder D, Elgamal AA, et al. Neoadjuvant hormonal therapy before radical prostatectomy decreases the number of positive surgical margins in stage T2 prostate cancer: interim results of a prospective randomized trial. J Urol 1995;154:429–434.

93. Labrie F, Cusan L, Gomez JL, et al. Downstaging of early stage prostate cancer before radical prostatectomy: the first randomized trial of neoadjuvant combination therapy with flutamide and a leutinizing hormone-releasing hormone agonist. Urology 1994;44:29–37.

94. Wieder JA, Soloway MS. Incidence, etiology, location, prevention and treatment of positive surgical margins after radical prostatectomy for prostate cancer. J Urol 1998;160:299–315.

16 Endocrinology of Epithelial Ovarian Cancer

Vicki V. Baker, MD

CONTENTS

INTRODUCTION

Epithelial ovarian carcinoma occurs as a consequence of multiple genetic mutations of the ovarian surface epithelial cell (EC). The vast majority of these cases (>90%) are sporadic rather than familial. Although the pathogenesis of epithelial ovarian cancer (OC) has not been fully defined, a growing body of evidence indicates that endocrinologic factors exert significant influences on both the development and the progression of this disease.

OVARIAN SURFACE EC

The ovarian surface epithelium (OSE) is a single, focally stratified layer of modified peritoneal cells that is separated from the underlying ovarian stroma by a distinct basement membrane *(1)*. The ovarian surface EC layer is contiguous with the mesothelial cell layer of the peritoneal cavity, but these cell populations can be differentiated on the basis of biochemical and functional differences *(2,3)*.

Histochemical studies have revealed the presence of glycogen and mucopolysaccharides within the cells that cover the surface of the ovary *(1,4)*. These cells weakly express E-cadherin and CA-125 *(5-7)*. In addition, cellular membrane receptors are present for estrogen and gonadotropins (Gns) *(8,9)*. Ovarian surface ECs also exhibit 17-β-hydroxy-steroid dehydrogenase activity *(4)*.

From: *Contemporary Endocrinology: Endocrine Oncology*
Edited by: S. P. Ethier © Humana Press Inc., Totowa, NJ

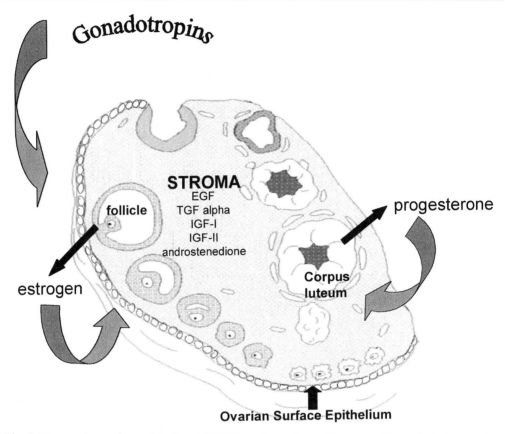

Fig. 1. The ovarian surface epithelium (OSE) lines the surface of the ovary. The underlying ovarian stroma and germ cell compartment, consisting of developing follicles and the corpus luteum, provide the OSE with exposure to a steroid hormones and GFs.

Unlike the peritoneal mesothelium, the EC layer of the ovary (e.g., the ovarian mesothelium) exhibits a much higher incidence of malignant transformation. Extraovarian primary papillary peritoneal carcinoma accounts for only about 10% of cases presumed to be of ovarian origin, based upon intraoperative findings (10). Although primary OC and extraovarian papillary peritoneal cancer can be differentiated pathologically, there are few, if any, differences in the epidemiology of these diseases (11). The proximity of the ovarian mesothelium to the underlying stroma provides a unique microenvironment for intercellular interactions (12). By virtue of this anatomic relationship, the OSE is subject to the effects of steroid hormones and growth factors produced by the stroma and germ cell compartment of the ovary (Fig. 1).

OVULATION

Epidemiologic studies have identified ovulation as a particularly important risk factor for the development of epithelial OC. Factors associated with uninterrupted ovulation (nulliparity) and a greater number of lifetime ovulatory cycles (early age at menarche and late age at menopause) are associated with an increased risk of OC. Conversely, factors that decrease the lifetime number of ovulatory events are associated with a decreased life-

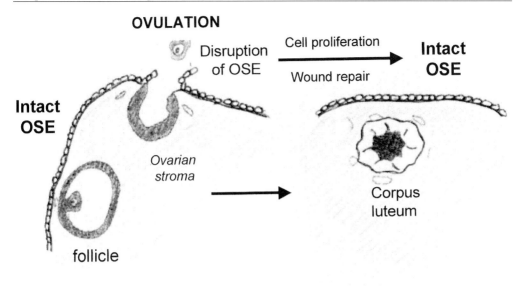

Fig. 2. During ovulation, extrusion of the ovum through the overlying OSE results in a surface epithelial defect. Repair of this defect or wound requires cellular proliferation, and introduces an opportunity for random genetic mutations to occur.

time risk of developing this disease. Oral contraceptive use and a reduced risk of OC is an established observation that is independent of study design and cohort selection *(13,14).*

Several hypotheses have been advanced to explain the association between ovulation and OC risk. Ovulation may lead to the formation of inclusion cysts, which are located within the stroma of the ovary. These cysts result from invaginations of the ovarian surface and are lined by ovarian surface ECs *(15).* Inclusion cysts are potential histologic precursor lesions of epithelial OC *(16,17).* The location of inclusion cysts within the ovarian stroma places ovarian surface ECs in a unique microenvironment, in which they are subject to the influence of growth factors (GF) and hormones.

A second hypothesis to explain the association between ovulation and OC risk focuses on the disruption of the OSE as a consequence of ovulation (Fig. 2). Repair of the epithelial defect requires proliferation of surrounding OSE cells, mimicking the process of wound repair *(18).* Proliferation of OSE cells provides an opportunity for genetic damage on the basis of chance alone. Because the fidelity of DNA replication is not 100%, there is a small chance that a random error may occur during the duplication of one or more critical genes, which may result in cellular transformation *(19).* The ovarian mesothelial cell is unique, because it behaves as a stem cell, yielding two daughter cells that both exhibit an equal potential for future proliferation, as opposed to terminal differentiation *(20).* Theoretically, this increases the probability that a mutation is propogated in subsequent generations of cells. The importance of proliferation to OSE cell transformation has been elegantly demonstrated by a series of experiments in which prolonged exposure of normal rat OSE cells to mitogens in vitro resulted in malignant transformation *(21).* When ovulation is inhibited, as with oral contraceptives, pregnancy, or breast-feeding, OSE cell proliferation is significantly reduced, and the likelihood of proliferation-related DNA damage is concomitantly diminished.

A third hypothesis to explain the protective effect of oral contraceptives is based on a progesterone-mediated effect. Oral contraceptive use has been associated with an increased rate of apoptosis of OSE cells, from a baseline of 5 to 25% *(22)*. Apoptosis is a mechanism to prevent the accumulation of single-cell genetic damage that contributes to transformation. Theoretically, an increase in apoptosis would be associated with a decreased risk of accumulating critical mutations that would lead to malignant transformation.

A relationship between ovulation and OC risk is generally accepted. However, this correlation is nonlinear, which suggests that factors distinct from ovulation influence neoplastic transformation of the OSE.

STEROID HORMONES

The ovary is the site of synthesis and a target organ for several steroid hormones, including estrogen, androgen, and progesterone. Estrogens induce proliferation of ovarian surface ECs. Estrogens also exert a direct effect on the ovarian stroma, and influence the synthesis of GFs as discussed below. However, the influence of estrogen therapy on lifetime OC risk is unclear. In one large prospective study of 240,073 peri- and postmenopausal women, with a 7-yr period of follow-up, every use of estrogen was associated with a rate ratio for fatal OC of 1.15 (CI 0.94–1.42). The risk increased with the duration of estrogen replacement therapy (ERT) *(23)*. However, other studies have failed to demonstrate an increased relative risk of OC with ERT. In one study, ERT was correlated with a reduction in lifetime risk. Differences in study design and cohort selection preclude meaningful comparisons of published data, and a significant relationship between ERT and risk of epithelial OC remains unproven.

The effect, if any, of ERT on disease progression and risk of recurrent ovarian carcinoma has also not been determined. Normal OSE cells are estrogen-receptor (ER)-positive. Epithelial OCs express the ER in 70% of cases and the progesterone receptor in 40% of cases *(24)*. In addition, a proportion of carcinomas exhibit aromatase activity, and can convert stromal androgen to estrogen *(25)*. In vitro, 17β-estradiol stimulates the proliferation of some, but not all, ER-positive cell lines *(26,27)*.

Because an estrogen effect cannot be predicated solely by the detection of the ER, it would be inappropriate to conclude that ERT is contraindicated for all patients with ER-positive neoplasms. ERT is often prescribed to women with advanced-stage epithelial OC, in the absence of recognized contraindications, such as venous thrombosis or a history of breast cancer. There are no published data based on prospective clinical trials to suggest that estrogen therapy adversely influences the biology of the disease or its clinical course. Theoretically, estrogen therapy may be beneficial by reducing serum Gn levels, which, in turn, may reduce tumor angiogenesis *(28)*. Estrogen also decreases invasive potential and cell motility in vitro *(29)*.

Antiestrogens, such as tamoxifen (TAM), inhibit the growth of normal OSE cells *(30)*. TAM can also inhibit the growth in vitro of ER-positive OC cells *(31)*. The antiproliferative effect of TAM is not restricted to cells that express the ER. Neoplastic OSE cells exhibit TAM-binding sites that are distinct from the ER, and occur in greater numbers than those found on normal OSE cells *(32)*. These in vitro observations have been tested in clinical trials. Disease stabilization or regression has been reported in approx 17–18% of women with advanced-stage disease treated with TAM as salvage therapy *(33,34)*. In vitro, TAM, in conjunction with cisplatin, exerts a synergistic antiproliferative effect on primary OC cells *(35)*. However, in one clinical study designed to address the efficacy of combined chemohormonal therapy, a beneficial effect was not apparent *(36)*.

Androgens may also play a role in the pathobiology of OC. The ovarian stroma is one site of androgen production, with androstenedione as the primary product *(37)*. Androgen synthesis is most apparent in women in postmenopause, which is also the time period when epithelial OC is typically diagnosed. Premenopausal women with polycystic ovarian disease, characterized by a relative androgen excess, may also be at increased risk of epithelial OC, based on the results of one preliminary study *(38)*. Although these observations support the hypothesis that androgens influence the biology of epithelial OC, a relationship between serum androgen levels and epithelial OC is controversial. One study has reported elevated levels of androstenedione and dehydroepiandrosterone sulfate *(39)*; other studies reported the opposite finding in women with OC *(40,41)*.

Laboratory evidence supporting a role for androgens in the etiology of OC is found in a study by Silva et al. *(42)*. The administration of testosterone to guinea pigs resulted in the growth of papillary excrescences of the OSE, ovarian cysts within the stroma, adenomas, and papillomas. Androgens also stimulate the growth of normal OSE cells in vitro *(30)*.

In contradistinction to a positive role for androgens in OC development, Thompson and Adelson *(25)* have hypothesized that the relatively high local concentration of androgen in the stromal compartment of the postmenopausal ovary may actually suppress its development. Using stable cell lines established from newly diagnosed cases of OC, an inhibitory effect of both testosterone and androstenedione on cell proliferation was demonstrated. This antiproliferative effect was steroid-receptor-independent.

Although limited data suggest that androgens may play a role in the pathogenesis of epithelial OC, there is no information to suggest that it plays a therapeutic role. The majority of epithelial ovarian carcinomas express the androgen receptor *(24,43)*. However, clinical trials of androgen therapy and antiandrogen therapy have failed to demonstrate a beneficial effect *(44,45)*.

GONADOTROPINS

Because epithelial OC is predominantly a disease of postmenopausal women, it has been suggested that elevated Gn levels may play a role in its pathogenesis *(46)*. Following menopause, serum levels of both follicle-stimulating hormone (FSH) and luteinizing hormone (LH) are markedly increased. A stimulatory effect of Gns upon the OSE is suggested by the more common occurrence of benign papillary excrescences of the OSE in postmenopausal, compared to premenopausal, women *(47)*.

Most of the tumor induction data based on animal models describes an association between chronically elevated Gn levels and granulosa cell tumors. A notable exception is the work of Blaaker et al. *(48)*. The Wx/Wv strain of mice exhibits a premature and rapid rise of serum Gn levels in response to spontaneous oocyte depletion at birth. As these animals age, they also exhibit an abnormally high incidence of bilateral complex tubular adenomas. Of particular interest, these OSE-derived lesions do not develop when Wx/Wv mice are treated with gonadotropin-releasing hormone (GnRH) agonist therapy to suppress Gn levels. When ovarian carcinoma cells are heterotransplanted into female nude athymic mice, castrate animals exhibit more rapid tumor growth and GnRH-agonist-treated mice exhibit less rapid tumor growth than control tumors in endocrinologically intact animals.

The mechanism of action of Gns in ovarian carcinogenesis has not been defined. Gn receptors for both FSH and LH are present on normal and malignant OSE cells *(9,49)*. When FSH binds to its receptor on a normal OSE cell, proliferation is stimulated *(50)*. FSH also causes an increase in cell proliferation of some, but not all, ovarian carcinoma cell lines *(28,51,52)*. Schiffernbauer et al. *(28)* have demonstrated that Gn stimulation of ovarian carcinoma spheroids implanted in nude mice is accompanied by neovascularization and elevated serum levels of vascular endothelial growth factor (VEGF). As discussed in the section below, VEGF is an important GF in OC.

Although GnRH agonist therapy should be of therapeutic benefit, based on the preceding data, this treatment strategy has not been particularly successful when tested in the clinical arena. Prospective, randomized clinical studies have failed to confirm the encouraging observations initially reported in small series and anecdotal case reports of patients with advanced stage OC who exhibited disease regression following GnRH agonist therapy *(53,54)*.

The relationship between Gns and epithelial OC is complex, and appears to involve multiple pathways. It is a puzzling paradox that elevated Gn levels are associated with OC, yet serum FSH levels (but not LH) are actually lower in postmenopausal women with OC, as compared to matched, postmenopausal controls *(39,41,55,56)*. These data suggest the presence of a tumor-specific inhibitor of FSH release, which results in lower serum FSH values in women with OC. Inhibin, an ovarian peptide belonging to the transforming growth factor β (TGF-β) superfamily, is a potential candidate for this role. Inhibin levels are elevated in some, but not all, women with advanced-stage OC *(41,57)*. Among epithelial ovarian carcinoma, mucinous cystadenocarcinoma is more likely to be associated with an increased inhibin value than the other histologic subtypes *(58)*.

OVARIAN STROMAL GFs

A contemporary discussion of the endocrinology of gynecologic cancer must extend beyond the boundaries of classical steroid biology, following the identification and characterization of peptide GFs. Through paracrine and autocrine mechanisms, GFs appear to exert an influence on the pathobiology of epithelial OC.

The ovarian stroma, which is located beneath the epithelial layer of ovarian mesothelial cells, and is separated from it by a basement membrane, is composed of spindle-shaped fibroblastic cells. The fibroblastic cells of the stroma differentiate into a variety of cell types, including follicular theca interna cells, enzymatically active stromal cells, smooth muscle cells, decidual cells, endometrial stromal-type cells, fat cells, and stromal Leydig cells *(59)*. After menopause, the volume and cellularity of the ovarian stroma decrease, although the stroma remains metabolically active.

Normal ovarian function, particularly ovulation, requires the participation of numerous interrelated GFs produced by the ovarian stroma via paracrine and autocrine pathways *(60)*. Alterations in the normal expression of GF receptors or growth-regulatory molecules may increase OSE cell proliferation or reduce the number of OSE cells that undergo programmed cell death. Abnormal expression of growth-regulatory molecules and mutations of GF receptors undoubtedly contribute to the progression of OC.

The epidermal growth factor receptor (EGFR) family of tyrosine kinase GF receptors plays a role in the growth regulation of normal OSE cells and epithelial ovarian carcinoma cells. OSE cells are weakly positive for the EGFR *(61)*. Neoplastic ovarian carcinoma cells overexpress the EGFR in approx 30% of cases.

The EGFR binds both EGF and TGF-α. These polypeptides exhibit 35% amino acid homology and similar structural conformations *(62)*. Both EGF and TGF-α are produced by the ovarian stroma in response to elevated Gn levels, particularly FSH *(63,64)*. Estradiol also increases TGF- α levels *(65)*. TGF-α is localized to the OSE and in the ECs that line inclusion cysts *(66)*. Both EGF and TGF-α stimulate OSE cells to proliferate *(67,68)*. Overexpression of either protein under the control of viral promoters in murine fibroblasts results in tumor formation in nude mice *(69,70)*.

The proliferation of transformed OSE cells can be inhibited with TGF-α antibodies *(71,72)*. Growth inhibition of OSE cells also occurs in response to TGF-β, which is expressed by normal and malignant ovarian ECs (73-75). Following malignant transformation, OC cells often lose the ability to respond to TGF-β (73,76). It has been suggested that alterations of the TGF-β pathway that result in the loss of normal inhibition of OSE cell proliferation may indirectly increase the likelihood of malignant transformation. The TGF pathways may also influence cancer progression following transformation. OC cells can acquire the ability to produce TGF-α (77) and stimulate their own growth through an autocrine pathway. Stromberg et al. (71) have provided evidence based on in vitro studies of 17 cell lines, in which an autocrine mechanism of TGF-α autocrine stimulation of the EGFR was demonstrated.

Insulin-like growth factor I (IGF-I) and IGF-II exert mitogenic effects on normal and transformed cells. These polypeptide hormones share 60% amino acid homology and 47% homology with insulin. IGF-I and its receptor (IGF-IR) are important regulators of OSE cell mitogenesis *(78)*. Transfection of normal OSE with IGF-IR induces transformation in vitro. In vitro, IGF-I and IGF-II alone exert little effect on the proliferative activity of established ovarian carcinoma cell lines *(67)*. However, when combined with EGF, a synergistic effect was observed, with either IGF-I or IGF-II, on proliferative activity.

Both the fluid of an ovarian follicle and corpora lutea extracts contain substances that exert a mitogenic effect on ovarian mesothelial cells. Corpora lutea extracts trigger proliferation of both ovarian surface ECs and peritoneal mesothelial cells *(79)*. The follicular fluid contains a steroidogenesis-inducing protein that is a potent mitogen for epithelial ovarian carcinoma cell lines *(80)*. This effect is potentiated by EGF, TGF-α, and IGF-I. Additional supporting work, using the rabbit model, has also been published *(68)*. Follicular fluid contains a number of GFs and hormonal substances, including IGF-I, IGF-II, EGF, TGF-α, relaxin, GnRH, proopiomelanocortin, prorenin, antidiuretic hormone, and atrial natriuretic peptide *(60)*. One or more of these substances undoubtedly induce a proliferative response in OSE cells.

The ovarian stroma also provides a microenviroment of elevated estrogen levels. Although it has not been investigated in epithelial ovarian carcinoma, studies in breast cancer demonstrate that elevations of local estrogen levels are sufficient to support local growth of MCF-7 cells in nude mice *(81)*. Because of the potential estrogen responsiveness of normal and transformed OSE cells, one may speculate that a similar phenomenon may occur in OC.

VEGF appears to play a role in tumor development by promoting neovascularization. VEGF also increases vascular permeability. It is normally produced by the ovary during ovulation *(82)*, and its levels are markedly elevated in ascites fluid from patients with OC *(83)*.

GENETIC MUTATIONS

Many genetic mutations have been described in sporadic epithelial OC *(84)*. Most published studies of genetic mutations in epithelial OC are based on analyses of advanced-stage cancer, and it is difficult to determine whether the mutations reflect causation or the inherent genomic instability of advanced-stage disease. The early genetic alterations associated with epithelial OC have been difficult to define. The study of stage I disease is limited by delay in diagnosis, with resulting advanced-stage disease, reflecting the absence of specific warning signs and screening tests.

The *BRCA1* and *BRCA2* genes have been the focus of considerable attention as important genes in the development of familial OC, which accounts for 5–10% of all cases of epithelial OC. Mutations of *BRCA1* increase the relative risk of OC approx 30-fold, and mutations of *BRCA2* increase the risk by a factor of 10.

The c-*fms* oncogene encodes the colony-stimulating factor receptor, and is abnormally expressed in approx 10% of advanced-stage OCs. It has been postulated that the c-*fms* gene product participates in an autocrine stimulatory pathway for transformed cells. However, there are no data to suggest that alterations of this gene play a role in the early events of ovarian EC transformation.

Loss or inactivation of p53 is an important event in neoplastic transformation. In a large number of unrelated in vitro and in vivo models, mutation of the *p53* gene is a central event in carcinogenesis. Inactivation of p53 contributes to malignant transformation by inhibiting apoptosis and permitting the accumulation of single-cell genetic damage *(85)*. Mutations of p53 can be detected in at least 50% of patients with advanced-stage OC *(86)*. Abnormalities in p53 can occur in ovarian inclusion cysts adjacent to invasive cancer, but are rare in benign tumors or borderline malignancies. Of particular note, there is a positive relationship between the number of lifetime ovulatory cycles and p53 mutations in epithelial OC *(87)*. The frequency of transitions, transversions, and deletions in sporadic cancer is consistent with spontaneous mutation arising from DNA deamination during replication, rather than from the activity of environmental carcinogens. The finding of spontaneous mutations of p53, rather than those induced by exogenous compounds, is consistent with the absence of epidemiologic data suggesting that environmental carcinogens play a role in the etiology of epithelial OC.

The EGFR is designated as the c-erbB oncogene product when its N-terminal extracellular sequences are deleted. The protein product of this mutated gene no longer binds EGF or TNF-α but is constitutively activated, providing a continuous intracellular signal for cellular proliferation. The Her-2/*neu* oncogene is amplified or overexpressed in 20–30% of epithelial OCs. It is an indicator of poor prognosis, and has been associated with resistance to platinum-based chemotherapy. There are no published data to suggest that alterations of this gene occur as an early event in the development of OC. Normal peritoneum of women with OC overexpresses HER-2/*neu*, but not EGFR *(88)*. The ErbB-2 protein is weakly expressed by OSE cells, and is strongly expressed by ovarian carcinoma cells *(61)*.

SUMMARY

The development of epithelial OC is facilitated by a variety of factors acting through interrelated and complex endocrine, paracrine, and autocrine pathways. Not only steroid hormones, but GFs synthesized by the ovarian stroma, stimulate proliferation of OSE cells. Following the occurrence of critical genetic mutations that result in transformation,

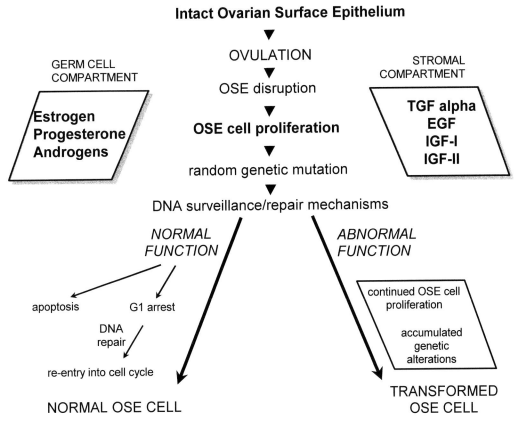

Fig. 3. Epithelial ovarian carcinoma is the result of accumulated genetic mutations. Repeated ovulation provides a stimulus for EC proliferation and the concomitant opportunity for random genetic mutations to occur. In the event of abnormal DNA repair mechanisms, these genetic mutations are passed to subsequent daughter cells. Over time, a sufficient number of mutations in critical genes may result in cellular transformation. Steroid hormones and GFs facilitate this process, through their positive effects on cellular proliferation.

these substances may further stimulate cellular proliferation and confer a growth advantage that favors the emergence of neoplastic clones and disease progression (Fig. 3).

REFERENCES

1. Mckay DG. The adult human ovary: a histochemical study. Obstet Gynecol 1961;18:13–39.
2. Blaustein A. Peritoneal mesothelium and ovarian surface cells: shared characteristics. Int J Gynecol Pathol 1984;3:361–375.
3. Nicosia SV, Johnson JH. Surface morphology of ovarian mesothelium (surface epithelium) and of other pelvic and extrapelvic mesothelial sites in the rabbit. Int J Gynecol Pathol 1984;3:249–260.
4. Blaustein A, Lee H. Surface cells of the ovary and pelvic peritoneum: a histochemical and ultrastructural comparison. Gynecol Oncol 1979;8:34.
5. Nouwen EJ, Hendrix PG, Dauwe S, et al. Tumor markers in the human ovary and its neoplasms. A comparative immunohistochemical study. Am J Pathol 1987;126:230–242.
6. Maines-Bandiera SL, Auersperg N. Increased E-cadherin expression in ovarian surface epithelium: an early step in metaplasia and dysplasia? Int J Gynecol Pathol 1997;16:250–255.
7. Sundfeldt K, Piontkewitz Y, Ivarsson K, et al. E-cadherin expression in human epithelial ovarian cancer and normal ovary.Int J Cancer 1997;74:275–280.
8. Hamilton TC, Davies P, Griffiths K, et al. Oestrogen receptor-like binding in the surface germinal epithelium of the rat ovary. J Endocrinol 1982;95:377–385.

9. Zheng W, Magid MS, Kramer EE, Chen YT. Follicle-stimulating hormone receptor is expressed in human ovarian surface epithelium and fallopian tube. Am J Pathol 1996;148:47–53.

10. Eltabbakh GH, Piver MS. Extraovarian primary peritoneal carcinoma. Oncology 1998;12:813–819.

11. Eltabbakh GH, Piver MS, Natarajan N, Mettlin CJ. Epidemiologic differences between women with extraovarian primary peritoneal carcinoma and women with epithelial ovarian cancer. Obstet Gynecol 1998;91:254–259.

12. Kruk PA, Uitto VJ, Firth JD, et al. Reciprocal interactions between human ovarian surface epithelial cells and adjacent extracellular matrix. Exp Cell Res 1994;215:97–108.

13. Whittemore AS, Harris R, Itnyre J. Characteristics relating to ovarian cancer risk: collaborative analysis of 12 U.S. case-control studies. II. Invasive epithelial ovarian cancers in white women. Am J Epidemiol 1992;136:1184–1203.

14. Franceschi S, Parazzini F, Negri E, et al. Pooled analysis of 3 European case-control studies. III. Oral contraceptive use. Int J Cancer 1991;49:61–65.

15. Radisklavejevic SV. The pathogenesis of ovarian inclusion cysts and cystadenomas. Obstet Gynecol 1977;49:424–429.

16. Clement PB. Nonneoplastic lesions of the ovary. In: Kurman RJ, ed. Blaustein's Pathology of the Female Genital Tract, 3rd ed. Springer, Berlin, New York, 1987, pp. 471–496.

17. Scully RE. Ovarian tumors. A review. Am J Pathol 1997;87:686–720.

18. Nicosia X, et al. In: Familiari G, Sayoko, M, Pietro M, eds. Ultrastructure of the Ovary. Klewer, The Netherlands, 1991, pp. 287–310.

19. Mendelsohn ML. The somatic mutational component of human carcinogenesis. In: Moolgavkar SH, ed. Scientific Issues in Quantitative Cancer Risk Assessment. Birkhaeuser, Boston, New York, 1990, pp. 22–31.

20. Hamilton TC. Ovarian cancer: part I: biology. Curr Probl Cancer 1992;16:1–57.

21. Godwin AK, Testa JR, Handel LM, et al. Spontaneous transformation of rat ovarian surface epithelial cells: association with cytogenetic changes and implications of repeated ovulation in the etiology of ovarian cancer. J Natl Cancer Inst 1992;84:592–601.

22. Rodriguez GC. Walmer DK, Cline M, et al. Effect of progestins on the ovarian epithelium of macaques: cancer prevention through apoptosis? J Soc Gynecol Invest 1998;5:271–276.

23. Rodriguez C, Calle EE, Coates RJ, et al. Estrogen replacement therapy and fatal ovarian cancer. Am J Epidemiol 1995;141:828–835.

24. Cardillo MR, Petrangeli E, Aliotta N, et al. Androgen receptors in ovarian tumors: correlation with oestrogen and progesterone receptors in an immunohistochemical and semiquantitative image analysis study. J Exp Clin Cancer Res 1998;17:231–237.

25. Thompson MA, Adelson MD. Aging and development of ovarian epithelial carcinoma: the relevance of changes in ovarian stromal androgen production. Adv Exp Med Biol 1993;330:155–165.

26. Langdon SP, Hawkes MM, Lawrie SS, et al. Oestrogen receptor expression and the effects of oestrogen and tamoxifen on the growth of human ovarian carcinoma cell lines. Br J Cancer 1990;62:213–216.

27. Hua W, Christianson T, Rougeot C, et al. SKOV3 ovarian carcinoma cells have functional estrogen receptor but are growth-resistant to estrogen and anti-estrogens. J Steroid Biochem Mol Med 1995;55:279–289.

28. Schiffernbauer YS, Abramovitch R, Meir G, et al. Loss of ovarian function promotes angiogenesis in human ovarian carcinoma. Proc Natl Acad Sci USA 1997;94:13,203–13,208.

29. Rochefort H, Platet N, Hayashido Y, et al. Estrogen receptor mediated inhibition of cancer cell invasion and motility: an overview. J Steroid Biochem Mol Biol 1998;65:163–168.

30. Hamilton TC, Davies P, Griffiths K. Steroid-hormone receptor status of the normal and neoplastic ovarian surface germinal epithelium. In: Greenwald GS, Terranova PF, eds. Factors Regulating Ovarian Function. Raven, New York, 1983, pp. 81–85.

31. Nash JD, Ozols RF, Smyth JF, Hamilton TC. Estrogen and anti-estrogen effects on the growth of human epithelial ovarian cancer in vitro. Obstet Gynecol 1989;73:1009–1016.

32. Batra S, Iosif CS. Elevated concentrations of antiestrogen binding sites in membrane fractions of human ovarian tumors. Gynecol Oncol 1996;60:228–232.

33. Ahlgren JD, Ellison NM, Gottlieb RJ, et al. Hormonal palliation of chemoresistant ovarian cancer: three consecutive phase II trials of the Mid-Atlantic Oncology Program. J Clin Oncol 1993;11:1957–1968.

34. Hatch KD, Beecham JB, Blessing JA, Creasman WT. Responsiveness of patients with advanced ovarian carcinoma to tamoxifen. A Gynecologic Oncology Group study of second-line therapy in 105 patients. Cancer 1991;68:269–271.

35. Scambia G, Ranelletti FO, Benedetti Panici P, et al. Synergistic antiproliferative activity of tamoxifen and cisplatin on primary ovarian tumours. Eur J Cancer 1992;28A:1885–1889.
36. Schwartz PE, Chambers JP, Kohorn EI, et al. Tamoxifen in combination with cytotoxic chemotherapy in advanced epithelial ovarian cancer. Cancer 1989;63:1074.
37. Rice BF, Savard K. Steroid hormone formation in the human ovary. IV. Ovarian stromal compartment: formation of radioactive steroids from acetate-I-14C and action of gonadotropins. J Clin Endocrinol 1966;26:593–609.
38. Schildkraut JM, Schwingel PJ, Bastos E, et al. Epithelial ovarian cancer risk among women with polycystic ovary syndrome. Obstet Gynecol 1996;88:554–559.
39. Helzlsouer KJ, Alberg AJ, Gordon GB, et al. Serum gonadotropoins and steroid hormones and the development of ovarian cancer. JAMA 1995;274:1926–1930.
40. Heinonen PK. Androgen production by epithelial ovarian tumors in post-menopausal women. Maturitas 1991;13:117–122.
41. Blaakaer J, Micic S, Morris ID, et al. Immunoreactive inhibin-production in postmenopausal women with malignant epithelial tumors. Eur J Obstet Gynecol Repro Biol 1993;52:105–110.
42. Silva EG, Tornos C, Fritsche HA, et al. The induction of benign epithelial neoplasms of the ovaries of guinea pigs by testosterone stimulation: a potential animal model. Modern Pathol 1997;10:879–883.
43. Kuhnel R, de Graaff J, Rao BR, Stolk JG. Androgen receptor predominance in human ovarian carcinoma. J Steroid Biochem 1987;26:393–397.
44. Kavanagh JJ, Wharton JT, Roberts WS. Androgen therapy in the treatment of refractory epithelial ovarian cancer. Cancer Treat Rep 1987;71:537,538.
45. Tumolo S, Rao BR, van der Burg ME, et al. Phase II trial of flutamide in advanced ovarian cancer: an EORTC Gynecologic Cancer Cooperative Study. Eur J Cancer 1994;30A:911–914.
46. Biskind MS, Biskin GS. Development of tumors in the rat ovary after transplantation into the spleen. Proc Soc Exp Biol Med 1944;55:176–179.
47. Makabe S, Iwaka A, Hafez ES, Motta PM. Physiomorphology of fertile and infertile human ovaries. In: Motta PM, Hafez ESE, eds. Biology of the Ovary. Nijhoff, The Hague, 1980, pp. 279–290.
48. Blaakaer J, Baeksted M, Micic S, et al. Gonadotropin-releasing hormone agonist suppression of ovarian tumorigenesis in mice of the Wx/Wv genotype. Biol Reprod 1995;53:775–779.
49. Al-Timimi A, Buckley CH, Fox X. An immunohistochemical study of the incidence and significance of human gonadotropin and prolactin binding sites in normal and neoplastic human ovarian tissue. Br J Cancer 1986;53:321–329.
50. Osterholzer HO, Streibel EJ, Nicosia SV. Growth effects of protein hormones on cultured rabbit ovarian surface epithelial cells. Biol Reprod 1985;33:247–258.
51. Feng Y, Zhang X, Gi B. Gonadotropins stimulate the proliferation of human epithelial ovarian cancer cells. Chin J Obstet Gynecol 1996;31:166–168.
52. Ohtani K, Sakamoto H, Satoh K. Stimulatory effects of follicular stimulating hormone on the proliferation of ovarian cancer cell lines in vitro and in vivo. Acta Obstet Gynecol Jpn 1992;44:717–724.
53. Emons G, Ortmann O, Teichert HM, et al. Luteinizing hormone-releasing hormone agonist triptorelin in combination with cytotoxic chemotherapy in patients with advanced ovarian carcinoma. A prospective double blind randomized trial. Decapeptyl Ovarian Cancer Study Group. Cancer 1996;78:1452–1460.
54. Erickson LD, Hartmann LC, Su JQ, et al. Cyclophosphamide, cisplatin, and leuprolide acetate in patients with debulked stage III and IV ovarian carcinoma. Gynecol Oncol 1994;54:196–200.
55. Blaakaer J, Djursing H, Hording U, et al. The pituitary-gonadal axis in women with benign or malignant ovarian tumors. Acta Endocrinol 1992;127:127–130.
56. Mahlck G, Grankvist K, Kjellgren O, Backstrom T. Human chorionic gonadotropin, follicle-stimulating hormone, and luteinizing hormone in patients with epithelial ovarian carcinoma. Gynecol Oncol 1990; 36:219–225.
57. Burger HG, Robertson DM, Cahirn N, et al. Characterization of inhibin immunoreactivity in postmenopausal women with ovarian tumors. Clin Endocr 1996;55:413–418.
58. Healy DL, Mamers P, Bangah M, Burger HG. Clinical and pathophysiological aspects of inhibin. Human Reprod 1993;8:138–140.
59. Scully RE. Tumors of the ovary and maldeveloped gonads. In: Atlas of Tumor Pathology, Second Series, Fascicle 16. Armed Forces Institute of Pathology, Washington, DC, 1979.
60. Giordano G, Barreca A, Minuto F. Growth factors in the ovary. J Endocrinol Invest 1992;15:689–707.
61. Wang D, Konishi I, Koshiyama M, et al. Immunohistochemical localization of c-erbB-2 protein and epidermal growth factor receptor in normal surface epithelium, surface inclusion cysts, and common epithelial tumors of the ovary. Virchows Arch A Pathol Anat 1992;421:393–400.

62. Marquardt H, Hunkapillar MW, Hood LE, Todaro GJ. Rat transforming growth factor alpha, structure and relation to epidermal growth factor. Science 1984;223:1079.

63. Roy SK, Greenwald GS. Immunohistochemical localization of epidermal growth factor-like activity in the hamster ovary with a polyclonal antibody. Endocrinology 1990;126:1309.

64. Kudlow JE, Kobrin MS, Purchio AF, et al. Ovarian transforming growth factor alpha gene expresion: immunohistochemical localization to the theca-interstitial cells. Endocrinology 1987;121:1577.

65. Simpson BJ, Langdon SP, Rabiasz GJ, et al. Estrogen regulation of transforming growth factor alpha in ovarian cancer. J Steroid Biochem Mol Biol 1998;64:137–145.

66. Jindal SK, Snoey DM, Lobb DK, Dorrington JH. Transforming growth factor alpha localization and role in surface epithelium of normal human ovaries and in ovarian carcinoma cells. Gynecol Oncol 1994;53:17–23.

67. Rodriguez GC, et al. Epidermal growth factor receptor expression in normal ovarian epithelium and ovarian cancer. III. Relationship between receptor expression and response to epidermal growth factor. Am J Oncol Gynecol 1991;164:745–750.

68. Pierroet E, Nicosia SV, Saunders B, et al. Influence of growth factors on proliferation and morphogenesis of rabbit ovarian mesothelial cells in vitro. Biol Reprod 1996;54:660–669.

69. Rosenthal A, Lindquist PB, Bringman TS, et al. Expression in rat fibroblasts of a human transforming growth factor alpha cDNA results in transformation. Cell 1986;46:301.

70. Stern DF, Hare DL, Cecchini MA, Weinberg RA. Construction of a novel oncogene based on synthetic sequences encoding epidermal growth factor. Science 1987;235:321.

71. Stromberg K, Collins TJ, Gordon AW, et al. Transforming growth factor-alpha acts as an autocrine growth factor in ovarian carcinoma cell lines. Cancer Res 1992;52:341–347.

72. Morishige K, Kurachi H, Amemiya X, et al. Involvement of transforming growth factor alpha/epidermal growth factor receptor autocrine growth mechanism in an ovarian cancer cell line in vitro. Cancer Res 1991;51:5951–5955.

73. Havrilesky LJ, Hurteau JA, Whitaker RS, et al. Regulation of apoptosis in normal and malignant ovarian epithelial cells by transforming growth factor beta. Cancer Res 1995;55:944–948.

74. Bartlett JM, Langdon SP, Scott WN, et al. Transforming growth factor-beta isoform expression in human ovarian tumours. Eur J Cancer 1997;33:2397–2403.

75. Nakanishi Y, Kodama J, Yoshiniouchi M, et al. The expression of vascular endothelial growth factor and transforming growth factor-beta associates with angiogenesis in epithelial ovarian cancer. Int J Obstet Gynecol Pathol 1997;16:256–262.

76. Hurteau J, Rodriguez GC, Whitaker RS, et al. Transforming growth factor beta inhibits proliferation of human ovarian cancer cells obtained from ascites. Cancer 1994;74:93–99.

77. Bauchnect T, Birmelin G, Kommoss F. Clinical significance of oncogenes and growth factors in ovarian carcinoma. J Steroid Biochem Mol Biol 1990;37:855–862.

78. Resnicoff M, Ambrose D, Coppola D, Rubin R. Insulin-like growth factor-1 and its receptor mediate the autocrine proliferation of human ovarian carcinoma cell lines. Lab Invest 1993;69:756–760.

79. Setrakian S, Oliveros-Saunders B, Nicosia SV. Growth stimulation of ovarian and extraovarian mesothelial cells by corpus luteum extract. In Vitro Cell Dev Biol Animal 1993;29A:879–883.

80. Khan SA, Matysiak-Zablocki E, Ball R, et al. Steroidogenesis-inducing protein, isolated from human ovarian follicular fluid, is a potent mitogen for cell lines derived from ovarian surface epithelial carcinomas. Gynecol Oncol 1997;66:501–508.

81. Huseby RA, Maloney TM, McGrath CM. Evidence for a direct growth-stimulating effect of estradiol on human MCF-7 cells in vivo. Cancer Res 1984;44:2654.

82. Gordon JD, Mesiano S, Zaloudek CJ, Jaffe RB. Vascular endothelial growth factor localization in human ovary and fallopian tubes: possible role in reproductive function and ovarian cyst formation. Clin Endocr Metabol 1996;81:353–359.

83. Barton DP, Cai A, Wendt K, et al. Angiogenic protein expression in advanced epithelial ovarian cancer. Clin Cancer Res 1997;3:1579–1586.

84. Baker VV. The molecular genetics of epithelial ovarian cancer. Obstet Gynecol Clin N Am 1994;21:25–40.

85. Wyllie AH. Apoptosis and carcinogenesis. Eur J Cell Biol 1997;73:189–197.

86. Berchuck A. Kohler MF, Marks JR, et al. The p53 tumor suppressor gene frequently is altered in gynecologic cancers. Am J Obstet Gynecol 1994;170:246–252.

87. Schildkraut JM, Bastos E, Berchuck A. Relationship between lifetime ovulatory cycles and an expression of mutant p53 in epithelial ovarian cancer. J Natl Cancer Inst 1997;89:932–938.

88. Jennings TS, Dottino PR, Mandeli JP, et al. Growth factor expression in normal peritoneum of patients with gynecologic carcinoma. Gynecol Oncol 1994;55:190.

17

Molecular Pathogenesis of Endometrial Cancer
The Role of Tamoxifen

Yukio Sonoda, MD and Richard R. Barakat, MD

CONTENTS

INTRODUCTION
EPIDEMIOLOGY
RISK FACTORS
TYPES OF ENDOMETRIAL CANCER
MOLECULAR BASIS OF ENDOMETRIAL CANCERS
ONCOGENES
TUMOR-SUPPRESSOR GENES
DNA REPAIR GENES
ROLE OF TAM IN ENDOMETRIAL CARCINOGENESIS
CONCLUSION
REFERENCES

INTRODUCTION

The molecular pathogenesis of a neoplasm is a multistep process in which a normal human cell undergoes a series of progressive changes, eventually resulting in a cancerous cell *(1)*. Genetic mutations are important etiologic factors in the development of cancer. More specifically, cancer is a consequence of the abnormal expression or function of specific cellular genes, oncogenes, and tumor-suppressor genes. These alterations are thought to occur by one of two routes: Mutations can occur somatically or through inheritance via the germline. These two routes correspond to the sporadic and hereditary classifications of cancers. The increased incidence of most human tumors in the older population suggests that several events must take place for this transformation to occur. A genetic model for tumorigenesis has been proposed that illustrates the multistep process in the development of colorectal cancer *(2)*. It is likely that this model can be applied to the study of other human neoplasms in which tumor development is less well defined, such as endometrial carcinoma. This application would in turn benefit researchers in defining the role of tamoxifen (TAM) in the development of endometrial cancer.

From: *Contemporary Endocrinology: Endocrine Oncology*
Edited by: S. P. Ethier © Humana Press Inc., Totowa, NJ

EPIDEMIOLOGY

Carcinoma of the endometrium is the most common gynecologic cancer in the United States. It is the fourth most common malignancy in females, ranking behind breast (BC), colon, and lung cancers. According to the American Cancer Society, there were an estimated 36,100 cases in United States in 1998, with 6300 deaths *(3)*. The relatively low death rate is, in large part, because of the early stage at which the majority of cases are diagnosed. In 75% of the cases, the tumor is confined to the uterine corpus (stage I) at the time of diagnosis, and uncorrected survival rates of 75% or more are expected *(4)*. In contrast, 63% of ovarian cancer cases are diagnosed in stages III or IV, with survival rates of just 22.9 and 14.3%, respectively *(5)*.

RISK FACTORS

In general, risk factors for the development of endometrial cancer have revolved around the theory of continuous stimulation of the endometrium by unopposed estrogen. Because of the associated peripheral conversion of androgens to estrogens, obesity ranks as the most significant risk factor *(4)*. Other high-estrogen states that have been associated with the development of endometrial cancer include early menarche, late menopause, nulliparity, and polycystic ovary syndrome. Hypertension and diabetes mellitus, two diseases often seen in conjunction with obesity, are considered risk factors *(4)*.

TYPES OF ENDOMETRIAL CANCER

Clinical and pathologic studies have suggested that two distinct forms of endometrial carcinoma exist *(6)*. Type I tumors comprise the classic estrogen-related carcinomas, usually of the endometroid subtype. They are frequently well-differentiated and associated with endometrial hyperplasias. Type I tumors are usually seen in the pre- and perimenopausal population, and carry a better prognosis. Type II tumors are more aggressive, and are usually seen in postmenopausal females. Serous, clear-cell, and poorly differentiated subtypes comprise this population, which does not seem to carry the strong correlation with unopposed estrogen, as with the Type I variety. It has been suggested that there is a molecular genetic basis for the existence of these two types of endometrial carcinomas, and recognition of such must be kept in mind as the search for their molecular and cellular etiologies continues *(7)*.

MOLECULAR BASIS OF ENDOMETRIAL CANCERS

Understanding of the molecular pathogenesis of endometrial carcinoma is still incomplete. It is evident that genetic alterations are responsible for the development of endometrial cancer, but its exact nature is still unclear. Early evidence for the role of genetic alterations was first demonstrated by DNA ploidy analysis. Those studies *(8)* revealed that 20% of endometrial cancers have increased DNA content (aneuploidy), compared to normal cells. Aneuploid endometrial cancers tend to be of more advanced stage, have adverse histologic features, and result in poorer survival, compared to the remaining 80% of endometrial cancers *(8)*. Gross chromosomal alterations of endometrial cancers have also been described in the literature *(9,10)*.

Supporting evidence for the genetic component of endometrial carcinogenesis comes from several sources. Although familial cancers comprise only a fraction of the endometrial cancers, these tumors are indicative of a genetic predisposition to their development. Examples of inheritable forms of endometrial cancer include site-specific endometrial cancer and those associated with the Lynch II syndrome. The site-specific form comprises approx 5% of endometrial cancers. This clustering of endometrial cancers occurs in families with no other evidence for neoplasms at other sites. An additional 5% of endometrial cancers are associated with Lynch II syndrome, and comprise the most common form of extracolonic neoplasm associated with this syndrome *(11)*.

Significant progress has been made in the molecular characterization of many human neoplasms, but a specific understanding of endometrial cancer is lacking. This chapter reviews the major findings thought to play a role in the molecular pathogenesis of endometrial neoplasms, as well as TAM's role in its development.

ONCOGENES

The oncogenes associated with endometrial cancer are subclassified, according to their biochemical activity, into three groups: peptide growth factors and their receptors, signal transducers, and nuclear transcription factors *(12)*.

Epidermal Growth Factors

The normal human endometrium is continuously undergoing change during the female's reproductive years. This change has been characterized in terms of the polypeptide cytokines and growth factors (GFs) regulating the endometrium *(13)*. It has been postulated that peptide GFs and their receptors may be activated to stimulate growth of the endometrium *(14)*. Epidermal growth factor (EGF) and its receptor (EGFR), which is coded by the ErbB gene, have been shown to be present in the normal endometrium. Estrogen treatment increases both the level of EGF and its receptor. However, their role in the pathogenesis of endometrial cancers still remains unclear. In other human neoplasms, high EGFR expression has been correlated with an unfavorable prognosis, but their prognostic value in endometrial cancers remains unknown. In contrast to the overexpression of the EGFR observed in some squamous cell carcinomas, endometrial neoplasms do not demonstrate this phenotype. In fact, endometrial carcinomas seem to have a decreased amount of receptor expression, compared to normal endometrium. Reynolds *(15)* used a radioreceptor assay to demonstrate that higher-grade endometrial cancers had progressively decreased amounts of EGFRs. From 34 total specimens (21 of which were normal endometrium), six grade 1 and 2 tumors exhibited a 34% decrease in EGFR expression, in contrast to seven grade 3 cancers, which had a 90% decrease. Loss of EGFR in endometrial cancers has also been demonstrated, using immunohistochemical staining. Berchuck et al. *(16)* examined 40 endometrial cancers for the presence of EGFR, and found only 67.5% to have EGFR expression, compared to 20 controls, of which 95% exhibited EGFR expression. Scambia et al. *(17)* also attempted to characterize the role, if any, of EGFR as a prognostic tool. They also used a radioreceptor assay, and reported that 26/60 tumors expressed EGFR. These tumors were associated with an unfavorable prognosis. Because of the contrasting data, the role of EGFR has yet to be determined.

Transforming Growth Factor α

Transforming growth factor α (TGF-α) is a GF related to EGF. It binds to the EGFR, and seems to function as an autocrine growth stimulator in cultured endometrial carcinoma cells *(7)*. TGF-α mediates estrogen action in the normal mouse uterus *(18)*, and has been noted to be increased in normal proliferative phase endometrium, compared to secretory endometrium *(7)*. It is overexpressed in endometrial cancers; thus, the deregulation of TGF-α expression may be an important event in endometrial carcinogenesis *(7)*.

HER-2/NEU

Like ERBB, *HER-2/neu* (ErbB-2), encodes for a receptor tyrosine kinase, and it too is found in the normal endometrium *(18)*. Amplification of this oncogene has been demonstrated in other cancers, and correlates with a poor prognosis. Its product has been shown to be overexpressed in 10–15 % of endometrial cancers. Hetzel et al. *(19)* studied 247 endometrial cancers for *HER-2/neu* expression. Their results revealed that expression of this oncogene was more prevalent in advanced-stage cases, and this correlated with poorer survival. Of the study population, 15% had high expression of *HER-2/neu*, 58% had moderate expression, and 27% had no expression. This translated into 56, 83, and 95% 5-yr progression-free survival, respectively. Similar results regarding *HER-2/neu* amplification were observed by Saffari et al. *(20)*. By using fluorescent *in situ* hybridization (FISH), those authors showed that endometrial cancers with amplification of the *HER-2/neu* gene correlated with shorter survival. Other studies *(18,21)* have also supported the association of *HER-2/neu* with poor clinical outcome.

FMS

The *fms* oncogene has also been studied in endometrial cancers. This gene encodes for a receptor tyrosine kinase for macrophage colony-stimulating factor (M-CSF). *fms* and M-CSF are co-expressed in endometrial cancers, and together may mediate an autocrine growth-stimulatory pathway *(22)*. In cell lines that express significant levels of *fms*, M-CSF increases their invasiveness, compared to cell lines that lack this expression. M-CSF levels seem to be elevated in patients with endometrial cancers. Expression of *fms* mRNA has been shown to correlate with high FIGO grade, advanced clinical stage of disease, and deep myometrial invasion, all of which are predictors of worse clinical outcome. M-CSF levels have been found to be increased in patients with endometrial cancer *(22,23)*.

Nuclear Transcription Factors

C-MYC

The c-*myc* oncogene encodes for a nuclear transcription factor that has been implicated in the development of human cancers. It has been shown to be expressed in normal endometrium, with a higher amount of expression in the proliferative phase, compared to the secretory phase *(24)*. The presence of c-*myc* has been demonstrated in endometrial cancers, and is associated with poor tumor grade. Borst et al. *(21)* identified 10/15 endometrial cancers with c-*myc* gene expression. The correlation of c-*myc* expression with higher tumor grade was also confirmed by others *(25)*. The intensity of immunostaining has been shown to increase from normal to hyperplastic to carcinomatous endometrium *(26)*.

G Proteins

RAS

The *ras* oncogene belongs to a family of guanine nucleotide-binding proteins known as G proteins, which function as physiologic switches that regulate the activity of target enzymes in response to a variety of signals *(27)*. G proteins have intrinsic GTPase activity, and are able to catalyze the exchange of guanosine triphosphate for guanosine diphosphate. When activated, Ras proteins are able to activate cytoplasmic serine/threonine kinases, which convey mitogenic stimuli to the nucleus *(12)*. The activation of the Ras protein is a common pathway that is activated after the binding of GFs to receptor tyrosine kinases. Point mutations in the *ras* gene at codons 12, 13, or 61, which result in activation, have been described in other cancers. As with c-*myc*, the Ras proteins are present in normal endometrium, and their clinical significance in endometrial cancer is under investigation.

The presence of ras mutations in endometrial cancers was first demonstrated in cell lines from 11 endometrial carcinomas. Codons 12, 13, and 61 of the H-*ras*, K-*ras*, and N-*ras* genes were screened for mutations. Sixty-four percent of cell lines exhibited mutations, with codon 12 of the K-*ras* containing the highest number (4/11) *(28–30)*. The occurrence of these mutations in premalignant lesions suggests that they comprise an early event in the multistep pathway of endometrial carcinoma. Sasaki et al. *(31)* found codon 12 mutations of K-*ras* in 14/89 (16%) of endometrial hyperplasias and 15/84 (18%) of endometrial carcinomas. Mutations were noted in simple, complex, and atypical hyperplasia, in addition to moderately and well-differentiated carcinomas. No mutations were noted in 20 type II carcinomas (poorly differentiated, clear-cell, or papillary serous). Duggan et al. *(32)* screened 60 endometrial cancer specimens, and identified nine (15%) occurrences of K-*ras* mutations. Adjacent areas of hyperplasia were also screened in the nine samples, but only those with hyperplastic areas, with nuclear atypia, contained the mutation. Thus, the K-*ras* mutation was felt to be an early oncogenic event in the multistep model of endometrial carcinogenesis.

Other Oncogenes

Bᴄʟ-2

The investigation of the Bcl-2 protein in endometrial cancers is relatively limited. It has been shown to prolong cell survival by preventing apoptosis *(33)*. Although previous studies of Bcl-2 focused on hematolymphoid malignancies, Bcl-2 protein has been detected in normal endometrium, where it peaks at the end of the proliferative phase, and disappears at the onset of the secretory phase *(34)*. Henderson et al. *(35)* demonstrated that Bcl -2 protein is downregulated in atypical hyperplasia and adenocarcinoma. Similar findings were reported by Zheng et al. *(36)*, who found that *bcl-2* staining diminished progressively from proliferative-phase endometrium to cancer. They hypothesized that early inactivation of *bcl-2* may provide an opportunity for accumulating genetic mutations, and lead to the evolution of endometrial carcinoma. Endometrioid cancers had a higher level of *bcl -2* staining than papillary-serous carcinomas, suggesting that deregulation of the *bcl-2* gene may play a larger role in this tumor type.

TUMOR-SUPPRESSOR GENES

p53

p53 was the second tumor-suppressor gene to be characterized. However, loss of its function is the single most frequent genetic alteration to be described in human cancers *(37)*. The presence of *p53* mutations in endometrial cancers has been extensively studied in the literature, and approx one-third of endometrial adenocarcinomas have abnormalities of *p53* by immunohistochemistry.

Kohler et al. *(38)* reported overexpression of mutant *p53* in 21% of 107 cases of endometrial cancers. Abnormal *p53* staining was frequent in more advanced-stage (III/IV) cancers (41%), compared to early-stage (I/II) cancers (9%). *p53* overexpression was associated with lower survival rates, in addition to poor-prognosis factors, including poor grade, nonendometrioid histology, and advanced stage. The authors subsequently sequenced eight cancers from the sample pool, and identified point mutations in all of the five cancers with *p53* overexpression, compared to no mutations in the three cancers with no *p53* staining. Endometrial hyperplasias have also been screened for *p53* mutations: The rarity of *p53* mutations in hyperlasias suggests that this is either a late event in the progression of type I tumors or an occurrence in type II endometrial carcinomas *(7,39)*.

PTEN/MMAC1

Recently, a potential tumor-suppressor gene, *PTEN/MMAC1*, was identified in endometrial cancers. Early studies *(40)* have reported the incidence of the *PTEN* mutation to be as high as 50%, which would make this the most commonly mutated gene in endometrial cancer. It has been shown that loss of heterozygosity exists on chromosome 10. However, it was only recently that the candidate-suppressor gene *PTEN* was mapped to chromosome 10 *(41)*. This discovery led to the search for *PTEN* mutations in endometrial cancer. Tashiro et al. *(40)* examined 32 primary endometrial carcinomas for *PTEN* mutations, and found 16 (50%) to contain this mutation. All were of the endometrioid subtype, and all grades exhibited mutations in *PTEN*. However, none of six serous tumors demonstrated *PTEN* mutations, leading the authors to conclude that *PTEN* mutations play a significant role in the pathogenesis of endometrioid-type endometrial cancer. Others have confirmed the frequency of *PTEN* mutations in endometrial cancers. Risinger et al. *(42)* found *PTEN* mutations in 24/70 (34%) endometrial carcinomas. *PTEN* mutations have also been identified in 27% of complex atypical hyperplasias (CAH) with synchronous endometrial cancers and 22% of isolated cases of CAH, thus supporting the role of *PTEN* in the pathogenesis of endometrioid adenocarcinoma *(43)*.

DNA REPAIR GENES

Microsatellite instability is a term for a replication error phenotype that may be a marker for cancer *(44)*. DNA mismatch repair genes are responsible for the correction of errors made during replication; thus, mutations in these genes can lead to errors in repetitive nucleotide sequences, or microsatellite repeats. This phenomenon was first observed in familial colorectal carcinomas of the hereditary nonpolyposis colorectal cancer (HNPCC) syndrome *(45,46)*. However, such an occurrence has also been reported in nonfamilial colorectal tumors, suggesting that both sporadic and inheritable cancers can exhibit microsatellite instability *(46)*. The search for errors in DNA repair capacity naturally carried over to endometrial cancers, which are the most common extracolonic cancers in the HNPCC syndrome. Risinger et al. *(47)* found that 75% of endometrial cancers associated with HNPCC and 17% of sporadic endometrial cancers contained microsatellite instability. Duggan et al. *(48)* also examined the occurrence of microsatellite instability in sporadic endometrial cancers. They reported 9/45 (20%) cases containing replication errors at three microsatellite loci. Of these nine, five (56%) had mutant k-ras alleles, compared to 5/36 (14%) cancers that did not exhibit microsatellite instability.

ROLE OF TAM IN ENDOMETRIAL CARGINOGENESIS

TAM is a nonsteroidal antiestrogen that has been used since 1978 for the treatment of patients with BC. It has demonstrated an improved recurrence-free and overall survival in both premenopausal and postmenopausal women. In addition, TAM may play a role in BC prevention in women at risk for the development of BC. Preliminary results from the Breast Cancer Prevention Trial *(49)* demonstrated a 45% reduction in BC incidence in women taking TAM, compared to placebo. Undoubtedly, an increase in the use of prophylactic TAM will be experienced in the near future, placing a large number of patients at risk for the associated side effects of the medication. One of the most significant complications of long-term TAM use is the possible development of endometrial cancer.

Clinical Evidence for Carcinogenicity of TAM

Killackey et al. *(50)* initially reported the occurrence of endometrial cancer in three BC patients receiving antiestrogens. Since that time, there have been multiple cases of TAM-associated endometrial cancer reported in the literature. Although many authors have attempted to examine the correlation between TAM use and endometrial cancer development, the results are controversial. Data from three large Scandinavian trials were pooled and analyzed. From the total patient population of 4914 individuals, the TAM-treated group had relative risk of 4.1 for the development of endometrial cancer, compared to controls *(51)*. Examining the National Surgical Adjuvant Breast and Bowel Project B14 trial data, Fisher *(52)* reported a relative risk of 7.5 in the TAM-treated group. Because of the unusually low incidence of endometrial carcinomas in the control population, this number was questioned by the authors. However, when SEER data were used in place of the control population, a relative risk of 2.2 was obtained in the TAM group. In support of the suspected increased risk for endometrial cancer, the preliminary results from the Breast Cancer Prevention Trial revealed that 33 patients taking TAM developed endometrial cancer, compared to 14 in the control population *(49)*.

Mechanisms of TAM-Associated Carcinogenesis

Although the clinical correlation between TAM and endometrial cancer has been widely examined, the mechanisms of TAM-associated endometrial carcinogenesis remain undetermined. Two theories have been postulated as to the carcinogenicity of TAM. The presence of a genotoxic mechanism has been investigated. This has been undertaken by a search for DNA adducts, covalent complexes between carcinogens or their metabolites and DNA. Measurement of these complexes are a reflection of the carcinogenic potential of a substance. DNA adduct formation has been detected in TAM-exposed rodents, illustrating its strong hepatocarcinogenic potential in these animals. In humans, however, no significant differences were noted in liver specimens from women on TAM, compared to controls *(53)*.

The potential of TAM to form DNA adducts in human endometrial tissue has been investigated, but results are inconclusive. Carmichael et al. *(54)* used thin-layer chromatography (TLC) and found that DNA adducts were not present in human endometrium cultures treated with TAM. They did report that α-hydroxytamoxifen, the metabolite implicated as the genotoxic intermediate in the rat liver, was detected in the endometrial cultures, but these were at levels too small to give rise to adducts. In contrast, Hemminki et al. *(55)* used high-performance liquid chromatography (HPLC) to detect the presence of DNA adducts in 5/7 patients treated with TAM. They commented on improved ability of HPLC over TLC in the detection of DNA adducts.

Other postulations on the carcinogenic potential of TAM center on its estrogen-agonist activity. Many epidemiologic studies concluded that the oral administration of estrogen is associated with the development of endometrial cancer *(56–58)*. As previously mentioned, many of the risk factors for endometrial cancer center around the concept of unopposed estrogen stimulation of the endometrium. TAM metabolites have been shown to have estrogen-agonist effects. Metabolite E, which is formed by the removal of the aminoethane side chain from TAM, is a weak agonist that binds to the estrogen receptor with low affinity. However, when the hydroxyl group destabilizes the ethylene bond, isomerization results in the E isomer, which is a potent estrogen agonist with high affinity for the estrogen receptor *(59)*. The clinical significance is controversial, since metabolite E has not been detected in women on TAM *(60)*.

4-hydroxytamoxifen, another metabolite, has also shown agonist effects in endometrial cancer cells. Gottardis et al. *(61)* transplanted endometrial cancer cells and BC cells to athymic mice and found that treatment with TAM stimulated growth of the endometrial cancer xenografts, but the BC xenograft was inhibited. Although the presence of an estrogenic pathway for TAM-mediated endometrial carcinogenesis has been questioned *(62)*, such a pathway could also be responsible for TAM's role in endometrial cancer development. The recent report that estrogens induce the expression of *HER-2/neu* in Ishikawa human endometrial cells may provide support for that hypothesis *(63)*.

Li et al. *(64)* have postulated that, in addition to being a carcinogen, TAM may exert indirect carcinogenic potential through enhancing the formation of endogenous DNA modifications. Barakat et al. *(65)* demonstrated that the frequency of K-*ras* mutations was similar in endometrial cancers occurring in BC patients, regardless of TAM treatment. They compared 14 cases of endometrial cancer patients, with prior TAM exposure, to 13 cases of endometrial cancers, with no prior TAM exposure, and found six cases of K-*ras* mutations in each group. However, among the patients whose endometrial cancers contained the K-*ras* mutations, TAM appeared to reduce the interval between the diagnosis of BC and endometrial cancer. These findings may provide support for the aforementioned hypothesis regarding TAM's role in the pathogenesis of endometrial cancer.

CONCLUSION

It is evident that human cancer development is a multistep process of genetic origin. Although the exact steps in the molecular pathogenesis of endometrial carcinomas are still not established, the genetic model of colorectal tumorigenesis has provided a paradigm on which to base the search. Recent evidence has provided clues to the genetic alterations associated with endometrial carcinomas. However, much is still unknown. Once a model for the development of endometrial neoplasia is established, it will undoubtedly illuminate TAM's role in endometrial carcinogenesis.

REFERENCES

1. Weinberg RA. Oncogenes, antioncogenes, and the molecular bases of multistep carcinogenesis. Cancer Res 1989;49:3713–3721.
2. Fearon ER, Vogelstein B. A genetic model for colorectal tumorigenesis. Cell 1990;61:759–767.
3. Landis SH, Murray T, Bolden S, Wingo PA. CA Cancer J Clin 1998;48:6–29.

4. Barakat RR, Park RC, Grigsby PW, Muss HD, Norris HJ. Corpus: epithelial tumors. In: Hoskins WJ, Perez CA, Young RC, eds. Principles and Practice of Gynecologic Oncology, 2nd ed. Lippincott-Raven, Philadelphia, 1997, pp. 859–896.

5. DiSaia PJ, Creasman WT. Clinical Gynecologic Oncology. 5th ed. Mosby, St. Louis, 1997, pp. 282–350.

6. Kurman RJ, Zaino RJ, Norris HJ. Endometrial carcinoma. In: Kurman RJ, ed. Blaustein's Pathology of the Female Genital Tract, 4th ed. Springer-Verlag, New York, 1994, pp. 439–486.

7. Boyd J. Estrogen as a carcinogen: the genetics and molecular biology of human endometrial carcinoma. In: Huff JE, Boyd J, Barrett JC, eds. Cellular and Molecular Mechanisms of Hormonal Carcinogenesis: Environmental Influences. Wiley, New York, 1996, pp.151–173.

8. Podratz KC, Wilson TO, Gaffey TA, Cha SS, Katzmann JA. Deoxyribonucleic acid analysis facilitates the pretreatment identification of high-risk endometrial cancer patients. Am J Obstet Gynecol 1993;168: 1206–1213.

9. Yoshida MA, Ohyashiki K, Piver SM, Sandberg AA. Recurrent endometrial adenocarcinoma with rearrangement of chromosomes 1 and 11. Cancer Genet Cytogenet 1996;20:159–162.

10. Fletcher JA, Aster JC. Morton CC. Association of trisomy 8 and squamous differentiation in an endometrial adenocarcinoma. Cancer Genet Cytogenet 1989;39:185–189.

11. Vasen HF, Offerhaus GJ, den Hartog Jager FC, Menko FH, Nagengast FM, et al. The tumour spectrum in hereditary non-polyposis colorectal cancer: a study of 24 kindreds in the Netherlands. Int J Cancer 1990;46:31–34.

12. Berchuck A, Evans AC, Boyd J. Alterations of oncogenes and tumor suppressor genes in endometrial cancer. In: Langdon SP, Miller WR, Berchuck A eds. Biology of Female Cancers. CRC, Boca Raton, 1997, pp. 205–217.

13. Tabibzadeh S. Human endometrium: an active site of cytokine production and action. Endocr Rev 1991; 12:272–290.

14. Mukku VR, Stancel GM. Regulation of epidermal growth factor receptor by estrogen. J Biol Chem 1985;260:9820–9824.

15. Reynolds RK, Talavera F, Roberts JA, Hopkins MP, Menon KM. Characterization of epidermal growth factor receptor in normal and neoplastic human endometrium. Cancer 1990;66:1967–1974.

16. Berchuck A, Soisson AP, Olt GJ, Soper JT, Clarke-Pearson DL, Bast RC Jr, McCarty KS Jr. Epidermal growth factor receptor expression in normal and malignant endometrium. Am J Obstet Gynecol 1989; 161:1247–1252.

17. Scambia G, Benedetti Panici P, Ferrandina G, Battaglia F, Distefano M, D'Andrea G, et al. Significance of epidermal growth factor receptor expression in primary human endometrial cancer. Int J Cancer 1994; 56:26–30.

18. Nelson KG, Takahashi T, Lee DC, Luetteke NC, Bossert NL, Ross K, Eitzman BE, McLachlan JA. Transforming growth factor-alpha is a potential mediator of estrogen action in the mouse uterus. Endocrinology 1992;131:1657–1664.

19. Hetzel DJ, Wilson TO, Keeney GL, Roche PC, Cha SS, Podratz KC. HER-2/neu expression: a major prognostic factor in endometrial cancer. Gynecol Oncol 1992;47:179–185.

20. Saffari B, Jones LA, el-Naggar A, Felix JC, George J, Press MF. Amplification and overexpression of HER-2/neu (c-erbB2) in endometrial cancers: correlation with overall survival. Cancer Res 1995;55: 5693–5698.

21. Borst MP, Baker VV, Dixon D, Hatch KD, Shingleton HM, Miller DM. Oncogene alterations in endometrial carcinoma. Gynecol Oncol 1990;38:364–366.

22. Kacinski BM, Carter D, Mittal K, Kohorn EI, Bloodgood RS, Donahue J, et al. High level expression of fms proto-oncogene mRNA is observed in clinically aggressive human endometrial adenocarcinomas. Int J Radiat Oncol Biol Phys 1988;15:823–829.

23. Leiserowitz GS, Harris SA, Subramaniam M, Keeney GL, Podratz KC, Spelsberg TC. The proto-oncogene c-fms is overexpressed in endometrial cancer. Gynecol Oncol 1993;49:190–196.

24. Odom LD, Barrett JM, Pantazis CG, Stoddard LD, McDonough PG. Immunocytochemical study of ras and myc proto-oncogene polypeptide expression in the human menstrual cycle. Am J Obstet Gynecol 1989;161:1663–1668.

25. Monk BJ, Chapman JA, Johnson GA, Brightman BK, Wilczynski SP, Schell MJ, Fan H. Correlation of C-myc and HER-2/neu amplification and expression with histopathologic variables in uterine corpus cancer. Am J Obstet Gynecol 1994;171:1193–1198.

26. Bai MK, Costopoulos JS, Christoforidou BP, Papadimitriou CS. Immunohistochemical detection of the c-myc oncogene product in normal, hyperplastic and carcinomatous endometrium. Oncology 1994;51: 314–319.

27. Cooper GM. Oncogenes, 2nd ed. Jones and Bartlett, Boston, 1995, pp. 222–242.
28. Boyd J, Risinger JI. Analysis of oncogene alterations in human endometrial carcinoma: prevalence of ras mutations. Mol Carcinog 1991;4:189–195.
29. Enomoto T, Inoue M, Perantoni AO, Buzard GS, Miki H, Tanizawa O, Rice JM. K-ras activation in premalignant and malignant epithelial lesions of the human uterus. Cancer Res 1991;51:5308–5314.
30. Mizuuchi H, Nasim S, Kudo R, Silverberg SG, Greenhouse S, Garrett CT. Clinical implications of K-ras mutations in malignant epithelial tumors of the endometrium. Cancer Res 1992;52:2777–2781.
31. Sasaki H, Nishii H, Takahashi H, Tada A, Furusato M, Terashima Y, et al. Mutation of the Ki-ras protooncogene in human endometrial hyperplasia and carcinoma. Cancer Res 1993;53:1906–1910.
32. Duggan BD, Felix JC, Muderspach LI, Tsao JL, Shibata DK. Early mutational activation of the c-Ki-ras oncogene in endometrial carcinoma. Cancer Res 1994;54:1604–1607.
33. Korsmeyer SJ. Bcl-2 initiates a new category of oncogenes: regulators of cell death. Blood 1992;80: 879–886.
34. Garcia I, Martinou I, Tsujimoto Y, Martinou JC. Prevention of programmed cell death of sympathetic neurons by the bcl-2 proto-oncogene. Science 1992;258:302–304.
35. Henderson GS, Brown KA, Perkins SL, Abbott TM, Clayton F. bcl-2 is downregulated in atypical endometrial hyperplasia and adenocarcinoma. Mod Pathol 1996;9:430–438.
36. Zheng W, Cao P, Zheng M, Kramer EE, Godwin TA. p53 overexpression and bcl-2 persistence in endometrial carcinoma: comparison of papillary serous and endometrioid subtypes. Gynecol Oncol 1996;61: 167–174.
37. Berchuck A. Kohler MF, Marks JR, Wiseman R, Boyd J, Bast RC Jr. The p53 tumor suppressor gene frequently is altered in gynecologic cancers. Am J Obstet Gynecol 1994;170:246–252.
38. Kohler MF, Berchuck A, Davidoff AM, Humphrey PA, Dodge RK, Iglehart JD, et al. Overexpression and mutation of p53 in endometrial carcinoma. Cancer Res 1992;52:1622–1627.
39. Kohler MF, Nishii H, Humphrey PA, Saski H, Marks J, Bast RC, et al. Mutation of the p53 tumor-suppressor gene is not a feature of endometrial hyperplasias. Am J Obstet Gynecol 1993;169:690–694.
40. Tashiro H, Blazes MS, Wu R, Cho KR, Bose S, Wang SI, et al. Mutations in PTEN are frequent in endometrial carcinoma but rare in other common gynecological malignances. Cancer Res 1997;57:3935–3940.
41. Steck PA, Pershouse MA, Jasser SA, Yung WK, Lin H, Ligon AH, et al. Identification of a candidate tumour suppressor gene, MMAC1, at chromosome 10q23.3 that is mutated in multiple advanced cancers. Nature Genet 1997;15:356–362.
42. Risinger JI, Hayes AK, Berchuck A, Barrett JC. PTEN/MMAC1 mutations in endometrial cancers. Cancer Res 1997;57:4736–4738.
43. Levine RL, Cargile CB, Blazes MS, van Rees B, Kurman RJ, Ellenson LH. PTEN mutations and microsatellite instability in complex atypical hyperplasia, a precursor lesion to uterine endometrial carcinoma. Cancer Res 1998;58:3254–3258.
44. Loeb LA. Microsatellite instability: marker of a mutator phenotype in cancer. Cancer Res 1994;54: 5059–5063.
45. Peltomaki P, Lothe RA, Aaltonen LA, Pylkkanen L, Nystrom-Lahti M, Seruca R, et al. Microsatellite instability is associated with tumors that characterize the hereditary non-polyposis colorectal carcinoma syndrome. Cancer Res 1993;53:5853–5855.
46. Thibodeau SN, Bren G, Schaid D. Microsatellite instability in cancer of the proximal colon. Science 1993;260:816–819.
47. Risinger JI, Berchuck A, Kohler MF, Watson P, Lynch HT, Boyd J. Genetic instability of microsatellites in endometrial carcinoma. Cancer Res 1993;53:5100–5103.
48. Duggan BD, Felix JC, Muderspach LI, Tourgeman D, Zheng J, Shibata D. Microsatellite instability in sporadic endometrial carcinoma. J Natl Cancer Inst 1994;86:1216–1221.
49. Smigel K. Breast Cancer Prevention Trial shows major benefit, some risk. J Natl Cancer Inst 1998;90: 647,648.
50. Killackey MA, Hakes TB, Pierce VK. Endometrial adenocarcinoma in breast cancer patients receiving antiestrogens. Cancer Treat Rep 1985;69:237,238.
51. Rutqvist LE, Johansson H, Signomklao T, Johansson U, Fornander T, Wilking N. Adjuvant tamoxifen therapy for early stage breast cancer and second primary malignancies. Stockholm Breast Cancer Study Group. J Natl Cancer Inst 1995;87:645–651.
52. Fisher B. Commentary on endometrial cancer deaths in tamoxifen-treated breast cancer patients. J Clin Oncol 1996;14:1027–1039.

53. Martin EA, Rich KJ, White IN, Woods KL, Powles TJ, Smith LL. 32P-postlabelled DNA adducts in liver obtained from women treated with tamoxifen. Carcinogenesis 1995;16:1651–1654.
54. Carmichael PL, Ugwumadu AH, Neven P, Hewer AJ, Poon GK, Phillips DH. Lack of genotoxicity of tamoxifen in human endometrium. Cancer Res 1996;56:1475–1479.
55. Hemminki K, Rajaniemi H, Lindahl B, Moberger B. Tamoxifen-induced DNA adducts in endometrial samples from breast cancer patients. Cancer Res 1996;56:4374–4377.
56. Mack TM, Pike MC, Henderson BE, Pfeffer RI, Gerkins VR, Arthur M, Brown SE. Estrogens and endometrial cancer in a retirement community. N Engl J Med 1976;294:1262–1267.
57. Jelovsek FR, Hammond CB, Woodard BH, Draffin R, Lee KL, Creasman WT, Parker RT. Risk of exogenous estrogen therapy and endometrial cancer. Am J Obstet Gynecol 1980;137:85–91.
58. Jick H, Watkins RN, Hunter JR, Dinan BJ, Madsen S, Rothman KJ, Walker AM. Replacement estrogens and endometrial cancer. N Engl J Med 1979;300:218–222.
59. Wolf DM, Jordan VC. Gynecologic complications associated with long-term adjuvant tamoxifen therapy for breast cancer. Gynecol Oncol 1992;45:118–128.
60. Langan-Fahey SM, Tormey DC, Jordan VC. Tamoxifen metabolites in patients on long-term adjuvant therapy for breast cancer. Eur J Cancer 1990;26:883–888.
61. Gottardis MM, Robinson SP, Satyaswaroop PG, Jordan VC. Contrasting actions of tamoxifen on endometrial and breast tumor growth in the athymic mouse. Cancer Res 1988;48:812–815.
62. Kuwashima Y, Kurosumi M, Kobayashi Y, Tanuma J, Suemasu K, Higashi Y, et al. Tamoxifen mediated human endometrial carcinogenesis may not involve estrogenic pathways: a preliminary note. Anticancer Res 1996;16:2993–2996.
63. Markogiannakis E, Georgoulias V, Margioris AN, Zoumakis E, Stournaras C, Gravanis A. Estrogens and glucocorticoids induce the expression of c-erbB2/NEU receptor in Ishikawa human endometrial cells. Life Sci 1997;61:1083–1095.
64. Li D, Dragan Y, Jordan VC, Wang M, Pitot HC. Effects of chronic administration of tamoxifen and toremifene on DNA adducts in rat liver, kidney, and uterus. Cancer Res 1997;57:1438–1441.
65. Barakat RR, Adhikari D, Saigo PE, O'Connor B, Banerjee D, Bertino JR. Mutation of c-Ki-ras in tamoxifen-associated endometrial carcinoma. Abstract 42. 27th SGO Annual Meeting. Gynecol Oncol 1996;60:108.

18

Structure and Function of *BRCA* Genes

Kenneth L. van Golen, MD
and Sofia D. Merajver, MD

CONTENTS

INTRODUCTION

The *BRCA1* and *BRCA2* genes fit the traditional description of tumor-suppressor genes, according to Knudson's classic two-hit model *(1,2)*. In familial cancers, an individual inherits a germline mutation, and thus this first hit is present in all cells of the body. A somatic mutation represents the second hit on a given cell, resulting in the loss of the wild-type (WT) allele, thus rendering both copies of the gene inactive *(3,4)*. In sporadic cancers, loss of function of a tumor-suppressor gene is accomplished by two somatic mutations that alter the alleles on both chromosomes (chrs). Knudson's model accurately accounts for the early onset of familial cancers caused by a pre-existing germline mutation; the accumulation of two somatic mutations in a single cell, a much less likely event, may occur once in several decades, giving rise to a sporadic cancer.

It is estimated that mutations in *BRCA1* account for 50% of all familial early-onset female breast cancers (BC) *(5)*; mutations in *BRCA2* may be responsible for up to 35% of the remaining hereditary BCs *(6,7)*. Several methods have been employed to screen for mutations in the *BRCA* genes, including direct sequencing of anomalous single-strand conformational polymorphism products *(8)*, heteroduplex analysis *(9,10)*, and protein truncation test *(9,11)*. During mutation screening, a host of polymorphisms have been identified for both the *BRCA1* and *BRCA2* genes *(12,13)*. Polymorphisms are missense alterations that cause either no change or a one-amino-acid substitution in the protein sequence. By definition, polymorphisms do not significantly modify the protein's function. Polymorphisms are found to varying degrees in the general population, and are typically not associated with obvious disease. It is possible, however, that certain missense

From: *Contemporary Endocrinology: Endocrine Oncology*
Edited by: S. P. Ethier © Humana Press Inc., Totowa, NJ

alterations cause subtle modifications of protein structure or expression, which may impact on function without causing overt clinical disease.

BRCA GENE STRUCTURE

It has long been recognized that a family history of BC is a contributing factor to the risk of developing this disease. In 1990, a BC susceptibility gene responsible for early-onset BC was localized to chr 17q21 *(14)*. A subsequent study confirmed this finding, and also implicated this hereditary BC gene in familial BC and ovarian cancer (OC) *(15)*. This gene, now known as *BRCA1*, was identified in 1994 by a combination of classical positional cloning and candidate gene strategies *(16)*. *BRCA1* is a large, well-characterized gene contained in an 81-kb segment of genomic DNA, which is rich in Alu-like repetitive sequences *(17)*. The intron lengths range in size from 403 bp to 9.2 kb, and a ribosomal protein pseudogene is contained within intron 13 *(17)*. Three polymorphic intragenic microsatellite markers, D17S1323, D17S1322, and D17S855, localize to introns 12, 19, and 20, respectively *(17)*.

The transcribed region of the *BRCA1* gene itself has 5651 nucleotides (nt) in 24 exons, 22 of which are coding exons: Almost half of the coding sequence is contained within exon 11. *BRCA1* encodes a 220-kDa cell cycle-regulated nuclear phosphoprotein composed of 1863 amino acids, with a zinc-finger domain near the N-terminus, typical of nucleic-acid-binding proteins *(18)*. The BRCA1 protein also has two functional nuclear localization motifs located at aa 503 and 607 *(19,20)*. Despite its nuclear localization, BRCA1 may also exhibit growth-inhibitory granin-like properties *(16,21,22)*.

Splice variants of *BRCA1* mRNA, which exist in normal breast cells *(23,24)*, have been identified. These alternatively spliced mRNAs code for truncated proteins; however, it is unknown whether these truncated proteins exhibit tumor-suppressor function or dominant-negative interactions. In BC-prone families, truncations of the BRCA1 protein result-ing from inherited mutations are correlated with a high mitotic index of breast tumor cells in the affected patients *(25)*.

One naturally occurring splice variant of BRCA1, which was isolated from breast tumor and colon epithelial cDNA libraries, has been useful in BRCA1 localization studies *(20)*. BRCA1-Δ11b, which is missing exon 4 and the majority of exon 11, has been shown to lose its ability to localize to the nucleus, and is subsequently confined to the cytoplasm. This variant of BRCA1 is expressed at similar levels in tissues, tumors, and cell lines, and, unlike the full-length BRCA1 protein, overexpression of the BRCA1-Δ11b protein is not toxic to the cell *(20)*, which suggests that this BRCA1 isoform has a role in cellular proliferation and differentiation. Two other naturally occurring splice variants of BRCA1, BRCA1a and BRCA1b, have been identified, and are found to code for 110-kDa and 100-kDa proteins, respectively *(26)*. The 110-kDa protein retains the amino-terminal region, and appears to function as a transcriptional activator. However, BRCA1b only retains the C-terminal end of the full-length protein, and may act as a negative regulator of transcriptional activity.

The *BRCA2* gene is notably similar to the *BRCA1* gene in its history and structure. *BRCA2* was localized to chr 13q12-13, using linkage analysis of cancer-prone kindreds *(27)*. Utilizing the lessons learned in cloning *BRCA1*, a partial sequence for *BRCA2* was reported less than 1.5 yr later *(28)*, almost simultaneously with the complete coding sequence of *BRCA2 (29)*. The *BRCA2* gene has 10,254 nt 27 exons, with a very large exon

11 containing almost half of the coding sequence *(29)*. Like *BRCA1*, *BRCA2* codes for a large, negatively charged protein with a putative granin domain *(30)*.

BRCA1 *and* BRCA2 *Homologs*

Cloning and sequencing of canine and murine *BRCA1* genes has demonstrated that the genes are highly homologous to each other and to the human *BRCA1* gene *(31)*. The human and canine genes are 84% identical at the nt level, and the human and murine genes are 72% identical. Key regions of the gene, such as the N-terminal and C-terminal ends, are greater than 80% identical in the three species, and significant homology exists in the areas that appear to have functional importance, such as the RING finger motif and the granin domain. The distribution of missense mutations associated with disease also peaks in areas that are highly conserved throughout species, such as the RING finger domain, lending support to the concept that these areas are crucial to the normal function of the gene product. In contrast, common polymorphisms tend to arise in regions of significantly lower interspecies homology *(31)*.

Using the human BRCA2 cDNA sequence as a guide, the mouse homolog was cloned *(32)*. At the nt level, human and murine BRCA2 cDNAs are 74% homologous. This is unlike other tumor-suppressor genes, such as *WT-1*, *NF-1*, and *APC*, which are, on average, 90% identical with their murine counterparts *(33–35)*. Murine BRCA2 has been localized to mouse chr 5, in a region syntenic with human 13q12-q13 *(32,36)*. Murine BRCA2 is 90 amino acids shorter than, and has a 59% overall homology to, its human counterpart.

The rat BRCA2 gene maps to rat chr 12, and has 58% identity and 73% similarity on the nt level with the human BRCA2 cDNA *(37,38)*. In the process of cloning the rat *Brca2* gene, various polymorphisms were detected in different strains of rats that exhibit different susceptibilities to carcinogen-induced tumors. The specific role that these polymorphisms play in the rat's susceptibility to carcinogenesis has yet to be determined. As in the case of BRCA1, several regions at the N-terminus, center, and the C-terminus of the murine, rat, and human BRCA2 proteins are conserved, with greater than 80% homology *(37,38)*. The *BRCA* genes are of mammalian origin, with highly conserved functional regions where disease-associated mutations have been identified in humans.

BRCA1 *Mutations in BC and Other Cancers*

Since its isolation in 1994, more than 100 mutations have been described in the *BRCA1* gene alone. The majority of these mutations were identified in individuals who belong to families with several generations affected with either BC or BC and OC *(4,12,39)*. Founder-effect mutations, common mutations presumably originating from a single ancestor within a historically isolated ethnic group, have been identified in several populations, such as Ashkenazic Jews *(40)*, French-Canadians *(41)*, Japanese *(42)*, Italians *(43)*, Swedes *(44)*, Finns *(45)*, Icelanders *(46)*, Belgians, and Dutch *(47,48)*. A salient example of these is the 185delAG mutation in individuals of Ashkenazic Jewish decent *(40,49–51)*.

This frame-shift mutation is a 2-bp deletion at base 185 in exon 2, which causes a premature truncation of the protein by producing a premature stop at codon 39 *(40)*. Other types of frame-shift mutations, caused either by deletions of 1–40 bp or insertions of up to 11 bp, have been identified, which also result in a premature stop codons *(52–54)*. Additionally, single-bp substitutions, resulting in missense, nonsense, or splicing mutations, have been described. Nearly 80% of mutations found so far in the *BRCA1* gene would produce a truncated protein *(12,39,55–58)*. In many cases, however, it is not known whether shorter or aberrant BRCA1 proteins are indeed expressed.

A different set of mutations occur in the regulatory regions of the *BRCA1* gene, such as methylatable CpG islands in promoters, enhancers, and repressors *(59,60)*. These mutations cause an alteration in the level of gene transcription, and are generally characterized by the absence of mRNA. Research is under way to better define the clinical significance of these mutations.

The role of *BRCA1* has been extensively investigated in sporadic BC and OC *(61–63)*. Several somatic mutations have been identified in the coding regions of *BRCA1* in sporadic ovarian tumors; however, until recently, none had been found in sporadic BCs *(64)*. Indications of involvement of the *BRCA1* gene in the formation of sporadic breast carcinomas derived from loss of heterozygosity (LOH) experiments *(61–63)*, putative loss of protein through unknown mechanisms *(64)*, and the observation that the promoter region of BRCA1 was hypermethylated in some invasive tumors *(65)*. Although loss of BRCA1 function occurs in sporadic BCs, neither the mechanism involved in this phenomenon nor its implications are known.

BRCA2 Mutations in BC and Other Cancers

Germline mutations in BRCA2 predispose female carriers to BC and OC, and male carriers to BC and possibly prostate cancer. The most common disease-associated mutations detected in the *BRCA2* gene of breast and ovarian patients have been microdeletions resulting in a frame-shift, with notably few point mutations, compared to BRCA1 *(8,13, 29,66,67)*. Founder mutations have also been identified in the *BRCA2* gene in members of defined ethnic groups *(68,69)*. This is once again well illustrated in the Ashkenazic Jewish population. A recurrent germline mutation, 6147delT, was detected in 8% of Ashkenazic Jewish women between the ages of 42 and 50 yr who were diagnosed with early-onset BC *(69)*. The 6147delT mutation is present in 1.5% of Ashkenazi Jews *(69)*.

LOH at the *BRCA2* locus has been observed in 30–40% of sporadic BC and OC *(70)*; however, very few somatic mutations or deletions have been found in the remaining allele *(67,71)*. This suggests that either *BRCA2* may be an infrequent target for somatic inactivation, or that intron or regulatory sequences may be the primary targets of somatic mutation. In a study of 45 unselected, grade 3, sporadic infiltrating ductal carcinomas, 21 cases demonstrated a concurrent LOH in the BRCA1 and BRCA2 loci *(72)*. This suggests a common pathway of tumorigenesis in familial and sporadic BCs that involves these two *BRCA* genes.

In addition to an increase in the risk of familial female BC and OC, mutations in the *BRCA2* gene are also associated with an increased risk of sporadic and familial forms of pancreatic *(73–75)*, hepatic *(76)*, prostate *(77,78)*, and, particularly, male BC *(13)*. Mutations in the *BRCA* genes that are found in these types of cancers are similar to those of breast and ovarian carcinomas, but no phenotype–genotype correlations have been established. In one study *(79)*, mutations in the central region of the *BRCA2* gene appear to carry higher risk of OC than mutations at either the 5' or 3' ends of the gene. This observation needs to be confirmed in studies of large numbers of BRCA2 carriers. Specific studies exploring the functional consequences of different mutations will be required before the phenotype–genotype correlations can be fully validated and applied in the clinic.

ADVANCES IN UNDERSTANDING BRCA1 AND BRCA2 FUNCTION

The role of BRCA1 in the regulation of cell growth has been investigated by studying its expression in diverse tissues. In adult human tissues, the highest expression of BRCA1 is seen in the testis and thymus, with moderate expression in the breast, ovary, uterus, lymph nodes, spleen, and liver *(16)*. BRCA1 expression levels in invasive cancers are 5–15-fold lower than in ductal carcinoma *in situ* or normal breast tissue *(80)*. Expression of BRCA1 appears to be directly upregulated by estrogen stimulation in estrogen-receptor (ER)-positive MCF-7 BC and BG-1 OC cells *(81,82)*, and by estrogen plus progesterone in ovariectomized mice *(83)*. However, recent evidence suggests that BRCA1 expression is not caused by direct induction of the gene, but rather by the mitogenic activity of estrogen *(84)*. The kinetics of BRCA1 expression are different from those expected of estrogen-inducible genes, such as *pS2*. Furthermore, treatment of ER-positive BC cells with insulin-like growth factor 1 or epithelial growth factor results in an increase in DNA synthesis and, subsequently, in BRCA1 upregulation *(84)*.

BRCA1 expression increases during puberty in the mouse mammary gland, and is associated with rapidly dividing cells of the mammary end bud, which differentiate during ductal morphogeneis *(83)*. Also, high levels of BRCA1 expression are seen during pregnancy in the differentiating aveolar buds *(83)*. In vitro transfection of WT *BRCA1* into lung, colon, breast, and ovarian tumor cells have demonstrated growth inhibition primarily in BC and OC cell lines *(85)*. *BRCA1* antisense oligo-nt introduced into primary mammary epithelial cell cultures, or *BRCA1* WT MCF-7 BC cells, accelerates the growth of the cells *(86)*. High levels of BRCA1 expression are also seen in rapidly dividing and differentiating cells of the mouse embryo *(83,87)*. Taken together, this evidence supports a tissue-specific role for BRCA1 in differentiation of breast and ovarian tissues.

A variety of experiments in animal models lend further support to the above findings. Mice homozygous for mutations in exons 5 and 6 of *BRCA1* (*Brca1$^{5-6}$*) were lethal at various embryonic stages; heterozygote mice were normal, and did not develop neoplasms *(88)*. *Brca1$^{5-6}$* mice died *in utero* at 4.5–6.5 d after gestation, with poorly developed embryonic tissues and an increase in expression of the CDK-inhibitor protein, p21. Furthermore, the embryonic stem cells from these mice appear nonviable. Similar cellular proliferation defects and embryonic lethality were observed in embryos carrying a 184-bp deletion of the 5'-portion of exon 11 of *BRCA1 (89)*. These studies indicate that at least one normal allele, coding for the full length protein, is required for normal embryonic development, and further supports the idea that BRCA1 not only has tumor-suppressor function, but also is essential for mammalian cell proliferation and embryo development. These findings led to investigations of the relationship of mutant *Brca1* with other key genes involved in cell differentiation and cell death.

Brca1$^{5-6}$ mutants showed a decrease in the expression of the p53 inhibitor mdm2, and an increase in the G1 cell-cycle inhibitor p21. To test whether embryonic lethality brought about by the *Brca1$^{5-6}$* mutation could be circumvented, double-mutant mice, which were *Brca1$^{5-6}$*-null, on either a p53-null (*p53$^-$*) or *p21*-null (*p21$^-$*) background, were produced *(90)*. Survival was prolonged in the *Brca1$^{5-6}$/p53$^-$* embryos from 7.5 to 9.5 d after gestation. And, although none of the *Brca1$^{5-6}$/p21$^-$* embryos survived past 10.5 d after gestation, they were developmentally similar to their WT litter mates. Therefore, because deletion of *p53* or *p21* was unable to completely rescue the *Brca1$^{5-6}$* embryos, a complex process of embryo development, involving interactions between several molecules, is postulated.

A recent study *(91)* demonstrated that mice that were heterozygous for *Brca1* (*Brca1$^{+/-}$*) and deficient for *p53* (*p53 $^{-/-}$*) had the same survival rate as mice that were *Brca1$^{+/+}$/ p53 $^{-/-}$*. However, mammary tumors developed in 4/23 *Brca1$^{+/-}$/p53 $^{-/-}$* mice, compared to only one *Brca1$^{+/+}$/p53 $^{-/-}$*. Although these data are suggestive of a trend of increased incidence of mammary tumors in *Brca1$^{+/-}$/p53 $^{-/-}$* mice, statistical significance was not reached.

In contrast to the *Brca1$^{5-6}$* null mice, homozygous exon 11 (*Brca1^{11}*) knockout embryos died at 9.5–13.5 d postgestation, because of severe neurological developmental defects seemingly brought on by rapid cellular proliferation and excessive cell death *(92)*. This experiment implicates Brca1 in differentiation of the murine central nervous system late in embryo development. The difference in phenotypes between *Brca1$^{5-6}$* and *Brca1^{11}* mutants suggests that alternate forms of the Brca1 protein, such as some of the naturally occurring truncated forms described previously, may have distinct functions in differentiating cells during embryo development.

Further studies *(93)* with *Brca1^{11}* demonstrated a hypersensitivity to γ-irradiation and massive abnormalities in chr structure and number, resulting from an increase in genetic instability when placed on a *p53*-null background. Accordingly, Brca1 appears to contribute to the maintenance of the integrity and stability of the genome during γ-irradiation. These findings in vivo correlate with a body of experimental evidence from in vitro studies.

Independent in vitro studies have shown that Brca1 co-precipitates with Rad51, the human homolog of the *Escherichia coli* RecA DNA repair protein *(94)*. Three potential nuclear localization motifs were identified in BRCA1 at aa 503, 606, and 651 *(19)*. Mutation of each of these individual motifs determined that the nuclear localization signals at aa 503 and 607 were needed for transporting BRCA1 to the nucleus; the nuclear localization motif at 651 was nonfunctional. Hence, the putative role of BRCA1 protein in DNA repair is supported by these data. It is reasonable to speculate that, in normal developing embryos, Brca1, acting in concert with Rad51, are able to effectively repair DNA damage. But, in homozygous *Brca1^{11-}* mutant embryos, the repair machinery is lost and a p53 cell-cycle checkpoint is induced. In the *Brca1^{11}/p53$^{-/-}$* mice, the checkpoint is lost, and severe chromosomal abnormalities can accumulate.

Paralleling the experiments on *Brca1* knockouts, *Brca2* knockout mice demonstrate that at least one normal copy of the *Brca2* gene is needed for normal embyrogenesis *(95,96)*. Likewise, mouse experiments have helped to correlate findings derived from human normal and tumor breast cells, which show cell cycle regulation of *BRCA2* corresponding to a general upregulation of mRNA during S-phase and mitosis *(97,98)*.

BRCA2 is also implicated in DNA repair *(93)*, as shown in experiments that introduced various mutations in the mouse *Brca2* gene by homologous recombination *(99)*. Mice were developed that had a disruption in exon 11 of the *Brca2* gene (*Brca2^{11}*). Some of the mice that were homozygous for this *Brca2* mutation were viable and lived to adulthood, but not beyond 5.5 mo of age. Fibroblasts cultured from the embryos of *Brca2^{11}* mutant mice overexpressed p21 and p53, which is reminiscent of the observation in the *Brca1$^{5-6}$* mice *(90)*. When the *Brca2^{11}* mutant fibroblasts were exposed to X-rays, the cells repaired double-stranded DNA breaks at a considerably slower rate than fibroblasts from WT *Brca2* mice, or from mice that were heterozygous for the exon 11 deletion mutation *(99)*.

The Role of BRCA1 and BRCA2 in DNA Repair

The *Brca1* knockout mouse data described above provide strong evidence that Brca1 has a role in double-stranded DNA repair *(100,101)*. BRCA1 and the human homolog of the bacterial RecA protein, Rad51, have been found to be associated both by in vivo and in vitro experiments *(94)*. Immunostaining of both meiotic and mitotic cells in S-phase demonstrated that BRCA1 and Rad51 co-localized in nuclear foci. Furthermore, the two proteins were co-immunoprecipitated from cells in S-phase. In vitro, BRCA1 and Rad51 formed complexes, and BRCA1 residues 768–1064 were identified to be key in the formation of these complexes with Rad51. Tissue culture experiments, which analyzed murine cells containing targeted truncated Brca2, demonstrated increased chromosomal abnormalities, and these cells had increased sensitivity to genotoxic agents, further implicating Brca2 in DNA repair *(102)*.

The human BRCA2 protein, like BRCA1, has been shown to associate with Rad51, and is therefore also involved in DNA repair *(103)*. Murine embryonic fibroblasts were generated *(104)* containing a *Brca2* gene with a C-terminal deletion at exon 27 *($Brca2^{27}$)*. These clones did not bind murine Rad51, and consequently were hypersensitive to γ-irradiation, suggesting a deficiency in DNA repair mechanisms. In addition, the *$Brca2^{27}$* mutant cells had decreased proliferation rates, and were prematurely senescent, presumably because of inefficient DNA repair. These data seem to indicate that the most distal portion of Brca2 downstream contains the Rad51 binding element, and is functionally important in DNA repair mediated by the Brca2–Rad51 complex. Multiple sites in BRCA2, termed BRC repeat motifs, interact with Rad51 *(105)*. The BRC repeat motifs are comprised of 59 amino acid residues, which are conserved in evolution, and are required for Rad51 interaction with BRCA2 *(103)*. In vitro experiments have demonstrated that interaction of Rad51 with these BRC repeat motifs of BRCA2 are critical for cellular response to DNA damage caused by genotoxic agents *(106)*. The identification of the specific regions of BRCA2 involved with binding to RAD51, and in effecting the DNA repair action of the complex, will assist in providing useful end points for functional assays. This experimental evidence will need to be reconciled with the possibility that truncation of the last 90–100 amino acids of the C-terminus of BRCA2 appears not to be associated with disease in humans.

BRCA1 and p53 Tumor-Suppressor Interactions

In vitro and in vivo experiments have shown that BRCA1 associates with another tumor-suppressor gene, *p53*, and regulates *p53*-responsive gene transcription *(107,108)*. Co-activation of *p53*-dependent genes by BRCA1 has been shown to be dependent on the presence of WT *p53 (107)* and WT *BRCA1 (107,108)*, suggesting a possible synergistic regulation of downstream genes by these two tumor suppressors. Investigation of the status of *p53* in breast tumors arising in *BRCA1* and *BRCA2* mutation carriers indicated that *p53* was mutant in 66% of the *BRCA*-related tumors, compared with only 35% of grade-matched non-*BRCA*-associated tumors *(109)*.

It has been suggested that the CDK-inhibitor p21 is transactivated by BRCA1 in a *p53*-dependent manner, therefore arresting cells before S-phase *(110)*. S-phase progression was inhibited by BRCA1 in cells that had WT p21, but not in either p21-null or BRCA1 transactivation-deficient mutant cells. Taken together, this evidence suggests that the tumor-suppressor action of BRCA1 with p53 may be mediated via cooperative BRCA1 regulation of WT p21.

BRCA1 Molecular Interactions

The BRCA1 protein has been shown to interact with various molecules throughout the cell cycle *(108,111–113)*, further implicating it in normal DNA recombination

(98) and activation of transcription, when BRCA1 is physically linked to RNA polymerase II *(114,115)*.

The expression pattern and subcellular localization of BRCA1 suggests that this protein may have a role in cell-cycle progression. BRCA1 protein levels are seen to fluctuate throughout the cell cycle, increasing in late G1 and reaching maximum levels during S-phase *(116)*. BARD1, a protein that binds and is structurally related to the NH_2-terminal RING domain of BRCA1 *(111)*, appears to co-localize with BRCA1 during in vivo S-phase in foci known as BRCA1 nuclear dots *(116)*. The ability of BARD1 to associate with BRCA1 is disrupted by BRCA1 tumorigenic mutations, such as the C61G mutation *(117)*, which replaces a key zinc-binding cysteine within the BRCA1 RING domain *(111)*. In addition, BARD1 missense mutations are accompanied by loss of the BARD1 WT allele in primary BC, OC, and uterine cancer *(118)*, further suggesting that loss of BARD1 function may play a role in BRCA1-mediated tumor suppression.

The C-terminal end of the BRCA1 protein contains tandem BRCA C-terminal (BRCT) domains at aa 1649–1736 and 1756–1855: These domains have been shown to interact in vivo with the C-terminal interacting protein (CtIP), a transcriptional co-repressor protein identified by its interaction with the C-terminal binding protein, CtBP, which was identified by its interacation with the transcriptional co-repressor protein, CtBP *(119)*. Tumor-associated mutations within the BRCT domains disrupt the BRCA1–CtIP interaction. Therefore, BRCA1 may have indirect tumor-suppression action through regulation of gene transcription via the CtBP pathway of transcriptional repression.

Several key proteins may be co-factors for BRCA1 in its tumor suppressor action. The exact pathways affected by these interactions of BRCA1 with its partners remain under study. Specific knowledge of which pathways are disturbed in different tumors may lead to novel therapeutic approaches based on modulating BRCA1 function.

Steroid Hormone Receptor Status of Tumors with Respect to BRCA1 and BRCA2 Mutations

The levels of expression of the ER and progesterone receptor (PR) in BC are important prognostic indicators, and modulate therapy for patients. Since work on animal models and tissue culture suggests that BRCA1 expression is, at least in part, hormonally regulated, research has been undertaken to explore the relationship between ER/PR status and BRCA1 expression in BC.

As previously described, the Ashkenazi Jewish population has four well-defined, recurrent heritable mutations in *BRCA1* and *BRCA2*, which result in an increased susceptibility to BC and OC. In a study of 149 unselected Ashkenazi Jewish women with BC, germline *BRCA1* and *BRCA2* mutation status was assessed *(120)*. Tumors from mutation carriers were compared with tumors from noncarriers, with respect to nuclear grade and steroid hormone receptor status. Tumors from women who harbored a *BRCA1* mutation were more often ER-negative and had a higher nuclear grade than the tumors form women without mutations. In contrast, tumors from four women harboring a *BRCA2* mutation were ER-positive.

Further studies on hereditary BCs have addressed this question outside of the well-defined Ashkenasic population *(121)*. It was found that breast tumors harboring BRCA1 mutations were predominantly ER-negative, compared with the tumors from other groups. Also, BRCA1-associated tumors had significantly lower expression of PR than those tumors from hereditary cases not related to *BRCA1* or *BRCA2*, but not lower than *BRCA2*-related tumors. Although larger studies are needed, these data suggest that diminution or loss of ER expression in breast cells containing a *BRCA1* mutation may attenuate the protective effects of antiestrogen preventive therapies such as TAM. Finally, familial male BC samples that were *BRCA2*-related did not have ER or PR levels different from non-*BRCA2*-related tumors. When assaying ER levels in a large number of sporadic BCs, it was found that loss or decrease of ER expression overwhelmingly coincided with LOH in the *BRCA1*, *BRCA2*, and *TP53* chromosomal regions *(122)*. Taken together, these data significantly link steroid hormone receptor status and the status of genes directly involved in the pathogenesis of BC and OC. The implications of these correlations for prognosis and survival of patients with BRCA-associated tumors are yet to be elucidated. It is still premature to apply these data to the chemopreventive management of *BRCA1* or *BRCA2* carriers with antiestrogens.

OVERVIEW

The idea that a tumor-suppressor gene may be responsible for early onset BC and OC led, through linkage analysis of families and classical positional cloning, to the identification of *BRCA1* and *BRCA2*. These genes are unique, because, aside from having weak homology to each other, they are quite unlike any other gene known. The importance of *BRCA1* and *BRCA2* mutations in familial BC and OC cannot be disputed. In less than 5 yr since both genes were cloned, more than 150 mutations have been described. Through analysis of homologs from other mammalian species, regions of these genes that have remained conserved throughout evolution have given insight into the functional domains of human BRCA1 and BRCA2, and are beginning to shed light on the impact that a mutation in these conserved regions may have on growth deregulation.

The functions of BRCA1 and BRCA2 are still under study. Results from experiments of yeast two-hybrid systems, interpreted in the context of results from knockout mouse experiments, point to the salient functions of these proteins. It is clear that both molecules have multiple functional domains that could allow interactions with several partners. Directed mutation of specific regions of either *BRCA1* or *BRCA2* in transgenic mice have resulted in specific phenotypes, which strongly implicate both genes in double-stranded DNA repair, cellular proliferation, and differentiation. In the case of BRCA1, the evidence of multiple functions and, presumably, independent interactions with several molecules may be reconciled with the identification of alternatively spliced forms of *BRCA1* mRNA, resulting in tissue-specific truncated proteins with different functions. Clearly, understanding of the roles of BRCA1 and BRCA2 in the cell and in human disease has greatly increased in the past few years. However, the major milestones in developing an in vitro molecular or cellular functional assay for these genes has not yet been achieved. That work is required for a better understanding of the possible impact of specific alterations in patients.

Although much progress has been made, the elucidation of the specific pathways of cell growth regulation that are altered by lack of BRCA expression still elude us. Such work is crucial to understand how loss of BRCA expression may participate in sporadic breast and ovarian carcinogenesis.

In addition to the advances in molecular carcinogenesis, the advent of BRCA1 and BRCA2 has fostered the development of comprehensive clinical risk evaluation programs, in the Americas, Europe, and some parts of Asia, of unprecedented proportions. The refinement of counseling methods for patients, the development of educational programs for patients and providers, and the creation of an ethical framework within which to translate these scientific advances to the clinic are critical achievements fostered by the study of these two genes and other familial cancer genes. The multidisciplinary teams at work on BRCA1 and BRCA2 throughout the world provide an invaluable paradigm for the theory and practice of translational research.

ACKNOWLEDGMENTS

This work was supported by grants from the U.S. Army (DAMD 17-94-J-4054 to SDM), the Susan G. Komen Breast Cancer Foundation (SDM and KvG), and the National Institutes of Health (P30-CA-46592 and T32-CA-09357).

REFERENCES

1. Rittling SR, Novick KE. Osteopontin expression in mammary gland development and tumorigenesis. Cell Growth Differ 1997;8:1061–1069.
2. Knudson AG. Mutation and cancer: statistical study of retinoblastoma. Proc Natl Acad Sci USA 1998; 68:820–823.
3. Smith SA, Easton DF, Evans DG, Ponder BA. Allele losses in the region 17q12-21 in familial breast and ovarian cancer involve the wild-type chromosome. Nat Genet 1992;2:128–131.
4. Merajver SD, Frank TS, Xu J, Pham TM, Calzone KA, Bennett-Baker P, et al. Germline *BRCA1* mutations and loss of the wild-type allele in tumors from families with early onset breast and ovarian cancer. Clin Can Res 1995;1:1–6.
5. Ford D, Easton DF, Bishop DT, Narod SA, Goldgar DE. Risks of cancer in *BRCA1*-mutation carriers. Breast Cancer Linkage Consortium. Lancet 1994;343:692–695.
6. Rebbeck TR, Couch FJ, Kant J, Calzone K, DeShano M, Peng Y, et al. Genetic heterogeneity in hereditary breast cancer: role of *BRCA1* and *BRCA2*. Am J Hum Genet 1996;59:547–553.
7. Krainer M, Silva-Arrieta S, Fitzgerlad MG, Shimada A, Ishioka C, Kanamaru R, et al. Differential contributions of *BRCA1* and *BRCA2* to early-onset breast cancer. N Engl J Med 1997;336:1416–1421.
8. Miki Y, Katagiri T, Kasumi F, Yoshimoto T, Nakamura Y. Mutation analysis in the *BRCA2* gene in primary breast cancers. Nat Genet 1996;13:245–247.
9. Gayther SA, Harrington P, Russel P, Kharkevich G, Garkavtseva RF, Ponder BA. Rapid detection of regionally clustered germ-line *BRCA1* mutations by multiplex heteroduplex analysis. Am J Hum Genet 1996;58:451–456.
10. Ozcelik H, Antebi YJ, Cole DE, Andrulis IL. Heteroduplex and protein truncation analysis of the *BRCA1* 185delAG mutation. Hum Genet 1996;98:310–312.
11. Lancaster JM, Cochran CJ, Brownlee HA, Evans AC, Berchuck A, Futreal PA, Wiseman RW. Detection of *BRCA1* mutations in women with early-onset ovarian cancer by use of the protein truncation test. J Natl Cancer Inst 1996;88:552–554.
12. Couch FJ, Weber BL. Mutations and polymorphisms in the familial early-onset breast cancer (*BRCA1*) gene. Breast Cancer Information Core. Hum Mutat 1996;8:8–18.
13. Couch FJ, Farid LM, DeShano ML, Tavtigian SV, Calzone K, Campeau L, et al. *BRCA2* germline mutations in male breast cancer cases and breast cancer families. Nat Genet 1996;13:123–125.
14. Hall JM, Lee MK, Newman B, Morrow JE, Anderson LA, Huey B, King MC. Linkage of early-onset familial breast cancer to chromosome 17q21. Science 1990;250:1684–1689.
15. Narod SA, Feunteun J, Lynch HT, Watson P, Conway T, Lynch J, Lenoir GM. Familial breast-ovarian cancer locus on chromosome 17q12-q23. Lancet 1991;338:82,83.
16. Miki Y, Swensen J, Shattuck-Eidens D, Futreal PA, Harshman K, Tavtigian S, et al. Strong candidate for the breast and ovarian cancer susceptibility gene *BRCA1*. Science 1994;266:66–71.
17. Smith TM, Lee MK, Szabo CI, Jerome N, McEuen M, Taylor M, Hood L, King MC. Complete genomic sequence and analysis of 117 kb of human DNA containing the gene BRCA1. Genome Res 1996;6: 1029–1049.

18. Chen Y, Farmer AA, Chi-Fen C, Jones DC, Chen P-L, Lee W-H. BRCA1 is a 220-kDa nuclear phosphoprotein that is expressed and phosphorylated in a cell cycle-dependent manner. Cancer Res 1996; 56:3168–3172.

19. Chen CF, Li S, Chen Y, Chen PL, Sharp ZD, Lee WH. Nuclear localization sequences of the BRCA1 protein interact with the importin-alpha subunit of the nuclear transport signal receptor. J Biol Chem 1996;271:32,863–32,868.

20. Wilson CA, Payton MN, Pekar SK, Zhang K, Pacifici RE, Gudas JL, et al. *BRCA1* protein products: antibody specificity. Nat Genet 1996;13:264,265.

21. Ruffner H, Verma IM. BRCA1 is a cell cycle-regulated nuclear phosphoprotein. Proc Natl Acad Sci USA 1994;94:7138–7143.

22. Jensen RA, Thompson ME, Jetton TL, Szabo CI, van der Meer R, Helou B, et al. *BRCA1* is secreted and exhibits properties of a granin. Nat Genet 1996;12:303–308.

23. Xu CF, Brown MA, Chambers JA, Griffiths B, Nicolai H, Solomon E. Distinct transcription state sites generate two forms of *BRCA1* mRNA. Hum Mol Genet 1995;4:2259–2264.

24. Lu M, Conzen SD, Cole CN, Arrick BA. Characterization of functional messenger RNA splice variants of *BRCA1* expressed in nonmalignant and tumor-derived breast cells. Cancer Res 1996;56:4578–4581.

25. Sobol H, Stoppa-Lyonet D, Bressac-de-Paillerets B, Peyrat J-P, Kerangueven F, Janin N, et al. Truncation at conserved terminal regions of *BRCA1* protein is associated with highly proliferating hereditary breast cancers. Cancer Res 1996;56:3216–3219.

26. Cui JQ, Wang H, Reddy ES, Rao VN. Differential transcriptional activation by the N-terminal region of BRCA1 splice variants BRCA1a and BRCA1b. Oncol Rep 1998;5:585–589.

27. Wooster R, Neuhausen SL, Mangion J, Quirk Y, Ford D, Collins N, et al. Localization of a breast cancer susceptibility gene, BRCA2, to chromosome 13q12-13. Science 1994;265:2088–2090.

28. Wooster R, Bignell G, Lancaster J, Swift S, Seal S, Mangion J, et al. Identification of the breast cancer susceptibility gene BRCA2. Nature 1995;378:789–792.

29. Tavtigian SV, Simard J, Rommens J, Couch F, Shattuck-Eidens D, Neuhausen S, et al. Complete *BRCA2* gene and mutations in chromosome 13q-linked kindreds. Nat Genet 1996;12:333–337.

30. Stratton MR. Recent advances in understanding of genetic susceptibility to breast cancer. Hum Mol Genet 1996;5:1515–1519.

31. Szabo CI, Wagner LA, Francisco LV, Roach JC, Argonza R, King MC, Ostrander EA. Human, canine and murine BRCA1 genes: sequence comparison among species. Hum Mol Genet 1996;5:1289–1298.

32. Sharan SK, Bradley A. Murine BRCA2: sequence, map position, and expression pattern. Genomics 1997;40:234–241.

33. Buckler AJ, Pelletier J, Haber DA, Glaser T, Housman DE. Isolation, characterization, and expression of the Murine Wilms' tumor gene (WT1) during kidney development. Mol Cell Biol 1991;11:1707–1712.

34. Hajra A, Martin-Gallardo A, Tarl'e SA, Freedman M, Wilson-Gunn S, Bernards A, Collins FS. DNA sequences in the promoter region of the *NF1* gene are highly conserved between human and mouse. Genomics 1994;21:649–652.

35. Su L-K, Kinzler KW, Vogelstein B, Preisinger AC, Moser AR, Luongo C, Gould KA, Dove WF. Multiple intestinal neoplasia caused by a mutation in the murine homolog of the APC gene. Science 1992;256:668–670.

36. Kozak CA, Bucan M, Goffinet A, Stephenson DA. Encyclopedia of the mouse genome V. Mouse *chromosome 5*. Mammalian Genome 1996;6:S97-S112.

37. Yamada S, Nakagama H, Toyota M, Ushijima T, Okada K, Sato K, Sugimura T, Nagao M. Cloning of rat BRCA2 and linkage mapping to chromosome 12. Mammalian Genome 1997;8:850–851.

38. McAllister KA, Haugen-Strano A, Hagevik S, Brownlee HA, Collins K, Futreal PA, Bennett LM, Wiseman RW. Characterization of the rat and mouse homologues of the BRCA2 breast cancer susceptibility gene. Cancer Res 1997;57:3121–3125.

39. Serova O, Montagna M, Torchard D, Narod SA, Tonin P, Sylla B, et al. A high incidence of *BRCA1* mutations in 20 breast-ovarian cancer families. Am J Hum Genet 1996;58:42–51.

40. Berman DB, Wagner-Costalas J, Schultz DC, Lynch HT, Daly M, Godwin AK. Two distinct origins of a common *BRCA1* mutation in breast-ovarian cancer families: a genetic study of 15 185delAG-mutation kindreds. Am J Hum Genet 1996;58:1166–1176.

41. Tonin PN, Mes-Masson AM, Futreal PA, Morgan K, Mahon M, Foulkes WD, et al. Founder BRCA1 and BRCA2 mutations in French Canadian breast and ovarian cancer families. Am J Hum Genet 1998; 63:1341–1351.

42. Katagiri T, Emi M, Ito I, Kobayashi K, Yoshimoto M, Iwase T, et al. Mutations in the *BRCA1* gene in Japanese breast cancer patients. Hum Mutat 1996;7:334–339.

43. Montagna M, Santacatterina M, Corneo B, Menin C, Serova O, Lenoir GM, Chieco-Bianchi L, D'Andrea E. Identification of seven new *BRCA1* germline mutations in italian breast and breast/ovarian cancer families. Cancer Res 1996;56:5466–5469.

44. Johannsson O, Ostermeyer EA, Hakansson S, Friedman LS, Johansson U, Sellberg G, et al. Founding *BRCA1* mutations in hereditary breast and ovarian cancer in southern Sweden. Am J Hum Genet 1996; 58:441–450.

45. Huusko P, Paakkonen K, Launonen V, Poyhonen M, Blanco G, Kauppila A, et al. Evidence of founder mutations in Finnish BRCA1 and BRCA2 families. Am J Hum Genet 1998;62:1544–1588.

46. Arason A, Jonasdottir A, Barkardottir RB, Bergthorsson JT, Teare MD, Easton DF, Egilsson V. A population study of mutations and LOH at breast cancer gene loci in tumours from sister pairs: two recurrent mutations seem to account for all BRCA1/BRCA2 linked breast cancer in Iceland. J Med Genet 1998;35:446–449.

47. Peelen T, vanVliet M, Petrij-Bosch A, Mieremet R, Czabo C, vandenOuweland A, et al. High proportion of novel mutations in BRCA1 with strong founder effects among Dutch and Belgian hereditary Breast and Ovarian Cancer Families. Am J Hum Genet 1998;60, 1041–1049.

48. Petrij-Bosch A, Peelen T, van Vliet M, van Eijk R, Olmer R, Drüsedau M, et al. BRCA1 genomic deletions are major founder mutations in Dutch breast cancer patients. Nat Genet 1997;17:341–345.

49. Offit K, Gilewski T, McGuire P, Schluger A, Hampel H, Brown K, et al. Germline *BRCA1* 185delAG mutations in Jewish women with breast cancer. Lancet 1996;347:1643–1645.

50. Tonin P, Serova O, Lenoir G, Lynch H, Durocher F, Simard J, Morgan K, Narod S. *BRCA1* mutations in Ashkenazi Jewish women letter. Am J Hum Genet 1995;57:189.

51. Friedman LS, Szabo CI, Ostermeyer EA, Dowd P, Butler L, Park T, et al. Novel inherited mutations and variable expressivity of BRCA2 I alleles including the founder mutation 185delAG in Ashkenazi Jewish families. Am J Hum Genet 1995;57:1284–1297.

52. Wu LC, Wnag ZW, Tsan JT, Spillman MA, Phung A, Xu XL, et al. Identification of a RING protein that can interact *in vivo* with the *BRCA1* gene product. Nat Genet 1996;14:430–440.

53. Weber BL. Types of mutations found in *BRCA1*. Cancer J 1996;2:302.

54. Swensen J, Hoffman M, Skolnick MH, Neuhausen SL. Identification of a 14 kb deletion involving the promoter region of BRCA1 in a breast cancer family. Hum Mol Genet 1997;6:1513–1517.

55. Couch FJ, Garber J, Kiousis S, Calzone K, Hauser ER, Merajver SD, et al. Genetic analysis of eight breast-ovarian cancer families with suspected *BRCA1* mutations. J Natl Cancer Inst Monogr 1995; 9–14.

56. Fitzgerald MG, MacDonald DJ, Krainer M, Hoover I, O'Neil E, Unsal H, et al. Germ-line *BRCA1* mutations in Jewish and non-Jewish women with early-onset breast cancer. N Engl J Med 1996;334: 137–142.

57. Neuhausen SL, Mazoyer S, Friedman L, Stratton M, Offit K, Caligo A, et al. Haplotype and phenotype analysis of six recurrent *BRCA1* mutations in 61 families: results of an international study. Am J Hum Genet 1996;58:271–280.

58. Struewing JP, Brody LC, Erdos MR, Kase RG, Giambarresi TR, Smith SA, Collins FS, Tucker MA. Detection of eight *BRCA1* mutations in 10 breast/ovarian cancer families, including 1 family with male breast cancer. Am J Hum Genet 1995;57:1–7.

59. Rodenhiser D, Chakraborty P, Andrews J, Ainsworth P, Mancini D, Lopes E, Singh S. Heterogeneous point mutations in the *BRCA1* breast cancer susceptibility gene occurs in high frequency at the site of homonucleotide tracts, short repeats and methlatable CpG/CpNpG motifs. Oncogene 1996;12: 2623–2629.

60. Rice JC, Massey-Brown KS, Futscher BW. Aberrant methylation of the BRCA1 CpG island promoter is associated with decreased BRCA1 mRNA in sporadic breast cancer cells. Oncogene 1998;17:1807–1812.

61. Cropp CS, Nevanlinna HA, Pyrhonen S, Stenman UH, Salmikangas P, Albertsen H, White R, Callahan R. Evidence for involvement of *BRCA1* in sporadic breast carcinomas. Cancer Res 1994;54:2548–2551.

62. Hosking L, Trowsdale J, Nicolai H, Solomon E, Foulkes W, Stamp G, Signer E, Jeffreys A. A somatic *BRCA1* mutation in an ovarian tumour. Nat Genet 1995;9:343,344.

63. Merajver SD, Pham TM, Caduff RF, Chen M, Poy EL, Cooney KA, et al. Somatic mutations in the *BRCA1* gene in sporadic ovarian tumours. Nat Genet 1995;9:439–443.

64. Zittoun RA, Mandelli F, Willemze R, de Witte T, Labar B, Resegotti L, et al. Autologous or allogeneic bone marrow transplantation compared with intensive chemotherapy in acute myelogenous leukemia.

European Organization for Research and Treatment of Cancer (EORTC) and the Gruppo Italiano Malattie Ematologiche Maligne dell'Adulto (GIMEMA) Leukemia Cooperative Groups. N Engl J Med 1995;332:217–223.

65. Dobrovic A, Simpfendorfer D. Methylation of the BRCA1 gene in sporadic breast cancer. Cancer Res 1997;57:3347–3350.

66. Phelan CM, Lancaster JM, Tonin P, Gumbs C, Cochran C, Carter R, et al. Mutation analysis of the *BRCA2* gene in 49 site-specific breast cancer families. Nat Genet 1996;13:120–122.

67. Lancaster JM, Wooster R, Mangion J, Phelan CM, Cochran C, Cumbs C, et al. *BRCA2* mutations in primary breast and ovarian cancers. Nat Genet 1996;13:238–240.

68. Thorlacius S, Olafsdottir G, Tryggvadottir L, Neuhausen S, Jonasson JG, Tavtigian SV, et al. Single *BRCA2* mutation in male and female breast cancer families from Iceland with varied cancer phenotypes. Nat Genet 1996;13:117–119.

69. Neuhausen S, Gilewski T, Norton L, Tran T, McGuire P, Swensen J, et al. Recurrent *BRCA2* 6174delT mutations in Ashkenazi Jewish women affected by breast cancer. Nat Genet 1996;13:126–128.

70. Cleton-Jansen A-M, Collins N, Lakhani SR, Weissenbach J, Devilee P, Cornelisse CJ, Stratton MR. Loss of heterozygosity in sporadic breast tumors at the BRCA2 lovus on chromosome 13q12-q13. Br J Cancer 1995;72:1241–1244.

71. Foster KA, Harrington P, Kerr J, Russell P, DiCioccio RA, Scott IV, et al. Somatic and germline mutations of the *BRCA2* gene in sporadic ovarian cancer. Cancer Res 1996;56:3622–3625.

72. Kelsell DP, DSpurr NK, Barnes DM, Gusterson B, Bishop DT. Combined loss of *BRCA1/BRCA2* in grade 3 breast carcinomas. Lancet 1996;347:1554,1555.

73. Schutte M, da Costa LT, Hahn SA, Moskaluk C, Hoque AT, Rozenblum E, et al. Identification by representational difference analysis of a homozygous deletion in pancreatic carcinoma that lies within the *BRCA2* region. Proc Natl Acad Sci USA 1995;92:5950–5954.

74. Goggins M, Schutte M, Lu J, Moskaluk CA, Weinstein CL, Petersen GM, et al. Germline *BRCA2* gene mutations in patients with apparently sporadic pancreatic carcinomas. Cancer Res 1996;56:5360–5364.

75. Ozcelik H, Schmocker B, Di Nicola N, Shi XH, Langer B, Moore M, et al. Germline BRCA2 6174delT mutations in Ashkenazi Jewish pancreatic cancer patients letter. Nat Genet 1997;16 :17–18.

76. Katagiri T, Nakamura Y, Miki Y. Mutations in the *BRCA2* gene in hepatocellular carcinomas. Cancer Res 1996;56:4575–4577.

77. Struewing J, Hartage P, Wacholder S, Baker SM, Berlin M, McAdams M, et al. Risk of cancer associated with specific mutations of *BRCA1* and *BRCA2* among Ashkenazi Jews. N Engl J Med 1997;336: 1401–1408.

78. Thorlacius S, Sigurdsson S, Bjarnadottir H, Olafsdottir G, Jonasson JG, Tryggvadottir L, Tulinius H, Eyfj'ord JE. Study of a single BRCA2 mutation with high carrier frequency in a small population. Am J Hum Genet 1997;60:1079–1084.

79. Gayther SA, Mangion J, Russell P, Seal S, Barfoot R, Ponder B, Stratton MR, Easton D. Variation of risks of breast and ovarian cancer associated with different germline mutations of the BRCA2 gene. Nat Genet 1997;15:103–105.

80. Thompson ME, Jensen RA, Obermiller PS, Page DL, Holt JT. Decreased expression of *BRCA1* accelerates growth and is often present during sporadic breast cancer progression. Nat Genet 1995;9:444–450.

81. Gudas JM, Nguyen H, Li T, Cowan KH. Hormone-dependent regulation of *BRCA1* in human breast cancer cells. Cancer Res 1995;55:4561–4565.

82. Romagnolo D, Annab LA, Thompson TE, Risinger JI, Terry LA, Barrett JC, Afshari CA. Estrogen upregulation of BRCA1 expression with no effect on localization. Mol Carcinog 1998;22:102–109.

83. Marquis ST, Rajan JV, Wynshaw-Boris A, Xu J, Yin GY, Abel KJ, Weber BL, Cho X. The development pattern of BRCA1 expression implies a role in differentiation of the breast and other tissues. Nat Genet 1995;11:17–26.

84. Marks JR, Huper G, Vaughn JP, Davis PL, Norris J, McDonnell DP, et al. BRCA1 expression is not directly responsive to estrogen. Oncogene 1997;14:115–121.

85. Holt JT, Thompson ME, Szabo C, Robinson-Benion C, Arteaga CL, King M-C, Jensen RA. Growth retardation and tumour inhibition by *BRCA1*. Nat Genet 1996;12:298–302.

86. Rao VN, Shao NS, Ahmad M, Reddy ESP. Antisense RNA to the putative tumor suppressor gene *BRCA1* transforms mouse fibroblasts. Oncogene 1996;12:523–528.

87. Lane TF, Deng C, Elson A, Lyu MS, Kozak CA, Leder P. Expression of BRCA1 is associated with terminal differentiation of ectodermally and mesodermally derived tissues in mice. [published erratum appears in Genes Dev 1996;10:365]. Genes Dev 1995;9:2712–2722.

88. Haken R, de la Pompa JL, Sirard C, Mo R, Woo M, Hakem A, et al. The tumor suppressor gene BRCA1 is required for embryonic cellular proliferation in the mouse. Cell 1996;85:1009–1023.

89. Liu CY, Flesken-Nikitin A, Li S, Zeng Y, Lee WH. Inactivation of the mouse BRCA1 gene leads to failure in the morphogenesis of the egg cylinder in early postimplantation development. Genes Dev 1996;10:1835–1843.

90. Haken R, de la Pompa J, Elia A, Potter J, Mak TW. Partial rescue of BRCA1$^{5-6}$ early embryonic lethality by *p53* or *p21* null mutation. Nat Genet 1997;16:298–302.

91. Cressman VL, Backlund DC, Hicks EM, Gowen LC, Godfrey V, Koller BK. Mammary tumor formation in p53- and BRCA1-deficient mice. Cell Growth Differ 1999;10:1–10.

92. Gowen LC, Johnson BL, Latour AM, Sulik KK, Koller BH. *BRCA1* deficiency results in early embryonic lethality characterized by neuroepithelial abnormalities. Nat Genet 1996;12:191–194.

93. Shen SX, Weaver Z, Xu X, Li C, Weinstein M, Chen L, et al. A targeted disruption of the murine BRCA1 gene causes gamma-irradiation hypersensitivity and genetic instability. Oncogene 1998;17:3115–3124.

94. Scully R, Chen J, Plug A, Xiao Y, Weaver D, Feunteun J, Ashley T, Livingston DM. Association of BRCA1 with Rad51 in mitotic and meiotic cells. Cell 1997;88:265–275.

95. Sharan SK, Morimatsu M, Albrecht U, Lim D-S, Regel E, Dinh C, et al. Embryonic lethality and radiation hypersensitivity mediated by Rad51 in mice lacking BRCA2. Nature 1997;386:804–810.

96. Suzuki A, de la Pompa JL, Haken R, Elia A, Yoshida R, Mo R, et al. BRCA2 is required for embryonic cellular proliferation in the mouse. Genes Dev 1997;11:1242–1252.

97. Vaughn JP, Cirisano FD, Huper G, Berchuck A, Futreal PA, Marks JR, Iglehart JD. Cell cycle control of *BRCA2*. Cancer Res 1996;56:4590–4594.

98. Scully R, Chen J, Plug A, Xiao Y, Weaver D, Feunteun J, Ashley T, Livingston DM. Association of BRCA1 with Rad51 in mitotic and meiotic cells. Cell 1997;88:265–275.

99. Connor F, Bertwistle D, Mee PJ, Ross GM, Swift S, Grigorieva E, Tybulewicz VLJ, Ashworth A. Tumorigenesis and a DNA repair defect in mice with a truncating BRCA2 mutation. Nat Genet 1997;17:423–430.

100. Gowen LC, Avrutskaya AV, Latour AM, Koller GH, Leadon SA. BRCA1 required for transcription-coupled repair of oxidative DNA damage. Science 1998;281:1009–1012.

101. Scully R, Chen J, Ochs RL, Keegan K, Hoekstra M, Feunteun J, Livingston DM. Dynamic changes if BRCA1 subnuclear location and phosphorylation state are initiated by DNA damage. Cell 1997;90:1–20.

102. Patel KJ, Yu V, Lee H, Corcoran A, Thistlethwaite F, Evans MJ, et al. Involvement of BRCA2 in DNA repair. Mol Cell 1998;1:347–357.

103. Wong A, Pero R, Ormonde P, Tavtigian SV, Bartel P. RAD51 interacts with the evolutionarily conserved BRC motifs in the human breast cancer susceptibility gene BRCA2. J Biol Chem 1997;272:31,941–31,944.

104. Morimatsu M, Donoho G, Hasty P. Cells deleted for BRCA2 COOH terminus exhibit hypersensitivity to *y*-radiation and premature senescence. Cancer Res 1998;58:3441–3447.

105. Katagiri T, Saito H, Shinohara A, Ogawa H, Kamada N, Nakamura Y, Miki Y. Multiple possible sites of BRCA2 interacting with DNA repair protein RAD51. Genes Chromosomes Cancer 1998;21:217–222.

106. Chen PL, Chen CF, Chen Y, Xiao J, Sharp ZD, Lee WH. BRC repeats in BRCA2 are critical for RAD51 binding and resistance to methyl methanesulfonate treatment. Proc Natl Acad Sci USA 1995;95:5287–5292.

107. Ouchi T, Monteiro AN, August A, Aaronson SA, Hanafusa H. BRCA1 regulates p53-dependent gene expression. Proc Natl Acad Sci USA 1998;95:2302–2306.

108. Zhang H, Somasundaram K, Peng Y, Tian H, Bi D, Weber BL, el-Deiry WS. BRCA1 physically associates with p53 and stimulates its transcriptional activity. Oncogene 1998;16:1713–1721.

109. Crook T, Brooks LA, Crossland S, Osin P, Barker KT, Waller J, et al. p53 mutation with frequent novel condons but not a mutator phenotype in BRCA1 and BRCA2-associated breast tumours. Oncogene 1998;17:1681–1689.

110. Somasundaram K, Zhang H, Zeng YX, Houvras Y, Peng Y, Wu GS, et al. Arrest of the cell cycle by the tumour-suppressor BRCA1 requires the CDK-inhibitor p21WAF1/CiP1. Nature 1997;389:187–190.

111. Wu LC, Wang ZW, Tsan JT, Spillman MA, Phung A, Xu XL, et al. Identification of a RING protein that can interact *in vivo* with the BRCA1 gene product. Nat Genet 1996;14:430–440.

112. Burke TF, Cocke KS, Lemke SJ, Angleton E, Becker GW, Beckmann RP. Identification of a BRCA1-associated kinase with potential biological relevance. Oncogene 1998;16:1031–1040.

113. Jensen DE, Proctor M, Marquis ST, Gardner HP, Ha SI, Chodosh LA, et al. BAP1: a novel ubiquitin hydrolase which binds to the BRCA1 RING finger and enhances BRCA1-mediated cell growth suppression. Oncogene 1998;16:1097–1112.

114. Scully R, Anderson SF, Chao DM, Wei W, Ye L, Young RA, Livingston DM, Parvin JD. BRCA1 is a component of the RNA polymerase II holoenzyme. Proc Natl Acad Sci USA 1997;94:5605–5610.

115. Anderson SF, Schlegel BP, Nakajima T, Wolpin ES, Parvin JD. BRCA1 protein is linked to the RNa polymerase II holoenzyme complex via RNA helicase A. Nat Genet 1998;19:254–256.

116. Jin Y, Xu XL, Yang MC, Wei F, Ayi TC, Bowcock AM, Baer R. Cell cycle-dependent colocalization of BARD1 and BRCA1 proteins in discrete nuclear domains. Proc Natl Acad Sci USA 1997;94: 12,075–12,080.

117. Brzovic PS, Meza J, King MC, Klevit RE. The cancer-predisposing mutation C61G disrupts homodimer formation in the NH2-terminal BRCA1 RING finger domain. J Biol Chem 1998;273:7795–7799.

118. Thai TH, Du F, Tsan JT, Jin Y, Phung A, Spillman MA, et al. Mutations in the BRCA1-associated RING domain (BARD1) gene in primary breast, ovarian and uterine cancers. Hum Mol Genet 1998;7: 195–202.

119. Xin Y, Wu LC, Bowcock AM, Aronheim A, Baer R. The C-terminal (BRCT) domains of BRCA1 interact *in vivo* with CtIP, a protein implicated in the CtBP pathway of transcriptional repression. J Biol Chem 1998;273:25,388–25,392.

120. Karp SE, Tonin PN, Begin LR, Martinez JJ, Zhang JC, Pollak MN, Foulkes WD. Influence of BRCA1 mutations on nuclear grade and estrogen receptor status of breast carcinoma in Ashkenazi Jewish women. Cancer 1997;80:435–441.

121. Loman N, Johannsson O, Bendahl PO, Borg A, Ferno M, Olsson H. Steroid receptors in hereditary breast carcinomas associated with BRCA1 or BRCA2 mutations or unknown susceptibility genes. Cancer 1998;83:310–319.

122. Schmutzler RK, Bierhoff E, Werkausen T, Fimmers R, Speiser P, Kubista E, et al. Genomic deletions in the BRCA1, BRCA2 and TP53 regions associate with low expression of the estrogen receptor in sporadic breast carcinoma. Int J Cancer (Pred Oncol) 1997;74:322–325.

19

Role of Apoptosis and its Modulation by Bcl-2 Family Members in Breast and Prostate Cancer

Venil N. Sumantran, PHD,
David R. Beidler, PHD, and Max S. Wicha, MD

CONTENTS

OVERVIEW AND RELEVANCE OF APOPTOSIS

Apoptosis

Apoptosis is a process critical to tissue homeostasis. The term describes a series of morphological changes that result in selective cell removal, but does not instigate a general inflammatory response (for review, *see* refs. *1* and *2*). Apoptotic responses are involved in numerous systems, including development, maintenance of the immune system, and host defense against invasion/injury. In breast tissue, this selective cell death and removal process is critical to the tissue-remodeling found during pregnancy, lactation, and involution, as well as alterations during normal menstrual cycling. In addition, epithelial cells (ECs) in the normal adult prostate continuously turn over, and the androgen-dependent glandular ECs undergo rapid apoptosis following castration. The first descriptions of these morphological changes were in the early 1970s, in which apoptosis was characterized by cell shrinkage, nuclear condensation, and cytoplasmic blebbing *(3)*.

From: *Contemporary Endocrinology: Endocrine Oncology*
Edited by: S. P. Ethier © Humana Press Inc., Totowa, NJ

During these events, membrane integrity was maintained, thus permitting the dismantling and removal of specific apoptotic cells, without the initiation of widespread inflammatory responses. As a result of vigorous recent research, many of the molecular components responsible for these early morphological observations have been revealed.

The Study of Apoptosis in Caenorhabditis elegans

One of the most valuable model systems for the study of apoptosis has been the nematode *Caenorhabditis elegans (4,5)*. During *C. elegans* development, 131/1090 somatic cells that are produced undergo apoptosis. Through a series of genetic analyses, the deletion of two genes, *ced3* and *ced4*, were found to prevent all 131 apoptotic events. In contrast, deletion of a third gene, *ced9*, was found to cause the majority of developing worm cells to die, resulting in embryonic lethality. These findings proved that cell death originated in a genetically defined pathway, and was not just a random byproduct of faulty growth. Finally, the fact that the *ced3*, *ced4*, and *ced9* genes of *C. elegans* had homologous mammalian counterparts confirmed that apoptosis was not only genetically controlled, but its components were highly conserved throughout evolution.

The identification of the mammalian counterparts of this evolutionarily conserved gene family has provided critical information in the control of apoptosis in mammals. The mammalian homologs of *ced3* comprise a family of at least 12 cysteine proteases, called caspases *(6)*. Caspases are present in the cell as inactive precursors, which, upon activation, are cleaved into smaller subunits to form active tetramers *(7)*. Caspases have been grouped according to the size of their prodomains: Large prodomain caspases are involved in the upstream initiation of caspase activity; small prodomain caspases are downstream effectors of caspase activity. Once active, these cysteine proteases cleave a subset of proteins, including caspases themselves. Therefore, the activation of upstream regulatory caspases initiate a cascade of downstream caspases, which are believed to bring about the morphological changes characteristic of apoptosis. The *ced4* homolog, apaf-1, has been found to localize to the outer mitochondrial membrane *(8)*. Upon activation, apaf-1 acts as an adapter protein to bind and subsequently activate an upstream caspase, caspase-9, by interacting with the N-terminal prodomain of caspase-9 through a caspase recruitment domain (CARD) *(9)*. The antiapoptotic *ced9* was found to be homologous to the Bcl-2 family of proteins, which also resides on the outer mitochondrial membrane *(10)*. The *bcl*-2 gene (B-cell lymphoma gene 2) was first discovered by its involvement in the t(14;18) chromosomal translocation common to B-cell lymphomas *(11)*. The members of the bcl-2 family are responsible for the positive and negative regulation of apoptosis. The Bcl-2 family proteins possess the ability to homo- and heterodimerize with other members of the bcl-2 family. As a result, the relative ratios of positive and negative apoptotic Bcl-2 family members determine a cells fate upon apoptotic insult.

Mouse Knockout Models

Mouse knockout studies allowed the assessment of the importance and/or redundancy of individual caspase and bcl-2 family members in several apoptotic events. The phenotypes resulting from knockout mice revealed, not only the necessity of each protein in the apoptotic pathway, but also the role of the apoptotic pathway in development, homeostasis, and reaction to insult/stress. Knockouts of the various caspase family members have revealed divergent roles for these family members. Targeted disruption of caspase-

1, -2, and –11, resulted in negligible effects on apoptotic responses in these mice; alterations in cytokine processing were observed *(12,13)*. However, caspase-8 $^{-/-}$ mice were embryonic lethal at d 11, with abnormal cardiac development *(14)*. Caspase-8$^{-/-}$ mice were also resistant to tumor necrosis factor receptor 1 (TNFR1) or CD95-induced apoptosis, but were sensitive to chemotherapeutic and dexamethasone-induced apoptosis. In contrast, knockouts of caspases-3 and -9 did not affect cardiac development, but had significant effects on brain development *(15–17)*. In contrast to caspase-8$^{-/-}$ mice, caspase-3$^{-/-}$ and -9$^{-/-}$ mice were found to be resistant to apoptosis induced by UV, γ-irradiation, and dexamethasone, but only caspase-3$^{-/-}$ and not caspase-9$^{-/-}$ mice were also resistant to TNF/CD95-induced apoptosis. The individual roles of the caspases were also found to be cell-type-specific; for example, caspase-3$^{-/-}$ ES cells were resistant to the stimuli mentioned above, but caspase-3$^{-/-}$ thymocytes were sensitive to all of these agents. Finally, caspase-9$^{-/-}$ thymocytes were resistant to apoptosis induced by γ-irradiation and dexamethasone, but not by apoptosis induced by UV irradiation. The dependency of a given caspase was found to be specific to the apoptotic stimuli. Therefore, although there is a measure of redundancy within the caspase family, it appears that distinct caspases (or caspase subsets) have distinct roles in apoptotic responses, and these roles are cell-type- and stimuli-specific.

Mice deficient in bcl-2 develop normally, which could indicate redundancy within the antiapoptotic family members *(18)*. Shortly after birth, however, defects appear in a subset of locations, including the kidney, immune system, and the small intestine. In contrast to bcl-2, bcl-XL knockout mice were embryonic lethal on d 13, and were characterized by elevated levels of apoptosis in the hematopoietic and central nervous systems *(19)*. Mice that had the proapoptotic protein, Bax, deleted, developed normally, but were found to have increased numbers of lymphoid cells, and Bax-deficient males were sterile because of gross abnormalities in the seminiferous tubules *(20)*.

Caspase and bcl-2 family knockouts produced abnormalities in a subset of organs during development, but mice deficient in apaf-1 demonstrated the central importance of this molecule in apoptosis, since virtually all developmental events that required apoptosis were affected *(8,20,21)*. However, not all apoptotic stimuli require apaf-1, because there were forms of apoptosis that were unaffected or partially inhibited by deletion of apaf-1 (such as Fas/CD95), which suggests that additional pathways independent from apaf-1 exist.

Role of Apoptosis in Tumor Progression

Not only does apoptosis play an important role in development, but it also has been shown to serve a vital function in tumor progression. The *bcl-2* gene was originally identified as a novel gene that was overexpressed in follicular lymphoma, as the result of a 14;18 chromosomal translocation *(22)*. This was the first description of an oncogene that did not deregulate cell division, but rather served to decrease the frequency of cell death. In addition, the regulation of apoptosis by bcl-2 family members was responsible for solid tumor progression in a mouse islet β-cell model of multistage carcinogenesis *(23)*. Although apoptotic levels were elevated in the early hyperplastic stage and peaked in the intermediate angiogenic stage, a significant reduction in apoptosis was necessary for progression into the final stage of solid tumor formation. A shift from low levels of Bcl-XL in the hyperplastic and angiogenic stages to higher Bcl-XL levels in the solid tumor stage was found to be responsible for the regulation of apoptosis throughout tumor progression. Also, the transition from small to large solid tumor formation required the continued elevation of Bcl-Xl levels in tumors, which suggested the regulation of apoptosis was the cause, not the effect, of tumor growth. Finally, a recent study concluded that, not only do caspase-9 and apaf-1 serve as essential downstream components of Myc-induced apoptosis, but deletion of either caspase-9 or apaf-1 enhanced the tumorgenicity of mouse embryo fibroblasts in immunocompromised mice *(24)*.

APOPTOTIC PATHWAYS

TNFR1/Fas/APO-1 Apoptotic Pathway

Much progress has been made on the apoptotic pathway(s) that mediates apoptosis induced by the cytokine surface receptors TNFR1/Fas/APO-1 *(25)*. TNFR1 and Fas/APO-1 are a family of surface receptors that are characterized by the presence of a cytoplasmic tail that contains a conserved region called the death domain. Ligand binding leads to receptor oligomerization, which triggers the recruitment of an adapter protein called Fas-associated death domain protein (FADD) via protein–protein interactions through the death domain. The result of these interactions is the formation of a protein complex, termed the death-inducing signaling complex (DISC) complex, in which caspase-8 is recruited by virtue of the binding of its prodomain to receptor-bound FADD, through a second protein interaction motif called the death effector domain. The DISC complex releases active caspase-8, which ultimately activates a cascade of downstream caspases that are responsible for the apoptotic response. The steps leading directly from receptor activation to caspase activation seem straightforward, but questions on the role of the antiapoptotic bcl-2 family members, as well as the role of mitochondria in TNF/Fas-induced apoptosis, remained unanswered.

Apoptotic Pathway Mediated Through Mitochondria

A second apoptotic pathway has recently emerged that involves a series of events located on the outer mitochondrial membrane, which ultimately leads to caspase activation by a series of protein–protein interactions *(26,27)*. Instead of receptor oligomerization found in the TNFR1/Fas/APO-1 pathway, this pathway is triggered by the release of the mitochondrial protein cytochrome C in response to mitochondrial insult. Once released from the inner membrane space, cytochrome C, along with adenosine triphosphate (ATP) or dATP, binds the adapter molecule, apaf-1, and induces a conformational change in apaf-1 that allows for caspase-9 binding through CARD domain interactions found on both proteins. As with caspase-8 in the DISC complex, the apaf-1–caspase-9 complex results in the release of active caspase-9, which in turn cleaves downstream caspases (caspase-3) to execute the apoptotic response (Fig. 1). In addition to the release of cytochrome C and subsequent caspase activation, the mitochondrial damage causes the disruption of the mitochondrial transmembrane potential (Ψ), which causes the increase of reactive oxygen species and loss of ATP levels. These widespread cellular insults may ultimately lead, not to a controlled apoptotic response, but to a spontaneous necrotic cell death. Therefore, the point of commitment to cell death (apoptotic or necrotic) may reside on the release of cytochrome C and the resulting disruption of mitochondrial transmembrane potential.

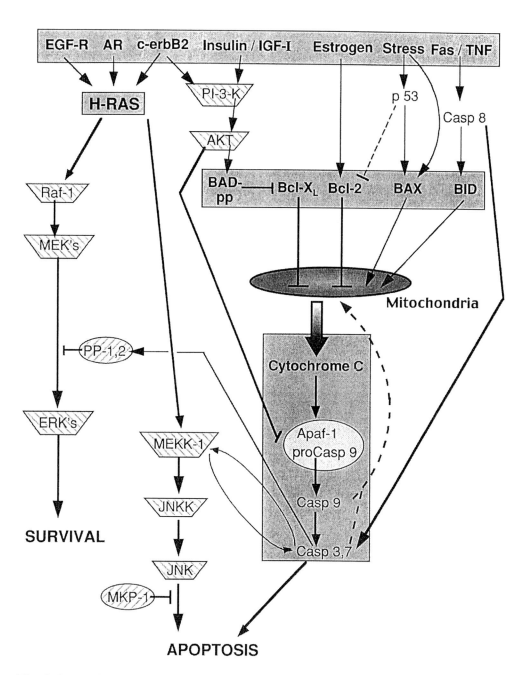

Fig. 1. Interactions between apoptosis and survival pathways in a BC or PC cell. The H-Ras-dependent MAPK pathway consists of kinase cascades that induce cell survival or apoptosis. The EGF, androgen, and c-erbB-2 receptors stimulate this pathway. This pathway interacts with specfic caspases, so that activation of caspase-3 and -7 is dependent on the MEKK-1 kinase. These caspases also activate protein phosphatases 1 and 2 (PP-1, -2) which in turn block the survival arm of the pathway (ERK). GF-induced PI-3-k promotes survival in two ways: blockade of caspase-9 activation and sequesteration of Bad, so that Bcl-xL remains active. Bcl-2 itself is induced by estrogen.

Role of bcl-2 Family in Apoptotic Pathways

How does the bcl-2 family fit into these apoptotic pathways? It appears that bcl-2 family members, which have been shown to reside on the outer mitochondrial membrane, govern the release of cytochrome C. Antiapoptotic members, such as Bcl-xL, have been shown to inhibit the release of cytochrome C in response to insult; proapoptotic members, such as BAX, in response to p53 induction, can stimulate the cytochrome C release. When it was found that the active caspase-8 could cleave Bid, a proapoptotic bcl-2 family member, and truncated Bid went on to release cytochrome C, a link between the TNFR1/ Fas/APO-1 and mitochondrial pathways was finally made *(28–30)*. The current models allow for two different modes of apoptosis that can be induced by TNFR1/Fas/APO-1 activation: one is characterized by abundant caspase-8, which can directly activate downstream caspases; a second mode involves the cleavage of Bid by caspase-8, which in turn activates the mitochodrial-based apoptotic response, with the release of cytochrome C *(31)*.

Therefore, the bcl-2 family members are responsible for the regulation of the release of cytochrome C, which in turn regulates the activation of the apaf-1 adapter molecule. Since apaf-1$^{-/-}$ mice were found to be deficient in virtually every apoptotic event required for development, this pathway must be the dominant pathway utilized during development. As a result, the relative proportions of proapoptotic and antiapoptotic bcl-2 members is of paramount importance in the regulation of apoptosis.

THE ROLE OF BCL-2 FAMILY
IN BREAST AND PROSTATE MALIGNANCIES

Expression Levels of bcl-2 Family Members
in Normal vs Neoplastic Mammary and Prostate Glands

Cyclic changes in bcl-2 expression occur within the mammary gland. Thus, high bcl-2 expression is observed in the resting and pregnant phases of the mammary gland. Bcl-2 expression peaks within the mammary epithelium, just before the gland enters the proliferative phase. By d 28, the proliferative rates, levels of estrogen, and bcl-2 decrease within the mammary gland *(32)*. During lactation and involution, bcl-2 levels drop sharply, but Bax levels are high *(32,33)*. Apoptosis occurs during the involution stage, which is consistent with in vitro studies showing that loss of attachment of normal mammary epithelium to the basement membrane induces apoptosis. Studies on immortalized human mammary epithelial MCF-10A cells show that bcl-2 expression is modestly increased by epidermal growth factor (EGF) and insulin, and that ectopic Bcl-2 expression protects these cells from apoptosis induced by growth factor (GF) removal *(34)*. Conversely, Bax expression is unaffected by these GFs, but high cell density correlates with increased Bax expression in these cells *(34)*.

Immunohistochemical studies show that bcl-2 or Bcl-xL are overexpressed in up to 80% of human breast cancers (BCs). Typically, bcl-2 overexpression occurs in estrogen receptor (ER)-positive tumors *(35)*; Bcl-xL overexpression occurs in the ER-negative late-stage cancers associated with poor prognosis *(36)*. Overexpression of bcl-2 is also common in metastatic and hormone-refactory prostate cancers (PCs) *(37,38)*. The mechanisms underlying overexpression of Bcl-2 and Bcl-xL proteins in breast and prostate tumor cells are not clear. Because these proteins confer resistance to cell death, tumor cells that overexpress them have a clear selective advantage during carcinogenesis. Tumors that overexpress Bcl-xL are often multidrug-resistant *(39)*.

In normal prostate and in androgen-dependent PC, the glandular epithelium depends on androgen for growth and survival, i.e., androgens inhibit cell death *(37,38)*. Upon castration, the normal prostate rapidly undergoes apoptosis, which is accompanied by elevated levels of c-myc and the tumor suppressor gene, *p53*, which can induce apoptosis *(37,38)*.

Regulation of the Apoptotic Threshold

The potential of a cell to undergo programmed cell death (apoptosis) in response to stress is defined as the apoptotic threshold. The Bcl-2 protein family primarily controls the apoptotic threshold, which is determined by the ratio of survival-promoting proteins (such as Bcl-2, Bcl-xL, Mcl-1, and Bag-1) to proteins that promote death (Bax, Bad, Bak, Bid, Bik, and so on) *(10,40)*. In some cases, the apoptotic threshold is regulated by apoptosis-inducing agents that directly alter levels of transcription of the *bcl-2*, *bax*, or *bcl*-x genes. In other cases, apoptosis-inducing agents regulate the apoptotic threshold by altering function of members of the Bcl-2 protein family.

The regulatory mechanisms that control the activities of Bcl-2 family members involve the H-Ras-dependent MAP-kinase (MAPK) pathway. As shown in Fig. 1, this pathway includes kinase cascades that bring about proliferation (H-Ras-Raf-ERKs) or apoptosis mediated by stress kinases (H-Ras-[MEKK]-[MEK]-[JNK]) *(41)*. These two arms of the H-Ras-dependent pathway play a major role in determining the apoptotic threshold. Thus, the functions of specific Bcl-2 family members and caspases are modulated by phosphorylation events mediated by serine (Ser) kinases in the MAPK pathway. Since phosphatases can attenuate the MAPK pathway *(41)*, the effects of mitogen-inducible phosphatases on Bcl-2 family members, caspases, and apoptosis are under investigation. In addition to the MAPK pathway, factors regulating growth of the mammary and prostate glands, such as insulin-like growth factor I (IGF-I), EGF, and steroid hormones, regulate cell survival and sensitivity to apoptosis *(32,42)*. The effects of IGF-I, EGF, and the H-Ras-dependent MAPK pathway, on the expression and function of Bcl-2 family members, will be discussed.

Thus, the apoptotic threshold depends on a dynamic balance between GF-dependent pathways, which signal mitoses and cell survival, and those inducing apoptosis. Transcriptional and posttranslational modulation of Bcl-2 family members, and key signaling molecules outside of the Bcl-2 family, affect the apoptotic threshold. A detailed discussion of each of these mechanisms follows.

Transcriptional Regulation of Bcl-2, Bcl-xL, and Bax in the Mammary Gland

Does the H-Ras–MAPK pathway affect Bcl-2 expression? Studies in hematopoietic cells expressing an inducible H-Ras show that interleukin 3 treatment inhibited apoptosis by transcriptional induction of bcl-2 and bcl-xL (but not bax), in a H-Ras-dependent manner *(43)*. There are lesions in BC that can constitutively and chronically activate H-Ras-dependent signaling in the absence of an activated H-*ras* oncogene. For example, erbB family members may be able to activate the H-Ras-dependent MAPK pathway, which may explain why there are BCs that exhibit constititive MAPK activation without H-ras mutation *(42)*. Overexpression of EGFR and/or erb-B2 can also lead to chronic activation of the H-Ras-dependent MAPK pathway, typically resulting in cell proliferation and/or survival *(42,44)*. This may cause constitutive bcl-2 expression, and may be manifested as resistance to apoptosis. R-Ras is reported to associate with Bcl-2 *(45)*.

Are bcl-2 family members transcriptionally regulated by GFs, tumor suppressor genes, and oncogenes? In vitro studies show that estrogen increases the ratio of bcl-2:bax in ER-positive MCF-7 BC cells, without altering bcl-xL *(46,47)*. This is consistent with data showing that estrogen withdrawal causes decreased growth and increased apoptosis in MCF-7 cell xenografts in vivo *(47)*. Subsequent treatment of estrogen-deprived cells with estrogen increased transcription of bcl-2, but not bax *(46,47)*. Prolonged co-culture of MCF-7 cells with estrogen and the antiestrogen, tamoxifen (TAM), did not alter the ratio of bcl-2:bax *(47)*. In fact, TAM treatment enhanced Bcl-2 expression and reduced tumor growth in ER-positive patients *(48)*. In several human BCs, the expression of Bcl-2 is inversely correlated with p53 expression. Overexpression of mutant p53 in MCF-7 cells was shown to induce downregulation of bcl-2 mRNA and protein *(49)*. It is not clear whether wild-type p53 has a similar effect on bcl-2 transcription.

Bax is the major proapoptotic member of the Bcl-2 family, which mediates cell death in response to several stresses, in a caspase-independent manner *(50)*. The p53 tumor suppressor gene induces bax transcription, and Bax-mediated apoptosis is p53-dependent *(51,52)*. Bax levels are high in normal breast epithelium, but decreased Bax-α expression is associated with resistance to apoptosis in response to combination chemotherapy (Chemo) in metastatic breast adenocarcinoma *(33)*. A large percentage of breast tumors with decreased Bax expression have lost Bcl-2 expression *(53)*. Conversely, overexpression of Bax can increase sensitivity to drug- and radiation-induced apoptosis *(50)*.

Transcriptional Regulation of Bcl-2 in the Prostate

In the normal prostate, Bcl-2 expression is negligible. Androgens induce bcl-2 expression in an androgen-dependent PC cell line, LNCaP *(32,37)*. However, high bcl-2 expression can persist after androgen withdrawal, thus permitting development of androgen-independent tumors, i.e,, androgen-independent tumors have elevated Bcl-2 expression *(32, 37)*. LNCaP cells are not tumorigenic in vivo, but overexpression of Bcl-2 in these cells results in rapid formation of tumors *(32,37)*. Mouse models of castration show that almost all PCs show decreased growth in response to androgen withdrawal, which is accompanied by an increased sensitivity to apoptosis in some, but not all, prostate tumor models *(32,37)*.

Posttranslational Modulation of Bcl-2 and Bcl-xL Function

Because Bcl-2 and Bcl-xL form ion channels that traverse the mitochondrial membrane *(54,55)*, changes in their three-dimensional structure can radically alter function. Posttanslational modification of these proteins provides an important mechanism to regulate their function. It has been reported that microtubule disrupters, such as taxanes (taxol, taxotere, and vincristine), phosphorylate and inactivate Bcl-2 and Bcl-xL in MCF-7 cells *(56,57)*. The H-Ras-dependent Raf-1 kinase may phosphorylate Bcl-2/Bcl-xL on Ser/threonine (Thr) residues in vivo *(56)*. Phosphorylation of Bcl-2 induced by taxol has also been reported in the androgen-independent PC-3 PC cell line. The phosphorylated Bcl-2 was inactive, to the extent that it was unable to form heterodimers with Bax *(57)*. Inactivation of Bcl-2/Bcl-xL may not be a necessary step in taxol-induced apoptosis, since the Bcl-2-negative DU-145 PC cell line is resistant to taxol *(57)*. The stress kinase p54-SAPK/JNK-β is activated by taxanes in MCF-7 cells, and can phosphorylate Bcl-2 when it is co-expressed with bcl-2 in COS cells *(58)*. Whether JNK-β phosphorylates Bcl-2 or Bcl-xL in response to these agents in BC and PCs in vivo is unknown.

The above data suggest that phosphorylation inactivates the survival-promoting function of Bcl-2/Bcl-xL. However, recent mutational studies show that an N-terminal cytoplasmic loop domain of Bcl-2 (and Bcl-xL) has critical phosphorylation sites required for the antiapoptotic function in HL-60 leukemia cells *(59)*. Thus, transfectants expressing Bcl-2 or Bcl-xL lacking the loop domain were sensitive to taxol-induced apoptosis; cells expressing full-length Bcl-2 /Bcl-xL were resistant to taxol *(59)*. However, this study also demonstrated that the loop domain is not required for the antiapoptotic function of Bcl-2 against ara-C- or etoposide-induced apoptosis. This is consistent with a report showing that Bcl-2 phosphorylation correlates with decreased apoptosis in Jurkat cells treated with the protein kinase C (PKC) activator Bryostatin-1 *(60)*.

These conflicting data on the effects of phosphorylation on Bcl-2 and Bcl-xL function may be dependent on which residues are phosphorylated. Thus, residues phosphorylated in response to taxanes vs Bryostatin-1 may differ, and result in opposite effects on Bcl-2/ Bcl-xL function. It is also possible that Bcl-2/Bcl-xL phosphorylation results in different effects on Bcl-2/Bcl-xL function in Jurkat cells and HL-60 cells, vs MCF-7 human BC and PC cells.

Regulating turnover of bcl-2 family members also affects expression levels and function of the Bcl-2 protein family. Thus, upon cleavage by caspases, both Bcl-2 and Bcl-xL can be converted into forms that induce apoptosis *(61,62)*. The stability of the Bax-α protein can be affected by Bcl-2 levels. A study in Jurkat cells showed that Bcl-2 over-expression causes stabilization of Bax *(63)*. Such posttranslational mechanisms may be a way to maintain the ratio of Bcl-2/Bax within a certain physiologically relevant range in BC and PC.

Posttranslational Modulation of Bad Function

The activity of another Bcl-2 family member has been shown to be primarily regulated by phosphorylation. Bad is a proapoptotic protein that acts by heterodimerizing preferentially with Bcl-xL and blocking its survival function *(64)*. Figure 1 shows that GFs, such as interleukin 3, insulin, and IGF-I, recruit and activate PI-3-kinase (PI-3-K), which in turn activates the AKT kinase. Active AKT phosphorylates Bad, so that it cannot dimerize with Bcl-xL. Thus, Bcl-xL is free to perform its survival function, and phosphorylated Bad is sequestered in the cytosol as a complex with 14-3-3, a Raf-1 kinase-binding protein *(65–67)*. Active Raf-1 kinase also mediates phosphorylation of Bad *(66,67)*. Immunohistochemical studies suggest that normal breast tissue and some PCs have high expression of Bad protein *(68)*. The significance of this is unclear. Whether the Bad protein is phosphorylated or not in vivo also remains to be determined.

Modulation of expression levels, function, stability, localization, and dimerization status of Bad, Bax, Bcl-2, and Bcl-xL has direct effects on the apoptotic threshold.

HORMONAL EFFECTS ON THE APOPTOTIC THRESHOLD

The general mechanisms regulating expression and activity of Bcl-2 family members have been discussed. The unique hormonal environments of the mammary and prostate glands modulate the apoptotic threshold by affecting bcl-2 family members and/or activity of the H-Ras-dependent signaling pathways. This subheading discusses the regulation of the apoptotic threshold in BCs overexpressing different hormone receptors. Androgen-dependent vs -independent PCs have varying apoptotic thresholds, and are also discussed.

ER Status and BC

Acquisition of estrogen independence is a crucial step that often leads to BC progression. Estrogen independence arises because of attenuated ER signaling and development of mechanisms of estrogen-independent growth. Expression of transfected ER in ER-negative cells produces transfectants with inhibited growth, in spite of the expression of certain estrogen-responsive genes *(42)*. Thus, overexpression of ER in an ER-negative cell is insufficient to restore patterns of GF signaling and sensitivity to apoptosis associated with an ER-positive BC cell. ER-negative cells often develop autocrine/paracrine activation of the EGFR or other receptor tyrosine kinases. The overexpression of certain oncogenes in BC cells with autoactivated EGFR (or other receptor tyrosine kinase signaling pathways, e.g., erb-B2), can result in tumors with very poor prognosis *(42)*.

Apoptotic Threshold in ER-Positive Cells

ER function can be altered by different signaling mechanisms. Because estrogen-mediated increase in the bcl-2:bax ratio occurs via the ER, it is important to note that ER function itself is regulated by phosphorylation. For example, cAMP and IGF-I modulate ER by phosphorylation, so that TAM's antiestrogen effects are blunted. This observation may in part explain why some tumors relapse after TAM therapy *(42)*. It will be interesting to determine whether the ER mutants and variants that have been discovered are capable of appropriately modulating the bcl-2:bax ratio in response to estrogen or TAM stimulation. PKC, which is activated during lactation, can downmodulate ER mRNA and phosphorylate the ER protein, so that it loses function *(42)*. This is consistent with the observation that PKC is activated in late-stage, drug-resistant, ER-negative, but not ER-positive, BC *(42)*.

Apoptotic Threshold in ER-Negative Cells

Typically, ER-negative BC cells are aggressive, invasive, and overexpress EGFR, and, in some cases, erb-B2. It has been hypothesized that ER-positive tumors with regulatable bcl-2 expression undergo deregulation of small subset of estrogen-dependent genes, resulting in tumors that are ER-negative, EGFR-positive, and multidrug-resistant *(42)*. Such aggressive cancers typically overexpress Bcl-xL, and are resistant to chemo-induced programmed cell death *(36,39)*. This is consistent with decreased rates of apoptosis measured in later stages of BC vs early stages *(23)*. A direct link between EGFR and Bcl-xL has been demonstrated. Thus, in human keratinocytes, both EGF and its homolog transforming growth factor α (TGF-α), stimulate the EGFR and induce Bcl-xL expression. Conversely, blockade of the EGFR resulted in induction of cell death *(69)*. TGF-α acts via the EGFR as a survival factor, and can block apoptosis during mammary gland involution in vivo *(42,70)*. TGF-α accelerates mammary carcinogenesis and prevents apoptosis in double-transgenic TGF-α/c-myc mice; c-myc single-transgenic mice form tumors that undergo apoptosis *(70)*.

The level of EGFR expression can determine whether EGF drives growth or apoptosis. In vitro studies show that EGF stimulates growth in ER-negative cells with low levels of EGFR, but induces apoptosis in cells with significant EGFR overexpression *(32,71)*. This induction of apoptosis is associated with a dramatic increase in c-myc expression *(32)*. Whether the levels of EGFR expression have similar effects in vivo remains to be determined.

c-erbB2/Her-2 + Status and Apoptotic Threshold

The c-*erb*B-2 gene codes for a receptor tyrosine kinase, which is amplified at the gene level in about 30% of BCs. Overexpression of c-ERBB-2 in MCF-7 cells was associated with upregulation of Bcl-2 and Bcl-xL *(72)*, suggesting that c-ERBB-2 overexpression affects the apoptotic threshold. These data are consistent with the observation that c-ERBB-2-overexpressing tumors are aggressive, metastatic, and refractory to agents that induce apoptosis, leading to drug resistance. Herceptin is a c-ERBB-2 protein-specific antibody (Ab) that is growth-inhibitory to c-ERBB-2-overexpressing cells only. This Ab synergized with drugs in phase II clinical trials on c-ERBB-2-positive patients with metastatic BC *(73)*. To date, herceptin has not been shown to induce apoptosis. However, introduction of an adenoviral vector, encoding a single-chain anti-erbB-2 Ab, prolonged survival of mice with solid tumors that overexpress c-erbB-2. This anti-erbB-2 Ab was shown to induce apoptosis within these tumors *(74)*.

The effects of heregulin, herceptin, and various c-ERBB-2-specific Abs on bcl-2 family members, erbB family receptors, PI-3-K, AKT, and the MAPK pathway, need to be investigated, in order to elucidate the pathways by which erb-2 signals and influences the apoptotic threshold. The ErbB-2 protein has been shown to be a potent activator of PI-3-K and the H-Ras-dependent MAPK pathways *(44,75)*.

Androgen Receptor Status and Apoptotic Threshold in PCs

A major step in PC progression is acquisition of androgen independence. The significance of this step is apparent when one considers androgen-dependent growth. Primary mediators of androgen-dependent growth are unknown, although induction of various cell cycle genes, transcription factors, and peptide GF receptors are associated with stimulation of the androgen receptor (AR). The GFs, IGF-I, EGF, keratocyte growth factor, fibroblast growth factor 7, and activated protein kinase A, can independently activate the AR signaling pathway *(38)*. This crosstalk between AR signaling and other GF signaling pathways may explain why androgen-deprived PC cells continue to grow and develop hormone-refractory tumors. The H-Ras–MAPK pathway is also induced by AR stimulation. v-Ki-ras transformation of immortalized prostate ECs induced EGF-independent growth and resistance to all trans retinoic acid (ATRA) *(76)*, suggesting a role for H-Ras-dependent signaling in acquisition of androgen-independent growth.

Androgen-dependent tumors are known to overexpress bcl-2. It is worth investigating whether the GF(s) that mimic AR signaling can modulate expression or function of individual bcl-2 family members in a manner that renders these tumors resistant to apoptosis. In addition, androgen-independent cancers proliferate slowly and do not respond to Chemo agents that primarily target cycling cells. Therefore, these tumors are often insensitive to Chemo-mediated induction of apoptosis in vivo *(37,38)*. However, agents that induce a sustained elevation of intracellular calcium do induce apoptosis in the hormone-refractory tumors *(32,77)*.

Hormone-independent BC and PCs may still be capable of apoptosis in response to anticancer therapies. However, the apoptosis pathways in these types of tumors are no longer hormonally modulatable *(32)*. The result is that hormone-independent cells survive and outgrow their hormone-dependent counterparts, and are largely responsible for the relapses observed in patients who have undergone hormone-based treatment for BC or PC.

MODULATION OF CASPASES BY PHOSPHORYLATION

GF signaling can affect the apoptotic threshold at several steps. The mechanisms by which GFs and the H-Ras-dependent signaling pathways modulate transcription, function, and subcellular localization of Bcl-2 family members are discussed in the subheading, Role of Bcl-2 Family in Breast and Prostate Malignancies. Specific mechanisms of regulation of apoptosis in BC and PC were discussed in the subheading, Hormonal Effects on Apoptotic Threshold. Recent data suggest that GFs can modulate the apoptotic threshold without directly affecting Bcl-2 family members. This subheading discusses mechanisms by which GF signaling via specific kinases and phosphatases directly regulate the activation of stress kinases and caspases, which in turn directly affect sensitivity to apoptosis.

Kinases Regulating Apoptosis

The PI-3-K–AKT pathway not only enhances cell survival, but can block activation of stress kinases. Thus, AKT inhibits caspase activity, which in turn blocks the caspase-dependent activation of stress kinase, p38, in HeLa cells (78). As shown in the Fig. 1, AKT can promote survival by blocking caspase-9 activation via specific phosphorylation (79). These data show that H-Ras-dependent kinases can directly influence the apoptotic threshold by regulating the activation of caspase-9, a crucial caspase in the apoptotic cascade.

Conversely, caspases may modify kinase activities, which in turn can lead to apoptosis. Thus, cleavage by caspases converts certain kinases into apoptosis inducers. The activities of the PKC isoforms, δ and φ, are regulated by caspases in this manner, and overexpression of the cleaved forms of PKC δ and φ induced apoptosis (80). Activation of the MEKK-1 kinase presents another interesting case: It is a Ser/Thr kinase in the H-Ras-dependent MAPK pathway that activates the JNK stress kinases in response to loss of contact with the extracellular matrix (ECM). MEKK-1 is a caspase substrate that is activated upon cleavage by caspase-3 and -7. Active MEKK-1 in turn further activates caspases-7/3, thus forming an amplification loop for caspase activation (81; Fig. 1). Cleavage-resistant or kinase-inactive mutants of MEKK-1 are inactive, and prevent complete activation of caspases-3 and -7. MEKK-2, -3, and -4 are not caspase substrates, and are poor inducers of apoptosis (80,81).

Phosphatases Regulating Apoptosis

The activities of major protein kinase signaling pathways are regulated by protein (Ser/Thr specific) phosphatases. Figure 1 shows that the proliferative arm of the MAPK pathway (H-Ras-Raf-ERK) is opposed by protein phosphatases 1 and 2 (PP-1 and PP-2); the MAP-kinase phosphatase-1 (MKP-1) can block activation of the JNK, the terminal kinase in the H-Ras-dependent stress kinase pathway.

Depending on the cell type, inhibitors of PP-1 and -2 inhibit or potentiate Chemo- and radiation-induced apoptosis. Thus, induction of MKP-1 protects cells from TNF- and UV-induced apoptosis by blocking sustained JNK activation. Conversely, phosphatase inhibitors, such as okadaic acid and calyculin A, augment TNF-induced apoptosis in BT-20 human BC cells, and in LNCaP human PC cells, respectively (82). These inhibitors have also been shown to induce Bcl-2 phosphorylation and apoptosis in BC and PC cells in vitro (82,83), suggesting that changes in phosphatase actvity can directly alter the apoptotic threshold. Indeed, two-hybrid studies suggest that Bcl-2 can associate with the phosphatase, calcineurin (PP-2B) *(83,84)*. However, the bcl-2–calcineurin interaction was not observed in vitro under physiological conditions *(85)*. Therefore PP-1, PP-2, and their inhibitors modulate sensitivity of cells to agents that induce apoptosis.

There is evidence showing that PP-2A is activated upon cleavage by caspase-3 *(86)*. Further, PP-2A activation appears to be necessary for Fas-induced apoptosis in Jurkat cells, since caspase inhibitors completely blocked Fas killing and PP-2A activation with similar kinetics *(86)*.

Key Ser/Thr kinases and phosphatases regulate H-Ras-dependent pathways, which control the balance between cell growth, death, and survival. The PI-3-K–AKT pathway can block activation of specific caspases. Conversely, the activities of crucial kinases and phosphatases, such as MEKK-1, p38, and PP-2A, are in turn regulated by caspases. It has been proposed that caspases coordinately turn on stress-activated pathways and shut off GF-activated signaling pathways that promote survival *(86)*. Whether GF-dependent kinases and phosphatases in turn alter the substrate specificity of caspases remains an interesting question.

ROLE OF ECM AND CELL–CELL CONTACT IN MODULATING APOPTOTIC THRESHOLD

Differentiation of the mammary gland requires the ECM proteins laminin-1, and the β1-integrins. Bcl-2 and Bax may be crucial intracellular mediators of apoptosis-inducing signals originating at the ECM *(34)*. Integrin-mediated suppression of apoptosis in normal mammary ECs grown on ECM occurs in part because of upregulation of bcl-2 and inhibition of interleukin-1 β-converting enzyme *(87)*. The integrins also affect survival by modulating the activities of the PI-3-K and MAPK pathways.

Cadherins are crucial players in mediating growth and survival signals associated with cell–cell contact in epithelial tumors. Studies on HSC-3 oral squamous carcinoma cells show that cadherins mediate cell–cell interactions that promote anchorage-independent growth and block apoptosis *(88)*. Monolayers and multicellular aggregates of these cells express high levels of bcl-2, and grow and survive; suspended single HSC-3 cells lack bcl-2 expression, and die *(88)*. This action of cadherins may not apply to normal cells, since normal keratinocytes in aggregates express cadherins, but fail to survive in suspension *(88)*. In BC, loss of E-cadherin is associated with increased invasiveness *(42)*.

Cadherin function may be more complex, because interactions with integrins and catenins occur. Mutants of β-catenin are found in certain cancers, and have been shown to disrupt E-cadherin–α-catenin interaction *(88)*. The result is decreased intercellular adhesiveness within the tumor. Since the EGFR and the Ras adapter protein, Shc, can interact with cadherin–catenin complexes *(28)*, cadherins may play an important role in anchorage-independent growth of BC and PC cells. In fact, alterations in E-cadherin/α-catenin-mediated cell–cell adhesions are reported to occur in 30% of PC cells, and may be important in the acquisition of metastatic potential *(89)*.

APOPTOSIS-BASED THERAPEUTIC STRATEGIES

Bcl-2 Antagonists

Antisense Bcl-2 oligonucleotides have been shown to sensitize some BC and PC cell lines to Chemo-induced apoptosis *(90)*. Antisense Bcl-2 oligonucleotides alone have been used in phase I trials of lymphoma patients, and have resulted in some antitumor response *(90)*. The proapoptotic protein, Bcl-xS, antagonizes Bcl-2 and Bcl-xL function *(91)*. Although the precise mechanism of Bcl-xS action is unknown, binding of Bcl-xS to Bcl-xL permits cytochrome C release into the cytosol, resulting in apoptosis *(92)*. The authors showed that an adenoviral bcl-xS vector, used to transiently overexpress Bcl-xS, induces programmed cell death in MCF-7 cells *(93)*, and partial tumor regression in a solid MCF-7 tumor model in nude mice in vivo *(94)*. Therefore, this vector has potential as a gene therapy agent for BC.

Anticancer Agents That Modulate Apoptotic Threshold

Both Chemo and radiation therapy are known to work mostly by induction of apoptosis in tumors; however, these anticancer therapies are also toxic to normal cells. Retinoids and carotenoids are two classes of related dietary compounds that have chemopreventive properties. However, some of these compounds have clinical potential, because they selectively induce apoptosis in epithelial tumor cell lines, but not in normal cells *(95,96)*. In this subheading, the actions of these compounds in BC and PC is discussed in further detail.

RETINOIDS

The retinoid, ATRA, primarily acts via growth inhibition, differentiation, or induction of apoptosis. Retinoids mediate their effects via different isoforms of retinoic acid receptors (RAR and RXR) *(97,98)*. In BCs, ATRA-induced apoptosis is mediated by RAR-β, and is independent of p53, bcl-2,and bax *(98,99)*. Retinoids differentially affect ER-positive vs ER-negative cells, in part because RAR-β expression is induced by retinoids in ER-positive, but not ER-negative, cells. RAR- β expression can also be induced by expression of RAR-α. RAR-β loss occurs in human BC, but not in normal breast epithelium *(100)*. Estrogen can also modulate sensitivity to retinoids by inducing levels of RAR-α *(101)*. For these reasons, ER-positive BCs are more sensitive to ATRA than ER-negative tumors.

Resistance to ATRA is a significant problem, and results from absence of RAR-β or lack of inducibility of RAR-β expression in ER-negative cells. In some cases, ATRA resistance may result from Bag-1, an antiapoptotic member of the Bcl-2 family. Thus, in the ER-positive cell lines, MCF-7 and ZR-75-1, Bag-1 prevented ATRA-dependent transriptional activation, by interfering with the binding of the RAR complex with specific retinoic acid response elements *(102)*. As mentioned above, ATRA resistance is observed in the v-Ki-Ras transformed pRNS-1-1/ras PC cell line *(76)*. In lieu of ATRA resistance, ATRA analogs are becoming important as potential anticancer agents. The analog, Fenretinamide (4-HPR) efficiently induces apoptosis in all human BC lines, regardless of receptor status (ER or RAR) *(97,98)*. In clinical trials, 4-HPR efficiently prevented BC recurrence in women who had resection of early-stage cancer *(103)*.

CAROTENOIDS

Carotenoids, such as the provitamin A carotenoid β-carotene, have significant chemopreventive activity in animal models of BC. However, over 90% of carotenoids are nonprovitamin A compounds, and are beginning to be studied. Lutein is a nonprovitamin A xanthophyll found in broccoli and spinach, which has been shown to have chemopreventive activity in vitro *(96,104)*. Lutein, as well as another carotenoid, zeaxanthin, accounted for a part of the decreased BC risk in women on high vegetable and fiber diets *(105,106)*. In addition, high plasma levels of lutein were associated with a favorable prognosis in women with newly diagnosed BC *(107)*.

The authors' data suggest a potentially new role for lutein in cancer Chemo. ATRA and lutein were found differentially modulate chemosensitivity in normal vs transformed human mammary ECs. Etoposide and cisplatin induced apoptosis in both cell types. However, lutein conferred significant protection from apoptosis induced by each of these agents in normal cells only. This was consistent with lutein's ability to increase the Bcl-2 + Bcl-xL:Bax ratio in normal cells, but not in transformed cells. Futher, lutein and high-dose ATRA each induce significant cell death in tumor cells, but not in normal mammary cells. A differential effect of certain carotenoids on proliferation in tumor cells vs normal cells has been reported *(96)*. Recently, the nonprovitamin A carotenoid, lycopene, has been associated with decreased PC risk *(108)*.

CONCLUSIONS AND PERSPECTIVES

Figure 1 attempts to illustrate the numerous regulatory components of the apoptotic threshold described in this review, but it is by no means a comprehensive illustration of the numerous models of cell death. As can be seen from the figure and the discussion in the text, the apoptotic threshold is the sum of a set of upstream components that eventually lead to the regulation of bcl-2 family members. These bcl-2 family members then govern the task of commitment to cell death through mitochondrial disturbances. If left to itself, this would provide a fairly straightforward explanation; however, numerous upstream factors (such as AKT and MEKK-1) can also regulate components downstream of bcl-2 activity. Furthermore, as with TNF/Fas receptor-induced apoptosis, additional cell death responses may altogether circumvent the regulatory importance of the bcl-2 molecules. What arises from these multiple levels of regulation is a tightly controlled means of cell removal. Considering the magnitude of the decision to commit to cell removal through apoptosis, this is no surprise. In terms of therapies to manipulate these apoptotic thresholds, equally sophisticated and tightly controlled strategies must be devised.

REFERENCES

1. Kaufmann SH. Apoptosis: Pharmacological implications and therapeutic opportunities. In: August JT, Anders MW, Coyle J. Advances in Pharmacology, Academic, New York, 1997.
2. Raff M. Cell suicide for beginners. Nature 1998;396:119–122.
3. Kerr JF, Wyllie AH, Currie AR. Apoptosis: a basic biological phenomenon with wide-ranging implications in tissue kinetics. Br J Cancer 1972;26:239–257.
4. Ellis HM, Horvitz HR. Genetic control of programmed cell death in the nematode C. elegans. Cell 1986;44:817–829.
5. Hengartner MO, Horvitz HR. Programmed cell death in Caenorhabditis elegans. Curr Opin Genet Dev 1994;4:581-586.
6. Yuan J, Shaham S, Ledoux S, Ellis HM, Horvitz HR. The C. elegans cell death gene ced-3 encodes a protein similar to mammalian interleukin-1 beta-converting enzyme. Cell 1993;75:641-652.
7. Salvesen GS, Dixit VM. Caspases: intracellular signaling by proteolysis. Cell 1997;91:443–446.
8. Cecconi F, Alvarez-Bolado G, Meyer BI, Roth KA, Gruss P. Apaf1 (CED-4 homolog) regulates programmed cell death in mammalian development. Cell 1998;94:727–737.
9. Li P, Nijhawan D, Budihardjo I, Srinivasula SM, Ahmad M, Alnemri ES, Wang X. Cytochrome c and dATP-dependent formation of Apaf-1/caspase-9 complex initiates an apoptotic protease cascade. Cell 1997;91:479–489.

10. Adams JM, Cory S. The Bcl-2 protein family: arbiters of cell survival. Science 1998;281:1322–1326.

11. Kroemer G. The proto-oncogene Bcl-2 and its role in regulating apoptosis. Nat Med 1997;3:614-620.

12. Li P, Allen H, Banerjee S, Franklin S, Herzog L, Johnston C, et al. Mice deficient in IL-1 beta-converting enzyme are defective in production of mature IL-1 beta and resistant to endotoxic shock. Cell 1995;80:401-411.

13. Kuida K, Lippke JA, Ku G, Harding MW, Livingston DJ, Su MS, Flavell RA. Altered cytokine export and apoptosis in mice deficient in interleukin-1 beta converting enzyme. Science 1995;267: 2000–2003.

14. Varfolomeev EE, Schuchmann M, Luria V, Chiannilkulchai N, Beckmann JS, Mett IL, et al. Targeted disruption of the mouse Caspase 8 gene ablates cell death. Immunity 1998;9:267–276.

15. Kuida K, Zheng TS, Na S, Kuan C, Yang D, Karasuyama H, Rakic P, Flavell RA. Decreased apoptosis in the brain and premature lethality in CPP32-deficient mice. Nature 1996;384:368–372.

16. Kuida K, Haydar TF, Kuan CY, Gu Y, Taya C, Karasuyama H, et al. Reduced apoptosis and cytochrome c-mediated caspase activation in mice lacking caspase 9. Cell 1998;94:325-337.

17. Hakem R, Hakem A, Duncan GS, Henderson JT, Woo M, Soengas MS, et al. Differential requirement for caspase 9 in apoptotic pathways in vivo. Cell 1998;94:339–352.

18. Veis DJ, Sorenson CM, Shutter JR, Korsmeyer SJ. Bcl-2-deficient mice demonstrate fulminant lymphoid apoptosis, polycystic kidneys, and hypopigmented hair. Cell 1993;75:229–240.

19. Motoyama N, Wang F, Roth KA, Sawa H, Nakayama K, Nakayama K, et al. Massive cell death of immature hematopoietic cells and neurons in Bcl-x-deficient mice. Science 1995;267:1506–1510.

20. Knudson CM, Tung KS, Tourtellotte WG, Brown GA, Korsmeyer SJ. Bax-deficient mice with lymphoid hyperplasia and male germ cell death. Science 1995;270:96–99.

21. Yoshida H, Kong YY, Yoshida R, Elia AJ, Hakem A, Hakem R, Penninger JM, Mak TW. Apaf1 is required for mitochondrial pathways of apoptosis and brain development. Cell 1998;94:739–750.

22. Cleary ML, Smith SD, Sklar J. Cloning and structural analysis of cDNAs for bcl-2 and a hybrid bcl-2/immunoglobulin transcript resulting from the t(14;18) translocation. Cell 1986;47:19–28.

23. Naik P, Karrim J, Hanahan D. The rise and fall of apoptosis during multistage tumorigenesis: down-modulation contributes to tumor progression from angiogenic progenitors. Genes Dev 1996;10:2105-2116.

24. Soengas MS, Alarcon RM, Yoshida A, Giaccia AJ, Hakem R, Mak TW, Lowe SW. Apaf-1 and caspase-9 in p53-dependent apoptosis and tumor inhibition. Science 1999;284:156–159.

25. Chinnaiyan AM, Dixit VM. Portrait of an executioner: the molecular mechanism of Fas/APO-1-induced apoptosis. Semin Immunol 1997;9:69–76.

26. Green DR, Reed JC. Mitochondria and apoptosis. Science 1998;281:1309–1312.

27. Green DR. Apoptotic pathways: the roads to ruin. Cell 1998;94:695-698.

28. Hoschuetzky H, Aberle H, Kemler R. Beta-catenin mediates interaction of the cadherin-catenin complex with the EGF-R. J Cell Biol 1994;127:1375-1380.

29. Li H, Zhu H, Xu CJ, Yuan J. Cleavage of BID by caspase 8 mediates the mitochondrial damage in the Fas pathway of apoptosis. Cell 1998;94:491–501.

30. Luo X, Budihardjo I, Zou H, Slaughter C, Wang X. Bid, a Bcl2 interacting protein, mediates cytochrome c release from mitochondria in response to activation of cell surface death receptors. Cell 1998; 94:481–490.

31. Scaffidi C, Fulda S, Srinivasan A, Friesen C, Li F, Tomaselli KJ, et al. Two CD95 (APO-1/Fas) signaling pathways. EMBO J 1998;17:1675-1687.

32. Denmeade SR, McCloskey DE, Joseph JK, Hahm HA, Isaacs JT, Davidson NE. Apoptosis in hormone responsive malignancies. Adv Pharmacol 1997;41:552–583.

33. Bargou RC, Daniel PT, Mapara MY, Bommert K, Waegner C, Kallinich B, Royer HD, Dorken B. Expression of the bcl-2 gene family in normal and malignant breast tissue: low Bax a expression in tumor cells correlates with resistance towards apoptosis. Int J Cancer 1995;60:854–859.

34. Merlo GR, Cell N, Hynes NE. Apoptosis is accompanied by changes in Bcl-2 and Bax expression, induced by loss of attachment, and inhibited by specific extracellular matrix proteins in mammary epithelial cells. Cell Growth Differ 1997;8:251–260.

35. Silvestrini R, Veneroni S, Daidone MG, Benini E, Borschi P. The Bcl-2 protein: a prognostic indicator strongly related to p53 protein in lymph node negative breast cancer patients. J Natl Cancer Inst 1994; 86:499–504.

36. Olufunmilayo I, Olopade MO, Adenyaju SAR, Hagos FH, Mick R, Thompson CB. Overexpression of Bcl-x protein in primary breast cancer is associated with high tumor grade and metastasis. Cancer J Sci Am 1997;3:230–237.

37. Tang DC, Porter AT. Target to apoptosis: a hopeful weapon for prostate cancer. Prostate 1997;322: 284–293.
38. Koivisto P, Kolmer M, Visakorppi T, Kallioniemi OP. Androgen receptor gene and hormonal therapy failure of prostate cancer. Am J Pathol 1998;1522:1–9.
39. Minn AJ, Rudin CM, Boise LH. Expression of Bcl-xL can confer a multidrug resistant phenotype. Blood 1995;86:11,903–11,909.
40. Oltvai ZN, Milliman CL, Korsmeyer SJ. Bcl-2 heterodimerizes in vivo with a conserved homolog, Bax, that accelerates programmed cell death. Cell 1993;74:609–619.
41. Hunter T. Oncoprotein networks. Cell 1997;80:333–346.
42. Dickson RB, Lippman ME. Growth factors in breast cancer. Endocr Rev 1995;16:559–589.
43. Kinoshita T, Yokota T, Arai K, Miyajima A. Regulation of Bcl-2 expression by oncogenic Ras protein in hematopoietic cells. Oncogene 1995;10:2207–2212.
44. Clark GJ, Derr CJ. Aberrant function of Ras signal transduction in human breast cancer. Breast Cancer Res Treat 1995;35:133–144.
45. Fernandes-Sabria MJ, Bischoff JR. Bcl-2 associates with the ras-related protein R-Ras p23. Nature 1993;366:274,275.
46. Texeira C, Reed JC, Pratt MAC. Estrogen promotes chemotherapeutic resistance by a mechanism involving Bcl-2 protooncoge expression in human breast cancer cells. Cancer Res 1995;55:3902–3907.
47. Huang Y, Roy S, Reed J, Ibrado A, Tang C, Nawabi A, Bhalla K. Estrogen increases intracellular p26Bcl-2 to p21Bax ratios and inhibits taxol-induced apoptosis of human breast cancer MCF-7 cells. Breast Cancer Res Treat 1997;42:73–81.
48. Johnston SR, MacLennan KA, Sacks NP, Salter J, Smith IE, Dowsett M. Modulation of Bcl-2 and Ki67 in oestrogen receptor-positive human breast cancer by tamoxifen. Eur J Cancer 1994;30A:1663–1669.
49. Haldar S, Negrini M, Monne M, Sabbioni S, Croce CM. Downregulation of bcl-2 by p53 in breast cancer cells. Cancer Res 1994;54:2095–2097.
50. Xiang J, Chao DT, Korsmeyer SJ. BAX-induced cell death may not require interleukin 1B-converting enyme-like proteases. Proc Natl Acad Sci USA 1996;93:14,559–14,563.
51. Zhan Q, Fan S, Bae I, Guillohf CA, O'Connor PM, Fornace AJJ, et al. Induction of bax by genotoxic stress in human cells correlates with normal p53 status and apoptosis. Oncogene 1994;9:3743–3751.
52. Yin C, Knudson CM, Korsmeyer SJ, Van Dyke T. Bax suppresses tumorigenesis and stimulates apoptosis in vivo. Nature 1997;385:637–640.
53. Reed J. Balancing cell life and death: bax apoptosis and breast cancer. J Clin Invest 1996;197:2403,2404.
54. Reed JC. Double identity for proteins of the Bcl-2 family. Nature 1997;387:773–776.
55. Vander Heiden MG, Chandel NS, Williamson EK, Schumacker PT, Thompson CB. Bcl-xL regulates the membrane potential and volume homeostasis of mitochondria. Cell 1997;91:627–637.
56. Blagosklonny MV, Schute T, Nguyen P, Trepel J, Neckers LM. Taxol-induced apoptosis and phosphorylation of Bcl-2 protein involves c-Raf-1 and represents a novel c-Raf-1 Signal transduction pathway. Cancer Res 1996;1996:1851–1853.
57. Haldar SJC, Croce C. Taxol induces bcl-2 phosphorylation and death of prsotate cancer cells. Cancer Res 1996;56:1253–1255.
58. Maundrell K, Antonsson B, Magnenat E, Camps M, Muda M, Chabert C, et al. Bcl-2 undergoes phosphorylation by the c-Jun terminal kinase/stress-activated protein kinase in the presence of the constitutively active GTP-binding protein Rac1. J Biol Chem 1997;272:25,238–25,242.
59. Fang G, Chang BS, Kim CN, Perkins C, Thompson CB, Bhalla KN. "Loop" domain is necessary for taxol-induced mobility shift and phosphorylation of Bcl-2 as well as for inhibiting taxol-induced cytosolic accumulation of cytochrome c and apoptosis. Cancer Res 1998;58:3202–3208.
60. May S, Tyler G, Takahito I, Armstrong DK, Qatasha KA, Davidson NE. Interleukin-3 and bryostatin-1 mediate hyperphosphorylation of Bcl-2 a in association with suppression of apoptosis. J Biol Chem 1994;269:26,865-26,870.
61. Clem RJ, Cheng EH, Karp CL, Kirsch DG, Ueno K, Hardwick JM. Modulation of cell death by Bcl-xL through caspase interaction. Proc Natl Acad Sci USA 1998;95:554–559.
62. Cheng EH, Kirsch DG, Clem RJ, Ravi R, Kastan MB, Bedi A, Ueno K, Hardwick JM. Conversion of Bcl-2 to a Bax-like death effector by caspases. Science 1997;278:1966–1968.
63. Miyashita T, Kitada S, Krajewski S, Horne WA, Delia D, Reed JC. Overexpression of the Bcl-2 protein increases the half-life of p21 Bax. J Biol Chem 1995;270:26,049–26,052.
64. Yang E, Zha J, Jockel J, Boise LH, Thompson CB, Korsmeyer SJ. Bad a heterodimeric partner for Bcl-XL and Bcl-2, displaces Bax and promotes cell death. Cell 1995;80:285-291.

65. del Peso L, Gonzalez-Garcia M, Page C, Herrera R, Nunez G. Interleukin-3-induced phosphorylation of BAD through the protein kinase Akt. Science 1997;278:687–689.
66. Zha J, Harada H, Yang E, Jockel J, Korsemeyer S. Serine phosphorylation of death agonist Bad in response to survival factor results in binding of 14-3-3 not Bcl-xL. Cell 1996;87:619–628.
67. Datta SR, Dudek H, Tao X, Masters S, Fu H, Gotoh Y, Greenberg ME. Akt phosphorylation of BAD couples survival signals to the cell-intrinsic death machinery. Cell 1997;91:231–241.
68. Kitada S, Krajewska M, Zhang X, Scudiero D, Shabaik A, Tudor G, et al. Expression and location of pro-apoptotic Bcl-2 family protein BAD in normal human tissues and tumor cell lines. Am J Pathol 1998;152:51–61.
69. Stoll SW, Benedict M, Mitra R, Hiniker ATEJ, Nunez G. EGF receptor signalling inhibits keratinocyte apoptosis: evidence for mediation by Bcl-xL. Oncogene 1998;16:1493–1498.
70. Amundadottir LT, Nass SJ, Berchem GJ, Johnson MD, Dickson RB. Cooperation of TGF-a and c-myc in mouse mammary tumorigenesis: coordinated stimulation of growth and suppression of apoptosis. Oncogene 1996;13:757–765.
71. Armstrong DK, Kaufmann SH, Ottavino YL, Furya Y, Buckley JA, Isaacs JT, Davidson NE. Epidermal growth factor mediated apoptosis of MDA-MB-468 human breast cancer cells. Cancer Res 1994; 54:5280–5283.
72. Kumar R, Mandal ML, Lipton A, Harvey H, Thompson CB. Overexpression of Her2 modulates Bcl-2, Bcl-xL, and tamoxifen induced apoptosis in human MCF-7 breast cancer cells. Clin Cancer Res 1996; 2:1215-1219.
73. Pegram MD, Lipton A, Hayes DF, Weber BL, Baselga J, Tripathy D, et al. Phase II study of receptor enhanced chemosensitivity using recombinant humanized anti-p185 Her2/neu monoclonal antibody plus cisplatin in patients with Her2/neu-overexpressing metastatic breast cancer refractory to chemotherapy treatment. J Clin Oncol 1998;16:2659–2671.
74. Deshane J, Grim J, Loechel F, Siegal GP, Alvarez RD. Intracellular antibody against erbB2 mediates targeted tumor cell eradication by apoptosis. Cancer Gene Ther 1996;3:89–98.
75. Kapeller R, Cantley LC. Phosphatidylinositol 3-kinase. Bioessays 1994;16:565-576.
76. Peehl DM, Wong ST, Sellers RG, Jin S, Rhim JS. Loss of response to EGF and retinoic acid accompanies the transformation of human prostatic epithelial cells to tumorigenicity with v-Ki-ras. Carcinogenesis 1997;18:11,643–11,650.
77. Issacs JT, Lundmo PI, Berges R, Martikainen P, Kyprianou N, English HF. Androgen regulation of programmed death of normal and malignant prostatic cells. J Androl 1992;13:457–464.
78. Berra E, Diaz-Meco MT, Moscat J. The activation of p38 and apoptosis by the inhibition of ERK is antagonized by the phophoinositide 3-kinase/AKT pathway. J Biol Chem 1998;273:10,792–10,797.
79. Cardone MH, Roy N, Stennicke HR, Salvesan GS, Franke TF, Stanbridge E, Frisch S, Reed JC. Regulation of cell death protease caspase9 by phosphorylation. Science 1998;282:1318–1321.
80. Kidd VJ. Proteolytic activities that mediate apoptosis. Ann Rev Physiol 1998;60:533–573.
81. Cardone MH, Salvesan GS, Widmann C, Johnsson G, Frosch SM. The regulation of anoikis: MEKK-1 activation requires cleavage by caspases. Cell 1997;90:315-323.
82. Wright SC, Zheng H, Zhong J, Torti FM, Larrick JW. Role of protein phosphorylation in TNF-induced apoptosis: phosphatase inhibitors synergize with TNF to activate DNA fragmentation in normal as well as TNF resistant variants. J Cell Biochem 1993;53:222–233.
83. Linette GP, Li Y, Roth K, Korsemeyer SJ. Cross-talk between cell death and cell cycle progression: Bcl-2 regulates NFAT-mediated activation. Proc Natl Acad Sci USA 1996;93:9545-9552.
84. Shibasaki F, Kondo E, Akagi T, McKeon F. Suppression of signalling through transcription factor NFAT by interactions between calcineurin and bcl-2. Nature 1997;386:728–731.
85. Otter I, Conus S, Raven U, Rager M, Olivier R, Monney L, Fabbro D, Borner C. The binding properties and biological properties of Bcl-2 and Bax in cells exposed to apoptotic stimuli. J Biol Chem 1998; 273:6110–6120.
86. Santoro MF, Anand RR, Robertson MM, Peng Y, Brady MJ, Mankovich JA, et al. Regulation of protein phosphatase 2A activity by caspase-3 during apoptosis. J Biol Chem 1998;273:13,119–13,128.
87. Boudreau N, Sympson CJ, Werb Z, Bissel MJ. Suppression of ICE and apoptosis in mammary epithelial cells by extracellular matrix. Science 1995;267:891–893.
88. Kantak SS, Kramer RH. E-cadherin regulates anchorage independent growth and survival in oral squamous carcinoma cells. J Biol Chem 1998;273:16,953–16,961.
89. Morton RA, Ewing CM, Nagafuchi A, Tsukita S, Issaccs WB. Reduction of E-cadherin levels and deletion of the alpa-catenin gene in human prostate cancer cells. Cancer Res 1993;53:3585-3590.

90. Reed J. Promise and problems of Bcl-2 antisense therapy. J Natl Cancer Inst 1997;89:988–990.
91. Boise LH, Gonzalez-Garcia M, Postema CE, Ding L, Lindsten T, Turka LA, et al. bcl-x, a bcl-2-related gene that functions as a dominant regulator of apoptotic cell death. Cell 1993;74:597–608.
92. Kharbanda S, Pandey P, Schoffield L, Israels S, Roncinske R, Yoshida K, et al. Role for Bcl-xL as an inhibitior of cytosolic cytochrome C accumulation in DNA damage induced apoptosis. Proc Natl Acad Sci USA 1997;94:6939–6942.
93. Sumantran VN, Ealovega MW, Nunez G, Clarke MF, Wicha MS. Overexpression of Bcl-xS sensitizes MCF-7 cells to chemotherapy induced apoptosis. Cancer Res 1995;55:2507–2510.
94. Ealovega MW, McGinnis PK, Sumantran VN, Clarke MF, Wicha MS. bcl-xs gene therapy induces apoptosis of human mammary tumors in nude mice. Cancer Res 1996;56:1965-1969.
95. Oridate N, Suzuki S, Higuchi M, Mitchell M, Hong WK, Lotan R. Involvement of reactive oxygen species in N-(4-hydroxyphenyl) retinamide-induced apoptosis in cervical carcinoma cells. J Natl Cancer Inst 1997;89:1191–1197.
96. Krinsky NI. Actions of carotenoids in biological systems. Annu Rev Nutr 1993;13:561–587.
97. Lotan R. Retinoids and apoptosis: implications for cancer chemoprevention and therapy. J Natl Cancer Inst 1995;87:1655-1657.
98. Muindi JRF. Retinoids in clinical cancer therapy. Cancer Treat Res 1996;87:3305-3342.
99. Liu Y, Lee MO, Wang HG, Li Y, Zhang XK. Retinoic acid receptor b mediates the growth inhibitory effects of retnoic acid by promoting apoptosis in human breast cancer cells. Mol Cell Biol 1996;16:1138–1149.
100. Swisshelm K, Ryan K, Lee X, Tsou HC, Peacocke M, Sager R. Down-regulation of retinoic acid receptor b in mammary carcinoma cell lines and its up-regulation in senescing normal mammary epithelial cells. Cell Growth Diff 1994;5:133–141.
101. Roman SD, Ormandy CJ, Manning DL, Blamey RW, Clarke CL. Estradiol induction of retinoic acid receptors in human breast cancer cells. Cancer Res 1993;53:5940–5945.
102. Liu R, Takayama S, Zheng Y, Froesch B, Chen G, Zhang X, Reed JC, Zhang XK. Interaction of BAG-1 with retinoic acid receptor and its inhibition of retinoic acid induced apoptosis in cancer cells. J Biol Chem 1998;273:16,985-16,992.
103. Atiba JO, Meyskens FL. Chemoprevention of breast cancer. Semin Oncol 1992;9:220–229.
104. Gerster H. Anticarcinogenic effect of common carotenoids. Int J Vit Nutr Res 1993;63:93–121.
105. Potischman N, McCullough CE, Byers T. Breast cancer and dietary and plasma concentrations of carotenoids and vitamin A. Am J Clin Nutr 1990;50:909–915.
106. Van Poppel G. Carotenoids and cancer: an update with emphasis on human intervention studies. Eur J Cancer 1993;29A:1335-1344.
107. Rock CL, Saxe GA, Ruffin MT, August DA, Schottenfield D. Carotenoids, vitamin A, and estrogen receptor status in breast cancer. J Nutr Cancer 1996;25:281–296.
108. Giovanucci E, Ascherio A, Rimm EB, Stampfer MJ, Colditz GAA, Willet WC. Intake of carotenoids and retinol in relation to prostate cancer. J Natl Cancer Inst 1995;87:1767–1776.

20   Transcriptional Coactivators in Cancer

Paul S. Meltzer, MD, PHD

CONTENTS

INTRODUCTION

The trophic effects of steroid hormones on hormone-dependent cancers are mediated by specific nuclear receptors (NRs), which act as transcriptional regulators. Androgen (AR), estrogen (ER), and progesterone (PR) receptors possess sequence-specific binding affinity for hormone response elements upstream of hormone-responsive genes. Thus, the principal mechanism of action of steroid hormones is the regulation of gene expression (1), with NRs acting as signal transducers. This simple concept encompasses a remarkably intricate biochemical mechanism, which involves numerous proteins in addition to the NRs themselves. Recently, efforts in a number of laboratories have begun to delineate the complex process by which signals impinging on steroid receptors regulate transcription.

Steroid receptors belong to the NR superfamily, and have a similar structure, containing distinct domains (regions A–F) (1). Transcriptional activation properties are associated with two regions, the ligand-independent N-terminal AF-1 domain, and the ligand-dependent C-terminal AF-2 domain. NRs bind to DNA as homo- or heterodimers, which form on ligand binding. Although ER, for example, can interact directly with components of the basal transcriptional apparatus (2,3), it has become increasingly apparent that NRs do not act in isolation to alter transcription at their response elements. Instead, they function as part of a multimeric protein complex that serves to transmit the hormone signal to the basal transcriptional machinery. Accessory factors, termed co-activators or co-repressors, regulate the effects of NRs on transcription, and are an essential part of the mechanism mediating hormone action. Disturbances in the integrity of this mechanism may be of critical importance to the biology of hormone-responsive cancers by affecting their sensitivity to endocrine signals and disrupting the integration of signaling pathways.

From: *Contemporary Endocrinology: Endocrine Oncology*
Edited by: S. P. Ethier © Humana Press Inc., Totowa, NJ

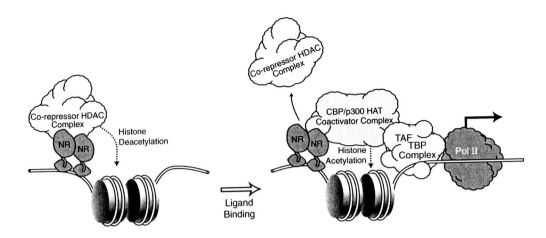

Fig. 1. The regulation of transcription by a NR at the promoter of a hormone-responsive gene involves changes in the co-regulator complex bound to chromatin. In the inactive state, the receptor is engaged with a co-repressor complex with histone deacetylase activity. On ligand binding, the receptor (NR) undergoes a conformational change, and binds co-activators with a histone acetyltransferase activity, and affinity for the basal transcriptional machinery favoring the initiation of transcription.

Recognition of the complexity of the apparatus mediating NR transcription has been driven by several biochemical approaches. Older studies, using reporter genes in transient transfection assays, demonstrated interference between NRs (squelching), which suggested the existence of limiting intermediary factors essential for NR transactivation. Using the yeast two-hybrid system, a long list of proteins that interact with NRs have been isolated. Supplementing this list are proteins that have been isolated by direct biochemical analysis of purified transcriptional complexes, as well as molecules that also have the ability to regulate viral oncoproteins and non-steroid signaling pathways, notably the E1A binding protein, p300, and the related molecule, CREB-binding protein (CBP).

The precise roles of several of these proteins remain to be determined. However, because ligand binding is the critical event in NR signaling, the subsequent discussion focuses primarily on the network of factors that associate with NRs on ligand binding (Fig. 1). A general picture has emerged in which NRs participate in multimeric protein complexes. In the nonliganded state, association with co-repressors leads to the formation of an inhibitory complex *(4,5)*. On receptor formation by ligand binding (or via ligand-independent pathways), an activating complex forms, which promotes transcription. Chromatin modification by histone acetylation and deacetylation has emerged as an important biochemical aspect of the process. The unliganded chromatin-bound NR co-repressor complex maintains a condensed chromatin state through its histone deacetylase activity. In contrast, liganded NRs recruit histone acetyltransferase (HAT) components of the co-activator complex. Decondensation of acetylated chromatin presumably facilitates access to the DNA template by transcriptional proteins. Ligand activation of receptor can be conceptualized as promoting HAT activity over histone deacetylase activity. The combinatorial utilization of various possible co-regulators in specific cell types establishes the pattern of hormone responsiveness. In addition to complexes with HAT activity, multimeric complexes with an adenosine triphosphate (ATP)-dependent nucleosome remodeling activity (notably the SWI/SNF complex) function to enhance NR-dependent transcription. Recently, two proteins, originally described because of their ubiquitin ligase activity, have been demonstrated to co-activate NRs *(6)*. Additionally, numerous proteins with ligand-independent NR-binding activity have been isolated. These last categories have not been directly related to cancer, and are not considered further in this chapter. Finally, several large multimeric transcription complexes have been described and characterized to varying degrees.

HAT CO-ACTIVATOR COMPLEXES

Assembly of the HAT co-activator complex depends on the interaction of NRs with members of the p160 co-activator family. This class of molecules, defined by steroid receptor co-activator 1 (SRC-1) is particularly well characterized. SRC-1 was originally isolated as an interactor of the PR ligand-binding domain *(7)*. This 160-kDa protein interacts with NRs in a ligand-dependent fashion, and co-activates several NRs in reporter-gene assays. SRC-1 defines a gene family including two closely related proteins, TIF2 *(8)* and amplified in breast cancer (AIB1) (also known as ACTR/RAC3/TRAM1) *(9–11)*. Each of these proteins has a domain structure that includes an N-terminal basic helix-loop-helix (bHLH)/Per-Arnt-Sim (PAS) domain. A number of transcription factors, such as the *Drosophila* clock protein, Period, and the aryl hydrocarbon nuclear transporter, contain PAS domains that function as protein-interaction domains *(12)*. Although highly conserved in SRC-1, deletion of the bHLH/PAS domain from SRC-1 does not interfere with its function in transient transfection, and its role remains undefined. SRC-1 family proteins also contain helical LXXLL motifs, which mediate the association of co-activator with receptor, and which are also found in other NR-interacting proteins *(13,14)*. In addition to these properties, SRC-1 interacts with CBP/p300 (*see* below), and recombinant SRC-1 protein has HAT activity *(15)*. SRC-1 has been shown to interact with and co-activate transcription factors outside the NR superfamily, including nuclear factor-κB and Jun/fos *(16–18)*, and microinjection experiments suggest a role for the mouse p160 (p/CIP) in CREB and STAT function *(19)*. However, the relative biological importance of p160 co-activator function to these various pathways remains to be established in vivo.

Mice homozygous for a null allele of SRC-1 are viable and fertile, but exhibit a blunted response to steroid hormones *(20)*. Some redundancy in the p160 family probably accounts for this mild phenotype. Knockouts for the remaining members of the p160 family have not yet been reported. One issue, yet to be fully resolved, is whether the three known p160 co-activators or their isoforms preferentially co-activate specific NRs. Biochemical and structural studies suggest that is likely to be the case *(21–25)*. According to this view, specific expression of varying combinations of p160 co-activators could regulate the pattern of hormone responsiveness in a tissue-specific manner. Recently, using chromatin immunoprecipitation techniques, it has been demonstrated that the p160 ACTR is itself acetylated on lysine residues flanking the LXXLL motifs *(26)*. This modification disrupts the NR–co-activator interaction, and accounts for the pulse of transcriptional activity observed on hormone stimulation.

An important component of the p160–NR complex, CBP, was originally isolated because of its interaction with CREB, a cyclic adenosine monophosphate-responsive transcription factor *(27)*. The closely related p300 was identified as a regulator of adenovirus E1A protein *(28)*. These molecules have potent HAT activity, and also recruit p/CAF, another HAT *(29,30)*. Through interactions with PolII-associated proteins, CBP/p300 can function as bridging factors between NRs and the basal transcriptional apparatus. In addition to binding to SRC-1 family proteins and NRs, CBP/p300 binds to and increases the activity of numerous sequence-specific transcription factors *(18,26,31–34)*. Because of this broad functional repertory, they have been termed "co-integrators." Partitioning limiting amounts of CBP/p300 among various promoters within a cell may be an important mechanism for balancing the effects of multiple signal transduction pathways. Although CBP/p300 interacts with SRC-1 family proteins, biochemical studies in T47-D cells suggest that the majority of CBP is not associated with SRC-1 in vivo *(35)*.

LARGE MULTIMERIC ACTIVATOR COMPLEXES

Several large transcriptional complexes have been identified in mammalian cells, including the SWI/SNF, vitamin D interacting proteins (DRIP), and thyroid-receptor-associated protein (TRAP) complexes. The SWI/SNF complex was first identified as a large (2 Mda) complex in *S. cerevesiae*, with an ATP-dependent nucleosomal remodeling activity *(36)*. Yeast SWI/SNF can functionally interact with NRs, and mammalian relatives of SWI/SNF proteins have been identified. One of these, brahma-related gene 1 (*BRG-1*) functions to co-activate ER and GR *(37,38)*. Several large multicomponent activator complexes have been described. With detailed characterization, they are tending to merge into a few distinct complexes. For example, the DRIP complex is very similar to the ARC complex (activating complex), which interacts with several sequence-specific activating transcription factors, including the vitamin D receptor and NF-κB *(39–41)*. The complexes TRAP and SRB/MED-containing co-factor complex are also identical *(42)*. A number of less completely defined activator complexes have been reported, and it is expected that additional complexes, with distinct or overlapping composition, remain to be described.

CO-ACTIVATORS AND CANCER

Several observations have drawn the attention of cancer biologists to the problem of transcriptional co-activation. Although not all of these results are directly related to hormone-responsive solid tumors, there is now enough information to strongly suggest that disturbances in the function of co-regulatory molecules are relevant to cancer progression, and that involvement of these mechanisms in cancer progression deserves close scrutiny. The regulation of gene expression is finely tuned. The quantities of certain co-activator molecules may be limiting, and competition for this limited supply between different signaling pathways is an essential aspect of transcriptional regulation. Varying the quantities of co-regulatory molecules of varying specificity, or altering them structurally, can result in major dysregulation of gene expression, with potentially catastrophic effects on the orderly processes of the cell cycle and cell differentiation.

The oncogenic potential of CBP and p300 is underscored by the involvement of these genes in chromosome translocations in acute myeloid leukemia. In each case, the translocation involves another transcription factor, and results in a fusion gene with presumptive oncogenic properties. Reported partner genes for CBP have been *MOZ* and *MLL* for *CBP* and *MLL* for p300 *(43–46)*. Remarkably, a fusion between *MOZ* and TIF-2 has also been observed *(47,48)*. CBP physically associates with PML, a consistent partner with RARA in chromosome translocations in acute promyelocytic leukemia *(49)*. The precise mechanism of leukemogenesis in any of these translocations remains to be determined, but almost certainly involves altered chromatin acetylation and gene expression. Although beyond the scope of this chapter, it is noteworthy that a number of leukemia fusion onco-protein transcription factors act to recruit co-regulator molecules, with a resultant disturbance in the normal process of hematopoiesis. Finally, a relationship between co-regulator molecules and the function of oncogenes, such as *myc*, and tumor suppressor genes, including *p53* and *RB*, has emerged *(34,50–54)*. Co-regulator molecules are involved in the function of these molecules, which fundamentally act as transcription factors. It is therefore possible that alterations in the cellular repertoire of co-regulators may disturb the normal function of these genes. Additionally, *p53* itself is a substrate for acetylation by CBP and p/CAF, with an increase in *p53*-dependent transcriptional activity as a result of this modification *(55)*.

Although chromosome translocations of genes encoding co-regulatory molecules have not been observed in solid tumors, other lines of evidence relate these genes to the evolution of solid tumors. These are derived from observations of patients with heredi-tary mutations in CBP and somatic alterations in co-activators in solid tumors. Mutations in only one of the known co-regulators, CBP, are known to cause a hereditary disease, the Rubinstein-Taybi syndrome (RTS), in an autosomal-dominant fashion *(56)*. This congenital malformation syndrome is associated with disturbed growth caused by haplo-insufficiency for CBP. RTS patients have a propensity for keloid development, and an apparent excess of benign and malignant tumors *(57,58)*. Malignant tumors in RTS have been diverse, including leukemia, medulloblastoma, neuroblastoma, and pheochromocy-toma. A mouse model for RTS exhibits anomalies in the heterozygotes, with embryonic lethality in the homozygotes *(59)*. A similar phenotype is observed in p300-null mice, with worsening embronic lethality in the compound heterozyogote with the CBP-null allele *(60)*. However, no propensity for tumors has been reported in either the p300 or CBP-null mice. Extensive searches for somatic mutations in co-regulator genes have not been reported. However, somatic mutations in CBP, resulting in amino acid substitutions with loss of the normal allele, have been observed in gastric and colorectal carcinomas *(61)*. Truncating mutations of the SWI/SNF component, hSNF5/INI1, have been observed in malignant rhabdoid tumor *(62)*.

The p160 co-activator, AIB1 (also known as ACTR, RAC3, TRAM1, and SRC-3), has been described as a target of gene amplification in breast cancer (BC) and ovarian cancer *(9–11,63,64)*. Gene amplification, with overexpression of the target gene, is a frequent mechanism of increased gene expression in solid tumors, notably including BC. Origi-nally described in the ER-positive BC cell lines, BT-474, MCF-7, and ZR 75-1, as well as in the ovarian carcinoma cell line BG-1, AIB1 amplification is also present in tumor samples *(9)*. The frequency of amplification in BC specimens was reported to be 9.5% by fluorescence *in situ* hybridization and 4.8% by Southern blot analysis, results that are consistent with the differences in these techniques *(65)*. Consistent with its function in steroid signaling, AIB1 amplification correlated positively with hormone receptor sta-tus. In cell lines, AIB1 gene amplification is associated with overexpression of AIB1 mRNA. AIB1 expression has not yet been studied by immunohistochemistry in BC specimens. However, high levels of AIB1 expression by mRNA *in situ* hybridization were considerably more frequent than AIB1 gene amplification.

Recently, a novel co-activator, designated AIB3/ASC-2, has been described *(66)*. The gene encoding this protein is amplified in 4.5% of BCs. AIB3/ASC-2 binds to ER, GR, TR, and RAR in a ligand-dependent fashion, and co-activates these receptors. It also binds to CBP and SRC-1, suggesting that it participates in co-activator complexes with these molecules. AIB3/ASC-2 and AIB1, which both map to different regions of 20q, are found co-amplified in BCs, raising the possibility that selection for overexpression of both genes is driven by their role in NR function. Amplification and overexpression of another LXXLL-containing NR co-activator in BC, termed "PBP/PPARBP" (also known as TRIP-2 and TRAP 220), has been described, extending further the concept that altered co-activator levels may provide enhanced tumor cell proliferation *(67–69)*.

How might overexpression of a co-activator, such as AIB1, AIB3, or PBP, provide a selective advantage to tumor clones bearing amplification of this gene? One possibility would be that increased abundance of co-activators increases the efficiency of signaling through critical NR-dependent pathways. This possibility is consistent with the association of ER/PR positivity and AIB1 amplification in BCs, and the fact that all the AIB1-amplified BC cell lines reported are ER-positive. An alternative explanation would consider the possibility that excess AIB1 is acting on nonsteroid signaling pathways, either directly or by altering the partition of limiting quantities of CBP/p300 between the multitude of pathways acted on by these proteins.

Given the occurrence of co-activator gene amplification in BC, it is notable that abnormalities of co-activators have not yet been reported in prostate cancer. Although a number of AR co-activators have been described, mutations or amplification of these genes have not been described. This contrasts with the observation of AR gene amplification in prostate cancer, which has recurred following androgen deprivation therapy *(70)*.

CONCLUSION

The regulation of the approx 100,000 or so genes in the human genome by developmental, physiologic, temporal, and environmental signals involves an complex network of transcriptional regulators. Although current concepts only partially describe the dynamic events occurring during hormone-responsive transcription, they do begin to identify the critical components of this system. Nonetheless, it is reasonable to propose that disturbances in the gene expression patterns of cells, as they evolve into malignant tumors, may be associated with genetic and epigenetic changes in the hormone-responsive transcriptional mechanism. The underlying complexity of these processes, and the large number of proteins involved, necessarily mean that current information on alterations in these genes during the evolution of hormone-dependent cancer is fragmentary.

Within this complex system, there are certainly opportunities to understand the mechanisms underlying the development of malignancies in hormone-responsive tissues, as well as important clinical phenomena, such as the evolution to the hormone-independent state. By defining the physical interactions of co-activator molecules with hormone receptors and the biochemical activities of co-activators, new opportunities are created for therapeutic intervention via the design of new molecules that disrupt these functions. Finally, by applying new technologies for the large-scale monitoring of gene expression, such as cDNA microarray analysis, it will be possible to unravel the effects of alterations in transcriptional function on the global pattern of gene expression in the tumor cell.

REFERENCES

1. Mangelsdorf DJ, Thummel C, Beato M, Herrlich P, Schutz G, Umesono K, et al. The nuclear receptor superfamily: the second decade. Cell 1995;83:835–839.
2. Ing NH, Beekman JM, Tsai SY, Tsai MJ, O'Malley BW. Members of the steroid hormone receptor superfamily interact with TFIIB (S300-II). J Biol Chem 1992;267:17,617–17,623.
3. Jacq X, Brou C, Lutz Y, Davidson I, Chambon P, Tora L. Human TAFII30 is present in a distinct TFIID complex and is required for transcriptional activation by the estrogen receptor. Cell 1994;79:107–117.
4. Chen JD, Evans RM. A transcriptional co-repressor that interacts with nuclear hormone receptors. Nature 1995;377:454–457.
5. Nagy L, Kao HY, Chakravarti D, Lin RJ, Hassig CA, Ayer DE, Schreiber SL, Evans RM. Nuclear receptor repression mediated by a complex containing SMRT, mSin3A, and histone deacetylase. Cell 1997;89:373–380.
6. McKenna NJ, Xu J, Nawaz Z, Tsai SY, Tsai MJ, O'Malley BW. Nuclear receptor coactivators: multiple enzymes, multiple complexes, multiple functions. J Steroid Biochem Mol Biol 1999;69:3–12.
7. Onate SA, Tsai SY, Tsai MJ, O'Malley BW. Sequence and characterization of a coactivator for the steroid hormone receptor superfamily. Science 1995;270:1354–7135.
8. Voegel JJ, Heine MJ, Zechel C, Chambon P, Gronemeyer H. TIF2, a 160 kDa transcriptional mediator for the ligand-dependent activation function AF-2 of nuclear receptors. Embo J 1996;15:3667–3675.
9. Anzick SL, Kononen J, Walker RL, Azorsa DO, Tanner MM, Guan XY, et al. AIB1, a steroid receptor coactivator amplified in breast and ovarian cancer. Science 1997;277:965–968.
10. Chen H, Lin RJ, Schiltz RL, Chakravarti D, Nash A, Nagy L, et al. Nuclear receptor coactivator ACTR is a novel histone acetyltransferase and forms a multimeric activation complex with P/CAF and CBP/p300. Cell 1997;90:569–580.
11. Takeshita A, Cardona GR, Koibuchi N, Suen CS, Chin WW. TRAM-1, a novel 160-kDa thyroid hormone receptor activator molecule exhibits distinct properties from steroid receptor coactivator-1. J Biol Chem 1997;272:27,629–27,634.
12. Huang ZJ, Edery I, Rosbash M. PAS is a dimerization domain common to Drosophila period and several transcription factors. Nature 1993;364:259–262.
13. Heery DM, Kalkhoven E, Hoare S, Parker MG. Signature motif in transcriptional co-activators mediates binding to nuclear receptors. Nature 1997;387:733–736.
14. Torchia J, Rose DW, Inostroza J, Kamei Y, Westin S, Glass CK, Rosenfeld MG. The transcriptional co-activator p/CIP binds CBP and mediates nuclear-receptor function. Nature 1997;387:677–684.
15. Spencer TE, Jenster G, Burcin MM, Allis CD, Zhou J, Mizzen CA, et al. Steroid receptor coactivator-1 is a histone acetyltransferase. Nature 1997;389:194–198.
16. Na SY, Lee SK, Han SJ, Choi HS, Im SY, Lee JW. Steroid receptor coactivator-1 interacts with the p50 subunit and coactivates nuclear factor kappaB-mediated transactivations. J Biol Chem 1998;273:10,831–10,834.
17. Lee SK, Kim HJ, Na SY, Kim TS, Choi HS, Im SY, Lee JW. Steroid receptor coactivator-1 coactivates activating protein-1-mediated transactivations through interaction with the c-Jun and c-Fos subunits. J Biol Chem. 1998;273:16,651–16,654.
18. Sheppard KA, Phelps KM, Williams AJ, Thanos D, Glass CK, Rosenfeld MG, Gerritsen ME, Collins T. Nuclear integration of glucocorticoid receptor and nuclear factor- kappaB signaling by CREB-binding protein and steroid receptor coactivator-1. J Biol Chem 1998;273:29,291–29,294.
19. Torchia J, Glass C, Rosenfeld MG. Co-activators and co-repressors in the integration of transcriptional responses. Curr Opin Cell Biol 1998;10:373–383.
20. Xu J, Qiu Y, DeMayo FJ, Tsai SY, Tsai MJ, O'Malley BW. Partial hormone resistance in mice with disruption of the steroid receptor coactivator-1 (SRC-1) gene. Science 1998;279:1922–1925.
21. McInerney EM, Rose DW, Flynn SE, Westin S, Mullen TM, Krones A, et al. Determinants of coactivator LXXLL motif specificity in nuclear receptor transcriptional activation. Genes Dev 1998;12:3357–3368.
22. Kalkhoven E, Valentine JE, Heery DM, Parker MG. Isoforms of steroid receptor co-activator 1 differ in their ability to potentiate transcription by the oestrogen receptor. EMBO J 1998;17:232–243.
23. Darimont BD, Wagner RL, Apriletti JW, Stallcup MR, Kushner PJ, Baxter JD, Fletterick RJ, Yamamoto KR. Structure and specificity of nuclear receptor-coactivator interactions. Genes Dev 1998;12:3343–3356.
24. Feng W, Ribeiro RC, Wagner RL, Nguyen H, Apriletti JW, Fletterick RJ, et al. Hormone-dependent coactivator binding to a hydrophobic cleft on nuclear receptors. Science 1998;280:1747–1749.

25. Shiau AK, Barstad D, Loria PM, Cheng L, Kushner PJ, Agard DA, Greene GL. The structural basis of estrogen receptor/coactivator recognition and the antagonism of this interaction by tamoxifen. Cell 1998;95:927–937.

26. Chen H, Lin RJ, Xie W, Wilpitz D, Evans RM. Regulation of hormone-induced histone hyperacetylation and gene activation via acetylation of an acetylase. Cell 1999;98:675–686.

27. Kwok RP, Lundblad JR, Chrivia JC, Richards JP, Bachinger HP, Brennan RG, et al. Nuclear protein CBP is a coactivator for the transcription factor CREB. Nature 1994;370:223–226.

28. Eckner R, Ewen ME, Newsome D, Gerdes M, DeCaprio JA, Lawrence JB, Livingston DM. Molecular cloning and functional analysis of the adenovirus E1A-associated 300-kD protein (p300) reveals a protein with properties of a transcriptional adaptor. Genes Dev 1994;8:869–884.

29. Bannister AJ, Kouzarides T. The CBP co-activator is a histone acetyltransferase. Nature 1996;384: 641–643.

30. Yang XJ, Ogryzko VV, Nishikawa J, Howard BH, Nakatani Y. A p300/CBP-associated factor that competes with the adenoviral oncoprotein E1A. Nature 1996;382:319–324.

31. Kamei Y, Xu L, Heinzel T, Torchia J, Kurokawa R, Gloss B, et al. A CBP integrator complex mediates transcriptional activation and AP-1 inhibition by nuclear receptors. Cell 1996;85:403–414.

32. Trouche D, Cook A, Kouzarides T. The CBP co-activator stimulates E2F1/DP1 activity. Nucleic Acids Res 1996;24:4139–4145.

33. Yang C, Shapiro LH, Rivera M, Kumar A, Brindle PK. A role for CREB binding protein and p300 transcriptional coactivators in Ets-1 transactivation functions. Mol Cell Biol 1998;18:2218–2229.

34. Avantaggiati ML, Ogryzko V, Gardner K, Giordano A, Levine AS, Kelly K. Recruitment of p300/CBP in p53-dependent signal pathways. Cell 1997;89:1175–1184.

35. McKenna NJ, Nawaz Z, Tsai SY, Tsai MJ, O'Malley BW. Distinct steady-state nuclear receptor coregulator complexes exist in vivo. Proc Natl Acad Sci USA 1998;95:11,697–11,702.

36. Pollard KJ, Peterson CL. Chromatin remodeling: a marriage between two families? Bioessays 1998;20: 771–780.

37. Khavari PA, Peterson CL, Tamkun JW, Mendel DB, Crabtree GR. BRG1 contains a conserved domain of the SWI2/SNF2 family necessary for normal mitotic growth and transcription. Nature 1993;366:170–174.

38. Fryer CJ, Archer TK. Chromatin remodelling by the glucocorticoid receptor requires the BRG1 complex. Nature 1998;393:88–91.

39. Rachez C, Lemon BD, Suldan Z, Bromleigh V, Gamble M, Naar AM, et al. Ligand-dependent transcription activation by nuclear receptors requires the DRIP complex. Nature 1999;398:824–828.

40. Rachez C, Suldan Z, Ward J, Chang CP, Burakov D, Erdjument-Bromage H, Tempst P, Freedman LP. A novel protein complex that interacts with the vitamin D3 receptor in a ligand-dependent manner and enhances VDR transactivation in a cell-free system. Genes Dev 1998;12:1787–1800.

41. Naar AM, Beaurang PA, Zhou S, Abraham S, Solomon W, Tjian R. Composite co-activator ARC mediates chromatin-directed transcriptional activation. Nature 1999;398:828–832.

42. Ito M, Yuan CX, Malik S, Gu W, Fondell JD, Yamamura S, et al. Identity between TRAP and SMCC complexes indicates novel pathways for the function of nuclear receptors and diverse mammalian activators. Mol Cell 1999;3:361–370.

43. Taki T, Sako M, Tsuchida M, Hayashi Y. The t(11;16)(q23;p13) translocation in myelodysplastic syndrome fuses the MLL gene to the CBP gene. Blood 1997;89:3945–3950.

44. Sobulo OM, Borrow J, Tomek R, Reshmi S, Harden A, Schlegelberger B, et al. MLL is fused to CBP, a histone acetyltransferase, in therapy-related acute myeloid leukemia with a t(11;16)(q23;p13.3). Proc Natl Acad Sci USA 1997;94:8732–8737.

45. Satake N, Ishida Y, Otoh Y, Hinohara S, Kobayashi H, Sakashita A, Maseki N, Kaneko Y. Novel MLL-CBP fusion transcript in therapy-related chronic myelomonocytic leukemia with a t(11;16)(q23;p13) chromosome translocation. Genes Chromosomes Cancer 1997;20:60–63.

46. Ida K, Kitabayashi I, Taki T, Taniwaki M, Noro K, Yamamoto M, Ohki M, Hayashi Y. Adenoviral E1A-associated protein p300 is involved in acute myeloid leukemia with t(11;22)(q23;q13). Blood 1997;90: 4699–4704.

47. Liang J, Prouty L, Williams BJ, Dayton MA, Blanchard KL. Acute mixed lineage leukemia with an inv(8)(p11q13) resulting in fusion of the genes for MOZ and TIF2. Blood 1998;92:2118–2122.

48. Carapeti M, Aguiar RC, Goldman JM, Cross NC. A novel fusion between MOZ and the nuclear receptor coactivator TIF2 in acute myeloid leukemia. Blood 1998;91:3127–3133.

49. Doucas V, Tini M, Egan DA, Evans RM. Modulation of CREB binding protein function by the promyelocytic (PML) oncoprotein suggests a role for nuclear bodies in hormone signaling. Proc Natl Acad Sci USA 1999;96:2627–2632.

50. Gu W, Shi XL, Roeder RG. Synergistic activation of transcription by CBP and p53. Nature 1997;387: 819–823.
51. Lill NL, Grossman SR, Ginsberg D, DeCaprio J, Livingston DM. Binding and modulation of p53 by p300/CBP coactivators. Nature 1997;387:823–827.
52. Lee CW, Sorensen TS, Shikama N, La Thangue NB. Functional interplay between p53 and E2F through co-activator p300. Oncogene 1998;16:2695–2710.
53. Scolnick DM, Chehab NH, Stavridi ES, Lien MC, Caruso L, Moran E, Berger SL, Halazonetis TD. CREB-binding protein and p300/CBP-associated factor are transcriptional coactivators of the p53 tumor suppressor protein. Cancer Res 1997;57:3693–3696.
54. Trouche D, Le Chalony C, Muchardt C, Yaniv M, Kouzarides T. RB and hbrm cooperate to repress the activation functions of E2F1. Proc Natl Acad Sci USA 1997;94:11,268–11,273.
55. Gu W, Roeder RG. Activation of p53 sequence-specific DNA binding by acetylation of the p53 C-terminal domain. Cell 1997;90:595–606.
56. Petrij F, Giles RH, Dauwerse HG, Saris JJ, Hennekam RC, Masuno M, et al. Rubinstein-Taybi syndrome caused by mutations in the transcriptional co-activator CBP. Nature 1995;376:348–351.
57. Siraganian PA, Rubinstein JH, Miller RW. Keloids and neoplasms in the Rubinstein-Taybi syndrome. Med Pediatr Oncol 1989;17:485–491.
58. Miller RW, Rubinstein JH. Tumors in Rubinstein-Taybi syndrome. Am J Med Genet 1995;56:112–115.
59. Tanaka Y, Naruse I, Maekawa T, Masuya H, Shiroishi T, Ishii S. Abnormal skeletal patterning in embryos lacking a single Cbp allele: a partial similarity with Rubinstein-Taybi syndrome. Proc Natl Acad Sci USA 1997;94:10,215–10,220.
60. Yao TP, Oh SP, Fuchs M, Zhou ND, Ch'ng LE, Newsome D, et al. Gene dosage-dependent embryonic development and proliferation defects in mice lacking the transcriptional integrator p300. Cell 1998; 93:361–372.
61. Muraoka M, Konishi M, Kikuchi-Yanoshita R, Tanaka K, Shitara N, Chong JM, Iwama T, Miyaki M. p300 gene alterations in colorectal and gastric carcinomas. Oncogene 1996;12:1565–1569.
62. Versteege I, Sevenet N, Lange J, Rousseau-Merck MF, Ambros P, Handgretinger R, Aurias A, Delattre O. Truncating mutations of hSNF5/INI1 in aggressive paediatric cancer. Nature 1998;394:203–206.
63. Li H, Gomes PJ, Chen JD. RAC3, a steroid/nuclear receptor-associated coactivator that is related to SRC-1 and TIF2. Proc Natl Acad Sci USA 1997;94:8479–8484.
64. Suen CS, Berrodin TJ, Mastroeni R, Cheskis BJ, Lyttle CR, Frail DE. A transcriptional coactivator, steroid receptor coactivator-3, selectively augments steroid receptor transcriptional activity. J Biol Chem 1998;273:27,645–27,653.
65. Bautista S, Valles H, Walker RL, Anzick S, Zeillinger R, Meltzer P, Theillet C. In breast cancer, amplification of the steroid receptor coactivator gene AIB1 is correlated with estrogen and progesterone receptor positivity. Clin Cancer Res 1998;4:2925–2929.
66. Lee SK, Anzick SL, Choi JE, Bubendorf L, Guan XY, et al. A nuclear factor, ASC-2, as a cancer-amplified transcriptional coactivator essential for ligand-dependent transactivation by nuclear receptors in vivo. J Biol Chem 1999;274:34,283–34,293.
67. Lee JW, Choi HS, Gyuris J, Brent R, Moore DD. Two classes of proteins dependent on either the presence or absence of thyroid hormone for interaction with the thyroid hormone receptor. Mol Endocrinol 1995;9:243–254.
68. Zhu Y, Qi C, Jain S, Le Beau MM, Espinosa R III, Atkins GB, et al. Amplification and overexpression of peroxisome proliferator-activated receptor binding protein (PBP/PPARBP) gene in breast cancer. Proc Natl Acad Sci USA 1999;96:10,848–10,853.
69. Yuan CX, Ito M, Fondell JD, Fu ZY, Roeder RG. The TRAP220 component of a thyroid hormone receptor-associated protein (TRAP) coactivator complex interacts directly with nuclear receptors in a ligand-dependent fashion. Proc Natl Acad Sci USA 1998;95:7939–7944.
70. Visakorpi T, Hyytinen E, Koivisto P, Tanner M, Keinanen R, Palmberg C, et al. In vivo amplification of the androgen receptor gene and progression of human prostate cancer. Nat Genet 1995;9:401–406.

INDEX

prolactin
  mitogenic signaling pathways,
    102–105, 103f
  transcriptional regulation, 359–360
Mammary gland cancer
  inhibition
    HCG, 126–127
    pregnancy, 126–127
  rodent
    GF, 146
    PRL, 106
Medical Research Council Study, 302–303, 303t
Medroxyprogesterone acetate (MPA), 41, 259
Men
  breast cancer
    incidence, 2
Metabolite E, 332
Mitochondria
  apoptotic pathways, 356
Mitogen-activated protein kinase (MAPK), 156
  breast cancer, 202
Mitogenic signaling pathways
  prolactin
    mammary tissue, 102–105, 103f
Mouse knockout models
  Bcl-2
    apoptosis, 354–355
Muellerian tumors
  malignant, 164
Myo-epithelial cells (ECs), 2

N

National Surgical Adjuvant Breast and
  Bowel Project (NSABP) B14, 313
National Surgical Adjuvant Breast and
  Bowel Project (NSABP) Protocol P-1,
    60, 61t, 62, 62t, 86, 88–90, 92
Neoadjuvant hormonal therapy
  prostate cancer
    early disease, 307–308
Neoplastic breast cells
  FGF8, 243–244
Neuregulins (NRGs)
  prostate cancer, 287
NGF1B, 266
Normal breast
  FGF8, 243–244
  FGFR, 246t, 247
  PR, 37–39
Normal mammary gland
  Bcl-2, 358–359

estrogen, development, 50
  PR, 37–39
Normal prostate epithelium
  IGF, 199
Normal prostate gland
  Bcl-2, 358–359
Novel therapeutic targets, 154t
Nuclear receptors (NRs), 373–375, 374f
Nur77, 266

O

Octreotide
  IGF-I, 204
Orchiectomy
  prostate cancer
    advanced disease, 294–295
Osteoporosis
  raloxifene, 93
  TAM, 89–90
Ovarian cancer, 166–170
  EGF-like peptides, 166–168
  EGF-receptors
    prognostic factors, 168–170
  epithelial. See Epithelial ovarian cancer
  erbB-2, 169
  erbB-3, 169
  IGF, 227
  incidence, 166
  TK type I receptors, 169t
Ovarian hormones
  serum levels, 125, 125f
Ovarian mesothelium, 313–314, 314f
Ovarian stromal growth factors
  epithelial ovarian cancer, 318–319
Ovarian surface epithelium (OSE),
    313–314, 314f
Ovaries
  HCG
    apoptotic gene expression, 132
  IGF-I, 227
Ovulation
  epithelial ovarian cancer, 314–316, 316f
Oxford Overview Analysis, 80–84, 84t, 95–96

P

P53, 53
  endometrial cancer, 329–330
  epithelial ovarian cancer, 320
  HCG, 131
P300, 376–377